Immunopharmacology of Joints and Connective Tissue

THE HANDBOOK OF IMMUNOPHARMACOLOGY

Series Editor: Clive Page
King's College London, UK

Titles in this series

Cells and Mediators

Immunopharmacology of Eosinophils
(edited by H. Smith and R. Cook)

Immunopharmacology of Mast
Cells and Basophils
(edited by J.C. Foreman)

Adhesion Molecules
(edited by C.D. Wegner)

Lipid Mediators
(edited by F. Cunningham)

Immunopharmacology of
Lymphocytes
(edited by M. Rola-Pleszczynski)

Immunopharmacology of
Neutrophils
(edited by P.G. Hellewell and
T.J. Williams)

Immunopharmacology of
Macrophages and Other
Antigen-Presenting Cells
(edited by C.A.F.M. Bruijnzeel-
Koomen, forthcoming)

Immunopharmacology of Platelets
(edited by M. Joseph, forthcoming)

Systems

Immunopharmacology of the
Gastrointestinal System
(edited by J.L. Wallace)

Immunopharmacology of the Heart
(edited by M.J. Curtis)

Immunopharmacology of Joints
and Connective Tissue
(edited by M.E. Davies and
J. T. Dingle)

Immunopharmacology of Epithelial
Barriers
(edited by R. Goldie)

Immunopharmacology of the Renal
System
(edited by C. Tetta)

Immunopharmacology of
Microcirculation
(edited by S. Brain)

Drugs

Immunotherapy for Immune-
related Diseases
(edited by W.J. Metzger,
forthcoming)

Immunopharmacology of AIDS
(forthcoming)

Immunosuppressive Drugs
(forthcoming)

Glucocorticosteroids
(forthcoming)

Angiogenesis
(forthcoming)

Immunopharmacology of Free
Radical Species
(forthcoming)

Immunopharmacology
of
Joints and
Connective Tissue

edited by

M. Elisabeth Davies
and John T. Dingle

Strangeways Research Laboratories, Cambridge, UK.

ACADEMIC PRESS

Harcourt Brace and Company, Publishers

London San Diego New York
Boston Sydney Tokyo Toronto

ACADEMIC PRESS LIMITED
24/28 Oval Road
London NW1 7DX

United States Edition published by
ACADEMIC PRESS INC.
San Diego, CA 92101

A catalogue record for this book
is available from the British Library

ISBN 0-12-206345-7

Typeset by Mathematical Composition Setters Ltd, Salisbury, Wiltshire
Printed and bound in Great Britain by The Bath Press, Avon

Contents

1. The Background to Autoimmunity 1

Warren M. Williams, Michael R. Ehrenstein *and* David A. Isenberg

2. Immunological Tolerance and its Implications for Autoimmunity

N.A. Mitchison

3. Peptide Blockade and Antigen-specific Modulation of Autoimmune Diseases

David C. Wraith

4. Monoclonal Antibody Therapy of Experimental Arthritis: Comparison with Cyclosporin A for Elucidating Cellular and Molecular Disease Mechanisms

M.E.J. Billingham

5. Anti-CD4 and Other Antibodies to Cell Surface Antigens for Therapy

Frank Emmrich, Hendrik Schulze-Koops *and* Gerd Burmester

6. Are Imbalances in Cytokine Function of Importance in the Pathogenesis of Rheumatoid Arthritis?

M. Feldmann, F.M. Brennan, E.R. Abney, A. Hales, Y. Chernajovsky, P. Katsikis, A. Corcoran, C. Haworth, A. Cope, D. Gibbons, C.Q. Chu, M. Field, B. Deleuran, R.O. Williams *and* R.N. Maini

7. Naturally Occurring Inhibitors of Cytokines

William P. Arend *and* Jean-Michel Dayer

8. Soluble Immunopeptides in Inflammatory Arthritis

Julian A. Symons *and* Gordon W. Duff

9. Inflammatory Reactions in Arthritis

Hans-Georg Fassbender

10. Connective Tissue Destruction in Rheumatoid Arthritis: Therapeutic Potential of Selective Metalloproteinase Inhibitors

Brian Henderson and Simon Blake

11. *Lysosomal Cysteine Endopeptidases in the Degradation of Cartilage and Bone*

David J. Buttle

Contributors

E.R. Abney, F.M. Brennan
Y. Chernajovsky, C.Q. Chu, A. Cope,
A. Corcoran, B. Deleuran, M. Feldmann,
M. Field, D. Gibbons, A. Hales,
C. Haworth *and* R.O. Williams
The Mathilda and Terence Kennedy
Institute of Rheumatology
(Incorporating The Charing Cross
Sunley Research Centre Trust),
Sunley Building,
1, Lurgan Avenue,
Hammersmith,
London,
W6 8LW,
UK

William P. Arend
Division of Rheumatology,
Box B-115,
University of Colorado Health Sciences Center,
4200 East Ninth Avenue,
Denver,
CO 80262,
USA

M.E.J. Billingham
Lilly Research Centre Limited,
Erl Wood Manor,
Windlesham,
Surrey,
GU20 6PH,
UK

Simon Blake
Maxillofacial Surgery and Oral Medicine Research Unit,
Institute of Dental Surgery,
University of London,
Eastman Dental Hospital,
256 Gray's Inn Road,
London,
WC1X 8LD,
UK

Gerd Burmester
Medizinische Klinik III,
Universität Erlangen-Nürnberg,
Krankenhausstrasse 12,
W-8520 Erlangen,
Germany

David J. Buttle
Department of Biochemistry,
Strangeways Research Laboratory,
Worts Causeway,
Cambridge,
CB1 4RN,
UK

Jean-Michel Dayer
Hôpital Cantonal Universitaire de Genève,
24 rue Micheli-du-Crest,
1211 Genève 4
Switzerland

Gordon W. Duff
Department of Medicine and Pharmacology,
The University of Sheffield,
Royal Hallamshire Hospital,
Glossop Road,
Sheffield,
S10 2JF,
UK

Michael R. Ehrenstein
Department of Rheumatology Research,
University College and Middlesex
School of Medicine,
London,
UK

Frank Emmrich
Max-Planck-Gesellschaft,
Klinische Arbeitsgruppe für Klinische Immunologie
und Rheumatologie der Universität
Erlangen-Nürnberg,
Schwabachanlage 10,
W-8520 Erlangen,
Germany

Hans-Georg Fassbender
Zentrum für Rheuma-Pathologie,
Breidenbacherstrasse 13,
6500 Mainz,
Germany

Brian Henderson
Maxillofacial Surgery and Oral Medicine Research Unit,
Institute of Dental Surgery,
University of London,
Eastman Dental Hospital,
256 Gray's Inn Road,
London,
WC1X 8LD,
UK

David A. Isenberg
Department of Rheumatology Research,
University College and Middlesex School of Medicine,
London,
UK

N.A. Mitchison
Deutsches Rheuma-Forschungszentrum Berlin,
Am Kleinen Wannsee 5,
D-1000 Berlin 39,
Germany

Hendrik Schulze-Koops
Max-Planck-Gesellschaft,
Klinische Arbeitsgruppe für Klinische Immunologie
und Rheumatologie der Universität
Erlangen–Nürnberg,
Schwabachanlage 10,
W-8520 Erlangen,
Germany

Julian A. Symons
Department of Medicine and Pharmacology,
The University of Sheffield,
Royal Hallamshire Hospital,
Glossop Road,
Sheffield,
S10 2JF,
UK

Warren M. Williams
Bloomsbury Rhematology Unit,
Arthur Stanley House,
40–50 Tottenham Street,
London,
W1P 9PG,
UK

D.C. Wraith
Department of Pathology,
University of Cambridge,
Tennis Court Road,
Cambridge,
CB2 1QP,
UK

Series Preface

The consequences of diseases involving the immune system such as AIDS, and chronic inflammatory diseases such as bronchial asthma, rheumatoid arthritis and atherosclerosis, now account for a considerable economic burden to governments worldwide. In response to this, there has been a massive research effort investigating the basic mechanisms underlying such diseases, and a tremendous drive to identify novel therapeutic applications for the prevention and treatment of such diseases. Despite this effort, however, much of it within the pharmaceutical industries, this area of medical research has not gained the prominence of cardiovascular pharmacology or neuropharmacology. Over the last decade there has been a plethora of research papers and publications on immunology, but comparatively little written about the implications of such research for drug development. There is also no focal information source for pharmacologists with an interest in diseases affecting the immune system or the inflammatory response to consult, whether as a teaching aid or as a research reference. The main impetus behind the creation of this series was to provide such a source by commissioning a comprehensive collection of volumes on all aspects of immunopharmacology. It has been a deliberate policy to seek editors for each volume who are not only active in their respective areas of expertise, but who also have a distinctly *pharmacological* bias to their research. My hope is that *The Handbook of Immunopharmacology* will become indispensable to researchers and teachers for many years to come, with volumes being regularly updated.

The series follows three main themes, each theme represented by volumes on individual component topics.

The first covers each of the major cell types and classes of inflammatory mediators. The second covers each of the major organ systems and the diseases involving the immune and inflammatory responses that can affect them. The series will thus include clinical aspects along with basic science. The third covers different classes of drugs that are currently being used to treat inflammatory disease or diseases involving the immune system, as well as novel classes of drugs under development for the treatment of such diseases.

To enhance the usefulness of the series as a reference and teaching aid, a standardized artwork policy has been adopted. A particular cell type, for instance, is represented identically throughout the series. An appendix of these standard drawings is published in each volume. Likewise, a standardized system of abbreviations of terms has been implemented and will be developed by the editors involved in individual volumes as the series grows. A glossary of abbreviated terms is also published in each volume. This should facilitate cross-referencing between volumes. In time, it is hoped that the glossary will be regarded as a source of standard terms.

While the series has been developed to be an integrated whole, each volume is complete in itself and may be used as an authoritative review of its designated topic.

I am extremely grateful to the officers of Academic Press, and in particular to Dr Carey Chapman, for their vision in agreeing to collaborate on such a venture, and greatly hope that the series does indeed prove to be invaluable to the medical and scientific community.

C.P. Page

Preface

It can be argued that the major advances in the treatment of inflammatory arthritic diseases that have occurred in the latter half of the twentieth century sprang from the discovery of corticosteroids. This led to the development of non-steroidal anti-inflammatory drugs and to research into the understanding and control of cellular catabolic enzyme activity. The search for agents controlling joint destruction gave rise to the recognition of the role of cytokines both in inflammation and in modulation of specific cellular functions and has provided a firm platform for pharmacological intervention. While the advances of the last decade have been based on the chemical control of inflammation, we would suggest that new treatment for arthritis in the first decade of the twenty-first century may prove to have developed from the immunopharmacological control mechanisms just beginning to be explored. It seems to us that the immunological approach to the modulation of the inflammatory mediators that initiate and maintain many of these mechanisms are targets likely to be readily accessible to pharmacological intervention.

The immunopharmacological approach to joints and connective tissue is new and we thank Dr Carey Chapman of Academic Press and Dr Clive Page, the series editor, for providing the challenge of assembling this volume, and for their support and encouragement.

The aims of the book are to provide an authoritative reference for academic and clinical research scientists and teachers with interests in immunology, inflammation and pharmacology and we are grateful to all the contributors who have presented the most up-to-date information available. We believe that the book will stimulate the concept of immunopharmacology as a true discipline of pharmacology with exciting avenues to be rapidly explored and which should lead to the alleviation of the destructive inflammatory arthritides.

M. Elisabeth Davies
John T. Dingle

Introduction

Rheumatoid arthritis remains a major medical problem and, in spite of prolonged and intensive investigation, its aetiology remains unknown. However, its pathogenesis is clearly inflammatory and brought about by immunological mechanisms. Indeed, it has been known for many years that lymphocyte depletion by prolonged thoracic duct drainage causes rheumatoid arthritis to go into remission. This therapeutic technique does not have widespread applicability nor indeed is it particularly safe, but it does demonstrate that lymphocytes (and probably particularly T cells) are involved not only in the initiation of the disease but in the maintenance of the inflammatory state.

In this book, Drs Davies and Dingle have recruited a team of authors to address the pathogenesis of rheumatoid arthritis and related diseases and to explore the prospects that an improved understanding of this pathogenesis may have for treatment. In so doing, they highlight the enormous progress that has been made in the last 25 years in the understanding of the immune responses underlying chronic inflammatory disease and of the molecular basis of the inflammatory reactions themselves. However, they also highlight how incomplete this understanding remains and how far there is still to go before a rational approach to the treatment of rheumatoid arthritis will become possible.

The immunological part of the book ranges from the highly theoretical – with Av Mitchison's challenging speculations on how the immune system ought to work – to the, so far quite empirical although very promising, attempts to modify the disease with monoclonal antibodies to lymphocyte surface antigens.

The section on cytokines and their inhibitors is a tribute to the transformation that molecular biology has brought to the study of inflammation. The number of these peptide mediators that have now been characterized, cloned and sequenced and whose existence was totally unsuspected a few years ago is both impressive and daunting. When the first two interleukins and α and γ interferon had been successfully cloned and shown to exist as genuine proteins rather than as activities of cell supernatants, there was a great optimism that the cellular "effector network" would rapidly be worked out to at least the same extent as its humoral counterpart, the complement system. Unfortunately this optimism was misplaced. These factors represent only a small minority of those that have since been described and it would be rash to assume that there are not yet more to come. Furthermore, and again to the investigators' initial surprise, the biological functions of most of these molecules are highly pleiotropic making the elucidation of their physiological roles and their pathological significance extraordinarily difficult. Because cytokines are not hormones which are secreted into the general circulation to have an effect at a distance, but are both produced and consumed within microenvironments, it has also proved difficult to measure their physiological (or pathophysiological) concentrations. The parenteral administration of cytokines as therapeutic agents (and for that matter of antibodies or inhibitors to them) has turned out to be far from straightforward. These problems are discussed in detail by the contributors to the cytokine section.

The final common pathway of inflammatory reactions is believed to lie in the generation or release of enzymes that destroy the intercellular matrix and damage cells. Various candidate enzymes for this function exist and are the topic of the final section. There is controversy whether oxygen and nitrogen radicals also contribute to a significant extent to inflammatory damage. This is yet another complex field and only time will tell whether the editors took the right option in excluding it from their survey of the immunopharmacology of joints.

The book provides an interesting and valuable progress report in an important, rapidly expanding and still far from clarified area. Those who are interested in autoimmunity, in inflammation and in arthritis will find much in it to stimulate them and to encourage them to continue their studies.

Peter Lachmann

1. The Background to Autoimmunity

Warren M. Williams, Michael R. Ehrenstein and David A. Isenberg

Immunopharmacology of Joints and Connective Tissue
ISBN 0–12–206345–7

1. Introduction

It is now well established that the clinical expression of autoimmunity is dependent upon the interaction of multiple factors. This chapter attempts to analyse the different components which have too often in the past tended to be viewed in isolation. It seems likely that many of the same components interact in different ways to produce what are clearly related diseases. Thus, very often one or more family members of a patient with one autoimmune disease will have a different autoimmune disorder. The role of autoantibodies and their idiotypes, the MHC, cytokines, infections, complement deficiency, hormones, age, nutrition, toxins and chemicals are thus reviewed to analyse their contribution to the auto-immune diseases. Despite the complexity of interactions that must occur before the onset of these diseases is clinically manifest, they are common. Up to 1 in 40 individuals is diagnosed as suffering from an autoimmune disease during his/her lifetime. These disorders are thus important and have economic implications.

2. Autoantibodies in Autoimmune Diseases

Ehrlich was the first to use the term "Horror autoxicus" to describe what he thought would be a key element in the development of the immune system, namely the ability to discriminate "self" from "non-self". The corollary of this was, he supposed, that the distinction would be absolute and no form of self "attack" could occur under normal circumstances. It is recognized, however, that a limited amount of autoimmunity is found in most healthy individuals as exemplified by the presence of natural antibodies.

2.1 NATURAL AUTOANTIBODIES

The term "natural antibodies" (NAbs) is used to describe those antibodies that may bind to a variety of antigens found in normal humans and healthy unimmunized animals. The existence of such antibodies was thought to result from a previous unsuspected antigenic challenge to the individual. However, many workers now believe that NAbs are formed independently of antigenic stimulation (Avrameas et al., 1983). Therefore, they have been redefined as antibodies found in the serum which do not require induction of B cells (such as by antigenic

challenge or mitogenic stimulation) for their synthesis. Moreover, NAbs may be thought of as part of the immune system, functioning as a first line of defence, and capable of destroying foreign agents on initial contact (Greenberg, 1985). During the past 20 years, NAbs reacting with various autoantigens have frequently been identified, and, in fact, a clear distinction between NAbs and natural autoantibodies (NAAbs) cannot be made.

NAAbs have been demonstrated in normal individuals. Avrameas and co-workers (1983) tested a pool of 800 healthy donors for antibodies against nine common self-antigens; tubulin, actin, thyroglobulin, myoglobulin, fetuin, transferrin, albumin, cytochrome c and collagen. The serum pool tested contained all nine autoantibodies which were shown to bind specifically to the antigens via the F(ab')2 fragments and not via the Fc portion. It was also demonstrated that these NAAbs were capable of binding cellular constituents.

In vitro experiments have shown that PBMCs from normal persons are capable of synthesizing autoanti-bodies in vitro. Cairns et al. (1984) showed that B cells from a normal individual were able to synthesize anti-DNA antibodies in vitro. They then produced hybridomas by fusing a human non-secreting myeloma cell line with tonsillar lymphoid B cells from a normal donor and found that, of 110 hybridomas, 13 (11.8%) produced anti-ssDNA antibodies. Rauch et al. (1987) demon-strated that human hybridoma-derived monoclonals from healthy individuals were both able to bind ssDNA and/or had lupus anticoagulant activity. These studies imply that genes coding for anti-DNA autoantibodies, similar to those produced in SLE exist in the genome of normal human B lymphocytes. Avrameas's group has found that 35% of human B lymphocytes immortalized by EBV secrete immunoglobulins with autoantibody reactivity. The vast majority of these clones, mostly IgG and IgA secretors, reacted with at least five of a panel of 13 test antigens. More than half of these antibodies also reacted with cellular antigens present in tissue sections. These results parallel those described amongst normal human polyclonal antibodies, in human paraproteins.

Taken together, these observations show that there exists a substantial population of B cells committed to the production of autoantibodies which are present in healthy normals. The autoreactive B cells can arise from germline precursors, possessing in their genome, genes coding for autoantibody synthesis, in other words these autoreactive clones are not produced by mutation or some other environmental changes, but rather constitute part of the normal B cell repertoire. It is postulated that a regulatory system exists to keep these autoreactive clones in check, and that failure of this regulatory mechanism causes autoimmune disease. However, the existence of autoantibodies in the serum of normal mice and humans, albeit in small amounts, shows that these autoreactive clones escape the normal controls, mature and produce anti-self-immunoglobulins.

Is there a population of B cells especially prone to produce NAAbs? A subset of B lymphocytes that express a cell surface marker normally associated with T cells (Ly-1$^+$, mouse; CD5+, human) has been identified, and it is evident this population is expanded in autoimmune diseases (Calvert et al., 1988). Analysis of PBL from a group of randomly chosen individuals has revealed a relatively constant frequency of B cells that express low levels (2–3%) of CD5; this corresponds to 20–30% of total B cells (Hardy et al., 1987). The consistency of the frequency with which these B cells are found in peripheral blood lymphocytes suggests that their numbers are controlled by genetic rather than environmental factors.

2.2 ORIGINS OF NAAbs

A number of ideas have been put forward to account for their presence. These NAAbs could be those produced by remaining autoreactive clones after those strongly reactive with important self-components had been "clonally deleted". These remaining autoantibodies (AAbs) are kept in check, by a suppressive system, at low levels and constitute NAAbs (Cunningham, 1976). It has been shown that in vitro and in vivo production of AAbs in response to PBAs differ, with a far greater response in vitro, inferring a regulatory mechanism in vivo (Dziarski, 1982). Neonatal thymectomy has been shown to lead to an increase in AAb production in response to PBA, implying that the regulatory mechanism is T cell dependent (Smith et al., 1982). Polyclonal activation of NAAb-producing B cells could result from infectious agents producing polyclonal activators in vivo.

The idea that AAb formation is the result of cross-reaction between foreign and self-determinants is well established. The autoantibodies against cardiac muscle myosin that occur in rheumatic fever and the antibodies that bind to both Trypanosoma cruzi and nervous system antigens are good examples (see also Section 8).

The concept that autoantibodies arise by cross-reaction between self- and non-self-epitopes can be extended to explain the appearance of NAAbs in normal individuals. Most studies indicate that the NAAb–antigen-combining region is polyreactive and capable of binding a number of structurally related but not identical ligands (Ortega et al., 1984). Therefore it is possible that the part of the B cell population that gives rise to the AAb carries a polyclonal receptor capable of binding several different antigenic determinants. The fixation of a foreign antigen

to this receptor would induce the B cell to undergo a series of divisions and mutations, which, under selective pressure of the antigen, would lead to the production of a highly specific antibody for that antigen. Thus natural polyreactive autoantibodies might constitute the antibodies secreted by these B cells before encountering foreign highly reactive antigens.

2.3 THE BIOLOGICAL ROLE OF NAAbs

The common observation of autoreactive B cells at relatively high frequency, expressing a wide variety of specificities in most healthy individuals, leads to the conclusion that they probably have an important physiological function which has led to their conservation as part of the immune system. One suggestion as to their possible role was made by Grabar (1983) who hypothesized that autoantibodies are formed as part of a physiological mechanism for cleansing the organism of self- and non-self-products. Those immunoglobulins reacting with metabolic products are classical antibodies, and those reacting with catabolic products are autoantibodies. An example of this mechanism was the finding of a NAAb, reacting with α-galactosyl residues on human RBC membrane (Galili et al., 1984). This AAb, which was found in the serum of all healthy individuals tested, is believed to be important in the process of degradation of senescent erythrocytes.

An alternative proposal by Cohen and Cooke (1986), views the NAAb synthesis as a mechanism for achieving self-tolerance. The NAAbs displaying low affinity for self-antigens may bind and mask self-antigens from recognition by self-reactive clones capable of producing a strong and damaging response. It is also postulated that these low-affinity NAAbs can mask the self-mimicking epitopes on invading microorganisms which may otherwise initiate a stronger autoimmune response. Cohen and Cooke (1986) suggested that NAAbs act as a filter that enables only non-self-antigens to induce a powerful immune response, while antigens masked by the preformed NAAbs fail to elicit an aggressive response. This theory has been criticized by Dziarski (1987) on the basis that IgM antibodies, which the majority of NAAbs are, have in some experiments been shown to specifically enhance humoral responses when administered with or without their respective antigen, whereas IgG antibodies suppress their responses. However, it should be emphasized that a substantial proportion of NAAbs are of the IgG class (Avrameas et al., 1983).

2.4 AUTOANTIBODIES IN HEALTHY SUBJECTS

Autoantibodies have been found in relatives of autoimmune patients, patients with plasma cell dyscrasia, individuals with infections and apparently healthy individuals. The range and frequency of these NAAbs have been studied by a number of groups. ANAbs were found in 6–13% of 1284 adult white people (Pandey *et al.*, 1979). In another study, the incidence of ANAbs was reported to be 4% (of 2838 subjects). Gender did not seem to affect the frequency. ANAbs were detected in only 4% (out of 2500) of healthy female blood donors aged 20–50 years (Fritzler *et al.*, 1985). However, age seemed to affect the incidence; it was increased to 16% in 56 males over age 40 years and to 18% (out of 279) in old people over the age of 65 years (Goodwin *et al.*, 1982; Moulias *et al.*, 1984). In a few studies the effect of sex on prevalence of autoantibodies was found to be higher among healthy females than males (Fritzler *et al.*, 1985).

2.5   ARE INDIVIDUALS WITH RELATIVELY HIGH LEVELS OF NAAbs DESTINED TO DEVELOP AUTOIMMUNE DISEASE?

Very little is known about the outcome of these normal subjects. Some of the previous long-term follow-ups reported in the literature support the theory that the presence of autoantibodies is associated with the development of autoimmune disorders. Swaak and Smeenk (1985) followed 441 subjects found to have antibodies to dsDNA for 8 years. Within 1 year, 69% of them fulfilled the American Rheumatism Association criteria for SLE.

Of the remaining 137 patients, 53% developed SLE within 5 years. They concluded that about 85% of individuals with anti-dsDNA antibodies in the circulation will develop SLE within a few years. Another 5-year follow-up was done by Weiner *et al.* (1987) on 44 patients with arthralgia and positive RF. They reported that 13.6% of their subjects developed RA within the 5-year follow up period, and concluded that the presence of RF in the serum may precede the overt disease by several years. However, the subjects reported in these two studies were not randomly selected healthy individuals, which biases the figures, and in a 5-year follow-up study of 60 healthy women with high titres of various antibodies, none developed clinically overt disease (Yadin *et al.*, 1989).

2.6   AUTOANTIBODIES IN AUTOIMMUNE DISEASES

Autoimmune diseases mediated by autoantibodies may be broadly divided into two categories. Disorders in the first group comprise diseases in which antibodies to a specific antigen are central to the pathology of the disease. Included in this category are myasthenia gravis and autoimmune thyroiditis (Hashimoto's thyroiditis and Graves' disease). The second comprises those diseases in which the immunizing antigen or inciting agent is not known. In this group are included SLE, RA and Sjögren's syndrome. The major autoantibody specificity in each disorder is shown in Table 1.1.

Table 1.1   Prominent autoantibodies found in organ-specific and non-organ-specific autoimmune diseases

Disease	Major organ/ system involved	Autoantibodies reactive with
Organ-specific		
Autoimmune haemolytic anaemia	Erythrocyte	Red cell surface antigen
Idiopathic thrombocytopenia purpura	Platelets	Platelet surface antigen
Hashimoto's thyroiditis	Thyroid	Thyroid surface antigen
Graves' disease	Thyroid	TSH receptor
Goodpasture's syndrome	Kidney	Glomerular basement membrane
Myasthenia gravis	Muscle	Acetylcholine receptor
Pernicious anaemia	Stomach	Intrinsic factor
Insulin-dependent diabetes mellitus	Pancreas	Pancreatic islet β cells
Primary biliary cirrhosis	Liver	Mitochondria
Non-organ-specific		
Rheumatoid arthritis	Joints, lungs, skin	IgG (rheumatoid factor) collagen,
SLE	Skin, joints, kidney, brain, heart, lungs	Polynucleotides, histones, extractable nuclear antigens, phospholipids
Sjögren's syndrome	Exocrine glands, notably lacrimal and parotid	Extractable nuclear antigens SS-A (Ro) and SS-B (La)
Polymyositis	Muscle, skin	Disease specific autoantibodies (e.g. anti-Jo-1)
Scleroderma	Skin, oesophagus, lungs, kidneys	Disease-specific kidney autoantibodies (e.g. Scl-70)

2.7 AUTOANTIBODIES INVOLVED IN ORGAN-SPECIFIC DISEASES

2.7.1 Autoimmune Haemolytic Anaemia

In this disease antibodies binding to antigens on the erythrocyte membrane are produced. This leads to premature erythrocyte destruction in a number of ways. The anti-erythrocyte antibodies, once bound, may activate the complement cascade leading to rupture of the erythrocyte membrane and haemoglobin release. In less severe cases the attached antibodies bind only some complement components, which then mediate immune adherence to macrophages with subsequent phagocytosis or opsonization resulting in morphological changes, changing the doughnut-shaped erythrocyte into a ball-shaped short-lived spherocyte which is soon removed from the circulation. *In vitro* experiments have revealed the existence of two types of red cell antibodies: warm reacting, those with optimum reactivity with red cells at 37°C, and cold reacting, those with optimum reactivity at close to freezing point.

The target of the warm autoantibodies appears to be the rhesus antigens and these antibodies may even be alloantigen specific. Most of these antibodies are of the IgG class and possess good opsonizing and immune adherence ability.

The cold autoantibodies or cold agglutinins attach to the red blood cells at cold temperatures and dissociate when the cells are rewarmed. They appear to be directed against either the I or the i blood group antigens which are carried by glycophorin, the major glycoprotein of human erythrocyte surfaces. It is not the antibody that is cold dependent but the antigen: the conformation of glycophorin alters with temperature, and at cold temperatures the I and i antigenic determinants are exposed, whereas at 37°C the determinants are hidden. Most cold autoantibodies are of the IgM isotype, and hence capable of binding complement and mediating haemolysis.

2.7.2 Idiopathic Thrombocytopenia Purpura (ITP)

Autoimmune thrombocytopenic purpura is characterized by the destruction of circulating platelets by auto-antibodies and/or by circulating immune complexes. Immunoglobulin may bind the platelets as specific antibodies reconizing antigens expressed on the platelet surface; the most common "targets" reside on glycoproteins which serve as important receptors for ligand-mediated aggregation and adhesion. Other immunoglobulins may bind as immune complexes bound through the Fc receptor, or as immunoglobulin bound non-specifically to the membrane fragments.

2.7.3 Hashimoto's Thyroiditis

In this disease autoantibodies are produced which, in concert with cytotoxic cells, cause destruction of thyroid cells, although it is not clear whether the autoantibodies of the cytotoxic cells initiate subsequent events. The autoantibodies in thyroiditis recognize certain cellular components of the gland. Thyroglobulin-specific antibodies are probably produced by plasma cells infiltrating the thyroid and are mostly of the IgG isotype. Other antibodies may specifically recognize microsomal cytoplasmic antigens, which occur in the thyroid and are lipoprotein. Second colloid antigen CA2, which is a fluid filling the thyroid follicles, and thyroid cell surface antigen, which is a component of the plasma membrane, may serve as targets for the destruction of the thyroid cells.

2.7.4 Graves' Disease

In the normal functioning of the thyroid, stimulatory signals are received from the pituitary gland in the form of TSH which binds to TSH receptors on the cell surface of the thyroid gland and activates the cell to synthesize and secrete thyroglobulin. In Graves' disease, antibodies are produced with the capacity to bind via their antigen-combining site to the TSH receptor in such a way as to trigger the cells to synthesize and secrete thyroglobulin. In effect the antigen-combining site on the antibody mimics the structure of TSH responsible for binding to the TSH receptor to such an extent that the two are indistinguishable in terms of ability to activate the thyroid cell. As the antibody is not under a negative feed-back regulation dependent on thyroglobulin levels, this stimulation continues as long as these antibodies are present, leading to overproduction of thyroglobulin.

2.7.5 Goodpasture's Syndrome

Antibodies bind to glomerular basement membrane of the glomerular capillaries inducing nephritis, and may also bind to alveolar membrane in the lung causing haemoptysis.

2.7.6 Myasthenia Gravis

Antibodies are present in the serum which are capable of binding to the AChR in an antigen-specific manner via the antigen-combining site of the antibody. The bound antibodies may (a) cross-link the receptors resulting in an increase of the AChR internalization, (b) induce complement-mediated lysis of the membrane, (c) cause direct blockage of the AChR site resulting in impairment of neuromuscular transmission.

2.7.7 Pernicious Anaemia

This form of anaemia results in the prevention of the body's uptake of vitamin B12 necessary for haemoglobin production by antibodies to intrinsic factor which mediates this uptake from the gastric lumen. Circulating antibody does not seem to be capable of inhibiting the activity of intrinsic factor and the antibody must be present in the lumen of the gastrointestinal tract to be effective. These antibodies can be identified in the gastric juices of these patients, synthesized by plasma cells in the gastric lesion.

2.7.8   Insulin-dependent Diabetes Mellitus

Antibodies are produced which bind to the pancreatic islet β cells. These mediate ADCC. They are IgG and specific for the endocrine pancreas cells.

2.7.9   Primary Biliary Cirrhosis

This is a chronic granulomatous inflammatory process causing progressive destruction of the intrahepatic biliary system. Almost all of these patients have detectable anti-mitochondrial antibodies.

2.8   Non-Organ-Specific Diseases

A variety of autoantibodies are present in non-organ-specific disease; some may be the most prevalent antibody perhaps mediating a particular disease but others are present at low concentration or titre and induce supplementary symptoms. A description of the major features of these diseases will be presented.

2.8.1   Rheumatoid Arthritis (RA)

The prevalent antibodies in this disease are the anti-globulin or RF antibodies. These are antibodies that react with autologous and heterologous immunoglobulins. The dominant class of RF are IgM, but IgG, and even IgA and IgE RFs have been detected. The antigenic binding site is usually located on the Fc portion and can be a genetic or structural determinant. The ability of these antibodies to bind other antibodies in solution leads to the formation of complexes which can be deposited in other organs. The synovium of joints may be heavily infiltrated with mononuclear cells often aggregated in the form of lymphoid follicles. Many plasma cells are present, of which a substantial proportion secrete RF antibodies. The joint space thus contains RF antibodies self-associated in complexes with complement. These complexes can mediate cartilage breakdown through different pathways.

Other autoantibodies have been found in RA patients: these include anti-collagen, anti-keratin, anti-nuclear, EBV-associated and anti-lymphocyte antibodies.

2.8.2   Systemic Lupus Erythematosus (SLE)

The prominent antibodies in this disease are reactive with nuclear components including DNA and histones, although a wide range of antibodies binding cell nuclear components has been described. The DNA antibodies may be specific for single- or double-stranded DNA or both. Anti-phospholipid antibodies may also be present as well as antibodies against cells including leucocytes, erythrocytes, platelets and neurones. The exact antigenic determinants are not known. Serum antibodies exhibit a range of cross-reactivity with other antigens.

2.8.3   Sjögren's Syndrome

Sjögren's is a chronic inflammatory autoimmune disorder characterized by a mixed cellular infiltration of exocrine glands, notably the lacrimal and salivary glands. This infiltration gives rise to dry eyes (xeropthalmia) and dry mouth (xerostomia). In many cases these clinical features are associated with RA, SLE and other autoimmune diseases. An array of autoantibodies may be detected in the serum of patients with both primary and secondary Sjögren's syndrome, and these may be organ-specific and non-organ specific. Those in the former category include antibodies to smooth muscle, salivary duct, gastric parietal cells, thyroglobulin-precipitating antibodies and thyroid microsomal antibodies. Those in the latter category are principally anti-SS-A (Ro) and anti-SS-B (La) reacting with Sjögren's syndrome antigens A or B.

2.8.4   Polymyositis

Of the autoantibodies present in polymyositis, perhaps the most disease-specific are the anti-Jo-1 antibodies. These recognize the Jo-1 antigen, which is the histidine tRNA synthetase subunit. It has been found in 30% of polymyositis patients, with adult onset myositis.

2.8.5   Scleroderma

A range of non-disease-specific autoantibodies are occasionally found, including RF, anti-salivary gland and anti-ssDNA antibodies. Antibodies to nuclear components, anti-centromere and anti-nucleolar antibodies appear to be more disease-specific, as is the more readily recognized anti-scl-70 antibody which is found in 25% of patients (the antigen is topoisomerase 1).

For a more detailed review of the role of autoantibodies in these different diseases, the reader is referred to "The Mosaic of Autoimmunity" (Shoenfeld and Isenberg, 1989).

2.9   Monoclonal Antibodies and Autoimmune Diseases

In the non-organ-specific autoimmune diseases, antibodies are commonly found to ubiquitous antigens. It was not known whether this reactivity was attributable to a range of individual antibodies, each specific for a single target antigen, or fewer antibodies capable of binding more than one antigen. The generation of monoclonal antibodies from patients with autoimmune disorders has shown that both types of antibody may be present. Shoenfeld *et al.* (1983a) generated a number of monoclonal antibodies from lupus patients; they found that in addition to binding dsDNA or ssDNA some antibodies bound both, and many additionally possessed other reactivities with polynucleotides and undefined antigenic determinants in tissue sections from different organs. These observations have been confirmed and established by Ravirajan *et al.* (1992) who examined the binding of human hybridoma supernatants to over 20 self- and foreign antigens.

3. Antibody Idiotypes in Autoimmune Disease

Antibodies are conventionally distinguished by the antigens which they bind. Another way of distinguishing antibodies serologically involves analysis of their idiotypes. Immunoglobulin idiotypes are essentially phenotypic markers of the V genes used to encode the "variable regions" of immunoglobulin molecules. These are the regions (sequences of amino acids) which are responsible for the antigen-binding function of the antibody, and their variable sequence enables this function. Essentially the seemingly infinite variability of the antigen-binding region of immunoglobulin molecules, which enables individual antibodies to be "custom made" to bind an individual antigen, is achieved by the construction of a "unique" antigen-binding region from a selection of evolutionarily conserved subunits. These subunits represent novel antigenic determinants and may be recognized in turn by anti-idiotypes. Thus an anti-idiotype may recognize an amino acid sequence of a heavy or light chain alone (a structural determinant) or a region where the conformation and proximity of these chains to one another forms a unique conformation (conformational determinant).

Anti-idiotypes that react only with the immunizing immunoglobulin define restricted or private idiotypes. Sharing of CRI between antibodies of the same or different specificities from different individuals may reflect common amino acid sequences within a framework region CDR.

The concept of an immune system evolving to recognize self-antigens rather than (or in addition to) foreign antigens was formulated by Jerne (1974). There is evidence that an idiotypic network exists in man (reviewed by Shoenfeld and Isenberg, 1989). Study of idiotypes may provide information about the genetic background of autoantibody-mediated disorders, and information about the mechanisms of autoantibody involvement in autoimmune conditions. The use of anti-idiotypic antibodies which identify idiotypes of interest can be used to analyse cellular interactions in these diseases, to examine the tissue distribution of the idiotypes and to explore the possibilities of a novel therapeutic intervention.

3.1 COMPARISON OF RESTRICTED CROSS-REACTIVE IDIOTYPES IN DIFFERENT AUTOIMMUNE DISEASES

Idiotypes associated with autoimmune diseases may be divided into those found in non-organ-specific diseases and those found in organ-specific diseases. The most frequently reported idiotypes associated with autoimmune disorders are shown in Table 1.2.

Table 1.2 Idiotypes in organ-specific and non-organ-specific autoimmune diseases

Autoantibody	Antigen specificity	Autoimmune disease	Idiotype	Reference
Organ-specific				
Anti-AChR	Acetylcholine receptor	Myasthenia gravis	MG/1	Lang et al. (1985)
Anti-AChR	Acetylcholine receptor	Myasthenia gravis	MG/2	Lang et al. (1985)
Anti-AChR	Acetylcholine receptor	Myasthenia gravis	MG/3	Lang et al. (1985)
Anti-AChR	Acetylcholine receptor	Myasthenia gravis	Fabγ3	Lefvert et al. (1982)
Anti-thyroglobulin (ART)	Rat thyroglobulin	Spontaneous autoimmune thyroiditis	BUF rat ART	Zanetti et al (1983)
IgG anti-thyroglobulin	Human thyroglobulin	Hashimoto's/ thyrotoxicosis	MOR	Delves and Roitt (1984)
IgG anti-thyroglobulin	Human thyroglobulin	Hashimoto's/ thyrotoxicosis	WAR	Delves and Roitt (1984)
IgG anti-thyroglobulin	Human thyroglobulin	Hashimoto's/ thyrotoxicosis	PAT	Delves and Roitt (1984)
IgM anti-thyroglobulin	Human thyroglobulin	(EBV B cell line)	E/JAR	Delves and Roitt (1984)
Non-organ-specific				
Mouse IgM RF	IgG Fc	Cryoglobulinaemia	Wa IgMRF	Agnello and Barnes (1986)
Mouse IgM RF	IgG Fc	Cryoglobulinaemia	Po IgMRF	Agnello and Barnes (1986)
Mouse IgM RF	IgG Fc	Cryoglobulinaemia	BLa IgMRF	Agnello and Barnes (1986)
Anti-La (SS-B)	La ribonucleoprotein	Sjögren's syndrome Sjögren's syndrome/SLE	E.P.W.	Horsfall et al. (1986)
Anti-DNA	DNA	SLE	16/6	Shoenfeld et al. (1983b)
Anti-DNA	DNA	SLE	134	Dudeney et al. (1986)
Anti-DNA	DNA	SLE	32/15	Shoenfeld et al. (1983b)

3.1.1 Non-organ-specific Diseases

Cross-reactive idiotypes on human monoclonal RFs were originally described using polyclonal anti-idiotypes by Kunkel and co-workers (1973) and subsequently by Agnello *et al.* (1980) and were classified into three main idiotypic groups, Wa, Po and Bla. By contrast, private idiotypes were reported as a more frequent finding using monoclonal anti-idiotypes (Posnett *et al.*, 1986). Studies by several investigators have revealed extensive DNA antibody idiotype sharing by both monoclonal and serum-derived anti-DNA antibodies in the MRL-lpr/lpr and (NZB/W) F1 lupus-prone mouse strains (reviewed by Rauch *et al.*, 1982). Idiotype sharing on DNA antibodies has also been found in man. Shoenfeld *et al.* (1983b) described two human anti-DNA monoclonal antibodies 16/6 and 32/15 with different antigen-binding profiles; anti-idiotypic studies showed that both the 16/6 and 32/15 idiotypes are at or very close to the antigen-binding site on DNA antibodies. In studies of serially collected sera, notable correlation of the 16/6 idiotype level with disease activity was found in 8 of 12 patients studied. In both these and subsequent studies, it was noted that the 16/6 idiotype level, sometimes reflected disease activity better than DNA binding. The subject is reviewed in detail elsewhere (Isenberg and Staines, 1990).

Several other groups have analysed DNA antibody idiotypes by purifying anti-DNA antibodies from the serum of SLE patients. The 3.I, 8.12 and AM idiotypes are framework determinants, whereas the TOF and PR4 idiotypes are binding-site-related. The distribution of the SLE idiotypes in patients, their healthy relatives and spouses is reviewed elsewhere (Watts and Isenberg, 1990). Although most of the DNA antibody idiotypes described in the literature are cross-reactive, others that are private have been identified.

In studies of idiotypes associated with antibodies to ribonucleoprotein antigens, three anti-idiotypes were raised against affinity-purified anti-La antibodies derived from three different patients with Sjögren's syndrome. Each anti-idiotype bound only to the immunizing antibody and recognized conformationally dependent idiotypic determinants which were associated with the antigen-binding site (Horsfall *et al.*, 1986). No CRIs could be demonstrated on autoantibodies to the La, Sm/RNP or DNA antigens in other patients. Similarly antibodies to the ribonucleoprotein antigen U1 RNP associated with mixed connective tissue were found to have private idiotypes (Satoh *et al.*, 1987).

By contrast, a CRI designated Y2 has been identified on a monoclonal anti-Sm antibody from an MRL-1pr/1pr mouse, and the idiotype has also been found in the sera of two autoimmune and several normal strains of mice. This idiotype has been detected in the sera of 41% of SLE patients, 27% of healthy first-degree relatives and 6% of healthy controls (Dang *et al.*, 1988).

3.1.2 Organ-specific Diseases

In experimental models of myasthenia gravis there is evidence for the existence of shared idiotypes. Idiotype sharing by 10 of 16 myasthenia gravis patients using a mouse monoclonal antibody against an isolated chain Fab fragment of affinity-purified anti-AChR antibody was shown by Lefvert *et al.* (1982). In contrast, polyclonal anti-idiotypes used by others failed to show evidence of site-related idiotype sharing between patients with anti-AChR antibodies (Lang *et al.*, 1985). Lefvert (1988) used monoclonal antibodies to define four idiotypes at or near the antigen combining site and two directed against framework determinants on anti-AChR antibodies. These monoclonals recognized idiotypes present on immunoglobulins from 14–60% of patients with myasthenia gravis. This indicates substantial sharing. These idiotypes were also found in patients with no detectable autoantibody activity in their serum. In all the patients studied, the levels of each idiotype fluctuated considerably during the course of the disease, regardless of clinical symptoms. This contrasts with the serial studies of the common DNA antibody idiotype 16/6 in patients with SLE (Isenberg *et al.*, 1984). However, it should be remembered that anti-AChR antibodies differ from anti-DNA antibodies in that there is poor correlation between the total concentration of serum autoantibodies and severity of disease symptoms. In thyroiditis, both public (Zanetti *et al.*, 1983) and private (Delves and Roitt, 1984; Ruf *et al.*, 1986) idiotypes have been reported. Ruf and colleagues (1986) have suggested that it is the private idiotypes that predominate.

3.1.3 Pathogenic Idiotypes of Autoantibodies

Immunocytochemical studies with anti-idiotypes have shown both local synthesis and deposition of idiotype-positive autoantibodies within pathological lesions. The cross-reactive anti-DNA antibody idiotype 16/6 has been found on tissue-bound immunoglobulins in kidney and skin biopsies from SLE patients. In one study, 42% of renal biopsies showed deposition of 16/6 idiotype-positive immunoglobulin, and in half of these patients another DNA idiotype, 32/15, was also detectable, whereas neither idiotype could be detected in healthy control kidney biopsies (Isenberg and Collins, 1985). In skin biopsies, 45% of SLE patients studied showed deposition of cross-reactive idiotypes at the dermal–epidermal junction. By comparison, 30% of discoid lupus biopsies shared the same idiotypes unlike any of 15 immunoglobulin-positive controls (Isenberg *et al.*, 1985a).

Pernis *et al.* (1984) found the RF cross-reactive idiotype Wa could be detected in plasma cells of synovial tissue of RA patients. Interestingly there were three times as many Id$^+$ cells as Ag-binding RF$^+$ cells. In salivary gland biopsies from patients with Sjögren's syndrome, idiotypes identical with those found on circulating and salivary IgG and IgA anti-La antibodies have been demonstrated in the cytoplasm of plasma cells and as peri-acinar deposits (Horsfall *et al.*, 1987).

Investigations have focused on whether certain idiotypes are more pathogenic than others (for instance, cross-reactive idiotypes more than private idiotypes) and if these idiotypes are directly involved in the pathogenesis of autoimmune disease. Mendlovic *et al.* (1988) performed an experiment to determine whether immunization of normal healthy mice with an autoantibody carrying an idiotype known to be strongly associated with autoimmune disease could induce a pathogenic effect. Human monoclonal antibody carrying the 16/6 idiotype (1µg) was immunized into mice followed by a booster injection. Later the mice developed an SLE-like disease and had sustained high titres of 16/6 idiotype as well as detectable anti-16/6 idiotype antibodies additional to antibodies normally associated with SLE. Immunizing NZB/W lupus-prone mice with the 16/6 idiotype accelerated the incidence of lupus-like disease (Mendlovic *et al.*, 1990).

However, an independent analysis failed to reproduce the model (Isenberg *et al.*, 1991), and the authors suggested that this failure implies that the idiotype alone is insufficient to cause the lupus-like disease and that unknown environmental factors must also be important. It has also been demonstrated by Datta *et al.* (1986) that the 16/6 idiotype that was present on non-anti-DNA antibodies in a patient in remission switched to expression on anti-DNA antibodies as the patient went into relapse. Thus idiotype shift could result in escape of autoantibodies from detection and modulation by anti-idiotype. Furthermore, the idiotype shift described might represent a shift of pathogenic idiotype in as much as active nephritis was noted when the first idiotype was present, whereas nephritis was not the predominant clinical manifestation when the second idiotype emerged.

3.1.4 V Gene Usage in Autoantibody Idiotypes

The study of idiotypy among monoclonal antibody populations using anti-idiotypes provides some clues to the genetic origins of these autoantibodies. Thus, CRIs present on autoantibodies from non-related individuals suggest the use of highly conserved germline genes which may have some evolutionary significance in protection for the host. The identification of primary amino acid sequences of known idiotypes and their position within fully sequenced V regions can enable the identification of families of V genes. For example, many monoclonal IgM antibodies with specificity for IgG Fc and DNA have a κ light chain belonging to the VKIIIb family and JK1 and JK2 gene families.

4. *Incidence of Autoimmune Disease in Families*

In almost all known autoimmune diseases there is a tendency for these conditions to run in families. This may occur in the form of an increased incidence of a given disorder in relatives of afflicted patients compared with a control population or in the form of an increased incidence of other autoimmune diseases in family members of patients with specific disorders.

A number of reports have described the detection of autoantibodies in family members of patients suffering autoimmune diseases. In 1960, Holman and Deicher reported hypergammaglobulinaemia in 11 of 57 relatives of SLE patients, belonging to 18 families. Furthermore, they found 14% of asymptomatic relatives had serological findings frequently detected in patients with RA, compared with 6% in the control group. Pollak *et al.* (1960) reported finding "anti-nuclear factor" in 19 of 36 first-degree relatives of 12 SLE patients, and in 5 out of 14 second-degree relatives. The control group included 50 patients with other diseases, all unrelated to SLE, of whom only one was found to be anti-nuclear factor positive, and 40 healthy subjects, all negative. In a later study, ANABs were found in 47 first-degree relatives of 43 SLE patients, and in 10 of 70 second-degree relatives (Pollak, 1964). Overt autoimmune disease (SLE or scleroderma) developed in three families, amongst relatives who were asymptomatic at the time of autoantibody detection. An increased prevalence of anti-cardiolipin antibodies amongst lupus family members has also been reported by Mackworth-Young *et al.* (1987).

Leonhart (1957) reported a family in which three siblings, all sisters, two of whom were dizygotic twins, out of 14 had developed SLE. These three lupus patients and one other sister had very high γ-globulin levels. In addition, a further three sisters and one brother also had a more moderate hypergammaglobulinaemia. Leonhardt envisaged the hypergammaglobulinaemic state as a phase preceding the development of overt SLE, and postulated the existence of an environmental or hereditary factor common to all the siblings, which induced their hypergammaglobulinaemia and in some eventually SLE.

Lippman *et al.* (1982) examined 10 families belonging to two large kindreds where more than one member was found to suffer from an autoimmune disease, and found that 21% of the 70 first-degree relatives of the patients also had an autoimmune disorder such as haemolytic anaemia, chronic immune thrombocytopenia, SLE, autoimmune thyroid disease, or RA. In a study of 985 patients with definite or classical RA attending an arthritis clinic, Wolfe *et al.* (1988) found that 10.9% of unrelated patients had one or more first-degree relatives affected with definite or classical RA.

In 1973, Spector *et al.* described two pairs of brothers who had SLE. They pointed out that as the disease is known to be less prevalent in males than females, its appearance specifically in pairs of brothers supports the significance of hereditary factors in its pathogenesis. However, the different clinical presentations in the brothers suggest that other factors are important. Arnett and Shulman (1976) described eight families with two SLE patients in each, and reviewed 31 similar families from the literature. They reported significant clinical concordance between two identical twins, as well as in parent–offspring couples, whereas the clinical presentation of non-identical siblings was quite different. The authors suggest that this finding further supports the significance of hereditary factors in the pathogenesis of autoimmune diseases.

4.1   AUTOIMMUNITY STUDIES IN TWINS

Studies of twins, primarily monozygotic twins, contribute greatly to our understanding of hereditary factors in the pathogenesis of autoimmune disorders. Mackay and Myrianthopoulos (1966) described the appearance of multiple sclerosis in twins with a concordance rate of 20.6% in monozygotic twins, as well as the development of the disease amongst their relatives, with an incidence of 1.7% in their parents, 1.4% in their offspring, 6.4% in their siblings and only 0.4% in cousins and more distant family members. The influence of genetic factors on the concordance rates in twins was shown by Johnston *et al.* (1983) who found concordance rates for insulin dependent diabetes was about 70% if twins were DR3/DR4 positive but only 40% if they were not.

Block *et al.* (1975) reported 12 pairs of twins with SLE, including seven definite monozygotic and three definite dizygotic pairs; similar clinical presentation was found in four of the seven monozygotic twins (57%). Serological similarity was also found, with ANAbs present in both twins in each of the monozygotic couples. All monozygotic pairs examined were raised in the same environment, and four of them were never separated for an extensive period of time prior to development of their disease. Amongst close relatives (parents and siblings), ANAbs were found in 28%, hypergammaglobulinaemia in 33% and overt autoimmune disease in one of the 34 relatives tested. The authors claimed that the incidence of clinical concordance amongst monozygotic twins with SLE is higher than that seen amongst other pairs of first-degree relatives. Furthermore, the same authors quoted a report of twins, separated at 14 months of age and subsequently raised in different separate environments. At the age of 14 years, within 1 month, they were both diagnosed to be suffering from SLE, with identical clinical presentations. Despite the fact that this report strengthens the claim of a genetic aetiology, the possibility of exposure to an environmental factor during early childhood or sooner, possibly during gestation, cannot be excluded. A more recent study by Deapen *et al.*

(1986) using a survey of 138 twins, in which the proband had SLE, found a concordance rate of only 23% in 66 same-sex monozygotic twins, compared with only 9% of 44 same-sex dizygotic twins. On balance, however, the published data strongly support the genetic influence in the aetiology of SLE.

4.2   GENETIC VERSUS ENVIRONMENTAL FACTORS

Much of the study in this area has focused on the detection of autoantibodies in patients, their blood relatives and spouses, and their prolonged exposure to common environments, i.e. cohabitation. De Horatius and Messner (1975) detected increased frequency of anti-lymphocyte and anti-RNA antibodies in relatives of SLE patients, when compared with control families. The authors suggested that these data signified exposure of patients and their families living in the same environment. However, with respect to anti-DNA antibodies, no major difference between SLE family members as a whole and close household contacts, was found. In a similar attempt to differentiate between hereditary and environmental factors, Lowenstein and Rothfield (1977) examined the sera of 27 patients with SLE and 16 patients with discoid lupus for the presence of various serological markers including ANAbs and compared the results with those of 21 first-degree relatives who lived in the same household as the patients, 19 first-degree relatives who did not live in the patients' environment, 15 spouses of the patients, and 26 control subjects, 20 of whom worked in the hospital laboratories which handled sera from the SLE patients. Both high titres and a statistically significant increase in incidence of ANAbs were found in the sera of healthy relatives of SLE patients, compared with their spouses or controls. The high incidence was independent of the household contact. This finding implies that genetic factors are more important than environmental ones. On the other hand, close household contacts of patients with discoid lupus, either blood relatives or spouses, were found to have a high incidence of immunoglobulin precipitins and complement components in the dermal–epidermal junction of clinically healthy/normal skin, a finding that supports the significance of environmental factors.

Antibody idiotypes, phenotypic markers of the antigen-binding variable region genes of immunoglobulin (discussed in more detail earlier in this chapter) have also been studied to elucidate any correlations of genetic or environmental factors. The presence of two idiotypes, designated 16/6 and 32/15 (initially identified on ssDNA-binding monoclonal antibodies), and found at high incidence in patients with SLE, RA and other autoimmune diseases, were found to be prevalent in the sera of relatives of patients with SLE. Of 147 relatives of 48 SLE patients, 24% and 7% carried the idiotypes 16/6 and 32/15 compared with 4% and 1% of normals

(Isenberg *et al.*, 1985b). Shoenfeld *et al.* (1986) also reported finding six members of a family of eight with high levels of the 16/6 idiotype. This family was characterized by C4 deficiency and two sisters developed SLE. An additional SLE idiotype, 134, originally identified on a human hybridoma antibody binding dsDNA (as opposed to ssDNA) was detected in a high titre in 45% of 31 SLE patients, and 30% of 50 first-degree relatives of the same patients. Only 1 of 40 control subjects, not known to have any autoimmune disease, had the idiotype (Dudeney *et al.*, 1986). Similar results with other common anti-DNA antibody idiotypes have been reported by other groups (Halpern *et al.*, 1985; Harkiss *et al.*, 1986).

In summary, most of these studies support the notion that genetic influences are important in the production of autoantibodies in asymptomatic subjects, in relatives of patients with autoimmune diseases and in the patients themselves. However, there is no doubt that the hereditary factor alone is insufficient to induce disease, and additional triggers must exist in order for overt disease to develop.

5. *Autoimmune Disease and the MHC/HLA*

The MHC is found on chromosome 17 in the mouse. The analogous region in man, known as the HLA, is in chromosome 6. HLAs are expressed at the cell surface and classified into two groups, class I and class II, based on structural and functional characteristics. The genes which code these "antigens" are in close proximity and generally inherited as a haplotype, that is a gene combination of the same single chromosome. The gene products from the two classes are structurally similar. The HLAs are characterized by a wide variance amongst unrelated individuals (allotypic polymorphism). The class I molecules are detected on the membranes of nucleated cells and blood platelets. These molecules are glycoproteins containing a heavy chain (molecular mass 43 kDa) which is anchored in the cell membrane, and a light chain (11 kDa) termed β_2-microglobulin which is not anchored to the cell membrane and is encoded by genes located on chromosome 15. The class II antigens are encoded on genes in the HLA-D region, specifically the DR, DQ and DP. In addition to these, there are class II antigens, termed DW, which can be identified by means of MLC. The class II molecules are detected on macrophages and dendritic cells, and other cells which present antigen to the immune system, activated T and B lymphocytes. The molecules in this class consist of two glycoprotein chains, α and β, with an average molecular mass of 33 and 28 kDa respectively. The antigens present on the cell membranes as dimers bound non-covalently (Shackelford *et al.*, 1982).

The HLAs play an important role in the regulation of the immune system. T cells can identify certain antigens only when presented, together with self-antigens of HLA classes I or II, on macrophage surfaces. Thus, as far as the T cells are concerned, a foreign antigen is a complex consisting of the antigen and HLA molecules of class I or II (Zinkernagel and Doherty, 1980). The T helper cells identify the antigen in combination with class II HLA markers, whereas cytotoxic T cells identify antigen associated with class I HLA molecules. Thus qualitative and quantitative changes in the degree of HLA expression serve as controls for the general immune response.

A number of factors that control the expression of class I or II HLA molecules have been identified. For example, interferon stimulates expression, whereas prostaglandin E and fetoproteins inhibit the production, of class II HLA molecules (Heron *et al.*, 1978). It appears that alterations in HLA expression in tissues, resulting from immune dysfunction, may be related to the pathogenesis of certain autoimmune diseases. Bottazzo *et al.* (1983) showed that, in Hashimoto's disease, the thyroid gland is infiltrated by cytotoxic T cells, and class II HLA antigens appear on the surface of affected thyroid cells, whereas normal thyroid epithelium does not exhibit these antigens. The appearance of these class I or II HLAs is controlled, as mentioned above, by active biological factors such as interferons. Pujol-Borrell *et al.* (1983) suggested that the interferon released as a result of a "silent" viral infection of the thyroid gland causes class II antigenic expression on the thyroid cells. These cells then present normal constituents of thyroid cells as foreign antigens and then serve as a stimulus for an autoimmune reaction.

In Graves' disease, it is thought that class II HLAs and their reactions with T cells play an important role. The disease is characterized by the production of antibodies directed against TSH receptors on the thyroid cell surface. The assumption is that any lesion of the thyroid cells, e.g. by viral infection, leads to an inflammatory response and T cell infiltration. The thyroid cells acquire the class II HLAs upon their surfaces by T cell induction or via IFNγ, TNF or some combination which may be produced by the T cells. Class II HLA molecules localize beside the TSH receptors on the cell surface so that a functional unit is formed. This unit simplifies presentation of the receptor to the T helper cells. As a result, a wide range of anti-TSH receptor antibodies is produced.

Similarly class I HLAs are absent from normal hepatocytes, but can appear on bile duct cells during inflammatory diseases, or diseases with an assumed autoimmune origin such as primary biliary cirrhosis (Daar *et al.*, 1984) or on pancreatic cells in type 1 diabetes mellitus (Bottazzo *et al.*, 1985). Class I HLAs have been found on most striated muscle cells in inflammatory myopathies and dystrophies but not in healthy muscles (Isenberg *et al.*, 1986).

5.1   HLA AND AUTOIMMUNE DISEASES

Where a relationship exists between autoimmune disease and HLA, it appears that the majority of diseases are related to class II HLAs. This may be due to the fact that class II HLAs are identified by helper T cells. In a number of autoimmune diseases, there are significant statistical relationships with HLAs, B8 and DR3 or both (DeVries and Van Rood, 1988). Other HLAs are linked to specific diseases by either over- or under-representation (e.g. in type 1 diabetes it is rare to find DR2 or DR5 (Maclaren *et al.*, 1988)). RA is linked to DR4 (Husby *et al.*, 1979) in many patient studies but to DR1 in others (Woodrow, 1988a). A variety of DR4 subtypes associated with varying susceptibility for RA in different ethnic groups have been identified. Unlike RA, SLE is linked to DR4 and DR3 (Woodrow, 1988b). Thus closely related diseases induced by different pathophysiological mechanisms are related to different HLAs. This confirms that the contribution of HLA to the development of a particular autoimmune disease is only partial, and other factors must be involved. Although DR3 is more common in a number of autoimmune diseases, most people with DR3 are healthy. However, these antigens are related to immunoregulatory dysfunction even in healthy individuals: for example, healthy women with HLA-B8 phenotype, when tested in an *in vitro* lymphocyte proliferation assay after T cell mitogen stimulation, showed abnormal proliferative response. In families of patients with autoimmune diseases, HLA-B8 is the most common phenotype observed in healthy family members who produce autoantibodies. Additionally, lymphocytes *in vitro* from healthy individuals with HLA-B8 react more strongly to common antigens than do individuals without HLA-B8 (Osaba and Falk, 1978). T suppressor cell activity was found to be deficient in healthy subjects with HLA-DR3 and, as a result, the number of antibody-producing cells was increased relative to subjects without HLA-DR3.

The most commonly associated HLA and autoimmune disease is HLA-DR3. In general, it is evident that DR3-positive individuals show a strong and rapid humoral immune response, but tend to be low responders in a number of tests in which accessory cells and T cells interact. The DR3 allele is also related to a disturbance in phagocytosis by monocytes, primarily when it is related to certain Gm allotypes. Thus one cause of the DR3 phenomenon is that antigens (e.g. bacteria and viruses) might bind more easily to class II molecules in individuals whose accessory cells express the DR3 haplotype. A second possibility is that the DR3-positive antigen-presenting cells might be quantitatively or qualitatively different in some way. These two possibilities are not mutually exclusive and both mechanisms might work in the thymus to generate a different repertoire of antibodies. The effects might also occur during an ongoing immune response and lead to increased activation of helper T cells.

There have also been claims of links between HLA and mycobacterium infection, which may lead to auto-immune disease. In one population studied, an increased frequency of individuals who were DR3-positive was present in responders to mycobacterial preparations (Van Eden *et al.*, 1983). An association has been found between HLA DR4 and mycobacterium tuberculosis. In particular, this allele, compared with others tested, is linked to an increased response to *Mycobacterium tuberculosis*-specific antigens (Bahr *et al.*, 1989).

The strong relationship between HLA-B27 and ankylosing spondylitis (individuals bearing this phenotype are 100 times more likely to develop the disease) is apparently not based on an autoimmune mechanism. A number of researchers have reported a cross-reaction between HLA-B27 molecules of these patients and bacteria, notably *Klebsiella* antigens (see Section 8). Elucidating the relationships between HLA and disease has proved useful at the population/genetic level, providing insights into possible associations, e.g. type 1 (insulin-dependent) diabetes mellitus is clearly associated with certain HLA haplotypes whereas type 2 is not. In contrast, at the individual level, knowledge of the HLA haplotype has provided only limited information. Its use as a diagnostic tool, for example, is generally insufficient to be of any practical value.

5.2   TREATMENT DIRECTED AGAINST HLAs

As the gene products of particular haplotypes have been strongly implicated in the aetiology of autoimmune disease, it has been tempting to speculate that blocking these products might have beneficial effect. Experiments performed in mice using reagents that recognize determinants in the MHC (analogous to the HLA-D region in man) have shown in some circumstances that prevention of disease can be achieved (Adelman *et al.*, 1983). However, in primates, application of the treatments with homologous antibodies led to disseminated intravascular coagulation (Kolb and Toyka, 1984), thus any further studies must wait until the nature of this serious complication is understood.

6.   *The Gm Allotype System and Autoimmune Disease*

Gm is an immunoglobulin constant region marker, encoded for by genes and phenotypically expressed as allotypic markers on certain immunoglobulins. Some heavy and light chain isotopes bear genetic markers that are inherited in typical Mendelian fashion. These alternative forms at a given genetic locus are called allotypes.

The allotypes associated with γ chains are called Gm. Those associated with α chains are termed Am and those associated with ϰ light chains are called Km. The contribution of Gm to inherited predisposition in chronic inflammatory disease is less well defined than HLA. This may be the result of limitations inherent in Gm as a polymorphism for use in population genetics. The Gm system has fewer alleles than HLA, stronger linkage disequilibrium between loci, is less readily and less widely measured in the laboratory and has not, unlike HLA, been the focus of major international workshops.

A relationship between the immune response and Gm has been shown, by correlating primary responses to Gm and HLA phenotypes with immune response to bacterial antigens. The association between the humoral response and Gm allotypes could be based on linkage disequilibrium between the Gm genes and genes that specify the idiotypic structure of the immunoglobulin. Because of this linkage, the binding ability of immunoglobulin is dependent on the presence of certain Gm allotypes. There are several reports that support this hypothesis (Weitkamp *et al.*, 1975; Rose and Mackay, 1985). Although HLA and Gm are both located on chromosome 6 (Bender *et al.*, 1979), there is no evidence for a close linkage between them in family studies. The association between Gm and the various autoimmune diseases has been studied in several disorders. Among the various autoimmune diseases, a statistically significant relationship with Gm was detected in patients with Graves' disease, Hashimoto's thyroiditis, diabetes mellitus type 1, SLE, RA, multiple sclerosis and myasthenia gravis.

Why are Gm allotypes associated with autoimmunity? There are several plausible explanations for the association between the Gm allotypes and autoimmune diseases. All these theories suggest that the Gm genes *per se* are not necessary for the development of the autoimmune diseases, but rather that these genes are in linkage disequilibrium with the others that are related to the immune response genes (Ir). One of these theories suggests linkage disequilibrium between the Gm allotypes and the genes that control idiotype regulation. Because of this linkage, it may be that certain Gm allotypes are related to the production of autoantibodies. The finding that certain Gm allotypes are associated with MG, RA and diabetes mellitus type 1, only in patients who had autoantibodies against the acetycholine receptor, collagen type II and insulin respectively supports this theory.

Several studies have reported an association between the Gm allotypes, HLA and autoimmune diseases. In one study of chronic active hepatitis, the relative risk for the disease was increased 39 times above the risk for individuals who did not carry the particular combination of HLA and Gm allotypes. It also appeared from the study that the Gm genes augment the risk of development of disease and in the absence of the HLA allotype the Gm genes appeared to be inactive (Whittingham

et al., 1981). The mechanism of the HLA and Gm interaction is still uncertain. One mechanism suggests that MHC genes are linked to genes that regulate the level of overall immunoglobulin synthesis, but the Gm-linked genes may determine the proportion of this response devoted to a particular autoantibody, so, in the presence of certain HLA and Gm allotypes, high levels of autoantibodies are produced.

7. Cytokines and Autoimmunity

Cytokines are potent polypeptides that mediate much of the intercellular signalling required for a coordinated immune response. Not only can these proteins induce a destructive response from a variety of effector cells, including cells from outside the immune system, but they themselves can be cytotoxic to a whole variety of cell types, thus acting as the final effector mechanism. Recently, the picture has been complicated further as it has been appreciated that some cytokines inhibit immune reactions, whilst others have apparently conflicting effects.

The cytokines are divided into a number of families (Table 1.3). The lymphokines are products of lymphocytes and participate in the processes of immune reaction, inflammation and haematopoiesis. Together with cytokines produced from monocytes, they have been designated interleukins, and those whose biological properties and amino acid sequences are known have been assigned a number; so far 12 have been identified. The other major cytokines are the interferons, which were originally identified by their ability to inhibit viral replication, and tumour necrosis factor, which was initially shown to be cytotoxic to many different cell types. In addition there are a number of growth factors which will not be discussed further.

In the next section we will review the evidence that links cytokines with autoimmunity as a fuller discussion of cytokines appears elsewhere. By understanding how these peptides are involved in these self-destructive diseases we can learn to modulate the immune reaction. It is simpler to understand the actions of cytokines in

Table 1.3 Outline of cytokine families

Family	Examples of members
Interleukins	IL-1 – IL-12
Lymphokines	
Monokines	
Interferons	IFNα, IFNβ, IFNγ
Tumour necrosis factors	TNF-α, TNF-β
Colony-stimulating factors	GM-CSF
Other growth factors	TGF

different diseases by looking at them individually. However, only by examining the interactions between them and their combined effects (sometimes antagonistic) can their full potential be appreciated. Although there are many autoimmune diseases, we will concentrate on two: RA and SLE, which represent examples of organ-focused and -non-focused diseases respectively.

7.1 INTERLEUKIN-1

IL-1 was originally thought to be produced by monocytes alone but it is now known to be synthesized by a range of cells. IL-1 seems to function both as a short- and long-range messenger and acts on many different cell types. Many of the pathological phenomena observed in RA can be explained in part by the observed elevation of IL-1 in serum and its increased production by synovial tissue, which has been shown to be related to disease activity (Shore *et al.*, 1986). For instance, IL-1 upregulates the expression of adhesion molecules on cultured vascular endothelium which *in vivo* would lead to increased traffic of immune cells into sites of inflammation. IL-1 also causes fibroblast proliferation and collagen synthesis leading to pannus formation. It activates osteoclasts resulting in the absorption of bone and leads to the release of proteinases and proteoglycanases from chondrocytes. By these various mechanisms, the unrestricted release of IL-1 can cause much tissue damage. Indeed the injection of IL-1 into rabbit joints can initiate a chronic arthritis (Pettipher *et al.*, 1986).

Patients with autoimmune conditions such as SLE have been shown to have defective production of IL-1 (Takei *et al.*, 1987) although, more recently, Aotsuka and colleagues (1991) have found that IL-1 is elevated in patients with SLE and other connective tissue disorders when anti-ribonucleoprotein antibodies are present. Others have demonstrated decreased IL-1 responsiveness of lymphocytes from patients with SLE (Alcocer-Varela *et al.*, 1984). Thus different workers have obtained apparently contradicting findings relating to the level of IL-1 in different diseases depending on the methods used. However, it is becoming clear that the level of IL-1 and its biological effects vary according to the presence of other cytokines. From studies on RA (Alvaro-Gracia *et al.*, 1990), IFNγ and TNF-α induce IL-1 production. Moreover, TNF-α and IL-1 enhance each other's effect. However, IFNγ inhibits the activity of TNF-α but not IL-1, whereas IL-6 inhibits the production of both (see below). As more studies of interactions are performed, the complexities relating to their role in health and disease increase.

7.2 INTERLEUKIN-2

IL-2 is probably the best characterized of the interleukins. It plays a pivotal role in the antigen specific response and its production reflects a commitment event

in T cell activation representing the final outcome of various immunological triggering stimuli. Thus it may lead to a breakdown of peripheral tolerance and eventually autoimmune disease. Andreu and co-workers (1991) reported that neonatal thymectomized mice develop autoimmunity characterized by the development of anti-DNA antibodies and the presence of interstitial nephritis when inoculated with an IL-2 vaccinia virus that produces large amounts of IL-2. This is associated with the conversion of double-negative T cells into CD4+ or CD8+T cells. However, introducing the human IL-2 genes into normal mice does not result in fulminant autoimmune disease. Moreover, patients who receive IL-2 do not develop fulminant autoimmune disease, rather they display transient autoimmune phenomena mainly manifesting in the thyroid. Thus it appears that IL-2 can only trigger autoimmune disease that is mediated by a non-deleted T cell repertoire. Antagonizing the IL-2/IL-2R system by administration of IL-2R-targeted drugs prevents, postpones or mitigates the development of autoimmune diseases in virtually any animal model studied, but has limited effects on already established autoimmune diseases (Kroemer *et al.*, 1991).

In marked contrast with its ability to induce autoimmune phenomena, IL-2 exerts a beneficial effect on MRL/1pr mice and results in the almost complete disappearance of cells bearing the 1pr phenotype: CD3+CD4−LD8−B220− (Gutierrez-Ramos *et al.*, 1990). A connection can be drawn between this and the experiment with neonatally thymectomized mice, that is the conversion of double-negative T cells into CD8+ or CD4+T cells. Thus IL-2 might re-equilibrate or aggravate whatever imbalance is present in the tolerance-preserving process. Further complicating the effects of IL-2 on the immune system are the mediators released by IL-2 administration. TNF-α and IFN-γ are both produced by lymphocytes after IL-2 stimulation which are able to prevent or accelerate autoimmunity (*vide infra*).

Not only is the production and bioavailability of IL-2 tightly controlled by a variety of mechanisms, but the resulting immune response is regulated by its receptor (IL-2R) which in turn can be up- or down-regulated by different mechanisms. Upon *in vitro* activation, T cells not only produce a surface IL-2R but also shed a soluble IL-2R. Elevated concentrations of IL-2 and the soluble IL-2R (sIL-2R) are encountered in various body fluids in a variety of conditions such as RA, SLE and Sjögren's syndrome (Kroemer *et al.*, 1991). It may be that the raised level of sIL-2R is secondary to elevated IL-2 which induces the release of sIL-2R.

Studies of freshly isolated lymphocytes (from patients with a variety of autoimmune diseases) *in vitro* have revealed a reduced production of IL-2. This apparent contradiction may be explained by the observation that lupus T cells have an enhanced ability to secrete IL-2 after a period of preculture (Huang *et al.*, 1986). In other words, the reduction in IL-2 synthesis may reflect a transient exhaustion of *in vivo*-activated IL-2-producing cells. Hishikawa and co-workers (1990) demonstrated that the defect in IL-2 production is correlated with the presence of activated T cells, and that, with a period of pre-culture, these T cells diminish in number. However, this phenomenon has not been observed with synovial cells in rheumatoid joints where "resting" the cells before culture did not reverse the defect in IL-2 production (Aaron and Paetkau, 1991). Studies on B cells from patients with SLE have revealed that they are already maximally stimulated and that the addition of IL-2, IL-4 and IL-6 does not increase immunoglobulin production *in vitro* (Pelton *et al.*, 1991). This would be compatible with the notion that B cells in SLE patients are already stimulated *in vivo* by these cytokines. Attempts to correlate IL-2 production with disease activity have not been rewarding.

Studies of RA have revealed reduced (Miyasaka *et al.*, 1984), normal (McKenna *et al.*, 1986) and raised (Cathely *et al.*, 1986) levels of IL-2 secretion. Kitas *et al.* (1988) could not find a clear association with disease activity. One explanation for these conflicting reports may be the lymphocyte products induced by IL-2. In addition, functional assays used to detect IL-2 are also affected by IL-4 and possibly also IL-7 (Londei *et al.*, 1990).

The correlation of sIL-2R with disease activity has been equally unrewarding. In RA no significant correlation between sIL-2R and 15 different clinical variables could be established (Keystone *et al.*, 1988). However, longitudinal studies revealed that peak levels coincide with active disease phases (Rubin *et al.*, 1990). Measurements of sIL-2R in SLE reveal that sIL-2R correlates well with levels of anti-dsDNA and the third and fourth components of complement, but not with a disease activity index (TerBorg *et al.*, 1990). The physiological significance of sIL-2R is a matter of debate. Some have postulated that it acts as an IL-2 antagonist, while others maintain that it is a transport protein for IL-2, releasing it in the vicinity of membrane-bound IL-2R which has an affinity for IL-2 three orders of magnitude higher than its soluble counterpart (Keystone *et al.*, 1988).

7.3   INTERLEUKIN-4

Several laboratories have evaluated mitogen-induced production of IL-4 by T cells from mice with SLE-like disease. Upland *et al.* (1989) reported that concavalin A-stimulated spleen cells from old (6–7-month) MRL/lpr mice produce only about a third of the amount of IL-4 produced by controls. In contrast, Davidson and co-workers (1991) reported that lymph nodes from C3H/lpr mice secrete significantly more IL-4 following stimulation with anti-TCRαβ antibodies plus PMA than lymph nodes from control C3H/+ mice.

Overexpression of IL-4 in transgenic mice leads to an increased level of IgG1 and IgE antibodies, and the occurrence of an allergic inflammatory blepharitis (Tepper *et al.*, 1990). IL-4 is a B cell stimulatory factor and may play a role in the B cell hyperactivity seen in SLE. An increase in IL-4 is seen in older Palmerston North mice (a murine lupus model), and this is associated with an increase in IgG1 anti-DNA antibodies (Handwerger, 1989). IL-4 is known to be an inhibitor of other cytokines, in particular IL-1β and TNF-α (TeVelde *et al.*, 1990).

7.4   INTERLEUKIN-5

IL-5 is a T helper cell-derived B cell stimulatory factor that may also play a role in B cell hyperactivity seen in SLE. Tominaga and co-workers (1991) reported that when transgenic mice carrying the mouse IL-5 gene were injected with cadmium-containing saline, IL-5 production increased approximately 5-fold. This was associated with the appearance of a variety of autoantibodies including anti-DNA antibodies. In addition, these mice have a massive increase in the number of eosinophils in many tissues including the peripheral blood and spleen.

7.5   INTERLEUKIN-6

IL-6 was originally characterized and isolated as a T cell-derived factor that caused the terminal maturation of activated B cells to immunoglobulin-producing cells. It is now known that IL-6 has a wide variety of biological functions, with target cells not restricted to normal B cells (Kawano *et al.*, 1988). Houssiau and co workers (1988) found that IL-6 activity was significantly elevated in the synovial fluid and serum from patients with RA and other inflammatory arthritides, as compared with that in a group of patients with osteoarthritis. In those patients where the serum IL-6 was elevated, there was a significant correlation between serum IL-6 activity and serum levels of C-reactive protein (as well as other acute-phase response proteins), supporting the notion that IL-6 might reflect disease activity in patients with RA. Moreover, Hazenburg *et al.* (1989) have shown the simultaneous induction of IL-6 release and flare up of arthritis. Several other cytokines, such as IL-1 and TNF which are also present in the synovial fluid (see above), are also potent inducers of IL-6. In contrast, Mihara *et al.* (1991) have shown that IL-6 inhibits the development of adjuvant arthritis. It has also been demonstrated that IL-6 suppresses the production of IL-1 and TNF, indicating the presence of negative feedback on these cytokines (Aderka *et al.*, 1989).

IL-6 has also been shown to be elevated in other autoimmune diseases such as psoriasis and Castleman's disease, which is characterized by lymphadenopathy and hypergammaglobulinaemia. In this rare disease, the raised IL-6 levels have been shown to be linked to raised levels of agalactosyl IgG (Nakao *et al.*, 1991). IL-6 has also been found to mediate the paraneoplastic autoimmunity seen in cardiac myxoma (Jourdan *et al.*, 1990). Most recently, IL-6 has been shown to be elevated in SLE and correlates well with disease activity (Linker-Israeli *et al.*, 1991). They also demonstrated that IL-4 inhibited the production of IL-6 in SLE whereas TNF-α and IL-1 enhanced this production. There is, however, an unresolved paradox in these observations, as CRP, which is induced by IL-6, is not elevated in SLE. This may be explained by an abnormality in the IL-6 receptor.

Studies with NZB/W F1 mice have shown that the addition of IL-6 increased IgG and IgM anti-DNA antibody production by splenic B cells. This production was enhanced by IL-5 which on its own only increased IgM anti-DNA production (Mihara and Ohsugi, 1990).

7.6 INTERLEUKIN-8

IL-8 has been characterized as a neutrophil chemo-attractant factor and has been found to be elevated in sites of inflammation such as the rheumatoid joint (Brennan *et al.*, 1990). However, no correlation was found by Brennan and co-workers between IL-8 levels in RA and chemotactic activity. This may be explained by the recent finding that IL-8 can markedly inhibit neutrophil recruitment to sites of inflammation (Hechtman *et al.*, 1991). It seems that IL-8 can act either as a pro-inflammatory or anti-inflammatory depending on whether it is produced extravascularly or intra-vascularly. IL-8 has also been found to cause rapid neutrophil-mediated cartilage degradation in RA (Elford and Cooper, 1991).

7.7 TNF

Several lines of evidence suggest that TNF is involved in the mediation of disease. TNF mRNA is overexpressed in the kidneys of NZB/WF1 mice (Boswell *et al.*, 1988). In patients with SLE, spontaneous production of TNF by peripheral blood monocytes is higher than in healthy controls (Malavé *et al.*, 1989). TNF is one of the most abundant cytokines seen in the rheumatoid synovium, and, although it is also found in osteoarthritis, it is thought not to be biologically active in osteoarthritis, as it does not induce IL-1 production (Brennan *et al.*, 1989b). Many of the effects of TNF can be related to the pathology seen in RA (cf. IL-1). These include cartilage breakdown, bone resorption, synovial cell growth and fibroblast proliferation. In rabbits, TNF causes transient synovitis after intra-articular injection (Henderson and Pettipher, 1989). In diabetes, TNF is a potent class II inducer on human islet β cells and disintegrates pancreatic islets (Pukel *et al.*, 1987).

In sharp contrast, a number of authors have suggested that several autoimmune diseases are associated with a deficient production of TNF. As compared with normal controls, NOD mice (which are a model for diabetes)

have a low level of TNF, and treatment with TNF prevents the development of diabetes (Jacob *et al.*, 1990). Treatment of NZB/W F1 hybrids with high doses of TNF can postpone the development of lupus nephritis, though not indefinitely (Jacob and McDevitt, 1988). It has been suggested that the effect of high doses may be related to the non-specific immunosuppressive effect on accessory cells, T cells and NK lymphocytes (Gordon and Wofsy, 1990). However, at lower doses TNF accelerates the disease and mortality in these mice (Brennan *et al.*, 1989a).

7.8 INTERFERONS

Interferons are a heterogeneous group of proteins originally divided into type I and type II. Type I interferons (IFNα and β) are produced when cells, particularly leucocytes and fibroblasts, are infected with a virus. In contrast, IFNγ is produced exclusively by lymphocytes when stimulated by antigen or mitogen.

A large number of patients with a variety of autoimmune diseases have raised levels of circulating IFN (Hooks *et al.*, 1979, 1982). Thus an elevated IFN level and/or IFN response has been reported in SLE, RA, Sjögren's syndrome, scleroderma, multiple sclerosis, vasculitis and other autoimmune diseases. Lackovic *et al.* (1984) found that IFNα levels showed a better correlation in SLE with clinical activity than IFNγ. Schattner (1983) has suggested that the lymphopenia of SLE may be mediated at least in part by IFN. This hypothesis was later confirmed by Kim *et al.* (1987). Furthermore, Schattner *et al.* (1986) showed that the production of a clinically important common anti-DNA idiotype (16/6 Id) is preferentially enhanced by IFNα.

Studies have shown that IFN therapy in oncology patients may be complicated by a variety of autoimmune phenomena including thyroid disease, haemolytic anaemia and thrombocytopenia (Quesada *et al.*, 1986). In addition anti-DNA antibodies have been documented in patients treated with IFNα (Ehrenstein *et al.*, 1991) as well as one case of SLE (Ronnblom *et al.*, 1991). Several of the side effects experienced by patients treated by IFNα are similar to some of the manifestations of SLE (Table 1.4). In contrast, Davignon *et al.* (1990) showed that treatment of normal mice with IFNγ, whilst causing profound changes in the immune system, did not induce autoimmunity.

In both autoimmune disease and animal models of autoimmune disease, IFNγ has been shown to augment disease. IFNγ-treated (NZB/W)F1 mice display an accelerated development of fatal immune complex glomerulonephritis compared with sham-treated controls (Jacob *et al.*, 1987). However, dependent on the timing of anti-IFNγ mAb injection, rat adjuvant arthritis is suppressed or augmented (Wiesenberg *et al.*, 1989). Intraperitoneal injection of rat recombinant IFNγ augments both myelin-induced and T cell line-mediated

Table 1.4   SLE manifestations that might be mediated by IFN

(1) Fever
(2) Malaise
(3) Myalgia
(4) Alopecia
(5) Lymphopenia
(6) Increased $\beta2$ microglobulin
(7) Increased 16/6 Id production
(8) MHC class II expression
(9) Decreased NK cell activity
(10) Polyclonal B cell activation
(11) Decreased delayed-type cutaneous hypersensitivity

experimental neuritis in Lewis rats, and *in vivo* adminis-tration of a mAb to IFNγ suppresses the disease (Hartnung *et al.*, 1990). In contrast, intraventricular administration of IFNγ completely suppresses clinical signs of experimental allergic encephalitis, and intra-peritoneal injection of anti-IFNγ just before the onset of clinical signs results in a more severe disease course in Lewis rats (Voorthuis *et al.*, 1990).

IFNγ can have conflicting effects in human auto-immune diseases. In multiple sclerosis and SLE, IFNγ can exacerbate the disease (Panitch *et al.*, 1987; Machold and Smolen, 1990). However, in a prospective 2-year follow-up of IFNγ therapy in RA, over half of the patients had a sustained clinical benefit after 1 year and 26% after 2 years (Cannon *et al.*, 1990). IFNγ causes an increase in the expression of MHC class II on synoviocytes and the adhesion molecule ICAM-1 (Chin *et al.*, 1990). In addition, it also causes moderate synovial proliferation. However, Alvaro-Gracia *et al.* (1990) have demonstrated that IFNγ antagonizes the synovial proliferation induced by TNF-α leading to pannus formation and collagenase production. They point out that IFNγ is present in low concentrations in the rheumatoid joint and thus allows the effects of TNF-α to occur unchecked. The benefits of IFNγ are limited, perhaps because of the effects of IFNγ on MHC expression and because IFNγ does not antagonize the effects of IL-1 present in abundance in the rheumatoid synovium.

The induction of MHC class II antigens by IFNγ may be an important mechanism in the induction of auto-immune disease. This has been demonstrated in several diseases including RA, thyroid disease and diabetes (Yu *et al.*, 1980; Klareskog *et al.*, 1982; Bottazzo *et al.*, 1983). An attractive hypothesis is that IFNγ could initiate an anti-self-immune reaction by inducing MHC class II on tissue cells, leading to activation of auto-reactive T cells, as proposed for Graves' disease (Bottazzo *et al.*, 1983), RA (Klareskog *et al.*, 1982) and diabetes (Bottazzo *et al.*, 1985). Monoclonal anti-Ia antibodies seem able to suppress experimental murine SLE, experimental allergic encephalomyelitis and myasthenia gravis (Adelman *et al.*, 1983) However, others have argued that the increase in MHC class II expression may activate T suppressors and protect against autoimmunity (Iwatani *et al.*, 1985). Thus IFNγ can exert ambiguous effects on autoimmunity, and therefore conditions deter-mining whether positive or negative effects on ongoing disease processes follow need to be established.

8.   Autoimmunity and Infection

The *raison d'être* of the immune system is to resist infection. Its ability to discern self from non-self is central to this function. Autoimmune phenomena occur when this distinction is blurred. With the stresses that an infection puts on the immune system, this blurring is more likely to occur. Some infectious organisms use the fine distinction between self and non-self to their advantage, masking under the protection of tolerance to self. In an attempt to clear the infection, tolerance is broken and the infection is unmasked. However, this process may be achieved at the price of self antigens becoming the target of immune effector cells. A detrimental immune response directed against host tissues or at other elements of the immune response may ensue. A key element in the loss of tolerance is thought to be molecular mimicry, i.e. parts of a foreign antigen mimic those in the host and thus elude an immune response. However, the microbe is not always successful, with detrimental consequences both to itself and to the host.

Perhaps the best example of molecular mimicry is the cross-reactivity between cardiac tissue and *Streptococcus* polysaccharides leading to rheumatic fever. Several host antigens have been identified that cross-react with streptococcal antigens: particularly the M proteins found in the streptococcal cell wall. Types 5, 6 and 19 M proteins contain epitopes that cross-react with human myocardial tissues and types 1 and 12 share epitopes with renal glomeruli (see Introduction and Gulizia *et al.*, 1991). It may be that there are only one or two epitopes shared between the M proteins that are cross-reactive with the human tissues. In a recent study monoclonal antibodies reactive against streptococcal antigens were shown to cross-react with cardiac myocytes, smooth muscle cells and cell surface and cytoplasm of endothelial cells lining the valves (Gulizia *et al.*, 1991). Myosin, vimentin and elastin were all targets for these antibodies, but collagen was unreactive. In addition to human heart tissues and kidney, cross-reactivity has also been demonstrated with basal brain nuclei in patients with Sydenham's chorea and most recently with articular cartilage and synovium: Dale and co-workers showed that the M5 protein cross-reacts with chondrocytes, cartilage and synovium (Baird *et al.*, 1991). Part of this cross-reactivity was due to vimentin; collagen was unreactive. These findings are in accord with the heart studies and suggest that the same antibody recognizes homologous epitopes in different tissues.

Molecular mimicry is, however, not the complete explanation for the pathogenesis of rheumatic fever for a number of reasons. Firstly, cross-reactive antibodies are associated with streptococci that cause dental caries but not rheumatic fever. It does not explain why it only follows pharyngeal infections and not for instance skin infections. Moreover, no cross-reactive antigens have been seen in the pericardium, a common site of pathology. No animal models have been convincingly demonstrated: injections of these cross-reactive M proteins into animals do not induce disease or cross-reactive antibodies (Baird *et al.*, 1991) For all these reasons, it cannot be a simple matter of breakdown of self-tolerance. Indeed it is notable that autoimmune reactions occur after many diseases, but only rarely do they manifest as autoimmune disease. Thus many other factors also play a role in the induction of autoimmune disease.

Not only has molecular mimicry been used to explain, in part, the phenomenon of autoimmunity occurring during infectious disease such as rheumatic fever but also in autoimmune disease without any identified cause. Examples of this latter include rheumatic diseases such as AS and RS. Some 95% of patients with AS and more than 80% with RS carry the HLA-B27 allele, compared with less than 7% of the general population. Six consecutive amino acids (QTDRED) are identical between the hypervariable domain of HLA-B27 and *Klebsiella pneumoniae* nitrogenase. Sera from a significant proportion of HLA-B27 individuals with RS (18 of 34) or AS (7 of 24), but not from appropriate controls, reacted with a synthetic peptide containing the homologous region of HLA-B27.1. As expected, sera from AS and RS patients also reacted with a peptide derived from the *K. pneumoniae* nitrogenase (CNSR*QTDRED*ELI) (summarized by Oldstone, 1987). These observations suggest that RS and AS might be autoimmune diseases directed against HLA-B27. Induction might be due to a microbe(s) encoding a protein with sequence homology to HLA-B27 (variable region). The disease might be related to an unusual concentration of HLA in particular tissues, including the joints.

More recently the concept of molecular mimicry has been applied to a certain group of highly conserved proteins called HSP. These are produced by prokaryote or eukaryote cells by stresses such as heat, infections, toxins and clearly have a protective role in normal physiology. The function of HSPs include the folding of many proteins and the chaperoning of proteins moving within the cell. In immunological terms, these proteins are highly potent, for instance they are one of the major antigens of pathogenic mycobacteria stimulating a strong humoral and cellular immune response (Young, 1990). Much attention has been focused on HSP 65 and its possible role in RA. Antibodies (Tsoulfa *et al.*, 1989; van

Eden *et al.*, 1991) and T cells (Holoshitz *et al.*, 1989) from patients with RA (and reactive arthropathies) react with mycobacterial and human HSP 65. However, mycobacterial infection in humans often leads to the production of a range of autoantibodies (e.g. rheumatoid factor, anti-nuclear antibodies) as well as autoreactive T cells, but normally no autoimmune disease manifests. Moreover, some normal individuals have autoantibodies to HSP 65. It is more likely that a further event is required to trigger autoimmune disease such as the upregulation of the endogenous HSPs following exposure to exogenous HSPs. Upregulation of HSP 90 has been demonstrated in a subset of patients with SLE (Norton *et al.*, 1989).

Other factors linking infection and autoimmunity have emerged in the last few years. It has been demonstrated for example that abnormalities in the glycosylation of IgG, i.e. an increased percentage of oligosaccharide chains attached to the C_H2 domain, lacking galactose (Gal 0) and terminating in *N*-acetylglucosamine, are restricted to just a few conditions, notably RA, Crohn's disease and tuberculosis (Parekh *et al.*, 1989). It seems very likely that an increase in Gal 0 is probably an indication of the presence of chronic T cell-mediated tissue damage accompanied by an acute phase response. Diseases in which either response occurs alone, e.g. sarcoidosis and acute rheumatic fever respectively, are not associated with a raised Gal 0.

8.1   Autoantibodies Produced by Patients with Infections

Sera from patients with autoimmune disease have frequently been reported to have higher titres of antibodies recognizing particular microbes. These reports are detailed later in this section. However, it is important to consider that this association might simply be circumstantial and not aetiological. For example, patients with an autoimmune disease might be chronically exposed to an infectious agent. Patients with an autoimmune disease are often on long-term immunosuppressive treatment which predisposes to infection. Alternatively the immune system might "over-react" to a given microbe, because of a defect within the system (Venables, 1988). Finally, recognition of an infecting antigen might be based upon a chance cross-reaction.

A wide range of autoantibodies have been observed in leprosy against a variety of organ- and non-organ-specific antigens. Antibodies to both nerves and skin, the two main sites of pathology, have been found in the sera of leprosy patients as well as antibodies to type II collagen, a major constituent of joint cartilage (Choi *et al.*, 1988). This last autoantibody is also found in RA but there is not thought to be any aetiological connection, as it is also found in other chronic inflammatory conditions such as GVHD and probably represents an epiphenomenon secondary to generalized disturbed immunoregulation. Autoantibodies to several nuclear antigens have also been identified in leprosy sera (Choi *et al.*, 1988).

A great diversity of autoantibodies has been reported in the sera of subjects infected with other bacteria, viruses and parasites. For example, Epstein EBV infection has been associated with the appearance of all autoantibodies to cytoskeletal proteins, immunoglobulins (rheumatoid factor) and red blood cells (Fong *et al.*, 1981; Schooley *et al.*, 1981). Similarly, infection with mumps or measles virus may be followed by the appearance of anti-vimentin antibodies and antibodies directed against the islet cells of the pancreas (Bodansky *et al.*, 1984); occasionally these infections may be followed by overt diabetes mellitus. The production of these antibodies may simply reflect the destruction of islet cells releasing previously "hidden" antigens into the circulation. However, the association of diabetes with Coxsackie B viruses is thought to be due to cytolytic infection of the islet cells with no link to autoimmunity (Yoon, 1990), although this would only cause a temporary disturbance.

Hepatitis B virus infection has been associated with the emergence of anti-DNA antibodies whose titre was correlated with the severity of the liver damage (Villarejos *et al.*, 1979). Chronic active hepatitis, a form of autoimmune disease of the liver, may follow these types of infections. Rabbits infected with the rinder-pest virus develop autoantibodies to dsDNA and nucleohistones (Imaoka *et al.*, 1990). However, these antibodies rapidly disappear despite continued infection with the virus suggesting that other factors are needed to prolong the breakdown in tolerance to nuclear antigens.

The most popular explanation for the *de novo* appearance of autoantibodies during infection is the polyclonal activation of B lymphocytes by constituents of the invading organism (Kobayakawa *et al.*, 1979). However, other mechanisms may be responsible. Damage to the immune system itself may occur by invasion of lymphocytes by lymphotropic viruses such as EBV (Fong *et al.*, 1981; Schooley *et al.*, 1981). Alternatively, infection could induce anti-lymphocyte antibodies as in the case of lepromatous leprosy and AIDS both characterized by hypergammaglobulinaemia and a variety of autoantibodies. The elimination or inhibition of a subset of lymphocytes (e.g. T suppressor cells) could lead to faulty regulation of the immune response and unleash the production of autoantibodies. However, the autoantibodies associated with overt infections do not usually produce the effects noted in classical autoimmune diseases. Thus infection more often induces autoimmune phenomena but not with the clinical expression of an autoimmune disease. This reinforces the idea that infection may act as a trigger for autoimmunity but that other mechanisms lead to the breakdown of tolerance and the activation of immune effector mechanisms causing tissue damage.

8.2   HIV INFECTION AND AUTOIMMUNITY

It has become apparent that AIDS is inextricably linked with autoimmunity. Initially, it was observed that many classical autoimmune reactions occurred in patients with AIDS, and now more recently evidence has accumulated suggesting that at least part of the devastating immunosuppression present in these patients is due to autoimmune mechanisms.

The key to the immunosuppression seen in AIDS is the selective loss of CD4+T helper cells and it is known that HIV, the agent responsible for the disease, binds to the CD4 molecule itself. However, only 1:1000 T cells or even fewer have been shown to be infected with the virus (Schnittman *et al.*, 1989). While some cells are destroyed by a variety of mechanisms linked to direct invasion such as syncytial formation, accumulation of unintegrated viral DNA and direct lysis by replicating virus, evidence in favour of autoimmune mechanisms has accumulated.

Investigators have demonstrated the presence of anti-lymphocyte antibodies in AIDS patients. Stricker *et al.* (1987a,b) found the presence of autoantibodies that bound to an 18 kDa antigen on CD4+T cells and that the presence of this antibody correlated with the clinical status of the individual. Other studies have found antibodies directed against class II MHC molecules. Beretta *et al.* (1987) described a cross-reaction between a monoclonal antibody raised against gp120 (the envelope glycoprotein that binds to CD4) and monocytes involved in antigen presentation. However, this antibody was not found in the sera of patients with lymphadenopathy and AIDS.

More intriguing are the experiments from Hoffman's group (Kion and Hoffman, 1991) in which B6 mice that had been treated with lymphocytes from the CBA strain developed antibodies against gp120 and another protein characteristic of HIV, gp24. Neither mouse strain had been exposed to HIV in any form. Hoffman argued that these antibodies are generated against foreign class II molecules which bear a close similarity to gp120. Thus infection with HIV results in the immune effector system being directed against MHC class II-bearing cells, i.e. T cells; this has been named the "civil war" scenario between two armies of T cells.

It appears that, whereas infection with HIV is necessary, it is not sufficient to cause AIDS. Further support for this hypothesis comes from experiments on macaque monkeys with the simian analogue of HIV called SIV (Stott, 1991). Stott found that an antibody response against foreign T cells and not an anti-HIV response protected against developing AIDS. Indeed AIDS patients have high quantities of anti-HIV antibodies as well as a strong anti-HIV cytotoxic response. This immune response is destructive; Hoffman argues that a beneficial response would be the development of tolerance towards HIV or at least the MHC-mimicking parts of HIV.

In addition to the evidence for autoimmunity playing a major role in the pathogenesis of AIDS, there are also several other autoimmune perturbations recorded in AIDS patients. These include the presence of anti-nuclear antibodies as well as other antibodies to a variety of self-antigens, including actin, DNA, tubulin, thyroglobulin, albumin and myosin (Matsiota *et al.*, 1987) and circulating anticoagulants (Bloom *et al.*, 1986; Cohen *et al.*, 1986). This and the presence of other autoantibodies described above suggests some similarity to SLE. There are many similarities between AIDS and SLE which are summarized in Table 1.5.

Parallels to other autoimmune rheumatic diseases have also been made including descriptions of myositis and Sjögren's syndrome. The most notable joint manifestations however, have been the description of RS (Forster *et al.*, 1988) and other seronegative arthritides including an atypical non-erosive arthritis (Rowe *et al.*, 1989). In the latter syndrome described in nine HIV-positive patients, the joint symptoms were severe, persistent and unresponsive to non-steroidal anti-inflammatory drugs. However, in a study involving 556 patients with HIV infection the incidence of Reiter's disease and other seronegative arthritides was no higher than in a population of homosexual men without HIV infection (Fernandez *et al.*, 1991). The authors conclude that the type of rheumatic disease seen in AIDS is more related to the risk factors for HIV infection than HIV itself. Despite this, it remains clear that for the rarer rheumatic syndromes seen in AIDS, such as myositis and Sjögren's syndrome there is a definite association with HIV.

9.   Complement Deficiency and Autoimmunity

The complement system comprises a series of rapidly acting plasma glycoproteins including several proenzymes and components that exist in the non-active state in the serum. The system is triggered by domains on the C_H2 region of antigen-bound IgG or IgM. The complement system has a vital role in the inflammatory process helping to defend the organism against infectious agents. It may be activated by either the classical or alternative pathways (Fig. 1.1). The classical pathway components are C1 including the subunits C1q, C1r and C1s; C4 and C2. The alternative pathway includes factors B, D, P (properdin) and the so-called membrane-attack complex which is the final common pathway whichever mode of activation occurs and consists of C5, C6, C7, C8 and C9. Activation by the classical pathway is dependent upon a specific humoral immune reaction involving mostly IgG antibodies and sometimes IgM, which bind to the antigen and consequently undergo structural changes. The sequence of events is shown in Fig. 1.1. The alternative complement pathway is activated non-specifically on the surface of various molecules including polysaccharides and lipopolysaccharides on the outer membranes of fungi, parasites, bacteria and viruses. The series of steps involved is also shown in Fig. 1.1.

The inheritance of the components of the classical complement pathway are usually more recessive. The components C4, C2 and BF are unique in that they are encoded by three structural genes. This group of genes designated MHC class III is situated between the class I and class II genes on the short arm of chromosome 6. Component C4 is encoded by two closely linked highly polymorphic genes which give rise to the isotypic forms designated C4A and C4B. Only 60% of the population have four functioning C4 genes making partial deficiency of C4 the commonest immune deficiency in man. Properdin, an important component of the alternative pathway is coded on the X chromosome.

Since the description thirty years ago by Silverstein (1960) of hereditary homozygous C2 deficiency, great interest has been sustained in the links between auto-immunity and complement component deficiencies (Morgan and Walport, 1991). The major clinical associations are shown in Table 1.6. The most frequently reported abnormality is that of homozygous C2

Table 1.5   Similarities between SLE and AIDS

	SLE	AIDS
Multisystem disease	+	+
Fever	+	+
Neurological findings	+	+
Arthritis	+	+
Virus	Type -C(?) HTLV-1(?)	HIV
Hypergammaglobulinaemia	+	+
Autoantibodies to:		
Nuclear components	+	+
RBCs	+	+
Leucocytes	+	+
Lymphocytes	+	+
(Lymphocytotoxic)	+	+
Platelets	+	+
Lupus anticoagulant	+	+
Lymphopenia	+	+
Defect in NK cell	+	+
Natural autoantibodies: actin, DNA, tubulin, thyroglobulin, albumin and myosin	+	+
Reduced T suppressor nos.	+	−
Reduced CD4/CD8 ratio	−	+
Increased IFNα	+	+
Reduced IL-1 and IL-2	+	+
Increased β2 microglobulin	+	+
DTH reaction	+	+
T cell response to mitogen	+	+
HLA B8, DR2, DR3	+	+/−
F/M ratio	10 : 1	M > F

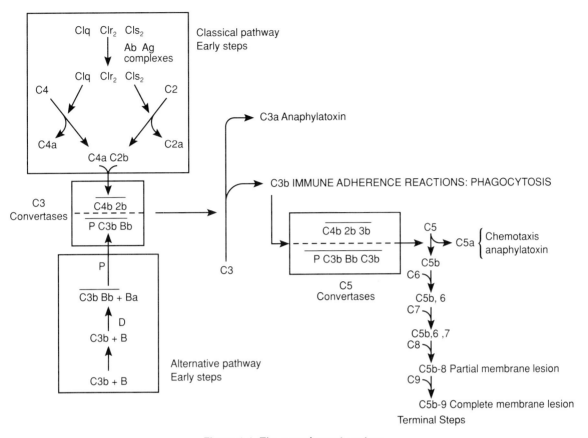

Figure 1.1 The complement system.

Table 1.6 Complement deficiency and disease

Component	Number of cases	Disease association
C1q	≈ 50	SLE + pyogenic infections
C1r/C1s	≈ 10	SLE + pyogenic infections
C4	≈ 15	SLE + pyogenic infections
C2	> 100	SLE + pyogenic infections (but most affected individuals are healthy)
Factor D	1	Neisserial infections
Properdin	≈ 50	Neisserial infections
C3	≈ 15	SLE/glomerulonephritis/ pyogenic infections
C5	≈ 20	Neisserial infections, rarely SLE
C6	> 50	Neisserial infections, rarely SLE
C7	≈ 25	Neisserial infections, rarely SLE
C8	≈ 8	Neisserial infections, rarely SLE
C9	≈ 5 (Caucasian)	Neisserial infections, rarely SLE

deficiency with SLE. Approximately 50% of the patients with this deficiency develop the disease. Considerable interest has also focused on the question of whether or not HLA DR3, which has long been linked to SLE, is actually associated with the disease because it is in linkage disequilibrium with a C4 null allele. Thus Latchman and Walport (1987) suggested that homozygous C4 deficiency alone might be a sufficient cause for the development of SLE. Because of the linkage disequilibrium between DR3 and C4A in Caucasian populations it was initially difficult to distinguish between the effects of null genes for this complement component and DR3. However, Batchelor *et al.* (1987) described the study of 44 SLE patients selected because they were DR3-negative; 18 of the 30 Caucasian patients (60%) had a C4 null allele compared with 22 of 60 (37%) of a controlled panel of DR3-negative normal Caucasian subjects. The difference is statistically significant and supports the idea that null alleles of the C4A and C4B genes are themselves directly responsible for comparing their susceptibility to SLE.

Although the other complement components have been associated with SLE and some other autoimmune disorders, these reports have been sparse, especially deficiencies of the alternative complement pathway. (They will not be further described here as they have already been reviewed by Morgan and Walport (1991).)

The precise mechanism that explains the relationship between complement component deficiencies and auto-immune diseases remains a matter for debate. One suggestion was that in early component deficiencies the individual is exposed to prolonged specific viral infections which might induce immune complex disorders. Latchman and Walport (1987) suggested an alternative mechanism. In the absence of adequate complement function potentially insoluble immune complexes with little C4 or C3 will be formed. These large immune complexes will fail to be bound normally to the erythrocyte complement receptor and this will eventually result in the deposition of immune complexes in peripheral small blood vessels rather than in sinusoids of the liver and the spleen. This in turn will give rise to inflammation with the release of autoantigens and the formation of autoantibodies.

10. Hormonal Components

The very fact that virtually all autoimmune diseases occur far more frequently in women than men strongly suggests that hormones must in some way be implicated in the aetiopathogenesis of autoimmune diseases.

The mechanisms by which sex hormones might affect the immune system in general are clearly multiple. Sex hormones via receptors located on lymphocyte membranes act directly upon T cells, notably those carrying the cytotoxic or suppressor phenotype. Oestrogen has been shown to inhibit these cells, thus allowing increased production by B cells of antibodies including almost certainly autoantibodies. In contrast, androgens induce T suppressor/cytotoxic activity which inhibits B cell production of antibodies in general (Talal and Ahmed, 1987).

On the basis of a number of simple observations, the probability that sex hormones affect the immune system is considered to be very likely. Thus females are, in general, more resistant to infections and have higher serum levels of IgM and IgG antibodies. In addition, they exhibit a generally stronger humoral and cell-mediated immune response. In addition, a number of clinical observations, besides the increased prevalence of autoimmune diseases amongst females, have also pointed to an important role for sex hormones. For example, clinical activity in several autoimmune diseases fluctuates with varying patterns of sex hormone levels. Thus, during pregnancy, three-quarters of patients with RA go into remission, although virtually all of these will relapse within the 6 months during the puerperium. Whilst in the main SLE represents a greater threat to the fetus than to the mother, a proportion of SLE patients will relapse during pregnancy and the disease may, on occasion, commence either during pregnancy or immediately following gestation.

There have been many studies on the role of sex steroid metabolism in disease, but SLE is the condition that has been analysed the most comprehensively. There are many reports of high oestrogen levels in both males and females with this condition, although the majority of investigators have not found consistently elevated oestradiol levels in males with SLE. It has, however, long been established that male patients with Kleinfelter's syndrome (associated with the XXY chromosomal abnormality) have an increased predisposition to SLE and an increase in the hydroxylation of oestrone towards the more feminine metabolites 16α-hydroxyoesterone and oestriol (Lahita *et al.*, 1985). Lavalle *et al.* (1987) have reported that male patients with SLE have reduced resting levels of serum testosterone and dihydro-testosterone and increased levels of oestrone. Male hormonal levels were unaltered by exogenous injections with luteinizing hormone-releasing hormone. Furthermore, these male SLE patients also had increased basal levels with serum prolactin. The idea that prolactin affects lymphocytes gained further support with the demonstration of prolactin receptors on these cells (Russell *et al.*, 1985). There thus appears to be a fundamental disturbance of sex steroid metabolism in SLE patients and this abnormality may be exaggerated in female patients with clinically active disease.

Male patients with RA have been reported to have decreased serum concentrations of testosterone and dihydroepiandrosterone sulphate (Cutolo, 1988). This has sparked suggestions that androgenic metabolism might be abnormal in female rheumatoid patients, although confirmation of this notion is awaited.

10.1 ANIMAL MODELS AND SEX HORMONES

Many analyses have been undertaken of the effects of sex hormones on animal models of autoimmunity. Studies of a rat model of autoimmune thyroiditis (Ahmed and Penhale, 1982) have shown that castration of male rats led to the appearance of autoimmune thyroiditis identical in both incidence and severity with that seen in female rats. However, administration of testosterone to both castrated males and normal females led to clinical improvement. Furthermore, treatment with testosterone was clinically beneficial, occasionally leading to complete regression of the disease. Similar results have been reported by Gause and Marsh (1985) in autoimmune thyroiditis in Obese strain chickens.

Even more studies have been undertaken in SLE models. The work of Roubinian *et al.* (1977, 1978, 1979a,b) is widely quoted in this respect. Following the well-established observation that NZB/W F$_1$ mice develop SLE-like disease earlier and die younger than their male counterparts, they demonstrated that the administration of oestrogen to males led to a much shortened life span and greatly increased mortality at an earlier age. This administration dramatically increased the formation of IgM and IgG antibodies to DNA whereas antigen treatment suppressed and inhibited the appearance of these antibodies. Oestrogen treatment also accelerated glomerulonephritis whilst androgen treatment of females inhibited the development of renal disease. Castration of males before reaching sexual maturity accelerated the rate of development of disease, and death was observed sooner than in the female group. In contrast, castration of females before sexual maturity did not affect the time of disease onset or its severity. However, oestrogen treatment commenced immediately after castration accelerated the disease process.

As indicated above, it is clear that sex hormones act in a variety of ways to influence immune response and thus lead to autoimmunity. Oestrogen, for example, can inhibit the appearance of immune complexes by macrophages and other reticular endothelial cells whilst androgen accelerates this effect. It seems clear that, in general, oestrogen stimulates the immune system and acts to exacerbate autoimmune disease whereas androgens have an inhibitory effect in general terms. It seems very likely that there are subtle relationships between sex hormones and the thymus and, as indicated earlier, it has recently been shown that sex hormones, acting via receptors located on T suppressor cytotoxic cells, directly influence immunoregulation and antibody production. It is now known that sex hormones, like glucocorticoids, having entered the cell will dislodge HSP 90 which chaperones the hormone receptor. The hormone–receptor complex is able to pass from the cytoplasm to the nucleus and is there able to induce the transcription of RNA from DNA and ultimately, by translation, the production of particular proteins (reviewed by Dhillon *et al.*, 1991). These protein products are likely to include the lymphokines. It is thus of interest to know that mouse models of SLE demonstrate a decreased activity of IL-2 (the administration of androgen can increase the level of this interleukin).

Given the effects described, it is therefore not surprising that the hormonal modulation of autoimmune disease has been attempted. However, the subtleties that are likely to be involved have equally clearly not been fully appreciated, as, in the main, these attempts have been unsuccessful. Occasional case reports have appeared describing, for example, the beneficial affects of danazol and androgen (with reduced virilizing effects) on SLE patients. In addition, some patients with autoimmune thrombocytopenia have improved when given the same drug. In the main, however, it appears that more work needs to be undertaken before appropriate hormonal modulation is likely to prove successful in the treatment of autoimmune conditions.

10.2   THYMIC HORMONES AND AUTOIMMUNITY

The thymic hormones have a major role in regulating and controlling the immune reaction through their effects on T cell differentiation. A variety of thymic hormones exist including thymosin, thymopoietin and FTS, and links between thymic hormones and immunity have been suggested by a number of studies. These hormones may be modulated, for example, by steroid hormones. Thus, oestradiol injections decrease the size of the thymus, and there have also been reports of testosterone acting to suppress autoimmunity by thymic hormones (Melez *et al.*, 1987). Castration of young NZB/W F$_1$ mice when treated with thymosin led to a suppression in the expected rise of anti-DNA antibodies. The cellular basis for this process is uncertain, although it is interestingly one of the thymic hormones that has been shown to cause an increase in the serum corticosteroid level (Hall *et al.*, 1984).

Neonatal thymectomy of normal mice is followed by the appearance of autoantibodies by 2 months of age (Thivolet *et al.*, 1967). Thymectomy of adult mice is also associated with autoimmune phenomena. Thus thymectomy in obese strain chickens that develop a spontaneous form of thyroiditis has been shown to be accelerated. In addition, thymus transplant in some of these animals corrects some of these immune defects.

A variety of other experiments in animal models and some clinical observations have also linked the thymus with autoimmunity, although again the precise mechanisms remain uncertain. Thus a decrease in FTS-like activity has been noted in the sera of NZB/W mice before the development of autoimmune phenomena. The addition of various thymic hormones also seems able to partially correct some of the autoimmune phenomena seen in these mice. Furthermore, FTS treatment improved some autoimmune features in the NZB/W F$_1$ mouse. In contrast, such treatment appears to lead to an enhancement of DNA antibody production of glomerulonephritis (Bach and Dardenne, 1984). A coexistence of

SLE and myasthenia gravis has been recorded by several authors, but adult thymectomy does not alter the course of human SLE. The thymus is, however, closely related to another autoimmune disease myasthenia gravis. Thymectomy has proved to be very useful for many patients with this condition and intriguingly there have been reports of the development of SLE after thymectomy for myasthenia (Smolen, 1987).

11. Ageing

It is generally agreed that the immune response tends to decline with increasing age as the accumulative effects of senescence of both the cellular and humoral components of the response become more obvious. It has been estimated that 5% of the elderly population suffer from some form of autoimmune disease and up to 15% of apparently healthy people over 60 have a significant level of autoantibodies in their serum (discussed by Taylor and Rose, 1991). However, autoimmune diseases, notably SLE, insulin-dependent diabetes and myasthenia gravis, are far more frequently found before the menopause. In contrast, some diseases including RA and Sjögren's syndrome are almost as common after the menopause as before it.

Most studies of autoimmune phenomena in the elderly have focused on the prevalence of a variety of auto-antibodies with age. These are reviewed in Table 1.7. It will be seen that whilst there are some discrepancies, in the main, rheumatoid factor and anti-nuclear antibodies are reported more frequently in healthy elderly individuals (over the age of 60) compared with young persons. Overproduction of autoantibodies reflects abnormalities in B and T cell functions and the changes reported in the elderly are reviewed in Table 1.8.

Much controversy surrounds the mechanisms responsible for increased autoimmunity in the elderly. Some appear to believe that this phenomenon is associated with underdiagnosed diseases. It has been shown, for example, that anti-thyroglobulin antibodies are more frequent in individuals aged between 70 and 90 with various chronic disorders, although paradoxically these were not elevated in healthy subjects aged over 90. Furthermore, information obtained from routine autopsies has suggested a 2–3-fold increase in prevalence of focal thyroiditis in old adults (Williams and Doniach, 1962).

As discussed earlier in this chapter it has been suggested that autoantibodies may have a protective role against certain infections and therefore as the body ages so they tend to accumulate. Thus, if the production of IgM rheumatoid factor does indeed represent a first line of defence against bacterial or viral infections, it might therefore be more understandable that this type of rheumatoid factor is more frequently found in healthy aged subjects (Silvestris et al., 1985).

Another possible explanation for age-dependent high production of autoantibodies is an increased rate of somatic mutations. The most likely mechanisms associated with appearance of autoantibodies in the elderly are shown in Table 1.9.

Some adult studies show that, whereas old animals do possess T suppressor cells, their function is impaired because of the relative inability to produce IL-2. Others claim that prolonged exposure to self-antigen, which may or may not be altered, results from the normal catabolic processes inducing autoreactive lymphoid clones. Indeed, Antel et al. (1980) have suggested that increased autoimmunity associated with ageing may represent an intrinsic biochemical alteration in lymphoid cells. It has

Table 1.7 Autoantibodies found in healthy elderly normal individuals

Antibody	Comment
IgM – rheumatoid factor	Most, although not all, studies report an increased prevalence in elderly subjects (up to 42% in one study, but this seems unduly high)
Anti-nuclear antibody	Again most, although not all, studies report an increased prevalence in the elderly
Anti-ssDNA	Although the elderly do not have anti-dsDNA antibodies, at least one study has described an increased prevalence of these antibodies
Anti-thyroglobulin	One report of an increased prevalence of this antibody in the elderly. Two other studies reported trends in this direction which did not reach statistical significance

For a more detailed review, see Shoenfeld and Isenberg (1989).

Table 1.8 B and T cell changes reported in healthy elderly individuals

B Lymphocyte changes
  (i)   Increased polyclonal immunoglobulin response to pokeweed mitogen
  (ii) General reduction of antigen-specific and polyclonal responses
  (iii) Intrinsic defects in B cell maturation

T lymphocyte changes
  (i)   Reduction in both T helper and T suppressor cells
  (ii) Increase in non-T, non-B null cells
  (iii) Decline in mitogen-induced lymphocyte response
  (iv) Reduced production of growth factors and expression of specific cell receptors

Table 1.9 Probable mechanisms associated with the increased appearance of autoantibodies in the elderly

(i)   Exposure to autoantigens in increased amounts associated with increased somatic mutations
(ii) Altered self-antigens
(iii) Alterations in lymphocyte receptors to antigens

been shown, for example, that the ratio cAMP to cGMP in splenic T cells of old mice is five times lower than that observed in younger animals. The alterations in cAMP and cGMP levels can be explained by the so called free-radical theory of ageing: the excess of free radicals occurring in older mammals leading to activation of guanylate cyclase and an increase in cGMP which in turn causes activation of phosphodiesterase and a decrease in cAMP.

Taylor and Rose (1991) have described an ageing paradox in which the response to foreign antigens declines with age as a result of an increase in the non-specific suppressor cells (or factors) while the response to self-antigens is rising. This combined with a rise in the proportion of autoantigen-specific helper/inducer T cells compared with the autoantigen-specific suppressor cells may be the key to the increased number of autoantibodies and possibly some autoimmune diseases found in the elderly.

12. Nutrition and Autoimmunity

On the basis of the old aphorism that "we are what we eat", numerous studies in the past 20 years have focused on components of the diet that might be associated with the clinical expression of autoimmune diseases (Homsy et al., 1986). Not surprisingly, given the complexities of the human diet, the results have been hard to interpret, although some clear messages are emerging.

There seems little doubt, for example, that calorie restriction can reduce levels of circulating immune complexes and, in SLE-prone mice, reduce the complement C3 and immunoglobulin deposition in the kidneys. Studies in NZB/W F1 mice have shown that such restriction prolongs the life span of these animals (Fernandes and Good, 1979). In addition, there has been a claim in at least one report that a reduction in the symptoms of patients with RA was noted when they were put on to a calorie-restricted diet (Skoldstam et al., 1979).

Protein restriction has been shown to delay the appearance of autoimmune diseases in certain animals but does not appear to prolong the life span (Atkinson et al., 1988). It may, however, also reduce antibody production. Synthetic amino acid diets have been shown to prolong survival and decrease anti-nuclear antibody levels in autoimmune murine disease (Batsford et al., 1984) and diets low in phenylalanine and tyrosine may prolong

survival of NZB/W mice. Zinc deficiency delays the onset of autoimmune phenomena in NZB/W and MRL/l mice whilst selenium supplementation, in one study, was able to improve the survival of NZB/W female mice (O'Dell et al., 1988). In contrast, vitamin A deficiency aggravated autoimmunity in NZB mice, while there has been at least one claim that a vitamin E-enriched diet prolongs the survival of NZB/W mice.

The majority of work, however, in both animal and human studies have focused on the alteration of fat in the diet. There is now firm evidence to show that the effect of fat on autoimmunity is modulated by the synthesis of prostaglandins and leukotrienes (Homsy et al., 1986). A schematic diagram of prostaglandin and leukotriene synthesis from polyunsaturated fatty acids is shown in Fig. 1.2. The absence of arachidonic acid precursors in the diet as well as supplementation with eicosapentaenoic acid cause a significant improvement in the survival and pathology of SLE-prone mice. Low-fat diets also significantly prolong the survival and reduce the autoantibody levels in NZB/W mice (Morrow et al., 1985) and, more recently, a combination of low-fat diet with fish oil supplementation has been shown to significantly improve a variety of clinical features in patients with SLE in a double-blind crossover study (Walton et al., 1991). There have also been intermittent, but persistent, reports of improvement in some clinical and serological parameters in patients with RA treated with low-fat diets.

13. Ultraviolet Light and Autoimmunity

It is well established that ultraviolet light may cause a flare in the rash associated with both systemic and discoid lupus erythematosus. Less frequently, such exposure may induce a more generalized flare of SLE (Tuffanelli and Epstein, 1987). However, the mechanism by which ultraviolet light might induce disease remains uncertain. It is known that dsDNA may be rendered more immunogenic after irradiation with ultraviolet light of 254 nm wavelength; however, DNA treated in this fashion does not induce experimental lupus in animal models.

In vitro release of DNA from lymphocytes has been shown to occur in experimental SLE mice following UVA exposure (Golan and Borel, 1984). In addition, exacerbation and early death of BXSB lupus mice occurs after UVB exposure; however, the relevance of these observations to human SLE remains uncertain.

14. Toxins and Chemicals

Smoking, as well as its well-known hazards of inducing cancer, heart disease and chronic bronchitis has been shown to effect the clinical manifestations of patients

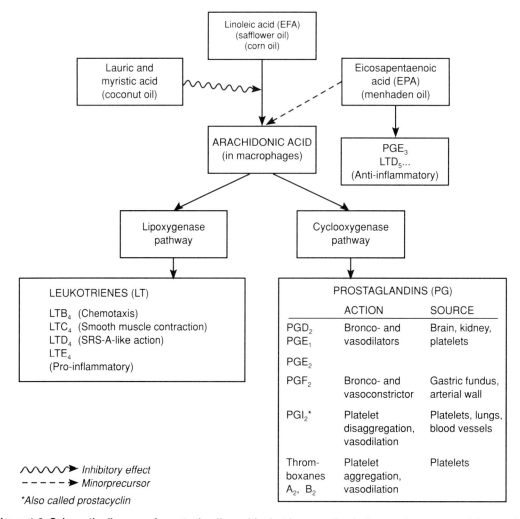

Figure 1.2 Schematic diagram of prostaglandin and leukotriene synthesis from polyunsaturated fatty acids.

with Goodpasture's syndrome (a combination of glomerulonephritis and haemoptysis) (Donaghy and Rees, 1983). Thus cigarette smokers with this syndrome were shown to be far more likely to suffer from lung haemorrhage compared with non-smokers.

Use of silicon implants in breast mammoplasty operations has lead in some unfortunate individuals to the development of various autoimmune phenomena including rheumatic symptoms. Of greater concern, however, was the so-called Spanish oil syndrome which appears to have resulted from the contamination of rape seed oil which was sold as cooking oil. A most unpleasant, and in many cases fatal, two-part illness developed in many individuals characterized by fever, rash, gastrointestinal upset and neurological complications in the early phase followed by more chronic disease in which the individuals developed Raynaud's phenomenon, indurated thickened skin, pulmonary hypertension, dryness of the eyes and mouth and arthritis (Spurzem and Lockey, 1984).

A scleroderma-like skin disease has been associated with a variety of chemicals notably polyvinyl chloride and a variety of other plastics and solvents including epoxy resins, methane, trichloroethylene, benzene and xylene.

15. Stress

Given the frequency with which stressful events such as marriage, divorce, work problems, bereavements etc., happen in everyday life, it is hard to ascertain a causal link between such an event and the onset or exacerbation of autoimmune disease. Nevertheless, many physicians have a distinct impression that flares in some autoimmune diseases, for example, multiple sclerosis and occasionally SLE, are associated with stressful events. Amongst the better established links between autoimmunity and stress are reports of the onset of insulin dependent diabetes in association with the death of a child's parent, divorce and separation of the parents immediately before disease onset (Vialettes *et al.*, 1986). Similarly, uveitis has been described in individuals who have recently lost spouses or undergone divorce, business losses or examination failure (O'Connor, 1983). Finally, the onset of Crohn's disease has been associated with a variety of stressful life events (Gerbert, 1980).

16. Summary

This chapter has emphasized the many different factors that are involved in the development of a clinically overt autoimmune disease. The precise modes of interactions are examined in other chapters of this book. The full complexity of these interactions is still being resolved but at least a picture of the components involved is now much more clearly identified.

17. References

Aaron, S. and Paetkau, V. (1991). Synovial secretion of IL-2 *in vitro*, a limiting dilutional analysis. Clin. Exp. Immunol. 9, 113–118.

Adelman, N., Watling, D. and McDevitt, H. (1983). Treatment of (NZB/W).F1 disease with anti-Ia monoclonal antibodies. J. Exp. Med. 158, 1350–1355.

Aderka, D., Le, J. M. and Vilcek, J. (1989). IL-6 inhibits lipopolysaccharide-induced tumor necrosis factor production in cultured human monocytes, U937 cells, and in mice. J. Immunol. 143, 3517–3523.

Agnello, V., Arbetter, A., de Kasep, G.I., Powell, R., Tan, E.M. and Joslin, F. (1980). Evidence for a subset of rheumatoid factors that cross react with DNA–Histone and have a distinct cross-idiotype. J. Exp. Med. 151, 1514–1527.

Ahmed, S.A. and Penhale, W.J. (1982). The influence of testosterone on the development of autoimmune thyroiditis in thymectomized and irradiated rats. Clin. Exp. Immunol. 48, 367–374.

Alcocer-Varela, J., Laffón, A. and Alarcón-Segovia, D. (1984). Differences in the production of and/or the response to interleukin-2 by T lymphocytes from patients with the various connective tissue diseases. Rheumatol. Int. 4, 39–44.

Alvaro-Gracia, J.M., Zvaifler, N.J. and Firestein, G.S. (1990). Cytokines in chronic inflammatory arthritis. V. Mutual antagonism between interferon-gamma and tumour necrosis factor-alpha on HLA-DR expression, proliferation, collagenase production, and granulocyte macrophage colony-stimulating factor production by rheumatoid arthritis synoviocytes. J. Clin. Invest. 86, 1790–1798.

Andreu, S.J., Moreno, d.A.I., Marcos, M.A., Sanchez, M.A., Martinez, A.C. and Kroemer, G. (1991). Interleukin 2 abrogates the nonresponsive state of T cells expressing a forbidden T cell receptor repertoire and induces autoimmune disease in neonatally thymectomized mice. J. Exp. Med. 173, 1323–1329.

Antel, J.P., Oger, J.F.J., Dropcho, E., Richman, D.P., Kuo, H.H. and Arnason, B.G. (1980). Reduced T-lymphocyte cell reactivity and function of human ageing. Cell. Immunol. 54, 184–192.

Aotsuka, S., Nakamura, K., Nakano, T., Kawakami, M., Goto, M., Okawa, T.M., Kinoshita, M. and Yokohari, R. (1991). Production of intracellular and extracellular interleukin-1 alpha and interleukin-1 beta by peripheral blood monocytes from patients with connective tissue diseases. Ann. Rheum. Dis. 50, 27–31.

Arnett. F.C. and Shulman, L.E. (1976). Studies in familial systemic lupus erythematosus. Medicine 55, 313–322.

Atkinson, M.A., Winter, W.E., Skordis, N., Beppu, H., Riley, W.M. and Maclaren, N.K. (1988). Dietary protein restriction reduces the frequency and delays the onset of insulin dependent diabetes in BB rats. Autoimmunity 2, 11–22.

Avrameas, S., Dighiero, G., Lymberi, P. and Guilbert, B. (1983). Studies on natural antibodies and autoantibodies. Ann. Immunol. 134, 103–113.

Bach, J.F. and Dardenne, M. (1984). In "Thymic Hormones and Lymphokines" (ed A.L. Goldstein), pp 593–600. Plenum Press, New York.

Bahr, G.M., Sattar, M.A., Stanford, J.C., Shaaban, M.A., Shimali, B.Al., Siddiqui, Z., Gabriel, M., Saffar, M.Al., Shahin, A., Chugh, T.D., Rook, G.A. and Behbahami, K. (1989). HLA-DR and tuberculin tests in rheumatoid arthritis and tuberculosis. Ann. Rheum. Dis. 48, 63–68.

Baird, R.W., Bronze, M.S., Kraus, W., Hill, H.R., Veasey, L.G., and Dale, J.B. (1991). Epitopes of group A streptococcal M protein shared with antigens of articular cartilage and synovium. J. Immunol. 146, 3132–3137.

Batchelor, R., Fielder, A.H.L., Walport, M.J., David, J., Lord, D.K., Davey, N., Dodi, I., Malasit, V., Berstein, R., Mackworth Young, C. and Isenberg, D.A. (1987). Family study of the major histocompatibility complex in HLA-DR3 negative patients with systemic lupus erythematosus. Clin. Exp. Immunol. 70, 364–371.

Batsford, S., Schwerdtfeger, M. and Rohrbach, R. (1984). Synthetic amino-acid diet prolongs survival in autoimmune murine disease. Clin. Nephrol. 21, 60–63.

Bender, K., Muller, C., Schmidt, A. Strohmaier, U. and Weinker, T.F (1979). Linkage studies on the human Pi, Gm, GL0 and HLA genes. Hum. Genet. 49, 159–166.

Beretta, A., Grass, F., Pelagi, M., Clivio, A., Parravicini, C., Giovinazzo, G., Andronico, F., Lopalco, L., Verani, P., Butto, S., Titti, F., Rossi, G.B., Viale, G., Ginelli, E. and Siccardi, A.G. (1987). HIV env glycoprotein shares a cross-reacting epitope with a surface protein present on activated human monocytes and involved in antigen presentation. Eur. J. Immunol. 17, 1793–1798.

Block, S.R., Winfield, J.B., Lockshin, M.D., D'Angelo. W.A. and Christain, C.L. (1975). Studies of twins with systemic lupus erythematosus, a review of the literature and presentation of 12 additional sets. Am. J. Med. 59, 533–552.

Bloom, E.J., Abrams, D.I. and Rodgers, G. (1986). Lupus anticoagulant in the AIDS. J. Am. Med. Assoc. 256, 491–493.

Bodansky, H.J., Littlewood, J.M., Bottazzo, G.F., Dean, B.M. and Hambling M.H. (1984). Which virus causes the initial islet cell lesion in type 1 diabetes? Lancet. 1, 401–402.

Boswell, J.M., Yui, M.A., Burt, D.W. and Kelley, V.E. (1988). Increased tumor necrosis factor and IL-1 beta gene expression in the kidneys of mice with lupus nephritis. J. Immunol. 141, 3050–3054.

Bottazzo, G.F., Pujol-Borrell, R., Hanafusa, T. and Feldman, M. (1983). Role of aberrant HLA-DR expression and antigen presentation in induction of endocrine autoimmunity. Lancet ii, 1115–1119.

Bottazzo, G.F., Dean, B.M., McNally, J.M., Mackay, E.H., Swift, P.G. and Gamble, D.R. (1985). In situ characterization of autoimmune phenomena and expression of HLA molecules in the pancreas in diabetic insulitis. N. Engl. J. Med. 313, 353–360.

Brennan, D.C., Yui, M.A., Wuthrich, R.P. and Kelley, V.E. (1989a). Tumor necrosis factor and IL-1 in New Zealand Black/White mice. Enhanced gene expression and acceleration of renal injury. J. Immunol. 143, 3470–3475.

Brennan, F.M., Chantry, D., Jackson, A., Maini, R. and Feldmann, M. (1989b). Inhibitory effect of TNF alpha antibodies on synovial cell interleukin-1 production in rheumatoid arthritis. Lancet ii, 244–247.

Brennan, F.M., Zachariae, C.O., Chantry, D., Larsen, C.G., Turner, M., Maini, R.N., Matsushima, K. and Feldmann, M. (1990). Detection of interleukin 8 biological activity in synovial fluids from patients with rheumatoid arthritis and production of interleukin 8 mRNA by isolated synovial cells. Eur. J. Immunol. 20, 2141–2144.

Cairns, E., Block, J. and Bell, D.A. (1984). Anti-DNA autoantibody–producing hybridomas of normal human lymphoid cell origin. J. Clin. Invest. 74, 880–887.

Calvert, J.E., Duggan Keen, M.F., Smith, S.W.G., Given, A.L. and Bird, P. (1988). The CD5+ B cell, a B cell lineage with a central role in autoimmune disease? Autoimmunity 1, 223–240.

Cannon, G.W., Emkey, R.D., Denes, A., Cohen, S.A., Saway, P.A., Wolfe, F., Jaffer, A.M., Weaver, A.L., Cogen, L., Gulinello, J., Kennedy, S.M. and Schindler, J.D. (1990). Prospective two-year follow up of recombinant interferon-gamma in rheumatoid arthritis. J. Rheumatol. 17, 304–310.

Cathely, G., Amor, B. and Fournier, C. F. (1986). Defective IL-2 production in active rheumatoid arthritis: association with active disease and systemic manifestations. Clin. Rheumatol. 5, 482–492.

Chin, J.E., Winterrowd, G.E., Krzesicki, R.F. and Sanders, M.E. (1990). Role of cytokines in inflammatory synovitis. The coordinate regulation of intercellular adhesion molecule 1 and HLA class I and class II antigens in rheumatoid synovial fibroblasts. Arth. Rheum. 33, 1776–1786.

Choi, E.K., Gatenby, P.A., McGill, N.W., Bateman, J.F., Cole, W.G. and York, J.R. (1988). Autoantibodies to type II collagen: occurrence in rheumatoid arthritis, other arthritides, autoimmune connective tissue diseases, and chronic inflammatory syndromes. Ann. Rheum. Dis. 47, 313–322.

Cohen, A.J., Philips, T.M. and Kessler, C.M. (1986). Circulating coagulation inhibitors in the AIDS. Ann. Intern. Med. 104, 175–180.

Cohen, I.R. and Cooke, A. (1986). Natural autoantibodies might prevent autoimmune disease. Immunol. Today 7, 363–364.

Cunningham, A.J. (1976). Selftolerance maintained by active suppressor mechanisms. Transplant Rev. 31, 23–43.

Cutolo, M. (1988). Sex hormone states of male patients with rheumatoid arthritis: evidence of low serum concentrations of testosterone at baseline and after human chorionic gonadotrophin stimulation. Arth. Rheum. 31, 1314–1317.

Daar, A.S., Fuggle, S.V., Fabre, J.W., Ting, A. and Morris, P.J. (1984). The detailed distribution of HLA-ABC antigens in normal human organs. Transplantation 38, 287–292.

Dang, H., Takei, M., Isenberg, D., Shoenfeld, Y., Backimer, R., Rauch, J. and Talal, N. (1988). Expression of an interspecies idiotype in sera of SLE patients and their first-degree relatives. Clin. Exp. Immunol. 713, 445–450.

Datta, S., Naparstek, Y. and Schwartz, R.S. (1986). In vitro production of anti-DNA idiotype by lymphocytes of normal subjects and patients with systemic lupus erythematosus. Clin. Immunol. Immunopathol. 38, 302–318.

Davidson, W.F., Calkins, C., Hugins, A., Giese, T. and Holmes, K.L. (1991). Cytokine secretion by C3H-lpr and -gld T cells. Hypersecretion of IFN-gamma and tumor necrosis factor-alpha by stimulated CD4+ T cells. J. Immunol. 146, 4138–4148.

Davignon, J.L., Cohen, P.L. and Eisenberg, R.A. (1990). Immunological effects of recombinant interferon gamma in vivo in normal mice: failure to induce autoantibodies. Int. J. Immunopharmacol. 12, 691–698.

De Horatius, R.J. and Messner, R.P. (1975). Lymphocytotoxic antibodies in family members of patients with systemic lupus erythematosus. J. Clin. Invest. 55, 1254–1258.

DeVries, R.R.P. and Van Rood, J.J. (1988). In "Perspectives on Autoimmunity" (ed I. Cohen), pp 2–17. CRC Press, Boca Raton, Florida.

Deapen, D.M., Weinrib, L., Langholtz, B., Horowitz, D.A. and Mack, T.M. (1986). A revised estimate of twin concordance in SLE, a survey of 138 pairs. Arth. Rheum. 29, S26.

Delves, P.J. and Roitt, I.M. (1984). Idiotypic determinants on human thyroglobulin autoantibodies derived from the serum of Hashimoto's patients and EB virus transformed cell lines. Clin. Exp. Immunol. 57, 33–40.

Dhillon, V.D., Latchman, D. and Isenberg, D.A. (1991). Heat shock proteins and systemic lupus erythematosus. Lupus 1, 3–8.

Donaghy, M. and Rees, A.J. (1983). Cigarette smoking and lung haemorrhage in glomerulonephritis caused by autoantibodies to glomerular basement membrane. Lancet ii, 1390–1393.

Dudeney, C., Shoenfeld, Y., Rauch, J., Jones, M., Mackworth-Young, C. and Tavassoli, M. (1986). A study of anti-poly(ADP-ribose) antibodies and an anti-DNA antibody idiotype and other immunological abnormalities in lupus family members. Ann. Rheum. Dis. 45, 502–507.

Dziarski, R. (1982). Preferential induction of autoantibody secretion in polyclonal activation by peptidoglycan and lipopolysaccharide. II. In vivo studies. J. Immunol. 128, 1026–1030.

Dziarski, R. (1987). Natural autoantibodies might prevent autoimmune disease. Immunol. Today 8, 132–137.

Ehrenstein, M.R., Swana, M., McSweeney, E., Goldstone, T. and Isenberg, D.A. (1993). Appearance of anti-DNA antibodies in patients treated with α interferon. Arthritis Rheum. 36, 279–280.

Elford, P.R. and Cooper, P.H. (1991). Induction of neutrophil-mediated cartilage degradation by interleukin-8. Arth. Rheum. 34, 325–332.

Fernandes, G. and Good, R.A. (1979). Alterations of longevity and immune function of B/W and MRL/1 mice by restriction of dietary intake. Fed. Proc. 38, 1370.

Fernandez, S.M., Cardenal, A., Balsa, A., Quiralte, J., del Arco, A., Pena, J.M., Barbado, F.J., Vazquez, J.J. and Gijon, J. (1991). Rheumatic manifestations in 556 patients with human immunodeficiency virus infection. Semin. Arth. Rheum. 21, 30–39.

Fong, S., Tsoukos, C.D., Frinke, L.A., Lawrence, S.K., Holbrook, T.L., Vaughan, J.H. and Carson, D.A. (1981). Age-associated changes in Epstein Barr virus-induced human lymphocyte autoantibody responses. J. Immunol. 126, 910–914.

Forster, S.M., Seifert, M.H., Keat, A.C., Rowe, I.F., Thomas, B.J., Taylor-Robinson, D., Pinching, A.J. and Harris, J.R. (1988). Inflammatory joint disease and human immuno-deficiency virus infection. Br. Med. J. 296, 1625–1627.

Fritzler, M.J., Pauls, J.D., Kinsella, T.D. and Bowen, T.J. (1985). Antinuclear, anticytoplasmic and anti-Sjögren's syndrome antigen A antibodies in female blood donors. Clin. Immunol. Immunopathol. 36, 120–128.

Galili, U., Rachmilewitz, E.A., Peleg, A. and Flechner, I. (1984). A unique natural human IgG antibody with anti-alpha-galactosyl specificity. J. Exp. Med. 160, 1519–1531.

Gause, W.C. and Marsh, J.A. (1985). Effects of testosterone on the development of autoimmune thyroiditis in two strains of chicken. Clin. Immunol. Immunopathol. 36, 10–17.

Gerbert, B. (1980). Psychological aspects of Crohn's disease. J. Behav. Med. 3, 41–58.

Golan, D.T. and Borel, Y. (1984). Increased photosensitivity to near-ultraviolet light in murine SLE. J. Immunol. 132, 705–710.

Goodwin, J.S., Searles, R.P. and Tung, K.S. (1982). Immuno-logical responses of a healthy elderly population. Clin. Exp. Immunol. 48, 403–410.

Gordon, C. and Wofsy, D. (1990). Effects of recombinant murine tumor necrosis factor-alpha on immune function. J. Immunol. 144, 1753–1758.

Grabar, P. (1983). Autoantibodies and the physiological role of immunoglobulins. Immunol. Today 4, 337–339.

Greenberg, A.H. (1985). Antibodies and natural immunity. Biomed. Pharmacother. 39, 4–6.

Gulizia, J.M., Cunningham, M.W. and McManus, B.M. (1991). Immunoreactivity of anti-streptococcal monoclonal antibodies to human heart valves. Evidence for multiple cross-reactive epitopes. Am. J. Pathol. 138, 285–301.

Gutierrez-Ramos, R.J., Andreu, J.L., Revilla, Y., Vinuela, E. and Martinez, C. (1990). Recovery from autoimmunity of MRL/lpr mice after infection with an interleukin-2/vaccinia recombinant virus. Nature (London) 346, 271–274.

Hall, N.R., McGillis, J.P., Spangels, B.L. and Goldstein, A.L. (1984). In "Thymic Hormones and Lymphokines" (ed A.L. Goldstein), pp 313–323. Plenum Press, New York/London.

Halpern, R., Davidson, A., Lazo, A., Solomon, G., Lahita, R. and Diamond, B. (1985). Familial SLE – presence of a cross reactive idiotype in healthy family members. J. Clin. Invest. 76, 731–736.

Handwerger, B.S. (1989). Abnormalities in interleukin-2 and interleukin-4 production in inbred Palmerston North (PN) mice. Arth. Rheum. 32, S91.

Hardy, R.R., Hayakawa, K., Shimizu, M., Yamasaki, K. and Kishimoto, T. (1987). Rheumatoid factor secretion from human Leu-1+ B cells. Science 236, 81–83.

Harkiss, G.D., Hendrie, F. and Nuki, G. (1986). Cross-reactive idiotypes in anti-DNA antibodies of systemic lupus erythematosus patients. Clin. Immunol. Immunopathol. 39, 421–430.

Hartung, H.P., Hughes, R.A., Taylor, W.A., Heininger, K., Reiners, K. and Toyka, K. (1990). T cell activation in Guillain-Barre syndrome and in MS: elevated serum levels of soluble IL-2 receptors. Neurology 40, 215–218.

Hazenberg, B.P., Van Leeuwen, M., Van Rijswijk, M., Stern, A. C. and Vellenga, E. (1989). Correction of granulo-cytopenia in Felty's syndrome by granulocyte-macrophage colony-stimulating factor. Simultaneous induction of interleukin-6 release and flare-up of the arthritis. Blood 74, 2769–2770.

Hechtman, D.H., Cybulsky, M.I., Fuchs, H.J., Baker, J.B. and Gimbrone, M.J. (1991). Intravascular IL-8. Inhibitor of polymorphonuclear leukocyte accumulation at sites of acute inflammation. J. Immunol. 147, 883–892.

Henderson, B. and Pettipher, E.R. (1989). Arthritogenic actions of recombinant IL-1 and tumour necrosis factor alpha in the rabbit: evidence for synergistic interactions between cytokines in vivo. Clin. Exp. Immunol. 75, 306–310.

Heron, I., Hoklund, M. and Berg, K. (1978). Enhanced expression of $\beta2$ microglobulin and HLA antigens on human lymphoid cells by interferon. Proc. Natl Acad Sci. USA. 75, 6215–6219.

Hishikawa, T., Tokano, Y., Sekigawa, I., Ando, S., Takasaki,Y., Hashimoto, H., Hirose, S., Okumura, K., Abe, M. and Shirai, T. (1990). HLA-DP + T cells and deficient interleukin-2 production in patients with systemic lupus erythematosus. Clin. Immunol. Immunopathol. 55, 285–296.

Holman, H., and Deicher, H.R. (1960). The appearance of hypergammaglobulinemia, positive serologic reactions for rheumatoid arthritis and complement fixation with tissue constituents in the sera of relatives of patients with systemic lupus erythematosus. Arth. Rheum. 3, 244–246.

Holoshitz, J., Koning, F., Coligan, J.E., De Bruyn, J. and Strober, S. (1989). Isolation of CD4- CD8- mycobacteria-reactive T lymphocyte clones from rheumatoid arthritis synovial fluid. Nature (London) 339, 226–229.

Homsy, J., Morrow, W.J.W. and Levy, J.A. (1986). Nutrition and autoimmunity: a review. Clin. Exp. Immunol. 65, 473–488.

Hooks, J., Moutsopoulos, H., Geis, S., Stahl, N., Decker, J. and Notkins, A. (1979). Immune interferon in the circulation of patients with autoimmune disease. N. Engl. J. Med. 301, 5–8.

Hooks, J., Jordan, G., Cupps, T., Moutsopoulos, H.M., Fauci, A.S. and Notkins, A.L. (1982). Multiple interferons in the circulation of patients with systemic lupus erythematosus and vasculitis. Arth. Rheum. 25, 396–400.

Horsfall, A.C., Venebles, P.J.W., Mumford, P.A. and Maini, R.N. (1986). Idiotypes on antibodies to the La (SS-B) antigen are restricted and associated with the antigen binding site. Clin. Exp. Immunol. 63, 395–401.

Horsfall, A.C., Venebles, P.J., Mumford, P.A., Allard, S.A. and Maini, R.N. (1987). Distribution of immunoregulatory idiotypes on anti-La (SS-B) antibodies in patients with Sjögren's syndrome. (Abstract). Br. J. Rheumatol. 26, 60.

Houssiau, F.A., Devogelaer, J.P., Van Damme, J., de Deuxchaisnes, C. and Van Snick, J. (1988). Interleukin-6 in synovial fluid and serum of patients with rheumatoid arthritis and other inflammatory arthritides. Arth. Rheum. 31, 784–788.

Huang, Y., Miescher, P. and Zubler, R. (1986). The interleukin 2 secretion defect *in vitro* in systemic lupus erythematosus is reversible in rested cultured T cells. J. Immunol. 137, 3515–3520.

Husby, G., Gran, J.T., Ostensen, M., Johannessen, A. and Thorsby, E. (1979). HLA-DRW4 and rheumatoid arthritis. Lancet i, 548–549.

Imaoka, K., Kanai, Y., Yoshikawa, Y. and Yamanouchi, K. (1990). Temporary breakdown of immunological tolerance to dsDNA and nucleohistone antigens in rabbits infected with rinderpest virus. Clin. Exp. Immunol. 82, 522–526.

Isenberg, D. and Collins, C. (1985). Detection of cross reactive anti-DNA antibody idiotypes on renal tissue bound immunoglobulins from lupus patients J. Clin. Invest. 76, 287–294.

Isenberg, D.A. and Staines, N.A. (1990). DNA antibody idiotypes – an analysis of their role in health and disease. J. Autoimmun. 3, 339–356.

Isenberg, D.A., Shoenfeld, Y., Madaio, M.P., Rauch, J., Reichlin, M., Stollar, B.D. and Schwartz, R.S. (1984). Anti-DNA idiotypes in systemic lupus erythematosus. Lancet ii, 417–422.

Isenberg, D.A., Dudeney, C., Wojnaruska, F., Bhogal, B.S., Rauch, J. and Schattner, A. (1985a). Detection of cross reactive anti-DNA antibody idiotypes on tissue bound immunoglobulins from skin biopsies of lupus patients. J. Immunol. 135, 261–264.

Isenberg, D.A., Shoenfeld, Y., Walport, M., Mackworth-Young, C., Dudeney, C. and Todd-Pokropek, A. (1985b). Detection of cross reactive anti-DNA antibody idiotypes in the serum of systemic lupus erythematosus patients and their relatives. Arth. Rheum. 28, 999–1007.

Isenberg, D.A., Rowe, D., Shearer, M., Novick, D. and Beverley, P.C. (1986). Localization of interferons and IL-2 in polymyositis and muscular dystrophy. Clin. Exp. Immunol. 63, 450–458.

Isenberg, D.A., Katz, D., Le Page, S., Knight, B., Tucker, L., Maddison, P., Hutchings, P., Watts, R., Andre-Schwarts, J., Schwartz, R.S. and Cooke, A. (1991). Independent analysis of the 16/6 idiotype lupus model. J. Immunol. 147, 4172–4177.

Iwatani, Y., Row, V. and Volpe, R. (1985). What prevents autoimmunity? Lancet ii, 839–840.

Jacob, C.O. and McDevitt, H.O. (1988). Tumour necrosis factor-alpha in murine autoimmune "lupus" nephritis. Nature (London) 331, 356–358.

Jacob, C.O., van der Meide, P. and McDevitt, H.O. (1987). *In vivo* treatment of (NZB X NZW).F1 lupus-like nephritis with monoclonal antibody to gamma interferon. J. Exp. Med. 166, 798–803.

Jacob, C.O., Aiso, S., Michie, S.A., McDevitt, H.O. and Acha, O.H. (1990). Prevention of diabetes in nonobese diabetic mice by tumor necrosis factor (TNF): similarities between TNF-alpha and interleukin 1. Proc. Natl Acad. Sci. USA 87, 968–972.

Jerne, N.K. (1974). Towards a network theory of the immune system. Ann. Immunol. (Inst. Pasteur) 125, 373–389.

Johnston, C., Pyke, D.A., Cudworth, A.G. and Wolf, E. (1983). HLA-DR typing in identical twins with insulin dependent diabetes, difference between concordant and discordant pairs. Br. Med. J. 286, 253–255.

Jourdan, M., Bataille, R., Seguin, J., Zhang, X.G., Chaptal, P.A. and Klein, B. (1990). Constitutive production of interleukin-6 and immunologic features in cardiac myxomas. Arth. Rheum. 33, 398–402.

Kawano, M., Hirano, T., Matsuda, T., Taga, T., Horii, Y., Iwato, K., Asaoku, H., Tang, B., Tanabe, O. and Tanaka, H. (1988). Autocrine generation and requirement of BSF-2/IL-6 for human multiple myelomas. Nature (London) 332, 83–85.

Keystone, E.C., Snow, K.M., Bombardier, C., Chang, C.H., Nelson, D.L. and Rubin, L.A. (1988). Elevated soluble interleukin-2 receptor levels in the sera and synovial fluids of patients with rheumatoid arthritis. Arth. Rheum. 31, 844–849.

Kim, T., Kanayama, Y., Negoro, N., Okamura, M., Takeda, T. and Inoue, T. (1987). Serum levels of interferons in patients with systemic lupus erythematosus. Clin. Exp. Immunol. 70, 562–569.

Kion, T.A., and Hoffmann, G.W. (1991). Anti-HIV and anti-anti-MHC antibodies in alloimmune and autoimmune mice. Science 253, 1138–1140.

Kitas, G.D., Salmon, M., Farr, M., Gaston, J.S. and Bacon, P.A. (1988). Deficient interleukin 2 production in rheumatoid arthritis: association with active disease and systemic complications. Clin. Exp. Immunol. 73, 242–249.

Klareskog, L., Forsum, U., Scheynius, A., Kabelitz, D. and Wigzell, H. (1982). Evidence in support of a self-perpetuating HLA-DR dependent delayed-type cell reaction in rheumatoid arthritis. Proc. Natl Acad. Sci. USA. 79, 3632–3636.

Kobayakawa, T., Louis, J., Izui, S. and Lambert, P.H. (1979). Autoimmune response to DNA, RBC and thymocyte antigens in association with polyclonal antibody synthesis during experimental African trypanosomiasis. J. Immunol. 122, 296–301.

Kolb, H. and Toyka, K.V. (1984). New concepts in immunotherapy. Immunol. Today 5, 307–309.

Kroemer, G., Andreu, J., Gonzalo, J., Gutuerrez-Ramos, J. and Martinez, A. (1991). Interleukin-2, autotolerance and autoimmunity. Adv. Immunol. 50, 147–235.

Kunkel, H.G., Agnello, V., Joslin, F.G., Winchester, R.J. and Capra, J.D. (1973). Cross idiotypic specificity among monoclonal IgM proteins with anti-G-globulin activity. J. Exp. Med. 137, 331–342.

Lackovic, V., Borecky, L., Rovensky, J., Zitnan, D., Lukac, J. and Matokova, M. (1984). Periodicity of interferon in the serum of patients with SLE. Arth. Rheum. 74, 597–598.

Lahita, R.G., Bucala, R., Bradlow, H.L. and Fishman, J. (1985). Determination of 16-alpha-hydroxysterone by radioimmunoassay in systemic lupus erythematosus. Arth. Rheum. 28, 1122–1127.

Lang, B., Roberts, A.J., Vincent, A. and Newsom-Davis, J. (1985). Anti-acetylcholine receptor idiotypes in myasthenia gravis analysed by rabbit anti-sera. Clin. Exp. Immunol. 60, 637–644.

Latchman, P.J. and Walport, M.J. (1987). In "Autoimmunity and Autoimmune Disease" (ed J. Whelan), pp 149–171. CIBA Foundation, Wiley and Sons, Chichester.

Lavalle, C., Logo, E., Paniagua, R., Bermudez, J.A., Herrera, J., Graef, A., Gonzalez-Barcena, D. and Fraga, A. (1987). Correlation study between prolactin and androgens in patients with systemic lupus erythematosus. J. Rheumatol. 14, 268–272.

Lefvert, A.K. (1988). Anti-acetylcholine receptor antibody idiotypes in myasthenia gravis. J. Autoimmun. 1, 63–72.

Lefvert, A.K., James, R.W., Alliod, C.A. and Fulpuis, B.W. (1982). A monoclonal anti-idiotypic antibody against anti-receptor antibodies from myasthenic sera. Eur. J. Immunol. 12, 790–792.

Leonhart, T. (1957). Familial hypergammaglobulinemia and systemic lupus erythematosus. Lancet ii, 1200–1203.

Linker-Israeli, M., Deans, R.J., Wallace, D.J., Prehn, J., Ozeri, C.T. and Klinenberg, J. R. (1991). Elevated levels of endogenous IL-6 in systemic lupus erythematosus. A putative role in pathogenesis. J. Immunol. 147, 117–123.

Lippman, S.M., Arnett, F.C. and Conley, C.L. (1982). Genetic factors predisposing to autoimmune diseases – autoimmune hemolytic anemia, chronic thrombocytopenic purpura and systemic lupus erythematosus. Am. J. Med. 73, 827–840.

Londei, M., Verhoef, A., Hawrylowicz, C., Groves, J., De, B. P. and Feldmann, M. (1990). Interleukin 7 is a growth factor for mature human T cells. Eur. J. Immunol. 20, 425–428.

Lowenstein, M.B. and Rothfield, N.F. (1977). Family study of systemic lupus erythematosus, analysis of the clinical history, skin immunofluorescence and serologic parameters. Arth. Rheum. 20, 1293–1303.

Machold, K.P. and Smolen, J.S. (1990). Interferon-gamma induced exacerbation of systemic lupus erythematosus. J. Rheumatol. 17, 831–832.

Mackay, R.P. and Myrianthopoulos, N.C. (1966). Multiple sclerosis in twins and their relatives. Arch. Neurol. 15, 449–462.

Mackworth-Young, C., Chan, J., Harris, N., Walport, M., Bernstein, R., Batchelor, R., Hughes, G. and Gharavi, A. (1987). High incidence of anti-cardiolipin antibodies in relatives of patients with SLE. J. Rheumatol. 14, 723–726.

Maclaren, N., Riley, W., Skordis, N., Atkinson, M., Spillar, R., Silverstein, J., Klein, R., Vadheim, C. and Rotter, J. (1988). Inherited susceptibility to insulin-dependent diabetes is associated with HLA-DR1, while DR5 is protective. Auto immunity, 1, 197–205.

Malavé, I., Searles, R.P., Montano, J. and Williams, R.J. (1989). Production of tumor necrosis factor/cachectin by peripheral blood mononuclear cells in patients with systemic lupus erythematosus. Int. Arch. Allergy. Appl. Immunol. 89, 355–361.

Matsiota, P., Chamaret, S., Montagnier, L. and Avrameas, S. (1987). Detection of natural autoantibodies in the serum of anti-HIV positive individuals. Ann. Inst. Pasteur Immunol. 138, 223–233.

McKenna, R., Ofosuh-Appiah, W., Warrington, R. and Wilkins, J.A. (1986). Interleukin-2 production and responsiveness in active and inactive rheumatoid arthritis. J. Rheumatol. 13, 28–32.

Melez, K.A., Deleeargyros, N. and Bellanti, J.A. (1987). Effect of partial testosterone replacement or thymosin on anti-DNA in castrated (NZB×NZW). F1 males. Clin. Immunol. Immunopathol. 42, 319–327.

Mendlovic, S., Brocke, S., Shoenfeld, Y., Ben-Bassat, M., Meshorer, A., Bakimer, R. and Mozes, E. (1988). Induction of a systemic lupus erythematosus-like disease in mice by a common human anti-DNA idiotype. Proc. Natl Acad. Sci. USA 85, 2260–2264.

Mendlovic, S., Brocke, S., Fricke, H., Shoenfeld, Y., Bakimer, R. and Mozes, E. (1990). The genetic regulation of the induction of experimental SLE. Immunology 69, 228–236.

Mihara, M. and Ohsugi, Y. (1990). Possible role of IL-6 in pathogenesis of immune complex-mediated glomerulonephritis in NZB/W F1 mice: induction of IgG class anti-DNA autoantibody production. Int. Arch. Allergy Appl. Immunol. 93, 89–92.

Mihara, M., Ikuta, M., Koishihara, Y. and Ohsugi, Y. (1991). Interleukin 6 inhibits delayed type hypersensitivity and the development of adjuvant arthritis. Eur. J. Immunol. 21, 2327–2331.

Miyasaka, N., Nakamura, T., Russell, I. and Talal, N. (1984). Interleukin-2 deficiencies in rheumatoid arthritis and systemic lupus erythematosus. Clin. Immunol. Immunopathol. 31, 28–32.

Morgan, B.P. and Walport, M.J. (1991). Complement deficiency and disease. Immunol. Today 12, 301–306.

Morrow, W.J.W., Ohashi, Y., Hall, J., Pribnow, J., Hirose, S., Shirai, T. and Levy, J.A. (1985). Dietary fat and immune function. I. Antibody responses, lymphocytes and accessory cell function in (NZB×NZW).F1 mice. J. Immunol. 135, 3857–3863.

Moulias, R., Proust, J., Wang, A., Congy, F., Marescot, M.R., Deville Chabrolle, A., Paris Hamelin, A. and Lesourd, B. (1984). Age related increase in autoantibodies. Lancet i, 1128–1129.

Nakao, N., Nishikawa, A., Nishiura, T., Kanayama, Y., Tarui, S. and Taniguchi, N. (1991). Hypogalactosylation of immunoglobulin G sugar chains and elevated serum interleukin 6 in Castleman's disease. Clin. Chim. Acta 197, 221–228.

Norton, P.M., Isenberg, D.A. and Latchmann, D.S. (1989). Elevated levels of glucocorticoid receptor associated 90 kDa hsp in a proportion of SLE patients with active disease. Autoimmunity 2, 187–195.

O'Connor, G.R. (1983). Factors related to the initiation and recurrence of uveitis. Am. J. Ophthalmol. 96, 577–599.

O'Dell, J.R., McGivern, J.P., Kay, H.D. and Klassen, J.W. (1988). Improved survival in murine lupus as the result of selenium supplementation. Clin. Exp. Immunol. 73, 322–327.

Oldstone, M.B.A. (1987). Molecular mimicry and autoimmune disease. Cell 50, 819–820.

Ortega, E., Kostovetzky, M. and Larralde, C. (1984). Natural DNP-binding immunoglobulins and antibody multi-specificity. Mol. Immunol. 21, 883–888.

Osoba, D. and Falk, J. (1978). HLA-B8 phenotype associated with an increased mixed leukocyte reaction. Immunogenetics 6, 425–429.

Pandey, J.P., Fudenberg, H.H., Ainsworth, S.K. and Loadholt, C.B. (1979). Autoantibodies in healthy subjects of different age groups. Mech. Aging Dev. 10, 399–404.

Panitch, H.S., Hirsch, R.L., Haley, A.S. and Johnson, K.P. (1987). Exacerbations of multiple sclerosis in patients treated with gamma interferon. Lancet i, 893–895.

Parekh, R.B., Isenberg, D.A., Rook, G., Roitt, I., Dwek, R. and Rademacher, T. (1989). A comparative analysis of disease associated changes in the galactosylation of serum IgG. J. Autoimmun. 2, 101–114.

Pelton, B.K., Speckmaier, M., Hylton, W., Farrant, J. and Denman, M. (1991). Cytokine-independent progression of immunoglobulin production *in vitro* by B lymphocytes from patients with systemic lupus erythematosus. Clin. Exp. Immunol. 83, 274–279.

Pernis, B., Bonagura, V., Posnett, O.N. and Kunkel, H.G. (1984). Idiotype expression in rheumatoid synovial plasma cells. Rheumatol. Int. 4 (Suppl)., 39–43.

Pettipher, E.R., Higgs, G.A. and Henderson, B. (1986). Interleukin 1 induces leucocyte infiltration and cartilage degradation in the synovial joint. Proc. Natl Acad. Sci. USA 83, 8742–8753.

Pollak, V.E. (1964). Antinuclear antibodies in families of patients with SLE. N. Engl. J. Med. 271, 165–171.

Pollak, V.E., Mandema, E. and Kark, R.M. (1960). Antinuclear factors in the serum of relatives of patients with systemic lupus erythematosus. Lancet ii, 1061–1063.

Posnett, D.N., Wisniewolska, R., Pernis, B. and Kunkel, H.G. (1986). Dissection of the human antigammaglobulin idiotype system with monoclonal antibodies. Scand. J. Immunol. 23, 169–181.

Pujol-Borrell, R., Hanafusa, T., Chiovato, I. and Bottazzo, G.F. (1983). Lectin-induced expression of DR antigen on human cultured thyroid follicle cells. Nature (London) 304, 71–73.

Pukel, C., Baquerizo, H. and Rabinovitch, A. (1987). Interleukin 2 activates BB/W diabetic rat lymphoid cells cytotoxic to islet cells. Diabetes. 36, 1217–1222.

Quesada, J.R., Talpaz, M., Rios, A., Kurzrock, R. and Gutterman, J.U. (1986). Clinical toxicity of interferons in cancer patients: a review. J. Clin. Oncol. 4, 234–243.

Rauch, J., Schwartz, R.S. and Stollar, B.D. (1982). In "Monoclonal Antibodies and T Cell Products" (ed D. Katz), pp 99–111. CRC Press, Boca Raton, Florida.

Rauch, J., Meng, Q. and Tannenbaum, H. (1987). Lupus anticoagulant and antiplatelet properties of human hybridoma autoantibodies. J. Immunol. 139, 2598–2604.

Ravirajan, C.T., Kalsi, J., Winska-Wiloch, H., Barakat, S., Tuaillon, N., Irving, W., Cockayne, A., Harris, A., Williams, D.G., Williams, W., Axford, J., Muller, S. and Isenberg, D.A. (1992). Antigen binding diversity of human hybridoma autoantibodies derived from splenocytes of patients with SLE. Lupus 1, 157–165.

Ronnblom, L.E., Alm, G.V. and Oberg, K. (1991) Autoimmune phenomenon in patients with malignant carcinoid tumors during interferon-alpha treatment. Acta-oncol, 30, 537–340.

Rose, N. and Mackay, I.R. (1985). In "The Autoimmune Diseases", pp 16–27. Academic Press, New York.

Roubinian, J.R., Papoian, R. and Talal, N. (1977). Androgenic hormones modulate autoantibody responses and improve survival in murine lupus. J. Clin. Invest. 59, 1066–1070.

Roubinian, J.R., Talal, N., Greenspan, J.S., Goodman, J.R. and Siiteri, P.K. (1978). Effect of castration and sex hormone treatment on survival, anti-nucleic acid antibodies and glomerulonephritis in (NZB/NZW).F1 mice. J. Exp. Med. 147, 1568–1583.

Roubinian, J.R., Talal, N., Greenspan, J.S., Goodman, J.R. and Nussenzweig, V. (1979a). Danazol's failure to suppress autoimmunity in (NZB/NZW).F1 mice. Arth. Rheum. 22, 1399–1402.

Roubinian, J.R., Talal, N., Siiteri, P.K. and Sadakian, J.A. (1979b). Sex hormone modulation of autoimmunity in NZB/NZW hybrid mice. Arth. Rheum. 22, 1162–1169.

Rowe, I.F., Forster, S.M., Seifert, M.H., Youle, M.S., Hawkins, D.A., Lawrence, A. G. and Keat, A.C. (1989). Rheumatological lesions in individuals with human immunodeficiency virus infection. Q. J. Med. 73, 1167–1184.

Rubin, L.A., Snow, K.M., Kurman, C.C., Nelson, D.L. and Keystone, E.C. (1990). Serial levels of soluble interleukin 2 receptor in the peripheral blood of patients with rheumatoid arthritis: correlations with disease activity. J. Rheumatol. 17, 597–602.

Ruf, J., Carayon, P. and Lissitsky, S. (1986). Idiotypic analysis of five xenogeneic antisera to anti-human thyroglobulin monoclonal antibodies. Immunol. Lett. 13, 39–44.

Russell, D.H., Kiber, R., Matrisian, L., Larson, D.F., Poulos, B. and Magun, B.E., (1985). Prolactin receptors on human T and B lymphocytes: antagonism of prolactin bindings by cyclosporin. J. Immunol. 134, 3027–3031.

Satoh, M., Hama, N. and Hirakata, M. (1987). Idiotypic analysis of auto-antibodies to U1RNP (Abstr). Clin. Exp. Rheumatol. 5, 22.

Schattner, A. (1983). Lymphopenia in SLE: possible role of interferon. Arth. Rheum. 26, 1415.

Schattner, A., Duggan, D., Naparstek, Y. and Schwartz, R.S. (1986). Effects of alpha interferon on the expression of a lupus idiotype in normal humans. Clin. Immunol. Immunopathol. 38, 327–336.

Schnittman, S.M., Psallidopoulos, M.C., Lane, H.C., Thompson, L., Baseler, M., Massari, F., Fox, C.H., Salzman, N.P. and Fauci, A.S. (1989). The reservoir for HIV-1 in human peripheral blood is a T cell that maintains expression of CD4. Science 245, 305–308.

Schoolcy, R.T., Haynes, B.F., Payling-Wright, C.R., Fauci, A.S. and Dolin, R. (1981). Development of suppressor T lymphocytes for Epstein Barr virus induced B lymphocyte outgrowth during acute infectious mononucleosis: assessment by two quantitative systems. Blood 57, 510–517.

Shackelford, D.A., Kaufman, J.F., Korman, A.J. and Strominger, J.L. (1982). HLA-DR antigens: structure, separation of subpopulations, gene cloning and function. Immunol. Rev. 66, 133–187.

Shoenfeld, Y. and Isenberg, D.A. (1989). "The Mosaic of Autoimmunity". Research Monographs in Immunology, vol. 12. Elsevier, Amsterdam.

Shoenfeld, Y., Rauch, J., Massicote, H., Datta, S.K., Andre-Schwartz, J., Stollar, B.D. and Schwartz, R.S. (1983a). Polyspecificity of monoclonal lupus autoantibodies produced by human–human hybridomas. N. Engl. J. Med. 308, 414–420.

Shoenfeld, Y., Isenberg, D.A., Rauch, J., Madio, M.P., Stollar, B.D. and Schwartz, R.S. (1983b). Idiotypic cross-reactions of monoclonal human lupus autoantibodies. J. Exp. Med. 158, 718–730.

Shoenfeld, Y., Brill, S., Weinberger, A., Pinkhas, J. and Isenberg, D.A. (1986). High levels of a common anti-DNA idiotype (16/6). A genetic marker for SLE. Acta Haematol. 76, 107–109.

Shore, A., Jaglal, S. and Keystone, E.C. (1986). Enhanced interleukin-1 generation by monocytes in vitro is temporally linked to an early event in the onset or exacerbation of rheumatoid arthritis. Clin. Exp. Immunol. 65, 293–302.

Silverstein, A.M. (1960). Essential hypocomplementemia; report of a case. Blood 16, 1338–1341.

Silvestris, F., Anderson, W., Goodwin, J.S. and Williams, R.C. Jr. (1985). Discrepancy in the expression of autoantibodies in healthy aged individuals. Clin. Immunol. Immunopathol. 35, 234–244.

Skoldstam, L., Larsson, L. and Lindstrom, F.D. (1979). Effects of fasting and lactovegetarian diet on rheumatoid arthritis. Scand. J. Rheumatol. 8, 249–255.

Smith, H.R., Green, D.R., Raveche, E.S., Smathers, P.A., Gershon, R.K. and Steinberg, A.D. (1982). Studies on the induction of anti-DNA in normal mice. J. Immunol. 129, 2332–2334.

Smolen, J.S. (1987). In "Systemic Lupus Erythematosus" (ed J.S. Smolen and C.C. Zierlinski), pp 170–196. Springer-Verlag, New York.

Spector, D.A., Jampol, L.M. and Hayslett, J.P. (1973). Report of the familial occurrence of systemic lupus erythematosus in male siblings. Arth. Rheum. 16, 221–224.

Spurzem, J.R. and Lockey, J.E. (1984). Toxic oil syndrome. Arch. Intern. Med. 144, 249–250.

Stott, E.J. (1991). Anti-cell antibody in macaques [letter]. Nature (London) 353, 6343.

Stricker, R.B., McHugh, T.M., Marx, P.A., Morrow, W.J.W., Levy, J.A., Shuman, M.A., Stites, D.P. and Neyman, P.D. (1987a). Prevalence of an AIDS-related autoantibody against CD4+ T cells in humans and monkeys. Blood 70, 127A.

Stricker, R.B., McHugh, T.M., Moody, D.J., Morrow, W.J.W., Stites, D.P., Shuman, M.A. and Levy, J.A. (1987b). An AIDS-related cytotoxic autoantibody reacts with a specific antigen or stimulated CD4+ T cells. Nature (London) 327, 710–713.

Swaak, T. and Smeenk, R. (1985). Detection of anti-dsDNA as a diagnostic tool; a prospective study in 441 non-systemic lupus erythematosus patients with anti-dsDNA antibody (anti-dsDNA). Ann. Rheum. Dis. 44, 245–251.

Takei, M., Kang, H., Tomura, K., Amaki, S., Hirata, M., Karasaki, M., Sawada, S. and Amaki, I. (1987). Aberration of monokine production and monocyte subset in patients with systemic lupus erythematosus. J. Clin. Lab. Immunol. 22, 169–173.

Talal, N. and Ahmed, S.A. (1987). Immunomodulation by hormones – an area of growing importance. J. Rheumatol. 14, 191–193.

Taylor, E. and Rose, N.R. (1991). Hypothesis: the ageing paradox and autoimmune disease. Autoimmunity 8, 245–249.

Tepper, R.I., Levinson, D.A., Stanger, B.Z., Campos, T.J., Abbas, A.K. and Leder, P. (1990). IL-4 induces allergic-like inflammatory disease and alters T cell development in transgenic mice. Cell 62, 457–467.

TerBorg, E., Horst, G., Limburg, P.C. and Kallenberg, C.G. (1990). Changes in plasma levels of interleukin-2 receptor in relation to disease exacerbations and levels of anti-dsDNA and complement in systemic lupus erythematosus. Clin. Exp. Immunol. 82, 21–26.

TeVelde, A., Huijbens, R.J., Heije, K., de, V.J. and Figdor, C.G. (1990). Interleukin-4 (IL-4) inhibits secretion of IL-1 beta, tumor necrosis factor alpha and IL-6 by human monocytes. Blood 76, 1392–1397.

Thivolet, J., Monier, J.C., Ruel, J.P. and Richard, M.H. (1967). Antinuclear autoantibodies in Swiss mice thymectomized at birth. Nature (London) 214, 1134–1136.

Tominaga, A., Takaki, S., Koyama, N., Katoh, S., Matsumoto, R., Migita, M., Hitoshi, Y., Hosoya, Y., Yamauchi, S., Kanai, Y., Miyazaki, J., Usaka, G., Yamamura, K. and Takatsu, K. (1991). Transgenic mice expressing a B cell growth and differentiation factor gene (interleukin 5) develop eosinophilia and autoantibody production. J. Exp. Med. 173, 429–437.

Tsoulfa, G., Rook, G.A., Van Embden, J., Young, D.B., Mehlert, A., Isenberg, D.A., Hay, F.C. and Lydyard, P.M. (1989). Raised serum IgG and IgA antibodies to myco-bacterial antigens in rheumatoid arthritis. Ann. Rheum. Dis. 48, 118–123.

Tuffanelli, D.L. and Epstein, J. (1987). In "Dubois Lupus erythematosus" (ed. D.J. Wallace and E.L. Dubois), pp 283–301. Lea and Febiger, Philadelphia.

Umland, S., Lee, R., Howard, M. and Martens, C. (1989). Expression of lymphokine genes in splenic lymphocytes of autoimmune mice. Mol. Immunol. 26, 649–656.

Van Eden, W., De Vries, R.R.P., Stanford, J.L. and Rook, G.A. (1983). HLA-DR3 associated genetic control of response to multiple skin tests with new tuberculosis. Clin. Exp. Immunol. 52, 287–293.

Van Eden, W., Hogervorst, E.J., Wauben, M.H., van der Zee, R. and Boog, C.J. (1991). Heat-shock proteins as antigens in autoimmunity. Biochem. Soc. Trans. 19, 171–175.

Venables, P. (1988). Epstein-Barr virus infection and auto-immunity in rheumatoid arthritis. Ann. Rheum. Dis. 47, 265–269.

Vialettes, B., Ozanon, J.P., Bernard, D., Vallo, J., Sauvage, E., Lassman, V. and Vague, P. (1986). Stress, immunity and type-I (insulin-dependent) diabetes. Diabetologia 29, A604.

Villarejos, V.M., Serra, J.C., Visona, K.A. and Eduarte, C.E. (1979). Antibodies to single stranded DNA: a diagnostic aid in chronic hepatitis B virus infections. J. Med. Virol. 4, 79–101.

Voorthuis, J.A., Uitdehaag, B.M., De Groot, C., Goede, P.H., van der Meide, P. and Dijkstra, C.D. (1990). Suppression of experimental allergic encephalomyelitis by intraventricular administration of interferon-gamma in Lewis rats. Clin. Exp. Immunol. 81, 183–188.

Walton, A.J.E, Snaith, M.L., Locniskar, M., Cumberland, A.G., Morrow, W.J.W. and Isenberg, D.A. (1991). Dietary fish oil and the severity of symptoms in patients with systemic lupus erythematosus. Ann. Rheum. Dis. 50, 463–466.

Watts, R. and Isenberg, D.A. (1990). DNA antibody idiotypes, an analysis of their clinical connections and origins. Int. Rev. Immunol. 5, 279–293.

Weiner, P., Landau, M. and Abu-Much, S. (1987). The presence of rheumatoid factor in patients with arthralgia, results of a 5 year follow up. Harefuah 112, 430–432.

Weitkamp, L.R., May, A.G. and Johnston, E. (1975). The linkage relationship of HLA with other genetic marker systems. Hum. Hered. 25, 337–345.

Whittingham, S., Matthews, J., Schanfield, M., Tait, B.D. and Mackay, I.R. (1981). Interaction of HLA and Gm in auto-immune chronic active hepatitis. Clin. Exp. Immunol. 43, 80–86.

Wiesenberg, I., van der Meide, P.H., Schellekens, H. and Alkan, S.S. (1989). Suppression and augmentation of rat adjuvant arthritis with monoclonal anti-interferon-gamma antibody. Clin. Exp. Immunol. 78, 245–249.

Williams, E.D. and Doniach, I. (1962). The post-mortem inci-dence of focal thyroiditis. J. Pathol. Bacteriol. 83, 255–264.

Wolfe, F., Kleinheksel, S.M. and Khan, M.A. (1988). Preva-lence of familial occurrence in patients with rheumatoid arthritis. Br. J. Rheumatol. 27 (Suppl. II), 150–152.

Woodrow, J.C. (1988a). Immunogenetics of rheumatoid arthritis. J. Rheumatol. 15, 1–2.

Woodrow, J.C. (1988b). Immunogenetics of SLE. J. Rheumatol. 15, 197–199.

Yadin, O., Sarov, B., Naggan, L., Slor, H. and Shoenfeld, Y. (1989). Natural autoantibodies in the serum of healthy women – a 5 year follow-up. Clin. Exp. Immunol. 75, 402–406.

Yoon, J. W. (1990). The role of viruses and environmental factors in the induction of diabetes. Curr. Top. Microbiol. Immunol. 164, 95–123.

Young, R. A. (1990). Stress proteins and immunology. Ann. Rev. Immunol. 8, 401–420.

Yu, T., Winchester, R., Fu, S.M., Gibofsky, A., Ko, H.S. and Kunkel, H.G. (1980). Peripheral blood Ia-positive cells. J. Exp. Med. 151, 91–100.

Zanetti, M., Barton, R.W. and Bigazzi, P.E. (1983). Anti-idiotypic immunity and autoimmunity. Cell. Immunol. 75, 292–299.

Zinkernagel, R.M. and Doherty, P.C. (1980). MHC-restricted cytotoxic T cells; studies on the biological role of polymorphic major transplantation antigens determining T-cell restriction specificity functions and responsiveness. Adv. Immunol. 27, 51–177.

2. Immunological Tolerance and its Implications for Autoimmunity

N.A. Mitchison

1. Introduction

This chapter deals with immunological tolerance, the subject which embraces the means by which the immune system discriminates between self and non-self. This is a central topic in immunology, and although there are still gaps in knowledge, the mechanisms which protect the body against attack by the immune system are now well understood in outline. Central to our understanding is the process of negative selection in the thymus. Accordingly this account begins with the reasons for focusing attention on the thymus, and then proceeds to describe the selection processes within that organ in some detail. It then describes tolerance mechanisms which can be implemented outside the thymus. These peripheral mechanisms, although of great experimental interest and potential therapeutic value, have as yet no definite role in the normal physiology of the immune system. The vexed area of cellular signals for tolerance is then discussed, and the conclusion drawn that more than one mechanism may be involved. The evolutionary constraints which tightly control negative selection are outlined. These constraints provide a background to autoimmunity, and demand an error-correction mechanism which is provided in the form of a suppression system. Tolerance among B cells and γδ-T cells is presented as a side issue. Finally, the connection between breakdown of tolerance and autoimmune disease is discussed.

An understanding of immunological tolerance is required for any theory of autoimmunity. Tolerance merits the extended treatment given it here because of the importance of autoimmunity in a variety of joint and

Immunopharmacology of Joints and Connective Tissue
ISBN 0–12–206345–7

connective tissue diseases, most notably in rheumatoid arthritis and SLE, but also in the rarer connective tissue diseases such as dermatomyositis. Reactive arthritis also may have an autoimmune component.

The present account departs somewhat from conventional presentations, in that it concentrates on the logic of the immune system rather than on summarizing research findings. Negative selection and the rest of the tolerance machinery can be seen to work as they do for understandable reasons. With natural selection at play, nothing is ever simple or straightforward, but one can claim with some confidence that the overall pattern is becoming clear. In the last section the presentation opens out to touch on such topics as the contribution to be expected from epidemiology.

This chapter could have been written from a rather different point of view, with a greater emphasis on the many recent findings made with transgenes, superantigens and cell lines (Arnold *et al.*, 1990). It could have concentrated on the various mechanisms of downregulation that these systems have revealed in T and B cells. The problem with this approach is that most of these mechanisms are still of uncertain status in the normal working of the immune system. Accordingly, the present account limits its scope to tolerance of self within the normal immune system.

2. The Immune System Avoids Reacting Against Self Mainly by Negative Selection of T Cells

The problem of tolerance has long attracted the attention of immunologists. Modern concepts trace back to the ideas formulated by Burnet and by Medawar (Billingham *et al.*, 1954) in the 1950s, at a time when the subject was first thrown open to experiment. Gradually it became clear that the immune system avoids reacting against self principally by deletion. Lymphocytes that have receptors able to bind self-epitopes become deleted during the course of their development, a process that is now termed negative selection (in contrast with positive selection; the two forms of selection are described below in detail). The result of negative selection is that individuals become unable to respond to their own macromolecules, a condition known as immunological tolerance. Along the way many alternative ideas were discarded, such as the hypothesis that the mature immune system does recognize self, but in doing so it also receives a signal to turn on suppression. Not all these possibilities have been entirely lost, as some of them turn up again in contemporary thinking as minor supplementary mechanisms, able to back up negative selection under appropriate circumstances. The extent to which the concept of negative selection has stood the test of

time and the new ideas that challenge it are assessed towards the end of this chapter (Section 11.1).

In this earlier era of research, recovery from experimentally induced tolerance provided the main evidence in favour of negative selection (Dresser and Mitchison, 1968; Howard and Mitchison, 1975). It was found that animals would recover spontaneously, provided (1) that the supply of the tolerance-inducing antigen ceased and (2) that the animal retained an intact thymus. These conditions were not met in animals that had been rendered "chimeric" by injection of viable allogeneic cells or in animals that had been thymectomized after tolerance induction. Under these circumstances, tolerance lasted indefinitely. Furthermore, the speed of recovery was related to the functional activity of the thymus: as thymus activity declined with age, so also did the speed of recovery. These observations imply that tolerance among mature lymphocytes is irreversible, and that recovery proceeds through the recruitment of new cells. They leave little room for such possibilities as temporarily switched-off cells or suppression by other cells.

Subsequent studies with superantigens and with animals transgenic for T cell receptors that recognize self-antigens have confirmed this conclusion. In certain cases, they dramatically demonstrate that T cells with the appropriate receptors, detectable by means of idiotypic antibodies, appear early in development but are subsequently deleted. (This finding has been made with superantigens rather than with receptor transgenes, possibly because in the latter case the receptors are expressed prematurely.)

The predominant importance attributed to T cells in negative selection rested originally on the common occurrence of potentially self-reactive B cells. These cells can be recognized in the normal immune system by their ability to bind, via their surface immunoglobulin receptors, such self-proteins as thyroglobulin. They can also be detected by their ability to make an anti-self-response in circumstances where help from T cells becomes available. For instance, mice genetically defective in production of the protein C5 (a complement component) contain C5-reactive T cells, as expected. When these cells are stimulated to respond to C5, in combination with B cells from normal mice, anti-C5 antibody is produced. Other self-proteins, such as F liver protein and thyroglobulin, are known to behave in much the same way (Griffiths *et al.*, 1987). The inability to make anti-self antibody can thus generally be attributed to the absence of T cell help, although some tolerance can be found among B cells, as is further discussed below.

As so often happens, a conclusion that was first reached on the basis of experimental evidence can now be deduced from fundamental principles. Under certain circumstances (while located within a germinal centre), a B cell hypermutates its expressed IgV genes, i.e. it encodes new antigen-combining sites at a frequency as high as one base substitution per V gene per cell generation (Jacob *et al.*, 1991; Apel and Berek, 1990). This process enables the affinity of antibody to rise progressively during an immune response. This is particularly valuable for its effect on the late memory phase of the immune response, as it enables low concentrations of antibody to work effectively. T cells do not hypermutate, and no doubt this can partly be attributed to the limited value of high affinity in the multipoint binding that these cells perform. But it also fits them for their role as guardians of self-tolerance, as their inability to generate new combining sites ensures that the gaps in their repertoire created by negative selection remain open. In a logical manner, the immune system has split in two, leaving one part responsible for self-tolerance, and thus permitting the other to evolve its mechanism of hypermutation.

This argument applies to helper T cells, which in general have the CD4, MHC class II-restricted phenotype. CD8, MHC class I-restricted cytotoxic T cells might be expected to behave more like B cells, as they are themselves under the partial control of helper T cells (von Boehmer and Haas, 1979; Mitchison, 1990). Indeed, certain experimental systems hint that CD8 cells may be more difficult to render tolerant (Waterfield *et al.*, 1983), although on the whole they seem to undergo negative selection in much the same way as helper T cells. Like CD4 T cells, CD8 T cells do not hypermutate. One concludes that their weaker control by helper T cells, coupled with their multipoint binding, probably prevents them from evolving in the B cell direction.

3. Negative Selection Occurs Mainly in the Thymus, at a Particular Stage of T Cell Development

Most of the important stages of T cell development occur within the thymus. A small stream of precursor cells enters the thymus, where they develop into mature T cells and later leave in a larger stream. Within the thymus these cells multiply and also die extensively, during the processes of positive and negative selection. As a result of these processes the mature T cells emerge with a highly selected repertoire of antigen-specific receptors, which endows the T cell compartment of the immune system with its unique properties of restriction by the MHC and immunological tolerance. The concepts of positive and negative selection are fairly new in their present formulation (von Boehmer and Kieselow, 1990; von Boehmer, 1991), but they trace back to much earlier experimental work. In particular, soon after it was first shown that T cells develop in the thymus, the small population of mature T cells which have not yet emigrated were found to be fully self-tolerant with respect to their reactivity with MHC antigens, in that they could react against allo- but not self-MHC. The complete process of tolerance induction must therefore have taken place within the thymus. This is now known to be true also of at least one soluble self-protein (Robertson *et al.*, 1992).

A detailed picture is beginning to emerge of when, where and how these selective processes operate. This is

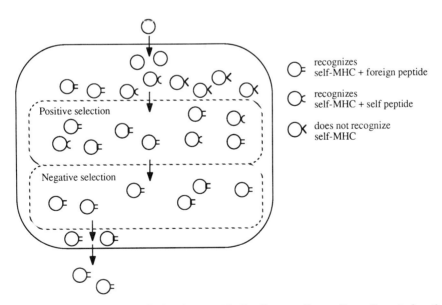

Figure 2.1 Selection of T cells during their development in the thymus. Progenitor cells entering the thymus do not express TCR. Then expression begins, and the cells develop an initial repertoire containing receptors which (i) recognize self-MHC + foreign peptide, (ii) self-MHC + self-peptide, and (iii) neither of these. Under positive selection, category (iii) is lost. At the next and final stage, negative selection eliminates cells which recognize self-MHC + self-peptides, leaving a mature population of self-MHC + foreign-peptide-recognizers which then exits from the thymus.

summarized in Figs 2.1–2.3, which should be looked at together. Figure 2.1 is concerned with the TCR, and shows how the developmental fate of T cells is determined by the specificity of this receptor. For functioning of the mature immune system, the only useful T cells are those that recognize self-MHC + foreign peptide, and the main purpose of the thymus is to make sure that this is the only type of cell that matures and finally emigrates. A second category of T cell recognizes self-MHC + self-peptide. These are dangerous cells, which it is the business of negative selection to eliminate. A third category does not recognize self-MHC at all, and their receptors presumably make up the majority of the initial repertoire that is generated by random V–D–J recombination. It is the business of positive selection to discard these from the population that finally matures; they are useless cells, although presumably not dangerous, and it is believed that most of the carnage that takes place in the thymus reflects the loss of these cells rather than that of the smaller category of dangerous self-recognizers.

The most useful surface markers for dissecting out developmental stages in the thymus are the CD4 and CD8 glycoproteins. These two accessory molecules bind respectively to constant parts of MHC class II and class I molecules, and the presence of either one is a safe guide to the class of MHC molecule (and hence type of antigen-presenting cell) with which a T cell can interact. Their distribution in the thymus is summarized in Fig. 2.2. The main puzzle here is why CD4 and CD8 are expressed simultaneously on T cells while they are located within the positive selection compartment, thus breaking

the general rule of alternative expression that holds in the periphery. It is now known that interaction during positive selection with MHC class I molecules instructs a T cell to switch off CD4 expression, and with class II to switch off CD8. The alternative possibility, which has been excluded by experiment, was that class I molecules selected cells that had previously come to express CD8 at random (Robey *et al.*, 1991). Thus joint expression of CD4 and CD8 provides a way of doubling the likelihood of a T cell surviving positive selection. A minor unsolved puzzle is why CD8 expression is turned on slightly before that of CD4. Robey's conclusion has been challenged in several subsequent studies, but confirmed at least once. The matter is therefore still under debate.

Another informative set of markers are the isoforms of CD45 (Lightstone and Marvel, 1990). These subdivide the CD4 and CD8 subsets in a way that is still not perfectly understood. After a good deal of debate it is now no longer believed that expression of CD45R0 versus CD45RA divides cells into those that have "helper versus suppressor" or "memory versus naive" function. The present view is rather that CD45R0 is a marker of activation. T cells in this condition are hyperreactive to antigen (and to stimulation with anti-CD3 monoclonal antibody), unlike resting CD45RA cells (Beverley, 1991; Lightstone *et al.*, 1992). Current information concerning the expression of these isoforms during development and activation is summarized in Fig. 2.3. The puzzle here is why the majority of cells in the thymus express CD45R0, although very early and at or soon after emigration they switch to the alternative CD45RA

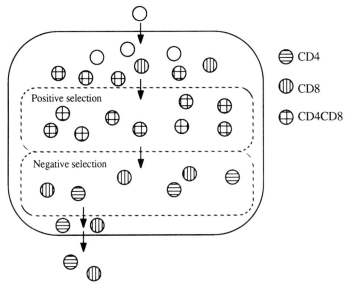

Figure 2.2 Expression of the accessory molecules CD4 and CD8 during development in the thymus. Cells entering the thymus do not express these molecules. They then turn on expression of CD8, followed shortly after by expression of CD4. These double-positive cells then undergo positive selection, during which they turn off expression of CD8 irreversibly if they contact MHC class II molecules, and of CD4 if they contact MHC class I. During subsequent negative selection they recognize MHC + self-peptide in the same way as do mature cells, using the appropriate accessory molecule in combination with their TCR.

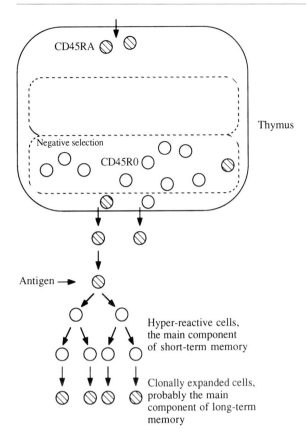

CD45RA

Thymus

Negative selection

CD45R0

Antigen →

Hyper-reactive cells, the main component of short-term memory

Clonally expanded cells, probably the main component of long-term memory

Figure 2.3 The kaleidoscopic expression of CD45 isoforms during T cell development and activation. The earliest T cells detectable in the thymus express CD45RA, and it is this type of cell which has repopulating activity in cell transfer experiments. Most cells then switch to expression of CD45R0, the majority phenotype within the thymus, and are believed to retain this activated phenotype during negative selection (the phenotype during positive selection is unknown). Mature T cells switch back to expressing CD45RA before or just after leaving the thymus, and continue to express this resting phenotype until they encounter antigen. After such encounter they switch to the CD45R0 phenotype, and become hyperreactive to the antigen. Later they come to rest again, switch back to CD45RA expression, and lose their hyperreactivity.

marker. Hyperreactivity provides a reasonable explanation, although not one that is fully substantiated. Suppose that the opposite were true, that T cells undergoing negative selection were not hyperreactive. Then some cells would emerge from the thymus in a condition such that they could not react against self-antigens while in the resting state, but upon activation would be able to do so. These would be dangerous cells, because any non-specific activation (for instance by a superantigen) could drive them into a state where they could initiate an autoimmune reaction. The thymus seems to exclude this possibility by ensuring that most or all cells undergoing

negative selection are in the hyperreactive CD45R0 state. On the other hand, hyperreactivity must not go too far. The thymus cannot afford to let T cells get so excited that they become refractory to tolerance induction, which can happen in the periphery as described below in Section 4 (Dresser, 1976).

Positive and negative selection occur at different developmental stages and sites in the thymus, and use different types of antigen-presenting cell. It makes sense to purge self-reactive T cells only after the main population of useless non-MHC-recognizing cells has been disposed of. Accordingly, positive selection occurs first, in the cortex, where T cell progenitors first enter the thymus. For presentation of MHC molecules, positive selection employs epithelial cells which have the unusual property of constitutively expressing MHC class II as well as class I molecules. Following positive selection, the developing T cells move on into the medulla and medulla–cortex border, where negative selection occurs. This type of selection occurs on dendritic cells, which closely match in their antigen-presenting properties the main presenters of the periphery, the interdigitating dendritic cells (Kyewski et al., 1986). Soon afterwards the T cells, now endowed with their mature repertoire, emigrate from the thymus to the periphery.

These two types of antigen presentation during the two processes of selection make good sense, and leave only one puzzle outstanding. In the periphery, T cells are likely, sooner or later, to encounter antigen presented not only by dendritic cells but also by B cells. Although interdigitating dendritic cells and B cells match fairly well in their antigen-processing properties, they do not do so exactly. B cells perform what is termed "vectored" or "protected" processing, by means of their surface immunoglobulin (Berzofsky, 1983; Manca et al., 1988). This characteristic has no counterpart in dendritic cells, and it is hard to see how negative selection mediated only by such cells would extend to all the epitopes that could later be presented by B cells. One possibility is that the 3% or so of B cells that do occur in the thymus take care of the problem (Isaacson et al., 1987; Inaba et al., 1991), although that hardly seems likely. A more attractive possibility, further discussed below in Section 9, is that self-tolerance among B cells may obviate the problem.

It should be emphasized that this account deals only with the main points in a complex developmental process which is still not fully understood. For instance, the exact location of selection in the thymus remains controversial, and a variety of cytokines of unknown significance are known to act within the organ.

4. Tolerance can be Induced Outside the Thymus

In some experimental systems, the presence of a thymus is not required for tolerance induction to occur.

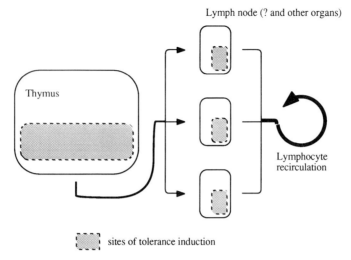

Figure 2.4 Tolerance can also be induced in organs other than the thymus. These include peripheral lymphoid tissue (lymph nodes and spleen), and perhaps also tissue sites such as pancreas islets. The exact sites within peripheral tissue where this occurs have not been identified, but are presumably located in areas where T cells make contact with antigen-presenting cells. Recirculation of lymphocytes is important for the process, and many passes through lymphoid tissue are required in order to achieve full tolerance of low concentration proteins. The Figure refers to "tolerance induction" rather than "negative selection", because anergy may also be involved (see text).

Evidently there are other compartments of the immune system where the process can take place, as illustrated in Fig. 2.4. The most direct demonstration comes from experiments in which serum proteins such as albumin or immunoglobulin from a foreign source are introduced into mice, some of which have been thymectomized (Zamoyska and Mitchison, 1989). These proteins readily induce tolerance, and the absence of a thymus has no detectable effect on the speed with which tolerance is induced. Figure 2.4 also illustrates a second point about peripheral tolerance: in order to undergo the process, CD4 T cells have to recirculate through lymphoid tissue, as would be expected from their dependence on antigen-presenting cells (Mitchison, 1968).

Similar conclusions have been reached from studies on transgenic mice, in which a neoantigen is expressed on cells in pancreatic islets, brain or other remote site (Lo et al., 1988; Arnold et al., 1990). A problem with this type of experiment is that transport of the neoantigen into the thymus is hard to exclude. A third line of argument comes from consideration of trophoblast proteins, such as chorionic gonadotrophin, which of course do not provoke an immune response during pregnancy, although one supposes that many T cells must escape from the thymus without ever having encountered them there.

One must be cautious about the mechanism of tolerance in these experiments. Sometimes there is no evidence of negative selection, and the T cells that one would have expected to be deleted are in fact still present, but unable to perform a normal immune response, a condition known as anergy (Lo et al., 1988; Schonrich et al., 1991; Arnold et al., 1990). Several forms of anergy have been encountered in the many transgene systems which have been devised. They range from complete failure of the affected T cell to respond, to a failure only of the late effector functions such as lymphokine secretion. Little purpose would be served by a detailed discussion of these conditions, as so far they have no known counterpart in the normal immune system, and there is no firm evidence that anergy plays a significant role in recovery from immunological disease. This situation may of course change, and research is now underway to define better the anergic phenotype, so as to enable this type of research to proceed. It should be added that some forms of extrathymic tolerance have a feature characteristic of negative selection, namely irreversible inactivation of specific T cells. This is evident in the permanent loss of reactivity in mice that have been thymectomized, after induction in adult life of tolerance to a foreign serum protein (Howard and Mitchison, 1975). Certainly the easiest interpretation of these findings is that negative selection is not confined to the thymus.

Tolerance induction in the thymus and periphery differs in one important respect. Activation of the peripheral immune systems by agents such as Freund's adjuvant (administered separately from antigen) inhibits tolerance induction, or at least masks it so that the net impact of an otherwise "tolerizing" antigenic stimulus becomes a positive immune response (Dresser, 1976). Cells in the thymus are evidently shielded from this kind of activation.

From the present point of view, perhaps the most exciting possibility is that extrathymic tolerance induction may provide a means of treating autoimmune disease. That hope inspires the present massive research effort on genetically manipulated models of tolerance.

5. Negative Selection Terminates in Apoptosis, but the Initiating Conditions are Controversial

The signals that bring about negative selection have long been a matter of debate, as summarized in Fig. 2.5. One possibility, first formulated by Lederberg (1959), is that what matters is the stage of development of the T cell. At an early stage, encounter with antigen causes the cell to die, while at a later stage the encounter causes proliferation and differentiation.

The most direct evidence in favour of the development-stage hypothesis comes from experiments in which antigen (Jenkinson *et al.*, 1989) or monoclonal anti-CD3 antibody (Smith *et al.*, 1989) is used to stimulate developing T cells. This form of stimulation gives a positive signal to mature T cells, causing them to proliferate and differentiate; but when given to thymus organ cultures, it causes T cells to go into apoptosis

(programmed cell death). Additional evidence comes from treatment of isolated CD4CD8 double-positive cells with the cellular antigen H-Y (the male-specific transplantation antigen), which also drives them into apoptosis (Swat *et al.*, 1991). The problem with this type of experiment is to distinguish between a signal that induces apoptosis and one that merely accelerates a process that has already been started.

Where the development-stage hypothesis runs into trouble is with soluble self-proteins. Such proteins evidently do normally induce tolerance within the thymus, but probably only because that is the first place where T cells encounter them. In terms of the dose–response curve, there is little if any difference in efficiency between thymic and post-thymic induction (Robertson *et al.*, 1992; further discussion in Section 6). It is true that the thymus is more efficient in the sense that one brief pass is all that is required, whereas peripheral lymphoid organs need many passes, as judged by the slow kinetics of post-thymic induction. These observations are better explained by the signal-deficit hypothesis, the other main contender for initiating negative selection.

The signal-deficit hypothesis was first proposed in terms of presentation of antigen to lymphocytes other than by macrophages, at a time when it was thought that all lymphocytes could recognize antigens in solution. That

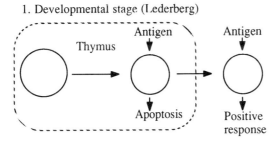

1. Developmental stage (Lederberg)

Apparently supported by apoptotic response of CD4+CD8+ T cell
to treatment with anti-CD3 antibodies, superantigens, H-Y antigen

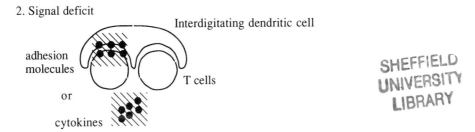

2. Signal deficit

Figure 2.5 Alternative hypotheses of tolerance. The first, formulated by Lederberg, holds that T cells become susceptible to negative selection at an immature stage of their development. It is supported (but perhaps only apparently, see text) by experiments with anti-CD3 and other forms of treatment. The second holds that a deficit in signalling (a form of "contextual discrimination", mentioned below in Section 11.1) causes negative selection. The deficit might lie in the presence or absence of some crucial adhesion or signalling glycoprotein, or of a cytokine.

is now inconceivable for T cells, and the hypothesis has been reformulated in terms of antigen presentation by cells that lack a "co-stimulator" present on "professional" antigen-presenting cells (Schwartz, 1990). The original idea of a signal deficit sprang from the tendency of adjuvant-free soluble protein antigens to induce tolerance in normal adult animals (Dresser and Mitchison, 1968). At present, each of these alternative hypotheses has difficulty in explaining all of the observations, and it is quite conceivable that both may apply, perhaps to different types of antigen.

This is not the place to pursue the argument in detail. Both hypotheses may turn out to be correct, as newly developed T cells might be defective with respect to one or more key signalling proteins. The outcome will probably depend on the discovery of any particular adhesion or signalling protein able to lend substance to the concept of a signal deficit. We might end with the validation of both mechanisms, perhaps one for CD8 T cells following the H-Y development-stage model, and the other for CD4 T cells with a signal defect as revealed by studies with soluble proteins. For present purposes, the latter is the more important category, as it includes the regulatory T cells that are critically important in autoimmune disease.

Note, in passing, how important a role apoptosis has come to play in immunology. It operates not only here in negative selection, but also in the selection of B cells within germinal centres (Liu et al., 1989) and in killing by cytotoxic T cells. Little is yet known about its intracellular pathways.

The action of cyclosporin A provides insight into signalling for negative selection, and has led to some interesting models of autoimmunity. This drug, like the other cyclophillins, is believed to block signal transmission in T cells at a late intranuclear stage. In effect it blindfolds the cell. Within the thymus it enables cells to escape negative selection, as has been demonstrated by the maturation under this treatment of T cells which would otherwise be deleted by endogenous superantigens (endogenous retroviral proteins; also known as "Vβ deletors") (Jenkins et al., 1988). The sensitivity of negative selection to inhibition by this agent underlines the fundamental similarity of positive and negative signalling. It also flags a hazard to be borne in mind in connection with the new specific immunotherapies. Consider, for instance, a patient under treatment for rheumatoid arthritis with a drug that blocks the HLA-DR4 molecule. Although no such drug is yet available, animal models suggest that this is a realistic possibility. The treatment would be expected to block the molecules within the thymus as well as in the peripheral immune system, and should therefore allow T cells to mature that would not be tolerant of DR4-presented self-epitopes. Such cells might become dangerous if the treatment were ever to stop. In the meanwhile the blindfolding effect of cyclosporin has been put to good use in a number of

animal models of autoimmunity (Sorokin et al., 1986; Sakaguchi and Sakaguchi, 1988). These models are valuable not only for experimentation, but also for demonstrating the importance of negative selection, although one cannot be quite sure that the drug really inhibits only this process.

6. Negative Selection is under Tight Evolutionary Constraint

In principle, one expects negative selection to be tightly controlled, so as to balance the need to preserve as much as possible of the receptor repertoire against the need to avoid autoimmune disease. This intuitive view is strongly supported by the new and increasingly powerful computer simulations of the immune system based on cellular automata (Celada and Seiden, 1992), which clearly show that preserving this balance is one of the fundamental principles governing the design of the immune system.

One way of looking at the balance is in terms of the number of epitopes that operate in negative and in peripheral positive selection (in this discussion it is hard to avoid using this rather clumsy term, to describe the "normal" positive response of mature T cells, in contrast with the quite different process of positive selection which goes on in the thymus). Recent research has made it abundantly clear that foreign proteins contain a surprisingly small number of epitopes recognized by T cells (Gammon et al., 1991a,b). This is in contrast with the enormous number of sequences of appropriate length which are potentially available. The process of epitope selection involves several steps, of which the most obvious is the need to fit the conformation of the peptide-binding groove in MHC molecules. Other constraints are imposed during the cleaving of antigens before presentation, which occurs within the late endosomes of antigen-presenting cells. Yet others are imposed by the availability of the corresponding T cell receptors, a limitation that itself results in part from negative selection. It is now becoming clear that, as expected, a similar degree of selection operates in negative selection. A recent study of hen egg lysozyme expressed off a transgene in mice illustrates the point (Cibotti et al., 1992). At low levels of expression, essentially only one epitope of the foreign protein manages to induce negative selection. As the level increases, the number of operative epitopes also increases, although without saturating the protein.

A second way of seeing the balance is in terms of the concentration of protein needed to operate negative and peripheral positive selection, as illustrated in Fig. 2.6 (the part of this Figure which refers to B cells will be discussed in Section 9). A recent study of F liver protein made the appropriate measurements, for the former in terms of the

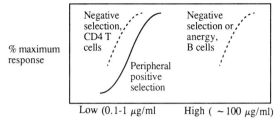

Figure 2.6 A schematic view of the dose–response thresholds of CD4 T cells (negative selection in thymus, and positive selection – the normal immune response – in the periphery) and B cells (tolerance mediated by negative selection or anergy). The threshold for negative selection of CD4 T cells is similar in the thymus and the periphery, as mentioned in the text.

concentration needed to obtain negative selection within thymus organ cultures, and for the latter in a conventional T cell proliferation assay (Robertson *et al.*, 1992). The thresholds for the two processes agree quite closely, with perhaps a slightly higher sensitivity to negative selection, as might be expected. The relationship shown in Fig. 2.6 seems to apply also to cellular antigens presented by MHC class I molecules, again with a somewhat higher sensitivity to negative selection (Pircher *et al.*, 1991).

A third view of the balance is in terms of the lack of access of some, perhaps many, self-proteins to the immune system. It has long been known that allogeneic cells can escape detection by the immune system if placed in certain anatomical sites, such as brain, cornea or in the pigmented layer of the skin (Medawar, 1948). Such sites are said to enjoy "immunological privilege". At first this was thought to reflect lack of access by lymphocytes, although nowadays a lack of access to antigen-presenting cells would seem at least equally important. As well as providing an immunological rationale for corneal transplantation, this consideration has inspired attempts to free other transplants of antigen-presenting cells, a procedure of some promise in the context of pancreas transplantation. Importantly for the purposes of this chapter, cartilage cells enjoy immunological privilege on account of the matrix in which they are embedded (Chesterman and Smith, 1968). Transgenic mice offer interesting possibilities for further exploring the phenomenon. A viral glycoprotein has been found to enjoy immunological privilege when expressed in the pancreas, whereas with the earlier privileged tissue allografts, immunization via a non-privileged route can procure rejection (Zinkernagel *et al.*, 1990). These experiments unequivocally demonstrate that tissue proteins can remain immunologically silent indefinitely, without eliciting either negative selection or auto-immunity. The ability of these proteins to do so clearly

reduces the impact of negative selection on the T cell repertoire.

These findings, in terms of epitopes and their concentrations, bear out the argument already made in connection with the CD45 isoforms. Negative selection needs to mimic peripheral positive selection, as otherwise potentially autoreactive T cells would emerge from the thymus. But it should not do much more than that, in order to preserve as much as possible of the TCR repertoire. Generalizing, not only T cells but also the cells that present antigen to them must mimic one another during the two types of selection. This applies not only to their morphological features, but also to their receptors and adhesion molecules. Any departure from mimicry is in principle likely to be either wasteful or hazardous.

An important consequence of this view is that, in a sense, every self-protein presents a hazard. Each contains many epitopes which did not operate during negative selection, and are therefore potentially able to mediate an autoimmune response. The immune system seems to have solved the problem, as so often happens in living organisms, by editing. The suppression system, which is discussed in the next section, can be regarded as a way of editing out the unfortunate consequences of the fine balance just described. Natural selection does not, of course, operate in quite such a simple manner. The editing process and the fine balance no doubt interact, so that the balance is continuously adjusted to the safety level set by the editing, and vice versa. Furthermore, as is argued below, it is likely that suppression has additional functions.

7. Suppression Prevents and Minimizes Autoimmunity

This is a large subject, which can be treated here in only a cursory fashion. A more detailed account can be found in recent reviews (Mitchison and Oliveira, 1986a; Mitchison, 1989). In this presentation the term suppression is used in a wide sense, to include such mechanisms as epitope capture and cytokine balance, rather than in the narrow sense of unique suppressor T cells with their "suppressor factors". It is best to present the subject from the genetic angle, as that is where the evidence of a protective role in autoimmune disease is clearest.

Immunological diseases often show HLA associations (a somewhat circular statement, as it is these very associations that often provide the strongest evidence of immunological involvement). Typically the frequency of HLA genes is determined in a group of cases, and compared with that in a group of controls. Any gene present at a significantly higher frequency among the cases is deemed to predispose for the disease, while any with a lower frequency is deemed to be protective. An analysis of this sort has its problems, such as the question of whether the marker gene itself is responsible, or another gene linked to it; and allowance needs to be made for a predisposing gene affecting the frequencies expected of other HLA genes. All the protective genes discovered so far are MHC class II genes, with a predominant representation of HLA-DQ, and they have no obvious physical features which distinguish them from predisposing genes (Ottenhof *et al.*, 1990; Kamikawaji *et al.*, 1991). Their best example for an autoimmune disease is in insulin-dependent diabetes (Baisch *et al.*, 1990). Limited evidence of their activity has been found in rheumatoid arthritis where HLA-DR2 (or perhaps the linked DQw6 allele) appear to exert a protective effect in the British (Jaraquemada *et al.*, 1986) and Japanese populations (Kawaharada, 1991), although these negative association data require recalculation to take account of the effect of predisposing genes mentioned above. Another candidate protective gene is HLA-DR4-Dw10 (Wordsworth *et al.*, 1989). Such genes have not been detected in SLE (Hartung *et al.*, 1991), although interestingly a negative association has been found for at least one of the SLE antibodies (Asherson *et al.*, 1992). There is evidence from diabetes that these genes, even when they fail to protect, can still moderate the course of the disease. As regards their mode of action, the most important genetic finding is that they are dominant in their effect. This implies that they do something actively, rather than fail to act.

The immunoinhibitory genes of mice share many features in common with the protective HLA genes, such as being MHC class II genes with dominant activity. By definition these genes inhibit, partially or almost completely, an immune response to some antigen. Even more clearly than the protective HLA genes, they can also act as classic immune response genes in conjunction with other antigens, so that one does better to refer to immunoinhibitory effects rather than immunoinhibitory genes. These effects bunch conspicuously, at H-2E (probably over a range of alleles) and at H-2A^b (Oliveira and Mitchison, 1989; Mitchison and Simon, 1990). The meaning of this bunching is unclear, although one guesses that it has to do with the location and level of expression of these genes rather than the structure of the glycoproteins that they encode. In certain cases they inhibit only one component of an immune response, such as the production of antibody (Pfeiffer *et al.*, 1991), an effect that could be regarded as diversionary rather than inhibitory.

Why do these protective and immunoinhibitory genes occur so frequently? One view is that pregnancy (and also spermatozoa in the female) poses an immunological threat that needs answering. Recent discussion has focused on two more likely possibilities. One, the "homunculus" theory illustrated in Fig. 2.7 (Cohen, 1990; Cohen and Young, 1991), proposes that the T cell repertoire is profoundly biased by certain immunodominant or

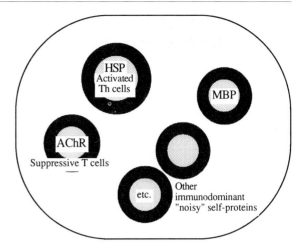

Figure 2.7 The "homunculus view" of the immune system. The T cell repertoire is biased towards recognition of certain self-proteins, such as heat shock proteins (HSP), myelin basic protein (MBP) and acetylcholine receptor (AChR), which can therefore be regarded as immunodominant. Even under normal conditions, without overt signs of autoimmunity, numerous helper T cells can recognize these proteins, but their activity is contained by T cells with suppressive function (anti-idiotypic or suppressive lymphokines), shaded more darkly.

"noisy" self-molecules, such as the heat-shock proteins (HSPs), myelin basic protein and the acetylcholine receptor (AChR; Sommer *et al.*, 1991). These proteins prime the immune system in normal individuals, and in some cases presumably also expand reactivity to related proteins present in infectious agents (Cohen and Young, 1991). Interestingly, type II collagen was at first thought to belong to this category, but it turns out that most of the T cell lines isolated from healthy donors in fact recognized a pepsin contaminant (Holmdahl *et al.*, 1990; Lacour *et al.*, 1990). The high level of T cell reactivity found *in vitro* towards these noisy proteins poses a problem for negative selection, which is further discussed in Section 11.1 below. So also do T cells with *in vitro* autoreactivity towards antigen-presenting cells of self origin, which constitute a long-standing immunological conundrum (Moeller, 1990). The need to control this reactivity may provide the selective force responsible for maintaining immunoinhibitory genes in human and animal populations. Another possibility is the evolutionary need to control hypersensitivity in chronic infectious disease, as exemplified by the value of immunosuppression in lepromatous leprosy (Mitchison and Oliveira 1986b; Ottenhof *et al.*, 1990).

These ideas point to the need for further study, not least in the difficult area of the population genetics of chronic tropical disease. One prediction of the "homunculus" theory has recently been verified, that bias should be detectable before exposure to

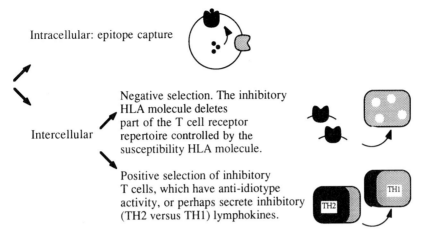

Intracellular: epitope capture

Intercellular

Negative selection. The inhibitory HLA molecule deletes part of the T cell receptor repertoire controlled by the susceptibility HLA molecule.

Positive selection of inhibitory T cells, which have anti-idiotype activity, or perhaps secrete inhibitory (TH2 versus TH1) lymphokines.

Figure 2.8 Possible ways in which an MHC molecule might exert an immunoinhibitory effect. The inhibitory molecule and the TCR repertoire which it controls are shaded more darkly as in Fig. 2.7.

microorganisms (the alternative possibility would be that the high level of reactivity towards HSPs results from cross-priming by microorganisms). A high level of reactivity to a mycobacterial HSP was in fact detected in cord blood (Fischer and Panayi, 1992).

These protective or immunoinhibitory genes offer an outstanding challenge to immunology, for in no case is their mode of action fully understood. The three major possibilities discussed below are illustrated in Fig. 2.8. One is that they act at the level of antigen presentation, by epitope capture. This would well explain the observed hierarchy of protective, susceptibility and neutral HLA class II genes (Nepom, 1990). The idea is simply that protective and susceptibility MHC molecules compete for the disease-inducing peptide, on the basis of relative affinity, within the same antigen-presenting cell. In addition one would have to postulate some sort of prior selection in the T cell repertoire which prevents the epitope, when captured by the protective gene product, from inducing disease.

Another possible mode of action is through negative selection. An MHC molecule might create holes in the repertoire which would eliminate reactivity towards a disease-inducing peptide. This idea has had its ups and downs, and contrary to earlier expectations it now seems unlikely to play much part in determining susceptibility to one of the better autoimmune disease models, collagen-induced arthritis in mice (Vidard et al., 1991). A recent study did demonstrate an effect of this sort, but only under the somewhat artificial circumstances of a known peptide immunogen chosen in conjunction with a known $V\beta$ deleter (Nanda et al., 1991).

There remains a third possibility, of positive selection of the T cell repertoire. The inhibitory or protective MHC molecule might enable a particular subset of T cells to develop and then to become activated by a particular antigen, where they would exert an inhibitory effect. Positive selection in this sense is tantamount to suppression, whether or not the same T cells could also drive a normal positive response to other antigens. Just how they might exert their suppressive effect is unknown. One possibility currently attracting attention is that they might secrete inhibitory cytokines, such as IFNγ, IL-4 or IL-10 (Mosmann and Coffman, 1989). In other words, the predisposing and protective MHC molecules would respectively restrict Th1 and Th2 cells. This is a flexible concept: the important point is that competing subsets of CD4 T cells may balance one another, while the precise cytokine profiles, and the extent to which restriction is biased towards particular MHC molecules, may vary from one case to another (and of course also between mouse and man). Another way that protective T cells might act is through the idiotypic network (Mitchison and Oliveira, 1986a; Cohen, 1991), a concept that finds support in recent animal models of T cell vaccination (Hashim et al., 1990; Offner et al., 1991).

It is important to remember that in most animal models suppressive mechanisms come into play only after the disease has started (Mathieson et al., 1991; Fowell et al., 1991). In much the same way tissue damage in man often gives rise to transient and harmless production of autoantibodies. In general, therefore, suppression should be regarded as a mechanism for righting a wrong, rather than for preventing one from starting up. As such, suppressive mechanisms can be expected to operate beneficially during the course of an autoimmune disease. Current research focuses on these mechanisms of cytokine balance and idiotypic control not only for their likely importance in prevention, but also because of the important role they may play in the development and response to treatment of ongoing autoimmune disease.

8. Negative Selection Operates on some but not all γδ T Cells

So far this chapter has dealt only with the major population of T cells which express the αβ T cell receptor. T cells expressing the γδ-TCR comprise a separate minor lineage with characteristics different from those of the classical αβ-TCR population (Moeller, 1991). They appear earlier, and leave the thymus in a series of discrete waves rather than in a continuous stream. They predominate in mucosal epithelium, with homogeneous TCRs which differ in skin, uterus and vagina, tongue, lung and intestine. Greater heterogeneity is found in lymphoid tissue, where these cells comprise a minor population. An interesting suggestion is that the epithelial populations are so homogeneous because, living where they do, they cannot expand clonally, and therefore do not need receptor diversity. The function of γδ cells is poorly understood, although it has proved relatively easy to generate, from lymphoid tissue, clones specific for (1) non-classic class I MHC products and (2) mycobacterial HSPs. This has given rise to the suggestion that these cells may exercise surveillance over stress proteins of self, and thus participate in resistance to infection.

If this really is their function, then they must escape, at least to an extent, the normal tolerance mechanisms. This question is addressed by an interesting experiment on γδ-TCR transgenes specific for a non-classic MHC molecule (Bluestone et al., 1991). In mice that possessed both the receptor transgenes and their target antigen, the thymus showed evidence of classic negative selection, whereas the epithelial γδ cells did not. It is therefore likely, but by no means certain, that tolerance plays some part in moulding the highly specialized but nevertheless valuable TCR repertoire of normal γδ T cells. It seems likely that, while lymphoid γδ cells participate in this and other ways in the adaptive immune system, epithelial γδ cells belong, along with macrophages and complement components, to the constitutive defence system.

A connection has been established between γδ T cells and arthritis, in that a high proportion of cells of this type with specificity for HSPs can be cloned out of synovia from patients with rheumatoid arthritis (Strober and Holoshitz, 1990). The starting populations of T cells are less strongly biased in this direction, however, and it has been suggested that γδ T cells accumulate selectively in joints for the same kind of (unknown) reason that they accumulate in epithelia, rather than as part of the disease process.

A historical note: although long superseded by the concept of negative selection, the idea was once current that self-cells might be positively flagged by a self-marker, which the immune system would recognize and take appropriate steps to avoid. Here, in the proposal that γδ T cells are selected to recognize self-stress proteins, the idea has been revived.

9. B Cells also become Tolerant, but only of Certain Categories of Self-Protein

The emphasis in this chapter has so far been on tolerance among T cells, and it has been argued that B cells could not be expected to assume responsibility for tolerance of self. Nevertheless, B cells clearly do naturally become tolerant of certain categories of self-proteins, and can be rendered tolerant of foreign antigens under certain experimental conditions.

The category of protein for which this form of self-tolerance is most clearly evident are the cell-membrane-attached glycoproteins. HLA molecules themselves, for instance, clearly establish tolerance within the B cell compartment, for the antibodies raised by alloimmunization recognize polymorphic but not ubiquitous epitopes. In other words, an immune system does not produce antibodies able to react with its own HLA molecules. The same applies to blood group antigens and to the large group of CD glycoproteins in man, and to polymorphic glycoproteins such as Thy1 in the mouse. This argument is indirect, and it is reassuring to find it fully confirmed by a recent study of a transgene-encoded anti-MHC antibody, in which deletion of self-reactive B cells was evident (Nemazee and Burki, 1989).

For soluble proteins, the position is less clear. Haemoglobin is often cited as an example of a soluble self-protein which establishes tolerance in the B cell compartment, on the basis of an old study in which rabbits were immunized against the human form of the protein (see Howard and Mitchison, 1975). They produced antibodies only against sequence epitopes not present in the rabbit's own haemoglobin. Recent quantitative studies with soluble protein antigens indicate that high concentrations of antigen (100–1000 μg/ml) delete B cells, while lower concentrations leave them present but anergic (Nossal, 1983; Nossal et al., 1989; see also Section 4). This confirms earlier studies showing that B cell tolerance requires treatment with high doses of antigen (see Howard and Mitchison, 1975). It is surprising that such high doses are needed, as during their development B cells pass through a stage when they can be inactivated by low concentrations (1 μg/ml) of antigen (Nossal, 1983). In fact, B cells may have not one but two windows of susceptibility to tolerance induction, one related to relatively early development and the other to later diversification in germinal centres (Nossal et al., 1989).

It is likely that the apparent difference between cell-bound and soluble proteins reflects simply their relative capacity to cross-link surface Ig receptors on B cells. The importance of cross-linking in downregulating B cells has long been recognized (Klaus et al., 1976). Soluble proteins may well need high concentrations in order to induce tolerance as a result of their low cross-linking activity. This mechanistic interpretation still leaves us with the question of what physiological function, if any, B cell tolerance may have. It seems unlikely that it could be protective in the same way as tolerance among T cells, as B cells are well able to respond positively to very low concentrations of antigen in the presence of T cell help. The curve on the right in Fig. 2.6 depicts this situation. One possibility is that this seemingly ineffective form of tolerance may prevent the otherwise dangerous processing of self-proteins by B cells. Processing initiated by pick-up of antigen via surface immunoglobulin receptors might end up by presenting neoepitopes, as described above (Section 3). These would be peptides not presented by dendritic cells, and therefore not inducers of negative selection. This idea has the attractive feature that it would be particularly effective in protecting against the most damaging type of autoantibody, namely that directed at the cell surface.

Nearly all our information about tolerance in the B cell compartment concerns classic B cells. The small population of non-classic B cells that bear the CD5 marker is also of interest (there may also be a "sister" population of similar non-classic B cells that lack the marker) (Herzenberg and Stall, 1989). These cells are over-represented among the producers of certain auto-antibodies, particularly among those that occur in bone and connective tissue disease (Maini et al., 1990). This may be related to a difference in tolerance threshold, or alternatively may reflect their failure to participate in the normal processes of peripheral selection by microbial antigens, and a consequent propensity to produce low-affinity cross-reactive antibodies.

In closing this somewhat speculative discussion, it is worth mentioning an elegant example of B cell tolerance in the context of rheumatoid arthritis. During the production of rheumatoid factors, B cells recognize many epitopes on self-Ig molecules. One set of epitopes which they do not, however, recognize, presumably as a result of self-tolerance, are those of their own allotype (Jones et al., 1988).

10. The Connection between Tolerance and Autoimmunity

It is almost a truism to say that while the causes of autoimmune disease are unknown, malfunction in the tolerance mechanism must somehow be involved. Ideas about the connection between tolerance and auto-immunity can be grouped as follows.

10.1 DEVELOPMENTAL ERROR

The main culprits are T cells which slip past the normal process of negative selection in the thymus. This possibility finds support in the animal models of auto-immunity referred to above, where treatment with cyclosporin A allows self-reactive T cells to slip through the thymus. The TCR+, CD4CD8 cell population within the thymus has attracted attention as possible instigators of autoimmunity (von Boehmer, 1991). These are cells that appear to express their TCR prematurely, and then accumulate at a developmental stage before negative selection (von Boehmer, 1991). Escape of such cells into the periphery might well constitute a hazard. However, one needs to be cautious in regarding any cell population of unknown function simply as a mistake.

10.2 MUTATION

Autoimmunity results from mutation of receptor V genes. This idea seems less attractive than it once did (Knight et al., 1986), now that T cells are given primacy in the initiation of autoimmune disease and their V genes are known not to hypermutate. In animal models disease susceptibility does not segregate with TCR V genes in the way predicted by the mutation hypothesis. Autoimmune diseases do not occur at random, as the mutation hypothesis predicts, but rather conform to a limited number of types, probably less than twenty, all told.

10.3 AUTOIMMUNITY EMERGES FROM THE LATENT REPERTOIRE

The problem is not that mistakes occur in the tolerance-inducing mechanism, but rather that the mechanism is set at a level such that self-proteins carry potentially dangerous epitopes. Under conditions of stringent immunization (which cannot at present be specified) these epitopes come into play. This idea takes us back to the discussion presented above in Section 6 of the balance between negative selection and the need to preserve as much as possible of the TCR repertoire. This possibility is in line with current ideas about the "cryptic" or "latent" repertoire, which are now securely based on experimental data (Gammon et al., 1991a,b; Mitchison, 1992). Indeed one can now ask why autoimmune diseases are not more ubiquitous in the structures that they attack.

10.4 AUTOIMMUNITY TRIGGERED BY INFECTION

Infection leads to autoimmunity, via the familiar cell–cell interactions of the immune system. Here a whole family of overlapping possibilities have been formulated, which include the following. (i) A virus or other intracellular infective agent introduces new T epitopes into a cell, which are recognized by helper T cells. These in turn help other lymphocytes (T or B) to react to endogenous epitopes of the infected cell (Leech and Mitchison, 1976; Lake *et al.*, 1988). (ii) A local infection activates T cells which then release IFNγ, and this in turn induces inappropriate expression of MHC class II molecules on neighbouring tissue cells. The tissue cells thus become able to present inappropriate epitopes (Bottazzo *et al.*, 1983; Salvetnick *et al.*, 1988). (iii) B cells that recognize Ig epitopes (i.e. that have rheumatoid factor specificity) bind and then process antibody–antigen complexes in which the antigen is derived from an infective agent. Helper T cells then recognize epitopes derived from the agent, and thus help the production of rheumatoid factors (Roosneck and Lanzavecchia, 1991). (iv) When T cells are cloned out of an infected individual, they commonly include a subset which recognizes normal (i.e. uninfected) antigen-presenting cells (Mustafa *et al.*, 1986). (v) Rats immunized against mycobacteria develop arthritis, and T cells can be cloned out of these animals that transmit the disease (Cohen, 1990; Strober and Holoshitz, 1990). The T cell response to bacterial HSPs correlates with the disease, and circumstantial evidence suggests that the T cell response to self-HSPs (which cross-react with bacterial HSPs, as mentioned above in Section 7) may be an important factor driving auto-immunity. (vi) As mentioned above (Section 6), immu-nization with whole virus can elicit immunological attack on an otherwise non-immunogenic viral glycoprotein expressed at a sequestered site (Zinkernagel *et al.*, 1990).

This is not the place to enumerate the many infectious agents that have been blamed for initiating auto-immunity. Suffice it to say that the view that infections (probably common ones) are likely to be important as causes or cofactors is widely held. A case can be made for the kind of large-scale prospective sero-epidemiological trial which might resolve the matter. Such a trial might be modelled on that carried out on EBV in Burkitt's lymphoma, although that one did prove both laborious and expensive (de The *et al.*, 1978).

10.5   CLUES FROM PROTECTION AND REMISSION

Immunology should help us to understand not only the genesis of autoimmunity, but also its prevention and remission. Learning about protection and recovery in immunological diseases must be worth while. The importance of protective HLA genes has already been discussed in Section 7. Autoimmune diseases, and indeed immunological diseases as a whole, tend to follow an erratic course characterized by intermittent exacerbations separated by intervals of stability or remission. This suggests that some kind of immunological conflict goes on, perhaps between T cell subsets secreting the mutually inhibitory cytokines as discussed above in Section 7. But we have to be careful. A large international trial of plasmapheresis combined with chemotherapy in SLE is

finding prolonged "normalization" following therapy, without any obvious signs of specific immunosuppression (Clark *et al.*, 1991). It will be hard to make progress in this area without more systematic epidemiology, which will take account not only of physical symptoms and laboratory tests, but also of psychological appreciation of the disease.

It is unsatisfactory to offer little more than a listing of ideas on this important subject, but nothing better is available at the present time. Let this section end, as it began, with a truism. The connection between tolerance breakdown and autoimmunity is simply not understood, largely because the disease-inducing epitopes have not yet been discovered. Once that gap has been filled, immunology will have more to contribute to the prevention and cure of autoimmune disease.

11.   New Ideas and Challenges

11.1   IMMUNOLOGICAL DECISIONS BASED ON CONTEXT

This account of immunological tolerance started from a position firmly rooted in negative selection, in which the overall decision whether or not to make a response depends simply on decisions made independently by individual lymphocytes on the basis of whether or not their receptors recognize a given protein. In the course of this account that position has been progressively eroded. In Section 3 we saw how T cells can be rendered hyper-reactive by prior exposure to antigen, and in Section 4 how they can be rendered anergic. Responsiveness is evidently not just a matter of possessing the right receptor, but is also deeply influenced by the past experi-ence of the cell. Section 6 described how highly selective is the T cell compartment with respect to the epitopes that it will recognize, so that clonal selection is not absolute, but rather a matter of thresholds and affinities. Section 7 mentioned the conundrum of autoreactive T cells and clones. Section 10 introduced an example (Zinkernagel *et al.*, 1990) of how exposure to an antigen during an infection can enhance the response. Above all, the noisy self-proteins identified in Section 7 challenge the concept of clonal selection, for here is a whole group of well-defined self-proteins for which reactivity to self has evidently not been eliminated.

These problems have inspired immunologists to formulate new ideas that supplement or even attempt to displace clonal selection (Janeway, 1989; Coutinho, 1989; Cohen, 1990; Cohen and Young, 1991; Grossman, 1992). Central to these is the concept of contextual discrimination (or "committee" or "distri-buted" decisions), which holds that the decision whether or not to make a response is made by groups of cells inter-acting with one another. This is rather the way a small

Swiss Canton makes its decisions, but in the immune system one has to imagine a Grossrat in which not only are all the members talking, but at the same time the minutes of previous meetings are being read and the agenda of future meetings decided. The transactions are thought to involve cell-clustering mediated by diverse adhesion molecules, cascades of cytokines, idiotypic networks and modification of cell response thresholds. The emphasis placed on these various forms of communication varies from author to author, and no consensus has yet been reached.

So has the time come to abandon the reductivist approach to immunology, and the negative selection theory in particular? I think not. For one thing, try to imagine an immune system devoid of negative selection: we might well be confronted not by a limited range of rare autoimmunities, but rather by the sort of catastrophe that the fate of young animals treated with cyclosporin hints at (Section 5). For another, negative selection has become increasingly well documented as a natural phenomenon, and it cannot simply be ignored, whereas its alternatives are still poorly understood. A more reasonable aim is to press on with the analysis of contextual discrimination, using for want of anything better the tried and trusted reductivist method. After all, there is still much to learn. For instance, how frequent are these noisy self-proteins, and do they all really map only on to the known autoimmune diseases? Just how does the hypothetical committee keep its more unruly members in order? Then there are important questions in pharmacology, discussed in the next section.

11.2 THREE CHALLENGES TO IMMUNOPHARMACOLOGY

In the course of this account problems have arisen that demand a specifically pharmacological approach. In any fast-moving subject, questions do not remain open for long and predictions are risky. This is particularly true of cellular immunology, which is moving rapidly under the impetus of genetic manipulation. At the beginning of 1992, when this was written, the following three challenges emerge as particularly important: (i) the nature of hyperreactivity on the part of T cells to antigenic stimulation (see Section 3 above), (ii) the nature of anergy (Sections 4 and 9 above) and (iii) the question of whether T cells undergo negative selection at a particular developmental stage, or because of a signal deficit, or for some other reason (Section 5 above).

By way of comment, the hyperreactivity problem would at first sight seem highly amenable to a transfection approach. In principle, one need only transfect one by one those genes that are overexpressed in the hyperreactive cell. Unfortunately this would encounter two difficulties, the combinatorial activity of signalling molecules, and the ability of a cell to adapt rapidly to

overexpression of a single molecule. The second challenge, of anergy, needs a systematic approach, to take account of the diversity of conditions subsumed under this name. As already mentioned in Section 4, a particularly urgent aspect of this problem is to find markers of anergy which would enable its physiological relevance to be assessed. The third challenge, of development stage versus signal deficit is more complicated, because it involves cell–cell interactions. Our investigative pharmacologist would need to forget about T cells as billiard balls, and have recourse to the microscope. At the end of the day, none of these challenges seem beyond the range of present technologies.

12. References

Apel, M. and Berek, C. (1990). Somatic mutations in antibodies expressed in germinal centre B cells early after primary immunization. Int. Immunol. 2, 813–819.

Arnold, B., Goodnow, C., Hengartner, H. and Hammerling, G. (1990). The coming of transgenic mice. Immunol. Today 11, 69–72.

Asherson, R.A., Doherty, D.G., Vergani, D., Khamashta, M.A., Hughes, G.R.V. (1992). Major histocompatibility complex associations with primary antiphospholipid syndrome. Arth. Rheum. 35, 124–125.

Baisch, J.M., Weeks, T., Giles, R., Hoover, M., Stastny P., Capra J.D. and Engle, N. (1990). Analysis of HLA-DQ genotypes and susceptibility in IDDM. N. Engl. J. Med. 322, 1836–1844.

Berzofsky, J.A. (1983). T-B reciprocity. An Ia-restricted epitope-specific circuit regulating T cell–B cell interaction and antibody specificity. Surv. Immunol. Res. 2, 223–229.

Beverley, P.C.L.B. (1991). Immunological memory in T cells. Curr. Opin. Immunol. 3, 355–360.

Billingham, R.E., Brent, L. and Medawar, P.B. (1954). Quantitative studies on tissue transplantation immunity. III. Actively acquired tolerance. Philos. Trans. R. Soc. London Ser. B. 239, 357–414.

Bluestone, J.A., Cron, R.Q., Barrett, T.A., Houlden, B., Sperling, A.I., Dent, A., Hedrick, S., Rellahan, B. and Matis, L.A. (1991). Repertoire development and ligand specificity of murine TcRγδ cells. Immunol. Rev. 120, 5–34.

von Boehmer, H. (1991). Positive and negative selection of the α-β T-cell repertoire *in vivo*. Curr. Opin. Immunol. 3, 210–215.

von Boehmer, H. and Haas, W. (1979). Distinct Ir genes for helper and killer cells in the cytotoxic response to M-Y ranges. J. Exp. Med. 150, 1134–1142.

von Boehmer, H. and Kieselow, P. (1990). Self-nonself discrimination by T cells. Science 248, 1369–73.

Bottazzo, G.F., Pujol-Borrell, R., Hanafusa, T. and Feldmann, M. (1983). Hypothesis: role of aberrant HLA-DR expression and antigen presentation in endocrine autoimmunity. Lancet ii, 1115–1119.

Celada, F. and Seiden, P.E. (1992). A computer model of cellular interactions in the immune system. Immunol. Today 13, 56–62.

Chesterman, P.J. and Smith, A.U. (1968). Homotransplantation of articular cartilage and isolated chondrocytes. An experimental study in rabbits. J. Bone Joint Surg. 50, 184–197.

Cibotti, R., Kanellopoulos, J.M., Cabaniols, J.-P., Halle-Panenko, O., Kosmatopoulos, K., Sercarz, E. and Kourilsky, P. (1992). Tolerance to a self-protein involves its immunodominant but not subdominant determinants. Proc. Natl Acad. Sci. USA 89, 416–420.

Clark, W.F., Dau, P.C., Euler, H.H., Guillevin, L., Hasford, J., Heer, A.H., Jones, J.V., Kashgarian, M., Knatterud, G., Lockwood, M.C., Pusey, C.D., Rifle, G., Robinson, J.A., Schroeder, J.O., Tan, E.M., Wallace, D.J. and Weiner, S.R. (1991). Plasmapheresis and subsequent pulse cyclophosphamide versus pulse cyclophosphamide alone in severe lupus: design of the LPSG trial. J. Clin. Apheresis 6, 40–47.

Cohen, I.R. (1990). A heat shock protein, molecular minimizing and autoimmunity. Isr. J. Med. Sci. 26, 673–676.

Cohen, I.R. (1991). Unresolved questions in clinical T cell vaccination. Br. J. Rheumatol. 30, Suppl. 2, 17–19.

Cohen, I.R. and Young, D.B. (1991). Autoimmunity, microbial immunity and the immunological homunculus. Immunol. Today 12, 105–110.

Coutinho, A. (1989). Beyond clonal selection and network. Immunol. Rev. 110, 63–87.

Dresser, D.W. (1976). Tolerance induction as a model for cell differentiation. Br. Med. Bull. 32, 147–151.

Dresser, D.W. and Mitchison, N.A. (1968). The mechanism of immunological paralysis. Adv. Immunol. 8, 129–181.

Fischer, H.P., Sharrock, C.E. and Panayi, G.S. (1992). High frequency of cord blood lymphocytes against mycobacterial 65 kDa heat shock protein. Eur. J. Immunol. 22, 1667–1669.

Fowell, D., McKnight, A.J., Powrie, F., Dyke, R. and Mason, D. (1991). Subsets of CD4+ T cells and their roles in the induction and prevention of autoimmunity. Immunol. Rev. 123, 37–64.

Gammon, G., Geysen, H.M., Apple, R.J., Pickett, E., Palmer, E., Ametani, A. and Sercarz, E.E. (1991a). T cell determinant structure: cores and determinant envelopes in three more major histocompatibility complex haplotypes. J. Exp. Med. 173, 609–617.

Gammon, G., Sercarz, E.E. and Benichou, G. (1991b). The dominant self and the cryptic self: shaping the autoreactive T cell repertoire. Immunol. Today 12, 193–195.

Griffiths, J.A., Mitchison, N.A., Nardi, N. and Oliveira, D.B.G. (1987). In "Immunogenicity of Protein Antigens: Repertoire and Regulation" (ed E. Sercarz and J. Berzofsky), Vol. II, pp 35–41. CRC Press, Boca Raton, Florida.

Grossman, Z. (1992). In "Theoretical and Experimental Insights into Immunology" (ed A.S. Perelson, G. Weisbuch and A. Coutinho). Springer-Verlag, New York, (in press).

Hartung, K., Coldewey, R., Krapf, F., Lang, B., Specker, C., Schendel, D., Schneider, P., Seuchter, S., Stangel, W., Albert, E. and Deicher, H. (1991). Hetero- and homozygosity of MHC class gene products in systemic lupus erythematosus. Tissue Antigens 38, 165–168.

Hashim, G.A., Vandenbark, A.A., Galang, A.B., Diamanduros, T., Carvalho, E., Srinivasan, J., Jones, R., Vainiene, M., Mollison, W.J. and Offner, H.J. (1990). Antibodies specific for VB8 receptor peptide suppress experimental autoimmune encephalomyelitis. J. Immunol. 144, 4621–4627.

Herzenberg, L.A. and Stall, A.M. (1990). Conventional and Ly-1 B-cell lineages in normal and μ transgenic mice. Cold Spring Harbor Symp. Quant. Biol. 54, 209–218.

Holmdahl, R.M., Andersson, M., Goldschmidt, T.J., Gustafsson, K., Jansson, L. and Mo, J.A. (1990). Type II collagen autoimmunity in animals and provocations leading to arthritis. Immunol. Rev. 118, 193–232.

Howard, J.G. and Mitchison, N.A. (1975). Immunological tolerance. Progr. Allergy 18, 43–96.

Inaba, M., Inaba, K., Hosono, M., Kumamoto, T., Ishida, T., Muramatsu, S., Masuda, T. and Ikehara, S. (1991). Distinct mechanisms of neonatal tolerance induced by dendritic cells and thymic B cells. J. Exp. Med. 173, 549–559.

Isaacson P.G., Norton, A.J. and Addis, B.J. (1987). The human thymus contains a novel population of B lymphocytes. Lancet ii, 1488–1491.

Jacob, J., Kelsoe, G., Rajewsky, K. and Weiss, W. (1991). Intraclonal generation of antibody mutants in germinal centres. Nature (London) 354, 389–392.

Janeway, C.A. (1989). Approaching the asymptote? Evolution and revolution in immunology. Cold Spring Harbor Symp. Quant. Biol. 54, 1–14.

Jaraquemada, D., Ollier, W., Awad, J., Young, A., Silman, A., Roitt, I.M., Corbett, M., Hay, F., Cosh, J.A. and Maini, R.N. (1986). HLA and rheumatoid arthritis: a combined analysis of 440 British patients. Ann. Rheum. Dis. 45, 627–636.

Jenkins, M.K., Schwartz, R.H. and Pardoll, D.M. (1988). Effects of cyclosporin A on T cell development and clonal deletion. Science 241, 1655–1658.

Jenkinson, E.J., Kingston, R., Smith, C.A., Williams, G.T. and Owen, J.J.T. (1989). Antigen induced apoptosis in developing T-cells: a mechanism for negative selection of the T cell repertoire. Eur. J. Immunol. 19, 2175–2177.

Jones, V.E., Puttick, A.H., Williamson, E.A. and Mageed, R.A. (1988). A new assay uses monoclonal anti-Rh(D) antibodies to determine rheumatoid factor specificity: reactivity to a monoclonal antibody of the GM allotype G3n(21) is most frequent in rheumatoid patients negative for G3n(21). Clin. Exp. Immunol. 71, 451–458.

Kamikawaji, M., Fujisawa, K., Yoshizumi, H., Fukunaga, N., Yasunami, M., Kimura, A., Nishimura, Y. and Sasazuki, T. (1991). HLA-DQ-restricted CD4+ T cells specific for streptococcal antigen are present in low but not in high responders. J. Immunol. 146, 2560–2567.

Kawaharada, T. (1991). The suppressive effect of HLA-DQw6 in collagen-induced arthritis in mice. Fukuoka Igaku Zasshi 82, 71–85.

Klaus, G.G.B, Howard, J.G and Feldmann, M. (1976). Mechanisms of B-cell tolerance. Br. Med. Bull. 32, 141–146.

Knight, J., Laing, P., Knight, A., Adams, D. and Ling, N. (1986). Thyroid-stimulating autoantibodies usually contain only λ-light chains: evidence for the "forbidden clone" theory. J. Clin. Endocrinol. Metab. 62, 342–347.

Kyewski, B.A., Fathman, C.G. and Rouse, R.V. (1986). Intrathymic presentation of circulating non-MHC antigens by medullary dendritic cells. An antigen-dependent microenvironment for T cell differentiation. J. Exp. Med. 163, 231–246.

Lacour, M., Rudolphi, U., Schlesier, M. and Peter, H.H. (1990). Type II collagen-specific human T cell lines established from healthy donors. Eur. J. Immunol. 20, 931–934.

Lake, P., Mitchison, N.A., Clark, E.A., Khorshidi, M., Nakashima, I., Bromberg, J.S., Brunswick, M.R., Szensky, T., Sainis, K.B., Sunshine, G.H., Favila-Castilo, L., Woody, J.N. and Lewohl, D. (1989). In "Cell Surface Antigen Thy-1: immunology, neurology and therapeutic applications" (ed A.E. Reif and M. Schlesinger), pp 367–394. Marcel Dekker, New York.

Lederberg, J. (1959). Genes and antibodies. Do antigens bear instructions for antibody specificity or do they select lines that arise by mutation? Science 129, 1649–1654.

Leech S.H. and Mitchison, N.A. (1976). Breakdown of tolerance. Br. Med. Bull. 32, 130–134.

Lightstone, E.B. and Marvel, J. (1990). CD45RA is detected in all thymocyte subsets defined by CD4 and CD8 by using three-colour flow cytometry. Immunology 71, 467–472.

Lightstone, E.B., Marvel, J. and Mitchison, N.A. (1992). Memory in helper T cells revealed *in vivo* by alloimmunizations in combination with Thy1 antigen. Eur. J. Immunol. 22, 115–122.

Liu, Y.-J., Joshua, D.E., Williams, G.T., Smith, C.A., Gordon, J. and MacLennan, I.C.M. (1989). Mechanism of antigen-driven selection of B cells in germinal centres. Nature (London) 342, 929–931.

Lo, D., Burkly, L.C., Widera, G., Cowing, C., Flavell, R.A., Palmiter, R.D. and Brinster, R.L. (1988). Diabetes and tolerance in transgenic mice expressing class II MHC molecules in pancreatic β-cells. Cell 53, 159–168.

Maini, R.N., Plater-Zyberk, C., Brown, C.M., Aghamohammadi, S., Brennan, F.M. and Feldmann, M. (1990). CD5+ B cells in rheumatoid arthritis and Sjögren's syndrome. Clin. Exp. Rheumatol. 8, Suppl. 5, 67–68.

Manca, F., Fenoglio, D., Kunkl, A., Cambiaggi, C., Sasso, M. and Celada, F.J. (1988). Differential activation of T cell clones stimulated by macrophages exposed to antigen complexed with monoclonal antibodies. J. Immunol. 140, 2893–2898.

Mathieson, P.W., Stapleton, K.J., Oliveira, D.B. and Lockwood, C.M. (1991). Immunoregulation of mercuric choride-induced autoimmunity in Brown Norway rats: a role for CD8+ T cells revealed by *in vivo* depletion studies. Eur. J. Immunol. 21, 2105–2109.

Medawar, P.B. (1948). Immunity to homologous grafted skin. III. The fate of skin homografts transplanted to the brain, to subcutaneous tissue, and to the anterior chamber of the eye. Br. J. Exp. Pathol. 29, 58–69.

Mitchison, N.A. (1968). Immunological paralysis induced by brief exposure of cells to protein antigens. Immunology 15, 531–547.

Mitchison, N.A. (1989). In "Progress in Immunology" (ed F. Melchers), Vol. VII, pp 845–852. Springer-Verlag, Berlin.

Mitchison, N.A. (1990). An exact comparison between the efficiency of two- and three-cell-type clusters in mediating helper activity. Eur. J. Immunol. 20, 699–702.

Mitchison, N.A. (1992). Latent help to and from H-2 antigens. Eur. J. Immunol. 22, 123–127.

Mitchison, N.A. and Oliveira, D.B.G. (1986a). In "Progress in Immunology" (ed B. Cinader and R.G. Miller), Vol. VI, pp 326–334. Academic Press, London.

Mitchison, N.A. and Oliveira, D.B.G. (1986b). Chronic infection as a major force in the evolution of the suppressor T cell system. Parasitol. Today 2, 312–313.

Mitchison, N.A. and Simon, K. (1990). Dominant unresponsiveness controlled by H-2A^b. A new pattern displayed by Thy-1 antigen and F liver antigen. Immunogenetics 32, 104–109.

Moeller, G. (1990). Autoreactive T cells and clones. Immunol. Rev. 116: *passim* 1–181.

Moeller, G. (1991) 'γδ' T cells. Immunol. Rev. 120: *passim* 1–204.

Mosmann, T.R. and Coffman, R.L. (1989). TH1 and TH2 cells: different patterns of lymphokine secretion lead to different functional properties. Annu. Rev. Immunol. 7, 145–173.

Mustafa, S.A., Kvalheim, G., Degre, M. and Godal, T. (1986). *Mycobacterium bovis* BCG-induced human T-cell clones from BCG-vaccinated healthy subjects: antigen specificity and lymphokine production. Infect. Immun. 53, 491–497.

Nanda, N., Apple, R. and Sercarz, E.E. (1991). Limitations in plasticity of the T cell receptor repertoire. Proc. Natl Acad. Sci. USA 88, 9503–9507.

Nemazee, D.A. and Burki, K. (1989). Clonal deletion of B lymphocytes in a transgenic mouse bearing anti-MHC class I antibody genes. Nature (London) 337, 562–566.

Nepom, G.T. (1990). A unified hypothesis for the complex genetics of HLA associations with IDDM. Diabetes 39, 1153–1157.

Nossal, G.J.V. (1983). Cellular mechanisms of immunological tolerance. Annu. Rev. Immunol. 1, 33–62.

Nossal, G.J.V., Karvelas, M. and Lalor, P.A. (1989). Immunological tolerance within the B-lymphocyte compartment: an adult tolerance model. Cold Spring Harbor Symp. Quant. Biol. 54, 893–898.

Offner, H., Hashim, G.A. and Vandenbark, A.A. (1991). T cell receptor peptide therapy triggers autoregulation of experimental encephalomyelitis. Science 251, 430–432.

Oliveira, D.B.G. and Mitchison, N.A. (1989). Immune supression genes. Clin. Exp. Immunol. 75, 167–177.

Ottenhof, T.H., Walford, C., Nishimura, Y., Reddy, N.B. and Sasazuki, T. (1990). HLA-DQ molecules and the control of *Mycobacterium leprae*-specific T cell nonresponsiveness in lepromatous leprosy patients. Eur. J. Immunol. 20, 2347–2350.

Pfeiffer, C., Murray, J., Madri, J. and Bottomly, K. (1991). Selective activation of Th1- and Th2-like cells in the *in vivo* response to human collagen IV. Immunol. Rev. 123, 65–84.

Pircher, H., Rohrer, U.H., Moskohidis, D., Zinkernagel, R.M. and Hengartner, H. (1991). Lower receptor avidity required for thymic clonal deletion than for effector T cell function. Nature (London) 351, 482–485.

Robertson, K., Schneider, S., Simon, K., Timms, E. and Mitchison, N.A. (1992). Tolerance of self induced in thymus organ culture. Eur. J. Immunol. 22, 207–211.

Robey, A., Fowlkes, B.J., Gordoin, J.W., Kioussis, D., von Boehmer, H., Ramsdell, F. and Axel, R. (1991). Thymic selection in CD8 transgenic mice supports an instructive model for commitment to a CD4 or CD8 lineage. Cell 64, 99–107.

Roosnek, E. and Lanzavecchia, A. (1991). Efficient and selective presentation of antigen–antibody complexes by rheumatoid factor B cells. J. Exp. Med. 173, 487–489.

Sakaguchi, S. and Sakaguchi, N. (1988). Thymus and autoimmunity. Transplantation of the thymus from cyclosporin-A treated mice causes organ-specific autoimmune disease in athymic nude mice. J. Exp. Med. 167, 1479–1485.

Sarvetnick, N., Liggitt, D., Pitts, S.L., Hansen, S.E. and Stewart, T.A. (1988). Insulin dependent diabetes mellitus induced in transgenic mice by ectopic expression of class II MHC and interferon-gamma. Cell 52, 773.

Schonrich, G., Kalinke, U., Momburg, F., Malissen, M., Schmitt-Verhulst, A.M., Malissen, B., Hammerling, G.J. and Arnold, B. (1991). Down-regulation of T cell receptors on self-reactive T cells as a novel mechanism for extrathymic tolerance induction. Cell 65, 293–304.

Schwartz, R.H. (1990). A cell culture model for T lymphocyte clonal anergy. Science 248, 1349–1356.

Seuchter, S.A., Knapp, M., Hartung, K., Coldeway, R., Kalden, J.R., Lakomak, H.J., Peter, H.H., Deichler, H. and Baur, M.P. (1991). Testing for association in SLE families. Genet. Epidemiol., 8, 409–416.

Smith, C.A., Williams, G.T., Kingston, R., Jenkinson, E.J. and Owen, J.J.T. (1989). Antibodies to the CD3/T-cell receptor complex induce death by apoptosis in immature T-cells in thymic cultures. Nature (London) 337, 181–183.

Sommer, N., Harcourt, G.C., Willcox, N., Beeson, D. and Newsom-Davies, J. (1991). Acetylcholine receptor-reactive T lymphocytes from healthy subjects and myasthenia gravis patients. Neurology 41, 1270–1276.

Sorokin, R., Kimura, H., Schroder, D.H. and Wilson, D.B. (1986). Cyclosporin-induced autoimmunity. Conditions for expressing disease, requirements for intact thymus, and potency estimations of autoimmune lymphocytes in drug-treated rats. J. Exp. Med. 164, 1615–1625.

Strober, S. and Holoshitz, J. (1990). Mechanisms of immune injury in rheumatoid arthritis: evidence for the involvement of T cells and heat-shock protein. Immunol. Rev. 118, 233–256.

Swat, W., Ignatowicz, L., von Boehmer, H. and Kiselow, P. (1991). Clonal deletion of immature CD4 + CD8 + thymocytes in suspension culture by extrathymic antigen-presenting cells. Nature (London) 351, 150–153.

de The, G., Geser, A., Day, N.E., Tukei, P.M., Williams, E.H., Beri, D.P., Smith, P.G., Dean, A.G., Bornkamm, G.W., Feorino, P. and Henle, W. (1978). Epidemiological evidence for causal relationship between Epstein-Barr virus and Burkitt's lymphoma from Ugandan prospective study. Nature (London) 274, 756–761.

Vidard, L., Roger, T., Bouvet, J.P., Couderc, J. and Seman, M. (1991). Resistance to collagen-induced arthritis in Biozzi mice is not associated with T cell receptor V beta gene polymorphism. Eur. J. Immunol. 21, 1783–1785.

Waterfield, J.D., King, I.D. and Dutton, R.W. (1983). Presence of host-reactive T cells in lymphohaematopoietic chimeries. Immunology 4, 219–227.

Wordsworth, B.P, Lanchbury, J.S.S., Sakkas, L.I., Welsh, K.I., Panayi, G.S. and Bell, J.J. (1989). HLA-DR4 subtype frequencies in rheumatoid arthritis indicate that DRB1 is the major susceptibility locus within the HLA cell II region. Proc. Natl Acad. Sci. USA 86, 10049–10053.

Zamoyska, R. and Mitchison, N.A. (1989). In "Perspectives on the Molecular Biology and Immunology of the Pancreatic β Cell" (ed D. Hanahan), pp 141–148. Cold Spring Harbor Laboratory, Cold Spring Harbor, NY.

Zinkernagel, R.M., Cooper, S., Chambers, J., Lazzarini, R.A., Hengartner, H. and Arnheiter, H. (1990). Virus-induced autoantibody responses to a transgenic viral antigen. Nature (London) 345, 68–71.

3. Peptide Blockade and Antigen-specific Modulation of Autoimmune Diseases

David C. Wraith

1. Introduction

Lymphocytes of the CD4 subtype play a central role in immune responses to foreign antigens (Schwartz, 1986). The control of immune responses is achieved through secretion of lymphokines which affect the growth, differentiation and activity of cells involved in the protective arms of the immune response.

A successful immune system will express a large repertoire of TCRs with specificity for countless foreign antigens and mechanisms for deleting or debilitating cells which carry receptors specific for self-antigens. Unfortunately no system is perfect; humans suffer from the evolution of a broad T cell repertoire by predisposition to autoimmune disease. CD4 + T cells have been implicated in numerous autoimmune conditions including juvenile diabetes, myasthenia gravis, rheumatoid arthritis and multiple sclerosis. A number of therapeutic approaches based on CD4 + T cell recognition have been described and are discussed briefly below. This chapter will analyse the rationale behind and experimental testing of two forms of therapy. The first takes MHC class II proteins as the target for peptide blockade. The second attempts to reinforce the normal state of self-tolerance by administration of autoantigens, and in particular autoantigenic peptides, by various non-conventional routes.

1.1 T CELL RECOGNITION AS THE TARGET FOR IMMUNE INTERVENTION IN AUTOIMMUNE DISEASE

The quaternary complex formed between TCR, CD4, the class II MHC and antigen in its processed fragmented form serves as the ideal target for immune intervention in

Immunopharmacology of Joints and Connective Tissue
ISBN 0-12-206345-7

autoimmune disease (Wraith *et al.*, 1989b). The aim is to achieve effective inhibition of the ongoing autoimmune response with, at the same time, a degree of specificity not possible with currently available immunosuppressive drugs. Each of these four targets has its own advantages and disadvantages.

The TCR is an ideal target given that antibodies to it are effective blockers (Acha-Orbea *et al.*, 1988), and blockade or removal of a small subset of T cells is unlikely to be immunosuppressive. However, there is some doubt as to whether autoimmune conditions in humans will display the limited heterogeneity in TCR usage noted in various experimental animal models (Hillert and Olerup, 1992; Steinman *et al.*, 1992). This debate will rage until more structural information concerning TCR usage in human conditions emerges. Furthermore, convincing data in this regard will be difficult to gather until the nature of each autoantigenic target is clarified.

Antibodies to CD4 molecules are potent immuno-suppressive agents (Waldmann, 1989). However, as CD4 molecules are surface markers of all Th cells their use will suffer from non-specificity and may thus increase the risk of infection.

Class II MHC molecules serve two important and not mutually exclusive roles. They shape the T cell repertoire by positive and negative selection of developing Th cells in the thymus and they present antigen to mature Th cells in the periphery. Class II molecules are encoded by I-A and I-E genes of the H-2 complex in mice and DP, DQ and DR genes of the HLA complex in man. There is increasing evidence in favour of mixed pairing between α and β chains of the various loci in rodents and humans (Matsunaga *et al.*, 1990; Lechler, 1988). Therefore, homozygotes will express a number of effective class II molecules for antigen presentation and heterozygotes correspondingly more. As autoimmune diseases in humans generally display strong MHC–disease associ-ation with specific class II isotypes (Nepom and Erlich, 1991), it is hoped that blockade of the predisposing MHC molecule will be possible without widespread immune suppression. MHC molecules serve as targets for both antibodies specific for their α-helical membrane-distal regions and peptides designed to compete with autoantigenic peptides for binding to the cleft formed by the two interfolded chains. For these approaches to be effective we must understand the way in which class II MHC molecules associate with antigenic peptides and present them to CD4 + T cells. This chapter will consider the cell biology of peptide association with class II MHC molecules and follow this with an account of recent attempts at immunotherapy with peptides.

2. *Antigen Processing*

TCRs on CD8 + cytotoxic T cells recognize antigenic peptides bound to class I MHC molecules while class II peptide complexes are detected by CD4 + cells (Yewdell and Bennink, 1990). Correlating with this diversification in function, class I molecules generally bind peptides derived from proteins synthesized by the presenting cell and thus are efficient in presenting fragments of viral proteins produced in an infected cell. By contrast, class II molecules are capable of presenting peptides derived from exogenous internalized proteins. These differences in presentation are not due to the specificity of binding, as some peptides can be presented by both class I and class II molecules (Perkins *et al.*, 1991). They are the result of class I and class II molecules binding antigenic peptides at distinct intracellular locations (Neefjes *et al.*, 1990).

Class II presentation of practically all exogenous antigens is abrogated by prior fixation of APC, which inhibits antigen uptake, and by treatment with lysosomotropic drugs (e.g. ammonium chloride, methylamine and chloroquine). These drugs raise the pH of intracellular compartments affecting both proteolytic activity and receptor recycling. Endogenously synthe-sized proteins (e.g. measles, hepatitis and influenza viral antigens) can be presented by class II molecules (Long and Jacobson, 1989). Class II presentation of some endogenously synthesized proteins (e.g. measles virus antigen) is chloroquine insensitive, whereas presentation of others can be inhibited by chloroquine. This implies that there are two separate pathways for class II presenta-tion of endogenous proteins, one of which (the chloroquine-sensitive) is more dependent on traffic through an acidic endosomal compartment.

2.1   THE ENDOCYTIC PATHWAY

The endocytic pathway, accessed by antigen internaliza-tion, consists of a sequence of increasingly degradative and acidified compartments that terminates with lyso-somes (Brodsky and Guagliardi, 1991). Early endosomes are characterized by pH 6–6.5, have cathepsin B and D and can fuse with newly formed plasma membrane vesicles and have a direct recycling route to the cell surface. These proteases have been implicated in both degradation of antigenic proteins and dissociation of the invariant chain associated with newly synthesized class II molecules. Late endosomes have a lower pH (5.5), are refractory to fusion from newly formed vesicles and do not have a direct recycling route to the cell surface. This compartment has also been called a prelysosomal compartment because it is the sorting compartment where lysosomal enzymes carried from the *trans*-Golgi by the mannose 6-phosphate receptor are dissociated from the receptor and sorted to lysosomes. The terminal endocytic compartment is the highly degradative lyso-some (pH 4.6–5.0) in which proteins are eventually reduced to single amino acids and dipeptides which are transported across the lysosomal membrane into the cytoplasm.

Most protein processing requires 20–30 min even though endocytosed proteins appear in the early endosome within 2–3 min. This delay could indicate the requirement for acid proteases not normally found in early endosomes, or it might reflect a requirement for entry into a compartment where newly synthesized invariant chain-free class II is present or alternatively it could imply the requirement for the generation of a finite number of class II–peptide complexes. Evidence in favour of the lysosome as a major site for antigen processing has been provided by liposome-loading experiments (Harding *et al.*, 1991).

The presence of mature carbohydrate side chains, terminal sialic acid, can be used to trace the biosynthesis of MHC glycoproteins (Neffjes *et al.*, 1990). There is a split in the pathways of class I and II molecules between the *trans*-Golgi reticulum and the cell surface. Class I molecules appear at the cell surface quickly, 2–3 h, whereas the class II pathway is slow, 8 h. Class I molecules do not pass through endosomes whereas class II molecules are detected in endosomes by 1 h in pulse–chase experiments.

2.2 THE INVARIANT CHAIN

Different routes of MHC glycoprotein traffic result from invariant chain binding to class II. Invariant chain is a type 2 glycoprotein with a single transmembrane domain and an N-terminal cytoplasmic tail. The N-terminal cytoplasmic tail has at least two separate targetting signals (Lotteau *et al.*, 1990). One is an ER retention signal. Another signal targets invariant chain and associated class II MHC to late endosomes/lysosomes. After leaving the ER, class I and II molecules traffic through the Golgi at similar rates. However, class I molecules arrive at the cell surface with a half-time of 30 min, whereas class II molecules have a half-time of 2–4 h (Neffjes *et al.*, 1990). The delay of class II molecules is between the Golgi and the plasma membrane and is accompanied by loss of invariant chain. This loss is a protease-dependent process probably involving cathepsins B and D. Isolated class II molecules will not bind peptides when complexed with invariant chain and biochemical release of invariant chain produces a protein which is more capable of binding peptides (Peterson and Miller, 1990).

Class II molecules leaving the low-pH environment of the late endosome in the absence of peptide fail to form a compact stable conformation. Addition of appropriate peptide to purified "floppy" molecules (63–67 kDa) at low pH promotes the compact (56 kDa) conformation (Sadegh-Nasseri and Germain, 1991). In pulse–chase studies, new class II chains do not form a compact conformation until dissociated from invariant chain (Germain and Hendrix, 1991). Compact dimers accumulate during a 4 h pulse implying that most newly formed class II MHC binds peptide in transit to the cell surface. However, some empty dimers do reach the cell surface.

The most likely pathway for class II antigen presentation is as follows. Endocytosed protein is gradually denatured and degraded in endosomes and lysosomes. Newly synthesized class II associates with invariant chain which serves as a "chaperone" to the late endosome/lysosome pool. In endosomes, invariant chain is attacked by proteases and separates from class II MHC leaving a "naked" groove available for peptide binding. Peptide binding stabilizes the conformation of the dimer, which might account for the slow off-rate for some peptide–MHC complexes. The elegance of this pathway is that MHC class II is available for peptide binding only in the cellular compartment loaded with exogenous antigens.

2.3 RECYCLING OF MHC CLASS II

For some time it was thought that class II MHC recycled from the cell surface, picked up antigen in endosomes/lysosomes and carried the antigen back up to the cell surface for presentation. However, early studies indicated that very low levels of class I molecules and only 3–10% of surface class II molecules internalize spontaneously (Neffjes *et al.*, 1990). It appears that the half-life of recycling to the cell surface is 2–3 min. How important is this for antigen presentation? In spite of the potential for peptide binding after class II internalization, the half-life of this process (2–3 min) means that recycled MHC will not reach late endosomes where conditions for degradation and binding are optimal. In the light of the convincing evidence that the export pathway of class II molecules contributes to their acquisition of peptides, the potential exchange of peptides after class II molecule internalization has to be considered an additional pathway for peptide binding, rather than the major mechanism.

3. *Peptide Blockade of MHC Molecules*

Crystallographic analysis of various MHC molecules has revealed the way in which the membrane-distal domains of both class I and class II molecules fold to form an antigen binding cleft (Bjorkman *et al.*, 1987; Brown *et al.*, 1988). An early indication that class II MHC molecules have a single binding site for antigen came from studies with synthetic copolymers. Presentation of GAT to GAT-specific T cell hybridomas could be inhibited by preincubation of APC with the hetero-logous copolymer GT (Rock and Bennacerraf, 1983). This evidence was extended at the cellular level using synthetic peptides (Lakey *et al.*, 1986; Guillet *et al.*, 1986) and was confirmed biochemically by direct antigen competition at the level of peptide binding to detergent-solubilized class II MHC proteins (Babbitt *et al.*, 1986).

3.1   IMPLICATIONS FOR THERAPY

Studies *in vitro* with detergent-solubilized protein have indicated that peptide binding to class II MHC generates stable, long-lived complexes. Furthermore, it appears that peptide binding contributes to the folding/stability of class II MHC molecules (Sadegh-Nasseri and Germain, 1992). For this reason, competitive peptide blocking of class II MHC would appear to be a tall order. How could one expect to block every available class II MHC protein in an individual?

Maybe one might not be able to displace autoantigenic peptide once bound. However, the battle to prevent new autoantigenic peptide binding then becomes a numbers game. Consider that the threshold for T cell activation is reached when 200–1000 cell surface peptide–MHC complexes are formed, corresponding to 0.1–1% of surface MHC on an APC (Demotz *et al.*, 1990; Harding and Unanue, 1990). It is generally difficult to achieve levels of MHC loading above this percentage, when using live APC, presumably because (a) there are numerous endogenous peptides which bind with higher affinity and (b) peptides associated with class II in APC may not necessarily display the infinite stability indicated by *in vitro* studies with solubilized class II. Therefore, to inhibit T cell activation it will be a matter of competing for binding such as to reduce the level of autoantigen presentation to below the threshold for activation. This should require blocking of only a small percentage of available MHC molecules. From the cell biology experiments, it becomes clear that we should (a) design peptides/drugs specifically to compete for binding at the site of processing, rather than at the cell surface, and (b) strive to create blockers with high affinity. The site of antigen processing, the enzymes involved and the mechanism of MHC loading are all crucial events which require further work.

3.2   PEPTIDE BLOCKADE *IN VIVO*

Adorini and co-workers have shown that it is possible to inhibit Th cell priming in mice by combination of a non-immunogenic peptide with an immunogenic peptide in the immunizing inoculum (Adorini *et al.*, 1988). Moreover, they have been able to demonstrate reduction in an immune response by administration of soluble peptides in slow-release capsules (Muller *et al.*, 1990). The immune response to a foreign antigen, a peptide from HEL, was inhibited by administration of a distinct peptide from the same protein in solution phase via an osmotic pump.

3.3   MHC-BLOCKING PEPTIDES IN IMMUNOTHERAPY

The work of Adorini and co-workers raises exciting possibilities for the treatment of autoimmune conditions. When the predisposing class II molecule has been identified in any one individual, it should be possible to treat the condition by administration of blocking peptides. Selective use of allele-specific blockers can also be seen as a means of identifying the restriction element for disease. Up to now, the use of MHC-binding peptides in blockade of an autoimmune response has been tested in three separate models of experimental autoimmune disease.

EAE is an induced autoimmune condition commonly used as a model for immunotherapy in rats and mice (Zamvil and Steinman, 1990). In mice, EAE can be induced by injection of an homogenate of spinal cord or by purified components of spinal cord, principally MBP and PLP, and more reproducibly by injection of the immunodominant peptides derived from these proteins. Mice of the H-2^s and H-2^u haplotypes are particularly susceptible to disease induction with synthetic peptides. In H-2^u mice there are two major epitopes of MBP, the acetylated N-terminal peptide 1–9 and the I-E-restricted epitope 33–45. In SJL (H-2^s) mice, peptide 84–96 serves as the major epitope from MBP and peptide 139–151 the immunodominant epitope from PLP.

The N-terminal peptide of MBP (Ac1–9) has been extensively analysed to identify determinants for binding I-A^u or interacting with encephalitogenic TCRs (Wraith *et al.*, 1989a). Single amino acid-substituted analogues were used to identify residue 4 as the determinant for MHC binding and residues 3 and 6 as determinants for TCR interactions. Acetylation of the N-terminal peptide is also required for optimal MHC binding. However, an extended version (amino acids 1–20 from rat MBP) of the minimal epitope can bind to I-A^u at a level sufficient to activate T cells specific for residues 9–20. Unacetylated peptide 1–20 is not recognized by Ac1–9-specific T cells which means that the N-terminal acetyl group must serve as an additional T cell determinant. Following this observation, Sakai and co-workers (1989) have shown that unacetylated peptide 1–20 reduces the incidence of disease in the acute EAE model.

The inhibition of EAE with an analogue of the autoantigenic epitope is difficult to interpret. Apart from simple MHC blockade, it is possible that this peptide modulates the immune response by generating suppressor T cells or inducing T cells of a distinct non-pathogenic phenotype. In order to avoid this criticism, it is possible to synthesize unrelated peptides with high affinity for the restriction element for disease. One such peptide has a core I-A binding sequence (VHAAHA) with additional lysine and methionine flanking sequences shown to increase resistance to degradation by proteases (Lamont *et al.*, 1990). The resulting peptide (KMKMVHAAHAKMKM) is a potent inhibitor of I-A^s-restricted antigen presentation *in vitro*. This KM-core extension peptide inhibited the induction of EAE in SJL

(I-A^s) mice on co-administration with an encephalitogenic dose of the immunodominant peptide from PLP. Furthermore, this peptide inhibited disease induction when administered at a separate site from the encephalitogen. The fact that the sequence of the KM-core extension peptide is unrelated to the encephalitogenic peptide means that its inhibitory activity must be due to a mechanism other than antigen-specific suppression.

The inhibitory effects of peptide 1–20 and the KM peptide in the H-2^u and H-2^s models of EAE have been interpreted as being due to direct competition for binding to the restriction element for disease. However, there is an alternative explanation. Both the 1–20 and KM peptides are highly immunogenic in their respective mouse strains, and it is conceivable that they inhibit disease by causing a dominant immune response to themselves rather than by straightforward competition for MHC binding. Ideally the design of MHC-binding antagonists should be based on the use of non-immunogenic peptides. The immune system is normally tolerant of self-proteins despite the fact that epitopes from such proteins can bind with high affinity to self-MHC restriction elements. Therefore, it is conceivable that certain non-immunogenic self-peptides will prove effective in inhibiting autoimmune conditions and may form the basis for improved immunotherapeutic agents.

The heart is a target organ in several autoimmune diseases, and cardiac myosin can be used to induce acute myocarditis in A/J mice (Smith and Allen, 1991). Smith and Allen used MHC-blocking peptides in order to identify the restriction element for disease in this model. When myosin was co-emulsified with peptide 49–62 from mouse lysozyme, the severity of myocarditis was reduced as the molar excess of blocking peptide increased. The 49–62 peptide is non-immunogenic due to self-tolerance and has been shown to bind strongly to I-A^k. An I-E^k-binding self-peptide from mouse haemoglobin failed to inhibit disease induction, thus identifying I-A^k as the restriction element for disease in this autoimmune myocarditis model.

In the latter case, however, a 1000-fold molar excess of blocking peptide was required to inhibit disease induction with myosin. This compares poorly with the 3 to 10-fold excess of inhibitors used in the EAE models described above. There are three possible explanations for this discrepancy. First, it could be that intact proteins such as myosin have an immunological advantage because of the requirement for antigen processing. Intact proteins require internalization into an acidic subcellular compartment where they are denatured, processed into fragments and loaded into the cleft of class II proteins. Future studies should be aware of the possibility that efficient blockers may require targeting to the same acidic subcellular compartment. As described above, some antigens are processed in the late endosomes/lysosomes so this

may be the compartment for targeting. Second, MHC-blocking studies in the EAE model have used immunogenic peptides as potential blocking agents. Further work with non-immunogenic peptides is required to substantiate the efficacy of MHC blockade especially in the reversal of ongoing disease. Third, it is possible that peptide analogues of autoantigens such as the unacetylated 1–20 peptide might interfere with T cell recognition of peptide Ac1–11 by antagonism at the level of the T cell receptor.

One recent study, in favour of the latter possibility, has provided compelling evidence to show that peptide analogues of peptide 307–319 of H, although non-stimulatory for T cell clones specific for haemagglutinin, nevertheless preferentially inhibit haemagglutinin-specific T cells in antigen-presentation assays (DeMagistris et al., 1992). Similar results were obtained using analogues of tetanus toxoid peptide 830–843 in competition for presentation of 830–843 but not in competition for haemagglutinin peptide 307–319. Direct binding and cellular experiments indicated that the mechanism responsible was distinct from competition for binding class II MHC molecules. The most likely mechanism for this effect is engagement of antigen-specific T cell receptors by MHC–peptide analogue complexes. The efficiency of this approach may stem from the fact that the antagonist would only have to occupy approximately 200 sites per APC to be effective (Demotz et al., 1990; Harding and Unanue, 1990), whereas MHC-blocking agents would have to fill 100% of available peptide-binding sites.

3.4 INHIBITION OF EAE BY PEPTIDE Ac1–11 [4A]

Substitution of lysine with alanine at position 4 of the dominant myelin basic protein epitope for H-2^u mice (Ac1–11) produces a heteroclitic analogue (Wraith et al., 1989a). The 4A peptide binds to I-A^u with a higher (10–100 times) affinity and is a potent stimulator of Ac1–11-immune cells in vitro. Surprisingly, this peptide proved to be non-immunogenic when injected into PL/J or (PL/J × SJL)F1 mice. As the peptide binds with higher affinity to I-A^u and yet is not immunogenic for Ac1–11-specific T cells in these strains, it was reasoned that it should block the encephalitogenic properties of Ac1–11. The 4A peptide was protective when co-administered with an encephalitogenic dose of Ac1–11. However, two recent observations indicate that Ac1–11[4A] is more than just a blocker. First, this peptide is itself encephalitogenic in B10.PL (H-2^u) mice (Wraith et al., 1992). Second, other analogues of Ac1–11, such as Ac1–11[3A,4A], which bind with similar affinity to I-A^u as Ac1–11[4A], fail to inhibit disease (Smilek et al., 1991). The ability of Ac1–11[4A] to modulate disease cannot be due simply to MHC blockade.

3.5   PEPTIDE COMPETITION FOR CLASS I-RESTRICTED PRESENTATION

Class I-restricted CD8+ cells are believed to play an important role in autoimmune diabetes (Miller *et al.*, 1988). Until recently, it seemed unlikely that exogenous peptides would be able to compete with endogenous peptides in the class I pathway. However, Zweerink and co-workers have demonstrated that a synthetic blocking peptide inhibited lysis of target cells in which endogenous peptide loading of class I MHC was achieved via a minigene coding for the target peptide (Gammon *et al.*, 1992). This remarkable finding confounds the current belief that peptides "from within" form irreversibly stable complexes with class I MHC and raises the possibility that class I may be used as a target for peptide therapy in appropriate cases.

4.   *Antigen-specific Modulation of Autoimmune Responses*

The ultimate aim of any therapeutic approach in auto-immunity is to reverse the disease process and to speci-fically target autoreactive cells. Many of the current approaches to immunotherapy are non-specific and generally immunosuppressive. The most specific approach will target only those T cells specific for the autoantigen in question: islet antigens in insulin-dependent diabetes, acetylcholine receptor in myasthenia gravis, synovial antigens in rheumatoid arthritis, spinal cord antigens in multiple sclerosis.

4.1   THE ROLE OF ADJUVANT

It has been known for some time that administration of antigen in the absence of appropriate adjuvant could lead to the induction of a state of unresponsiveness rather than immunity (Shaw *et al.*, 1962). In fact, EAE in guinea pigs could be treated with MBP in IFA even after the onset of disease. More recently we have attempted to reproduce these findings in the peptide-induced EAE model (Smilek *et al.*, 1991). Here we found that pretreat-ment of H-2^u mice with the encephalitogenic peptide Ac1–11[4K] inhibited disease induction, but when this peptide was administered after disease onset, it did not affect the resulting symptoms. However, a high-affinity MHC-binding analogue of Ac1–11 (Ac1–11[4A]) both prevented the induction of and inhibited progression to further disease when given at disease onset. Therefore, the high-affinity analogue can modulate the effects of autoreactive T cells both before and after priming.

Why should the administration of autoantigens in a mixture of oil and water (IFA) lead to non-responsiveness, whereas addition of heat-killed mycobacterium to the same inoculum (CFA) produces a highly immunogenic mixture? Heat-killed mycobacteria induce granuloma formation on subcutaneous injection and it is reasonable to believe that cells infiltrating the granulomatous region contribute to both antigen presentation and T cell activation. In the absence of such additional stimuli, potentially autoreactive T lymphocytes recognize antigen but are either inhibited from proliferating or default to non-responsiveness. This may be considered along the lines of the two-signal hypothesis (Bretscher and Cohn, 1970). This theory was proposed originally to explain B cell activation but has gained acceptance also as a frame-work for T cell activation (Jenkins, 1992). Thus, the first signal is provided by ligation of the antigen-specific receptor, surface immunoglobulin or TCR. The second signal, required to switch from anergy to activation, is a complex combination of different factors which are broadly defined as stimuli that promote cell division. There seems little doubt that a co-stimulatory signal is provided by cell–cell contact between T cells and APC, possibly by molecules such as CD28 on the T cell (Harding *et al.*, 1992) and B7 on the APC (Linsley *et al.*, 1991). This, in turn, promotes transcription of autocrine growth factors and supports cell division as long as space permits. T cell activation concomitantly results in the intracellular build-up of negative regulators that inhibit IL-2 transcription and produce anergy (Zubiaga *et al.*, 1991). These may be diluted out by cell division, hence explaining the need for space to escape anergy. It is likely that CFA stimulates the upregulation of co-stimulatory molecules on APC and/or enhances the infiltration of suitable (co-stimulator-positive) APC into the site of inoculation.

4.2   INTRAVENOUS ANTIGEN ADMINISTRATION

The immune response to both self- and foreign antigens, or antigenic peptides, may be modulated by inappropriate administration. There are various routes of antigen administration which tend to induce a state of partial or complete non-reponsiveness to the antigen. For example, foreign antigens may be administered intravenously in order to induce tolerance. A well-characterized model system for i.v. tolerance to a foreign antigen is HEL (Gammon and Sercarz, 1989). Adult mice injected i.v. with intact HEL become refractory to subsequent T cell priming with whole protein in CFA. Notably, the mice become tolerant to the immunodominant epitope of the protein. Nevertheless, immune responses to subdominant epitopes are elicited by immunization of tolerant mice with appropriate peptides in CFA. Administration of peptide epitopes of foreign antigens also leads to a state of epitope-specific hyporesponsiveness in the T cell pool (Scherer *et al.*, 1989).

The i.v. route of administration has been effective for reinforcing tolerance to self- as well as foreign antigens. EAT can be induced with relative ease in susceptible mouse strains by injection of mouse thyroglobulin with adjuvant, which leads to the development of autoantibodies and thyroiditis (Rose *et al.*, 1971). EAT can be prevented by i.v. treatment with soluble mouse thyroglobulin before treatment (Kong *et al.*, 1982).

What are the mechanisms of i.v. tolerance? It has been suggested that i.v. injection of foreign peptides or proteins leads to clonal anergy (Scherer *et al.*, 1989). When peptide epitopes of foreign antigens were injected into adult thymectomized mice, the state of hypo-responsiveness was not permanent (M. Gefter, personal communication). This argues against the induction of memory-suppressor cells, implies that clonal deletion had not taken place and leaves anergy as the only alternative. However, injection of autologous thyroglobulin i.v. in mice induces a state of suppression which can be transferred to irradiated syngeneic recipients and is specific for thyroglobulin (Parish *et al.*, 1988a). Injection of normal cells does not reverse this tolerance, also indicative of an active suppression. The suppressor cells may be deleted with anti-CD4 antibodies suggesting that suppression is mediated either by a CD4 + T suppressor cell or a CD4 + suppressor-inducer cell (Parish *et al.*, 1988b). Recent experiments have raised further questions about tolerance induction with thyroglobulin. Thus thyroiditis can be induced only with iodinated thyroglobulin and not with the iodine-free derivative when these are used as the primary stimulus (Champion *et al.*, 1987). Tolerance to thyroglobulin can be reinforced, however, by injection of the thyroxine-free protein, suggesting that one suppressor epitope of thyroglobulin is distinct from the epitope for thyroiditogenic T cells (Rayner *et al.*, 1992).

It is not clear why the injection of peptide epitopes should induce anergy whereas the injection of thyroglobulin induces suppression. Even more puzzling is the fact that injection of a foreign protein (HEL) does not induce tolerance to the whole protein, which one would expect to be a consequence of active suppression (Gammon and Sercarz, 1989). Could it be that the experiments with HEL peptides used an *in vitro* read-out system which might disrupt the immune architecture required for normal operation of suppressor cells? The fact that immunodominant epitopes were "tolerized" in the HEL system argues in favour of clonal anergy or deletion as a mechanism for tolerance to these epitopes. Without an immune response to these immuno-dominant epitopes, the normal immune response to intact antigen might be so disrupted as to prevent an *in vivo* response. This still fails to explain the transfer of suppression in the thyroglobulin experiments. Perhaps anergic cells can actively suppress an immune response *in vivo* even though they themselves are unable to proliferate. It will be interesting to test the effect of i.v.

administration of thyroglobulin T cell epitopes to test whether they alone are capable of inducing T suppressor/anergic cells.

4.3 ORAL ADMINISTRATION OF ANTIGEN

Oral tolerance is a highly complex phenomenon which may involve a wide range of immunoregulatory mechanisms. Although feeding protein tolerizes humoral and cellular immunity, there is general agreement that this is determined principally by T-cell unresponsiveness (Mowat, 1987). Thus, only T-dependent antigens can induce tolerance of the antibody response, and tolerance generated by feeding hapten–protein conjugates shows carrier specificity. Reactive B cells have been demonstrated directly in *in vitro* assays of T-cell-depleted lymphocytes from mice fed ovalbumin.

Mechanisms of induction of T-cell unresponsiveness are not yet clear but the eventual return of T cell activity indicates that clonal deletion is unlikely to be involved. As tolerance ensues rapidly after one feed of protein and is rarely preceded by a phase of systemic priming, it seems probable that the depressed function of Th cells partly reflects a direct interaction between Th and antigen (T cell anergy). Nonetheless, transfer experiments have suggested the presence of suppressor cells following protein feeding.

These findings have obvious implications for the prevention and possible reversal of autoimmune diseases (Thompson and Staines, 1990). With identification of the principal autoantigen, it may be possible to prevent or delay onset of disease in genetically predisposed individuals before attack or to reverse ongoing disease. This is a long-term aim relying on the identification of autoantigens, which remain obscure for the majority of human autoimmune diseases, careful consideration of dose and time of administration but most significantly clarification of the mechanism of tolerance induction.

Two groups have begun studies on EAE in rats. Bitar and Whitacre (1988) have shown that oral administration of MBP to Lewis rats before an encephalitogenic challenge resulted in total inhibition or a significant delay in the onset of EAE. *In vitro* lymphocyte proliferative responses to MBP were significantly decreased in rats fed MBP when compared with vehicle-fed controls. Suppression of EAE and *in vitro* proliferative responses to MBP were observed to be antigen specific, as oral feeding of a control protein exerted no suppressive effect. Moreover, the specificity of MBP-induced oral tolerance was shown to be species specific, as feeding guinea pig MBP or human MBP induced protection only against the induction of disease by protein derived from the same species. Most notably, these workers were unable to induce tolerance by oral administration of rat MBP. Weiner and co-workers have extended these findings to show that oral tolerance could be induced by administration of peptides derived from myelin basic protein by pepsin digestion (Higgins and Weiner, 1988). Notably, susceptibility to disease could be decreased by administration of either encephalitogenic or non-encephalitogenic fragments. The fact that non-encephalitogenic epitopes are as effective as encephalitogenic epitopes again points to distinct helper and suppressogenic epitopes within the same protein. Protection from EAE may be transferred with T cells (CD8+) (Lider *et al.*, 1989) and could involve antigen-driven bystander effects (Miller *et al.*, 1991a,b) mediated by the local production of TGFβ (Miller *et al.*, 1992).

4.4 ANTIGEN INHALATION

It is now clear that downregulation of immune responses in the gastrointestinal tract plays an important role in adaptive immunity (see above). The respiratory tract, being a similar mucosal surface continuously exposed to foreign antigens, might possess a similar protective mechanism (Holt and McMenamin, 1989). This was suggested by early experiments showing that intratracheal intubation with inorganic antigens in guinea pigs could lead to specific immunological unresponsiveness (Katz, 1980). Further work has shown that aerosol administration of a number of different antigens can result in specific immunological unresponsiveness to the inhaled antigen (Holt *et al.*, 1981; Fox and Siraganian, 1981; Stewart and Holt, 1987). Administration of serum from aerosol-exposed animals failed to transfer the state of tolerance whereas injection of T lymphocytes (CD8+ in the rat) proved successful (Sedgwick and Holt, 1985).

Recently this route of administration has been tested for the administration of autoantigenic peptides. Mice of the H-2^u haplotype develop acute or chronic relapsing EAE when injected with analogues of the N-terminal peptide of MBP. Mice pretreated with analogues of the N-terminal peptide by inhalation develop resistance to the induction of disease (Wraith *et al.*, 1992). Furthermore, high-affinity MHC-binding analogues of the peptide are more effective in suppressing the response and can prevent the development of relapsing disease.

5. Concluding Remarks

In this chapter, I have discussed two areas in which the use of synthetic peptides has contributed to advances in both our basic understanding of immunology and the development of peptide-based therapeutic strategies. The use of peptides as MHC-binding antagonists still poses theoretical challenges. How is it possible for sufficient agent to be administered to prevent T cell activation? Certain areas of future progress are evident. First, such

agents should be targeted to the correct intracellular compartment to optimize MHC binding; what is the correct compartment and how can peptides be modified to facilitate entry? Second, peptides should be easy to administer and stable *in vivo*. Third, their binding to MHC should be irreversible; the design of such reagents will be greatly assisted by knowledge of the three-dimensional structure of class II MHC molecules. Finally, these agents must be shown to reverse or halt the progression of ongoing disease.

With ever increasing information about autoantigenic epitopes in human autoimmune conditions the use of peptides as tolerogens has become an exciting prospect. We are faced with three realistic routes of administration, namely, aerosol, intravenous and oral. Unfortunately, the phenomena of aerosol, intravenous and oral tolerance are treated with disbelief and rancour by many investigators; their mechanisms will have to be carefully worked out. Much of the work in this field has used the intact antigen as tolerogen. This could be hazarduous in cases where B cells play a role in immunopathogenesis. It should be safer to use peptides as tolerogens, especially as it appears that high-affinity analogues are more potent tolerogens (Smilek *et al.*, 1991; Wraith *et al.*, 1992). The design of tolerogens requires a comprehensive knowledge of the autoantigenic epitope; or does it? A number of studies now implicate regulator or suppressor T (Ts) cells in the modulation of autoimmune responses following deviant autoantigen administration (Miller *et al.*, 1991a,b). Apparently, the induction of these cells is antigen specific and yet the effector phase is not (Miller *et al.*, 1992). Thus, one can generate bystander suppression and this can be induced by epitopes within the autoantigen, but distinct from the autoantigenic epitope itself. The possibility arises, therefore, of administering tolerogenic epitopes without fear of cross-reactivity with the autoantigenic epitope. Given that HLA-DR antigens are promiscuous in their association with antigenic epitopes (Sinigaglia *et al.*, 1988; Paninabordignon *et al.*, 1989), it might be possible to identify universal tolerogenic epitopes within autoantigens.

6. Acknowledgements

The author is a Wellcome Trust Senior Research Fellow and acknowledges support from the Wellcome Trust, the Multiple Sclerosis Society of Great Britain and Northern Ireland and Hoffmann La Roche, Basel, Switzerland.

7. References

Acha-Orbea, H., Mitchell, D.J., Timmermann, L., Wraith, D.C., Tausch, G.S., Waldor, M.K., Zamvil, S.S., McDevitt, H.O. and Steinman, L. (1988). Limited heterogeneity of T cell receptors from lymphocytes mediating autoimmune encephalomyelitis allows specific immune intervention. Cell 54, 263–273.

Adorini, L., Muller, S., Cardinaux, F., Lehmann, P.F., Falcioni, F. and Nagy, Z.A. (1988). *In vivo* competition between self peptides and foreign antigens in T-cell activation. Nature (London) 334, 623–625.

Babbitt, B.P., Matsueda, G., Haber, E., Unanue, E.R. and Allen, P.M. (1986). Antigenic competition at the level of peptide-Ia binding. Proc. Natl Acad. Sci. USA 83, 4509–4513.

Bitar, D.M. and Whitacre, C.C. (1988). Suppression of experimental autoimmune encephalomyelitis by the oral administration of myelin basic protein. Cell. Immunol. 112, 364–370.

Bjorkman, P.J., Saper, M.A., Samraoui, B., Bennet, W.S., Strominger, J.L. and Wiley, D.C. (1987). Structure of the human class I histocompatibility antigen, HLA-A2. Nature (London) 329, 506–612.

Bretscher, P. and Cohn, M. (1970). A theory of self-nonself discrimination. Science 169, 1042–1049.

Brodsky, F.M. and Guagliardi, L.E. (1991). The cell biology of antigen processing. Annu. Rev. Immunol. 9, 707–744.

Brown, J.H., Jardetzky, T., Saper, M.A., Samraoui, B., Bjorkman, P.J. and Wiley, D.C. (1988). A hypothetical model of the foreign antigen binding site of class II histocompatibility molecules. Nature (London) 332, 845–850.

Champion, B.R., Rayner, D.C., Byfield, P.G.H., Page, K.R., Chan, C.T.J. and Roitt, I.M. (1987). Critical role of iodination for T cell recognition of thyroglobulin in experimental murine thyroid autoimmunity. J. Immunol. 139, 2665–2670.

DeMagistris, M.T., Alexander, J., Coggeshall, M., Altman, A., Gaeta, F.C.A., Grey, H.M. and Sette, A. (1992). Antigen analogy–major histocompatibility complexes act as antagonists of the T cell receptor. Cell 68, 625–634.

Demotz, S., Grey, H.M. and Sette, A. (1990). The minimal number of class II MHC–antigen complexes needed for T cell activation. Science 249, 1028–1030.

Fox, P.C. and Siraganian, R.P. (1981). IgE antibody suppression following aerosol exposure to antigens. Immunology 43, 227–234.

Gammon, G. and Sercarz, E.E. (1989). How some T cells escape tolerance induction. Nature (London) 342, 183–185.

Gammon, M.C., Bednarek, M.A., Biddison, W.E., Bondy, S.S., Hermes, H., Mark, G.E., Williamson, A.R. and Zweerink, H.J. (1992). Endogenous loading of HLA-A2 molecules with an analog of the influenza virus matrix protein derived peptide and its inhibition by an exogenous peptide antagonist. J. Immunol. 148, 7–12.

Germain, R.N. and Hendrix, L.R. (1991). MHC class II structure, occupancy and surface expression determined by post-endoplasmic reticulum antigen binding. Nature (London) 353, 134–139.

Guillet, J-G., Lai, M.Z., Briner, T.J., Smith, J.A. and Gefter, M.L. (1986). Interaction of peptide antigens and class II major histocompatibility complex antigens. Nature (London) 324, 260–262.

Harding, C.V. and Unanue, E.R. (1990). Quantitation of antigen presenting cell MHC class II/peptide complexes necessary for T cell stimulation. Nature (London) 346, 574–576.

Harding, C.V., Collins, D.S., Slot, J.W., Geuze, H.J. and Unanue, E.R. (1991). Liposome-encapsulated antigens are processed in lysosomes, recycled, and presented to T cells. Cell 64, 393–401.

Harding, F.A., McArthur, J.G., Gross, J.A., Raulet, D.H. and Allison, J.P. (1992). CD28-mediated signalling co-stimulates murine T cells and prevents induction of anergy in T-cell clones. Nature (London) 356, 607–609.

Higgins, P.J. and Weiner, H.L. (1988). Suppression of experimental autoimmune encephalomyelitis by oral administration of myelin basic protein and its fragments. J. Immunol. 140, 440–445.

Hillert, J. and Olerup, O. (1992). Germ-line polymorphism of TCR genes and disease susceptibility – fact or hypothesis? Immunol. Today 13, 47–49.

Holt, P.G. and McMenamin, C. (1989). Defence against allergic sensitization in the healthy lung: the role of inhalation tolerance. Clin. Exp. Allergy 19, 255–262.

Holt, P.G., Batty, J.E. and Turner, K.J. (1981). Inhibition of specific IgE responses in mice by pre-exposure to inhaled antigen. Immunology 42, 409–417.

Jenkins, M.K. (1992). The role of cell division in the induction of clonal anergy. Immunol. Today 13, 69–73.

Katz, D.H. (1980). Recent studies on the regulation of IgE antibody synthesis in experimental animals and man. Immunology 41, 1–24.

Kong, Y.M., Okayasu, I., Giraldo, A.A., Beisel, K.W., Sundick, R.S., Rose, N.R., David, C.S., Audibert, F. and Chedid, L. (1982). Tolerance to thyroglobulin by activating suppressor mechanisms. Ann. N.Y. Acad. Sci. 392, 191–207.

Lakey, E.K., Margoliash, E., Flouret, G. and Pierce, S.K. (1986). Peptides related to the antigenic determinant block T cell recognition of the native protein as processed by antigen-presenting cells. Eur. J. Immunol. 16, 721–727.

Lamont, A.G., Sette, A., Fujinami, R., Colon, S.M., Miles, C. and Grey, H.M. (1990). Inhibition of experimental auto-immune encephalomyelitis induction in SJL/J mice by using a peptide with high affinity for I-A^s molecules. J. Immunol. 145, 1687–1693.

Lecher, R. I. (1988). MHC class II molecular structure permitted pairs? Immunol. Today 9, 76–78.

Lider, O., Santos, L.M.B., Lee, C.S.Y., Higgins P.J. and Weiner, H.L. (1989). Suppression of experimental allergic encephalomyelitis by oral administration of myelin basic protein. II. Suppression of disease and *in vitro* immune responses are mediated by antigen-specific CD8 + T lymphocytes. J. Immunol. 142, 748–752.

Linsley, P.S., Brady, W. and Grosmaire, L. (1991). Binding of the B cell activation antigen B7 to CD28 costimulates T cell proliferation and interleukin 2 mRNA activation. J. Exp. Med. 173, 721–730.

Long, E.O. and Jacobson, S. (1989). Pathways of viral antigen processing and presentation to CTL: defined by the mode of virus entry? Immunol. Today 10, 45–48.

Lotteau, V., Teyton, L., Peleraux, A., Nilsson, T., Karlsson, L., Schmid, S.L., Quaranta, V. and Peterson, P.A. (1990). Intracellular-transport of class-II MHC molecules directed by invariant chain. Nature (London) 348, 600–605.

Matsunaga, M., Seki, K., Mineta, T. and Kimoto, M. (1990). Antigen-reactive T cell clones restricted by mixed isotype $A\beta^d E\alpha^d$ class II molecules. J. Exp. Med. 171, 577–582.

Metzler, B. and Wraith, D.C. (1993). Inhibition of experimental autoimmune encephalomyelitis by inhalation but not oral administration of the encephalitogenic peptide: influence of MHC binding affinity. Int. Immunol. (in press).

Miller, A. Hafler, D. and Weiner, H. (1991a). Immunotherapy in autoimmune diseases. Curr. Opin. Immunol. 3, 936–940.

Miller, A., Lider, O. and Weiner, H.L. (1991b). Antigen-driven bystander suppression after oral administration of antigens. J. Exp. Med. 174, 791–798.

Miller, A., Lider, O., Roberts, A.B., Sporn, M.B. and Weiner, H.L. (1992). Suppressor T cells generated by oral tolerization to myelin basic protein suppress both *in vitro* and *in vivo* immune responses by the release of transforming growth factor β after antigen-specific triggering. Proc. Natl. Acad. Sci. USA 89, 421–425.

Miller, B.J., Appel, M.C., O'Neill, J.J. and Wicker, L.S. (1988). Both the Lyt-2+ and L3T4+ T cell subsets are required for the transfer of diabetes in non-obese diabetic mice. J. Immunol. 140, 52–58.

Mowat, A. Mc. (1987). The regulation of immune responses to dietary protein antigens. Immunol. Today. 8, 93–98.

Muller, S., Adorini, L., Juretic, A. and Nagy, Z.A. (1990). Selective *in vivo* inhibition of T cell activation by class II MHC-binding peptides administered in soluble form. J. Immunol. 145, 4006–4011.

Neefjes, J.J., Stollorz, V., Peters, P.J., Geuze, H.J. and Ploegh, H.L. (1990). The biosynthetic pathway of MHC class-II but not class-I intersects the endocytic route. Cell 61, 171–183.

Nepom, G.T. and Erlich, H. (1991). MHC class-II molecules and autoimmunity. Annu. Rev. Immunol. 9, 493–525.

Paninabordignon, P., Tan, A., Termijtelen, A., Demotz, S., Corradin, G. and Lanzavecchia, A. (1989). Universally immunogenic T-cell epitopes:- promiscuous binding to human class II and promiscuous recognition by T cells. Eur. J. Immunol. 19, 2237–2242.

Parish, N.M., Rayner, D., Cooke, A. and Roitt, I.M. (1988a). An investigation of the nature of induced suppression to experimental autoimmune thyroiditis. Immunology 63, 199–203.

Parish, N.M., Roitt, I.M. and Cooke, A. (1988b). Phenotypic characteristics of cells involved in induced suppression to murine experimental autoimmune thyroiditis. Eur. J. Immunol. 18, 1463–1467.

Perkins, D.L., Berritz, G., Wang, Y.S., Smith, J.A. and Gefter, M.L. (1991). Comparison of class I-restricted and II-restricted T-cell recognition of the identical peptide. Eur. J. Immunol. 21, 2781–2789.

Peterson, M. and Miller, J. (1990). Invariant chain influences the immunological recognition of MHC class II molecules. Nature (London) 345, 172–174.

Rayner, D.C., Champion, B.R. and Cooke, A. (1992). In "Monoclonal Antibody and Peptide Therapy in Autoimmune Diseases" (ed J.-F. Bach), pp 359–376. Marcel Dekker, New York.

Rock, K.L. and Benacerraf, B. (1983). Inhibition of antigen-specific T lymphocyte activation by structurally related Ir gene controlled polymers. J. Exp. Med. 157, 1618–1634.

Rose, N.R., Twarog, F.J. and Crowle, A.J. (1971). Murine thyroiditis: importance of adjuvant and mouse strains for the induction of thyroid lesions. J. Immunol. 106, 698–704.

Sadegh-Nasseri, S. and Germain, R.N. (1991). A role for peptide in determining MHC class II structure. Nature (London) 353, 167–170.

Sadegh-Nasseri, S. and Germain, R.N. (1992). How class II molecules work – peptide-dependent completion of protein folding. Immunol. Today 13, 43–46.

Sakai, K., Zamvil, S.S., Mitchell, D.J., Hodgkinson, S., Rothbard, J.B. and Steinman, L. (1989). Prevention of experimental encephalomyelitis with peptides that block interaction of T cells with major histocompatibility complex proteins. Proc. Natl. Acad. Sci. USA 86, 9470–9474.

Scherer, M.T., Chan, B.M.C., Ria, F., Smith, J.A., Perkins, D.L. and Gefter, M.L. (1989). Control of cellular and humoral immune responses by peptides containing T-cell epitopes. Cold Spring Harbor Symp. Quant. Biol. 54, 497–504.

Schwartz, R.H. (1986). Immune response (Ir) genes of the murine major histocompatibility complex. Adv. Immunol. 38, 31–201.

Sedgwick, J.D. and Holt, P.G. (1985). Induction of IgE-secreting cells and IgE-isotype-specific suppressor T-cells in respiratory tract lymph nodes of rats exposed to an antigen aerosol. Cell. Immunol. 94, 182–194.

Shaw, C.-M., Alvord, E.C., Fahlberg, W.J. and Kies, M.W. (1962). Specificity of encephalitogen-induced inhibition of experimental "allergic" encephalomyelitis in the guinea pig. J. Immunol. 89, 54–61.

Sinigaglia, F., Guttinger, M., Kilgus, J., Doran, D.M., Matile, H., Etlinger, H., Trzeciak, A., Gillessen, D. and Pink, J.R.L. (1988). A malaria T-cell epitope recognized in association with most mouse and human MHC class II molecules. Nature (London) 336, 778–781.

Smilek, D.E., Wraith, D.C., Hodgkinson, S., Dwivedy, S., Steinman, L. and McDevitt, H.O. (1991). Prevention of experimental autoimmune encephalomyelitis with a myelin basic protein peptide analog. Proc. Natl. Acad. Sci. USA 88, 9633–9637.

Smith, S.C. and Allen, P.M. (1991). Myosin induced acute myocarditis is a T cell mediated disease. J. Immunol. 147, 2141–2147.

Steinman, L., Oksenberg, J.R. and Bernard, C.C.A. (1992). Association of susceptibility to multiple sclerosis with TCR genes. Immunol. Today 13, 49–51.

Stewart, G.A. and Holt, P.G. (1987). The immunogenicity and tolerogenicity of a major house dust mite allergen, *Der p* I, in mice and rats. Int. Arch. Allergy Appl. Immunol. 83, 44–51.

Thompson, H.S.G. and Staines, N.A. (1990). Could specific oral tolerance be a therapy for autoimmune disease? Immunol. Today. 11, 396–399.

Waldmann, H. (1989). Manipulation of T-cell responses with monoclonal antibodies. Annu. Rev. Immunol. 7, 407–444.

Wraith, D.C., Smilek, D.E., Mitchell, D.J., Steinman, L. and McDevitt, H.O. (1989a). Antigen recognition in autoimmune encephalomyelitis and the potential for peptide-mediated immunotherapy. Cell 59, 247–255.

Wraith, D.C., McDevitt, H.O., Steinman, L. and Acha-Orbea, H. (1989b). T cell recognition as the target for immune intervention in autoimmune disease. Cell 57, 709–715.

Yewdell, J.W. and Bennink, J.R. (1990). The binary logic of antigen processing. Cell 62, 203–206.

Zamvil, S.S. and Steinman, I. (1990). The T-lymphocyte in experimental allergic encephalomyelitis. Annu. Rev. Immunol. 8, 579–621.

Zubiaga, A.M., Munoz, A. and Huber, B.T. (1991). Super-induction of IL-2 gene transcription in the presence of cycloheximide. J. Immunol. 146, 3857–3863.

4. Monoclonal Antibody Therapy of Experimental Arthritis: Comparison with Cyclosporin A for Elucidating Cellular and Molecular Disease Mechanisms

M.E.J. Billingham

1. Introduction

A major goal of research in the field of RA and other inflammatory arthritic diseases is to discover a treatment which selectively inhibits arthritis progression yet leaves the host defence mechanisms intact. This requires an intimate knowledge of the cells and mediator molecules which initiate, maintain and, in some circumstances, remit the arthritic process. Such definitive clinical research is made difficult, however, when the time of onset of human arthritis is usually unknown. One way of circumventing such problems is to resort to the use of experimental models to investigate the cellular and molecular events responsible for arthritis, in spite of their general lack of precise homology to human RA. Such use of experimental models of arthritis for unravelling disease mechanisms and attaining the above therapeutic goal has been reviewed recently (Billingham, 1990) where it was apparent that selective disease-modifying therapy remains elusive despite the considerable strides forward made in our understanding of the arthritic process. Potential therapies need to be evaluated in the human diseases

Immunopharmacology of Joints and Connective Tissue
ISBN 0–12–206345–7

before the predictive value of models is ascertained. This process is slow, and discoveries made today will take up to a decade to be translated into a therapeutic entity when the conventional path to drug discovery is explored, perhaps even longer.

Biological molecules such as cytokines and particularly mAbs are, however, entering clinical evaluation much more rapidly and are providing both an answer as to their therapeutic effectiveness and greater insight into the pathogenesis of disease processes. This is happening while medicinal chemical entities designed to inhibit similar cellular and molecular activities, often discovered before the biological agent, wend their slow way through the due process of toxicological evaluation and subsequent agreement for clinical trial in man. Examples of this phenomenon are the evaluation of anti-CD4 mAbs in RA (see Chapter 6 of this volume and Horneff et al., 1991) and the use of IRAP which has progressed very rapidly from discovery in 1990 to therapeutic trials in man (Eisenberg et al., 1990).

Biological molecules such as mAbs have considerable advantage, therefore, over conventional therapy based on medicinal chemistry, by virtue of their potential for great specificity and, at present, very rapid progression to clinical experimentation in man. Even our most useful agent for suppressing the immune system, CSA, is regarded as crude in comparison with the specificity of mAbs. Of all current agents, they most nearly attain the status of Ehrlich's "magic bullet". They have disadvantages, of course, particularly in relation to host response against a foreign protein, such as mouse mAb. Additionally, some of the most effective in achieving an antiarthritic effect, such as anti-CD4 mAbs, do so in a manner that could potentially compromise host defence and surveillance mechanisms. To counteract these problems, the host anti-mAb response is being vigorously addressed in terms of humanizing the mAbs currently raised in the rat or mouse (Riechmann et al., 1988), and the latter may be overcome by selecting a mAb that is directed to a cell target specific for a particular disease.

At present, there appear to be two broad schools of thought. There are those who believe that the problems surrounding the clinical use of mAbs are so great that they will only be used as tools for unravelling disease mechanisms, enabling better direction of conventional medical chemistry approaches. Others, however, are convinced that the problems associated with host anti-mAb responsiveness will be circumvented by humanizing strategies and that problems inherent in those mAbs that may compromise host defence and surveillance are potentially avoidable by suitable dosing strategies, such as those adopted for cancer chemotherapy. Either way the prospects of better therapy emerging for crippling inflammatory arthritic diseases are enhanced now that mAbs are available for study, initially by enabling further dissection and understanding of the cellular and molecular mechanisms involved in experimental arthritis models and later through translation of the knowledge gained into human therapy.

Although not ideal in the eyes of many in terms of precise mimicry of human arthritic disease, experimental models of arthritis do reflect key aspects of the human conditions. Their known time-course, the facility to transfer arthritis to naive hosts and a shared sensitivity with the human diseases to certain therapeutic agents, particularly mAbs and CSA, underscore their usefulness in a quest for insight and eventual conquest of RA (Hunneyball et al., 1989; Billingham, 1990).

Our current knowledge of the effectiveness of antibody therapy against experimental arthritis began in the late 1960s. Curry and Ziff (1968) made the observation that polyclonal anti-rat lymphocyte serum, raised in rabbits, could block the development of classical adjuvant arthritis in the rat. It was later found that the anti-inflammatory activity of anti-lymphocyte serum resided in both an immunoglobulin and an α-globulin fraction of the serum (Billingham et al., 1970), and there the matter lay for well over a decade. The next reports of the value of antibody therapy in arthritis models, although this time mainly with mAbs, emerged in the mid-1980s from the studies of Wooley et al., (1985b) and Ranges et al., (1985) on the model of type II collagen-induced arthritis in the mouse, together with Larsson et al., (1985) working on adjuvant arthritis in the rat. These later studies followed naturally from a number of earlier studies using mAbs against a variety of autoimmune disease models including experimental myasthenia gravis (Waldor et al., 1983), experimental allergic encephalomyelitis (Steinman et al., 1981; Sriram and Steinman, 1983) and lupus disease in (NZB × NZW)F1 mice (Adelman et al., 1983).

Since the mid-1980s a relatively small number of reports have appeared which describe the effect of mAbs in models of arthritis, in comparison with their use for immunocytochemical identification of cells in situ or by FACS analysis. In vivo experimentation is not a trivial task when 1–2 g of a particular mAb, prepared from ascites, may be required for treatment of several groups of rats. Such studies are resource intensive and those directed to understanding events associated with natural remission can take months to complete. It is not too surprising, therefore, that such reports number between 5 and 10 per year, orders of magnitude fewer than those concerning any popular cytokine studied by in vitro methods. Notwithstanding the value of what is learnt from in vitro studies, it is impossible to add every required factor to the culture melting pot and certainly not in the right sequence and concentration to mimic an in vivo disease process. Unravelling the complexities of the cellular and molecular mechanisms responsible for induction, maintenance and remission of arthritis necessitates the use of in vivo experimental models. Hopefully this review will encourage others to take up the challenge to answer definitively which cells and what cytokines dictate the various phases of arthritis.

Whilst several models of arthritis have been described in a number of rodent species, rabbits and occasionally larger mammals (see Billingham (1990) for review), studies involving the therapeutic use of mAbs have been largely restricted to the mouse model of type II collagen-induced arthritis, its counterpart in the rat, classical adjuvant arthritis, and the arthritis induced in the rat by SCWs. Most studies have investigated the effectiveness of mAbs directed against T lymphocyte antigens such as CD4, MHC gene products and IL-2R. A few studies have addressed the mechanisms associated with non-responsiveness and natural remission, again mostly in terms of T lymphocyte involvement. The macrophage, however, has essentially been neglected despite a proposed pivotal role in the maintenance of RA (Firestein and Zvaifler, 1990) and the recent discovery that erosive arthritis can occur through macrophage/mesenchymal interaction in the absence of T lymphocyte involvement (Shiozawa et al., 1992).

This chapter will discuss the therapeutic use of mAbs in experimental models of arthritis, plus their use in targeting cytotoxic agents to activated T lymphocytes involved in the arthritic process. Induction of tolerance to arthritis development with mAbs and their value in elucidating cells involved in the natural remission of arthritis will also be reviewed. Comparison will be made with the effect of CSA in the same experimental models where this has added to the understanding of disease mechanisms.

2.   Therapeutic Use of mAbs

Only a few of the available models of arthritis that are available (Billingham, 1990) have been used for studying the effect of mAbs. Such studies that have been performed are confined to the mouse and the rat. For the mouse this is essentially the type II collagen-induced model, although the flare up of antigen-induced arthritis has been investigated with mAbs (van den Broek et al., 1986). Type II collagen-induced arthritis in the rat has been investigated but to a much lesser degree than classical rat adjuvant arthritis induced by heat-killed Mycobacterium tuberculosis. Other models in the rat, such as SCW-induced arthritis and that induced by the non-immunogenic adjuvant "Avridene" (a lipoidal amine, Pfizer), have undergone limited investigation.

By far the most attention has been paid to the effect of anti-CD4 mAbs directed to T-helper lymphocytes and anti-Ia (MHC Class II) on antigen-presenting cells. mAbs to IL-2R and pan-T mAbs have attracted limited attention, as has the $\alpha\beta$ TCR, and, to date, there has only been one report of an effect of an anti-adhesion molecule mAb (to ICAM-1) in an arthritis model (Iigo et al., 1991).

In relation to the cellular interactions involved in the induction of a variety of models of arthritis, the most popular view is that of T lymphocyte interaction with an antigen-presenting cell leading to cell-mediated reactivity, although for many models the initiating antigen is unknown, with the exception of those induced by collagen. Springer (1990) has illustrated the main molecular interactions involved in this process (see Fig. 4.1), although there are other peripheral interactions which modulate the overall reactivity, for example with cytokines and their receptors such as IL-2/IL-2R.

It is now clear that a number of mAbs can interfere with the initiation of arthritis, and that several cell surface receptors/molecules are involved in the process. This, in itself, suggests a variety of therapeutic approaches towards treatment of arthritis, and certain of these are being evaluated in the clinic.

The effects of mAbs in the arthritis models will be discussed initially for the mouse and then for the various rat models where studies have included attempts to

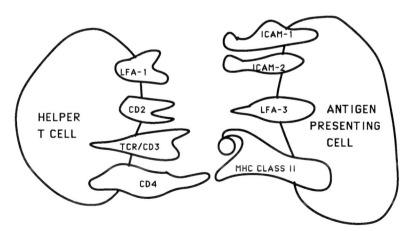

Figure 4.1 Molecular interactions involved in MHC class II-restricted antigen presentation to helper T lymphocytes. After Springer (1990).

elucidate disease mechanisms more comprehensively than with the mouse. Induction and measurement of the progression of arthritis in the models discussed here are not given in detail as these aspects have been described in a recent review (Billingham, 1990).

2.1 TYPE II COLLAGEN-INDUCED ARTHRITIS IN THE MOUSE

This model was originally described by Courtenay et al., (1980) and was subsequently found to be restricted to a small number of mouse strains (Wooley et al., 1981, 1985a). Susceptibility was found to be related to the MHC, as only mouse strains with the H-2^q and H-2^r locus developed arthritis (Wooley et al., 1981, 1985a); furthermore, this locus was associated with a high antibody response to type II collagen. Mapping of the H-2^q locus linked arthritis susceptibility to the I^q region leading Wooley et al. (1981) to postulate that Ia antigens on macrophages of I^q strains could effectively present type II collagen peptide antigens in such a fashion as to trigger an anti-self response leading to arthritis. The most antigenic epitopes of type II collagen for both cell-mediated and humoral responsiveness reside in the CB11 peptide (Andersson et al., 1991), and recognition of these arthritogenic epitopes is suggested to reside within Vβ gene segments coded on the TCR β chain (Chiocchia et al., 1991; Mori et al., 1992).

Initial experiments with mAbs probed the interaction between antigen-presenting cells and T lymphocytes responsible for class II MHC-restricted functions (Wooley et al., 1985b; Ranges et al., 1985).

2.1.1 mAbs Directed Towards T Lymphocytes

GK1.5 is a rat anti-mouse antibody that defines the L3T4 antigen (i.e. CD4) on the surface of T cells involved in MHC class II-restricted functions. Using GK1.5, Ranges et al. (1985) conducted an elegant series of experiments to define the role of these CD4+ T cells in collagen-induced arthritis. Two protocols were used to examine the effect of GK1.5 either on the induction of arthritis or when there was a vigorous response to collagen but no visible signs of arthritis. Both protocols caused a greater than 90% depletion of circulating L3T4+ T cells and also within lymph nodes and spleen; these returned to normal levels by 1 month after the last dose of GK1.5. A significant decrease in incidence and delay in onset of arthritis associated with markedly lowered IgG antibody titre to type II collagen was seen when the mAb was given the day before collagen immunization and the day after at 100 μg/mouse, followed by a further 100 μg at 14-day intervals until day 45, the normal time of arthritis development. Incidence dropped from 9/10 to 2/10 and the onset occurred at day 80 for the GK1.5-treated mice. If, however, the antibody was given at day 28 and 45 or days 23–50, at 100 μg/day per mouse, there was no

significant difference from control mice in terms of arthritis development. Ranges et al. (1985) concluded that L3T4+ helper T lymphocytes played an important role in the initiation of type II collagen-induced arthritis and in the generation of anti-(type II collagen) antibodies, but viewed the lack of effect of GK1.5 when given after day 23 as evidence that CD4 helper T lymphocytes were not particularly involved in the progression of arthritis.

A little later, Hom et al. (1988) re-addressed the role of CD4 helper T cells in the chronicity of type II collagen-induced arthritis in mice. They questioned whether the earlier experiments had produced sufficient depletion of this subset to prevent arthritis progression, a point conceded by Ranges et al. (1985). Hom et al. (1988) confirmed the previous results that GK1.5, the anti-L3T4 (CD4) mAb, was very effective against the induction phase of arthritis, using a protocol which involved giving 500 μg of antibody to mice on days −8, −4, 0, 7 and then twice a week for 1–2 months after collagen immunization. This reduced the L3T4+ population to less than 1% of normal levels in these mice, i.e. a more profound depletion than that produced by Ranges et al. (1985); in these circumstances incidence of arthritis was zero and no anti-collagen antibodies were detected. Such vigorous depleting regimes were, however, again unable to exert any effect against the established arthritis; in this instance, the mice were regrouped when the first signs of arthritis appeared, before treatment with anti-CD4 (GK1.5) commenced. Interestingly, Hom and her colleagues (1988) found that polyclonal anti-lymphocyte serum raised in rabbits caused a depletion in the L3T4+, Ly-2+ and Thy-1+ lymphocyte populations and reduced the severity of established collagen-induced arthritis in their mice, so they reasoned that some subset(s) of T cells alone, or in combination, was responsible for the disease chronicity.

Using the earlier experimental design of grouping mice with obvious signs of disease before treatment, neither depletion of Ly-2+ lymphocytes (a subset with cytotoxic activity) nor combined depletion of Ly-2+ and L3T4+ lymphocytes had any effect on progression of established arthritis. Hom et al. (1988) also looked at the effectiveness of anti-Thy-1 mAb, which defines a cell surface antigen on all mouse T cells, both alone and in combination with the anti-L3T4 mAb GK1.5. GK1.5 was combined with anti-Thy-1 in this instance for its ability, as an anti-CD4 mAb, to induce tolerance to both itself and anti-Thy-1, thereby enabling long periods of dosing without inducing an anti-rat IgG response in recipient mice (Benjamin and Waldmann, 1986). Anti-Thy-1 alone and in combination with GK1.5 (1 mg and 400 μg respectively, twice weekly for 1 month) both produced a complete depletion of Thy-1+ T lymphocytes, but only the combination inhibited the progression of the arthritis. The only other treatment found to prevent progression of established arthritis by Hom et al. (1988)

was high-dose CSA, at 50 and 75 mg/kg given daily. None of the above treatment regimens against the established arthritis, either antibodies or CSA, however, had a significant effect on antibody levels against type II collagen, regardless of an inhibitory effect against arthritis progression. The authors concluded that, whilst CD4+ T lymphocytes were vital for induction of arthritis, the progression of established disease involved a population expressing the pan-T marker, Thy-1. However, although T cell involvement in progression was implicated, additionally, by the sensitivity of established arthritis to CSA, this was at the very high dose levels of 50 and 75 mg/kg, virtually an order of magnitude higher than those used in the rat or man; at such levels a non-specific effect of the drug cannot be ruled out.

In relation to disease maintenance, it is now being realized that additional mechanisms, largely involving the macrophage, may be involved in the chronicity of arthritis, but at the time of the above studies, up to 1988, the omnipotence of T cells in human rheumatoid disease had yet to be challenged by Firestein and Zvaifler (1990). Furthermore, the studies of Shiozawa et al. (1992), demonstrating erosive arthritis development in transgenic mice overexpressing c-fos but without lymphocyte involvement locally within lesion sites, remained to be described. Chronicity of even mouse collagen arthritis is unlikely, therefore, to be totally dominated by the T cell and, when extrapolating to potential human therapy, it is equally unlikely that the degree of T cell depletion demonstrated to be necessary for success against established mouse arthritis (Hom et al., 1988) could ever be contemplated to be safe for man.

2.1.2   mAbs against the TCR

The finding that anti-CD4 mAbs could prevent the induction of type II collagen-induced arthritis in mice, inferring a T-cell-mediated pathology, led to the investigation of the TCR repertoire involved in the disease by several groups. Such studies were also encouraged by the earlier success of anti-V_β mAb therapy in the mouse model of EAE (Acha-Orbea et al., 1988; Burns et al., 1989), and that resistance to arthritis in SWR mice may be due to the genomic deletion of 50% of the V_β genes in this mouse strain (Banerjee et al., 1988a). The advantage of targeting the TCR, particularly specific chains, is that this approach may be less broadly immunosuppressive than targeting CD4 or Ia, as is also argued for the IL-2R on activated T lymphocytes (see below).

Goldschmidt et al. (1990) reported on the effect of rat mAbs directed to mouse V_β6 (44.22.1) and V_β8.1,2. (KJ16). Both antibodies produced a marked reduction in lymph node T cells bearing V_β6 and V_β8, particularly when given in combination with a mouse anti-rat kappa mAb (MAR 18.5) at a dose of 100 μg per mouse. Despite the fact, however, that a profound depletion of T cells bearing the respective TCR V_β antigens could be achieved at this level of mAb treatment, no effect was seen against

the development of type II collagen-induced arthritis. The antibodies were given as a single administration 1 h after immunization with collagen. In contrast, a mAb to CD4 (GK 1.5) efficiently abrogated development of arthritis, thereby providing a positive control for Goldschmidt et al. (1990).

Using the same mAbs to the above V_β antigens, but this time at much higher levels, Chiocchia et al. (1991) were able to profoundly inhibit arthritis development in the mouse. Their protocol involved administration of mAbs, 500 μg per mouse, 1 day before immunization with collagen and again at day 22 afterwards. mAbs to V_β2, 3, 5, 6, 8 and 11 were evaluated. mAb treatment produced a profound and long-lasting depletion of T cells bearing the respective TCR V_β chains (apart from V_β3), some of which had not returned to normal levels 90 days later. The most effective mAb at preventing development of arthritis was the anti-V_β8 (KJ16), which essentially prevented the appearance of arthritic symptoms. Anti-V_β2 and -V_β5 had a partial effect on incidence and time of onset, but mAbs against V_β6 and V_β11 were ineffective. Where mAbs were effective against development of arthritis, they also reduced the titre of anti-collagen antibodies. These studies narrowed down the potential CD4+ T lymphocyte population of the mouse to a minor arthritogenic V_β8+ subset which reacts, most likely, with an epitope(s) on the CB11 fragment of type II collagen.

The results of Chiocchia et al. (1991) emphasize the need to produce an adequate depletion, or inhibition of function, of the T cells in order to exert an effect against arthritis development. It is also interesting to observe that very few groups investigate mAbs in a pharmacological dose–response manner, which would eliminate some of the discrepancies in the literature. Overall, these results argue in favour of a limited expression of TCR V regions by arthritogenic clones of T cells, and in this respect reflect a similar circumstance in EAE where most encephalitic clones bear a V_β8.2 TCR (Burns et al., 1989).

2.1.3   mAbs against the IL-2R

The value of the IL-2R as a therapeutic target is that it is essentially expressed on the surface of activated T lymphocytes (Robb et al., 1981; Malek and Korty, 1986), although there are reports of its expression on both human (Hancock et al., 1987a) and rat macrophages (Hancock et al., 1987b). Targeting CD4 and Ia antigens, although effective therapeutically, has the potential disadvantage of broad immunosuppression of all immune responses, as these antigens are constitutively expressed (Banerjee et al., 1988a). Early experiments had shown that anti-IL-2R mAbs could prolong both cardiac (Kirkman et al., 1985) and skin allograft survival in mice (Granstein et al., 1986), so the stage was set for investigation of these mAbs in a wide range of autoimmune diseases.

Banerjee *et al.*, (1988b) used an IgM anti-IL-2R mAb, 7D4, raised in the rat, which bound to a site on the mouse IL-2R distinct from the IL-2-binding site, yet suppressed IL-2-driven T cell proliferation. A dose of 200 μg of this mAb was administered to mice daily from day −1 to 6 after challenge with type II collagen, with the aim of modulating the effectiveness of T cells expressing the IL-2R. This was found to lower the incidence of arthritis by about 50% and the severity, although the time of onset was not significantly affected. Total antibody to type II collagen was also reduced at day 14 after challenge, although this effect was lost by day 28, i.e. before arthritis had appeared. IgG2a and IgG2b were the isotypes most inhibited, these being the classes with the greatest association with arthritis severity (Watson and Townes, 1985) and which had been noted earlier by Wooley *et al.* (1985b) to be affected by anti-Ia mAbs used to inhibit arthritis.

In relation to the mechanism of arthritis inhibition afforded by anti-IL-2R mAb treatment, the authors suggested certain possibilities. mAb 7D4 could have caused a downregulation of T cell help to B cells involved in generating pathogenic anti-collagen antibodies, but these had reached control levels by day 28, before the arthritis was evident. Alternatively, the mAb could have suppressed effector T cell function and inhibited inflammatory lymphokine production within the mouse joints, or it could have caused the deletion of activated T cells bearing the IL-2R, by complement activation, antibody-dependent T cell cytotoxicity or phagocytosis by the reticuloendothelial system. Inhibition of IL-2 binding to its receptor was clearly not the mechanism involved in preventing arthritis.

The problem noted by Banerjee *et al.* (1988b) was that the mice developed anti-rat IgM antibodies by day 14 after the first administration, thereby negating the long-term use of anti-IL-2R therapy without some tolerizing protocol.

2.1.4   mAbs against MHC class II (anti-Ia)

The major study on the effect of anti-Ia sera on type II collagen-induced arthritis in mice has been that of Wooley and his colleagues (1985b). Earlier work by this group (Wooley *et al.* 1981, 1983) had shown that high antibody responses to type II collagen were associated with disease incidence and severity and that this antibody response was under immunoreactive gene control. Noting that susceptibility was associated with the $H-2^q$ I region and that the species source of type II collagen could also influence susceptibility, i.e. $H-2^r$ strains respond to bovine and not chick type II collagen, they investigated both polyclonal and monoclonal antibodies to relevant Ia antigens for suppression or a delay in the onset of arthritis; antisera to an irrelevant haplotype/s were also investigated.

Woolley and his co-workers (1985b) investigated two strains of mice which were respectively susceptible to chick type II collagen, B10. Q ($H-2^q$, I-A), or bovine type II collagen, B10. RIII ($H-2^r$, I-E). The Ia antigens expressed by the B10.Q mice were Ia 3, 5, 9, 10, 13 and 16, and those expressed by B10.RIII were 1, 3, 5, 7, 12, 17, 19, 22 and 24. Both polyclonal and monoclonal antibodies were obtained against some of these antigens and were given to mice at a level of 1−3 mg per mouse just before immunization with collagen.

For the B10.Q strain, polyclonal antisera to Ia 10 and 16 significantly reduced the incidence of arthritis, as did a mAB to I^q. Antibodies to irrelevant haplotypes, i.e. Ia 7, which is strongly expressed in the B10. RIII strain, were without effect on arthritis development in B10. Q mice. In the B10. RIII strain, a polyclonal antibody against Ia 1, 3, 7 profoundly inhibited the incidence of arthritis, and mAbs against the Ia 7(I) antigen were also effective. Antisera to other Ia 7 antigens and irrelevant Ia haplotypes were ineffective. Interestingly a mAb to Ia 22 induced 100% incidence and an earlier onset of arthritis together with a significant increase in antibody titre to type II collagen in the B10. RIII strain; clearly, not all antisera are protective!

Where Ia antibodies were protective against arthritis development, the onset was also delayed, and it was also noted that titres of antibody against type II collagen were generally lower than those in the arthritic control mice. This effect against anti-collagen antibodies was only apparent at day 14 after collagen immunization, becoming equivalent to the levels in control arthritic mice by day 28, as was also the case with anti-IL-2R treatment (above). These results are essentially in agreement with earlier studies of anti-Ia effects in EAE in which suppression of disease is associated with a reduction of antibody titres to myelin basic protein (Steinman *et al.*, 1981; Sriram and Steinman, 1983), although the overall effect of anti-Ia against collagen-induced arthritis was not as profound or long-lasting as that seen in other autoimmune diseases, e.g. EAE (Sriram and Steinman, 1983), experimental myasthenia gravis (Waldor *et al.*, 1983) or renal involvement in murine lupus (Adelman *et al.*, 1983).

In a later series of experiments, Cooper *et al.* (1988) evaluated the effect of a mAb, M5/114.15.2, which recognizes an allodeterminant shared between the two types of class II histocompatibility molecules (I-A and I-E) expressed by mice carrying the $H-2^{q, b, d, k, r}$ haplotypes; in this respect M5/114.15.2 encompassed all the haplotypes selectively targetted in the studies of Wooley *et al.* (1985b). Cooper *et al.* (1988) varied the time of administration of their mAb and also investigated the effect of enhancing the induction of Ia on synovial cells, by murine recombinant interferonγ (murine rINFγ) administration, on arthritic disease incidence and severity in their mice. Mice were either given 1 mg of M5 on day −2 and at days 3 and 10 after immunization with type II collagen, or on days 14, 21 and 28 after immunization to determine any effect against the arthritis. Only the protocol involving administration of M5 at the time of collagen immunization inhibited arthritis development; the later protocol was without effect. M5, as used, caused a modest depletion of Ia-positive cells, and, when this lowered the incidence and delayed the time of onset of arthritis, the titre of anti-collagen antibodies was also lowered.

Cooper *et al.* (1988) concluded that Ia-expressing cells played an important role in the initiation of type II collagen-induced arthritis in the mouse, although anti-Ia mAbs were only effective when given at the time of immunization. This was reinforced by experiments involving administration of murine rINFγ before challenge with collagen; this upregulated Ia expression on synovial and other cells and was associated with an enhanced incidence and earlier onset of arthritis, although it had no effect on anti-collagen antibody titres. The authors suggested that the effect of anti-Ia on arthritis was unlikely to be due to an influence on antibody production but that it may have affected antigen presentation at relevant sites.

2.2 POLYARTHRITIS MODELS IN THE RAT

A diverse collection of materials, both antigenic and non-antigenic, leads to the expression of polyarthritis in the rat which tends to have a broadly similar histopathology, regardless of the initiating arthritogen (Billingham, 1990). Pannus tissue forms within many of the articulating joints of the fore and hind feet leading to destruction of cartilage and bone in a manner similar to that seen in human rheumatoid arthritis, although over a period of just a few weeks. However, the most prominent reaction is a periostitis outside the joint, which occurs at sites of ligament and muscle insertion, resulting in bone loss and massive new bone and osteoid formation along the areas of periosteal reactivity; there is also profound bone removal and re-formation within the tarsal, metatarsals, carpals and metacarpals and other small bones of the wrists and feet. Similar bone remodelling also occurs in the spine, scapulae and skull, again at sites of ligament and muscle insertion.

This reactivity can be induced by many species of mycobacteria, certain streptococcal species, *Nocardia asteroides* and *Corynebacterium rubrum*, and is due to the peptidoglycan fraction which can be extracted from all these species and other Gram-positive bacteria. The key element for mycobacteria appears to be MDP (Kohashi *et al.*, 1980), which is non-antigenic, unlike the peptidoglycans and whole cell walls, but can induce an arthritis essentially identical with that produced by the intact mycobacteria, their cell walls and peptidoglycans. Most of these materials need to be suspended in an oil vehicle and injected intradermally to induce arthritis (see review by Billingham (1990) for details of the precise

methodology). A non-antigenic synthetic interferon inducer, CP20961 (Avridene, Pfizer: *NN*-dioctadecyl-*N′N′*-bis(2-hydroxyethyl)propanediamine), also induces a polyarthritis "morphologically identical" with classical adjuvant arthritis induced by mycobacteria (Chang *et al.*, 1980). Types II and XI collagens evoke a polyarthritis which has a similar histopathological appearance to the other polyarthritic models in the rat, involving considerable periostitis and new bone formation. It is a possibility, therefore, that a common pathological process is triggered in the rat by all these various arthritogenic materials. mAbs, particularly anti-CD4, have helped considerably to determine whether these materials all trigger arthritis via the same pathway, as well as demonstrating which cells are critical in the induction and remission of these models of polyarthritis in the rat.

2.2.1 Classical Adjuvant Arthritis

Adjuvant arthritis, the first and most extensively studied model of polyarthritis, was discovered nearly 40 years ago by Stoerk and his colleagues (1954) as an experimental accident. Whilst trying to produce immunity to spleen extracts emulsified in Freund's adjuvant, an arthritis developed in the immunized rats. This was later shown to be due solely to the mycobacterial component of Freund's adjuvant (Pearson, 1956). Newbould (1963) subsequently developed the model as a screening test for antirheumatic drugs, and it has remained popular ever since as a potential indicator of drug activity against RA in man.

Since that time, considerable progress has been made in our understanding of the pathogenesis of this experimental arthritis. Mention has already been made of the similarity of the histopathology of the disease produced by mycobacteria and MDP, the ultimate fragment with adjuvant properties. The key early experiments directed towards unravelling the disease process and its underlying mechanisms were those of Kohashi *et al.* (1980) who demonstrated the arthritogenicity of non-antigenic materials such as MDP, the ultimate fragment of mycobacteria, and Chang *et al.* (1980) with the synthetic adjuvant CP20961. These experiments brought into question the relevance of antigenic epitopes on mycobacterial cell walls, and the peptidoglycans contained within them, for the induction of arthritis. Comparison of the effect of MDP in euthymic rats with that in their athymic littermates demonstrated that the full polyarthritic syndrome, involving extensive periostitis, only developed in the euthymic rats (Kohashi *et al.*, 1982), clearly establishing a role for thymus-primed (T) lymphocytes in the pathogenesis of arthritis. T lymphocyte involvement was elegantly substantiated by the adoptive transfer of arthritis to naive hosts with lymphocytes obtained from rats primed with myco-bacteria or the non-antigenic arthritogen, CP20961 (Taurog *et al.*, 1983); such lymphocytes were of the CD4+ helper subset. Finally, the work of Holoshitz *et al.* (1983), demonstrating that T lymphocyte lines derived from rats primed with mycobacterial adjuvant could induce arthritis, further emphasized the requirement of T lymphocytes for establishment of classical adjuvant arthritis. All that remained was for anti-CD4 mAbs to finally confirm the T lymphocyte dependence of these models (see below).

One final point on pathogenesis should be discussed before describing the effects of mAbs in the various models of polyarthritis in the rat. This relates to the fact that non-antigenic materials such as MDP and CP20961 can induce an arthritis essentially identical with that produced by antigenic arthritogens, e.g. peptidoglycan and mycobacteria. This suggests that the arthritic antigen is an endogenous epitope, which may, amongst many other candidates, potentially be related to a bacterial antigen. Van Eden and his colleagues (1988) have suggested that this may reside on the cartilage link protein, which binds proteoglycan to hyaluronic acid in the cartilage matrix, as one nonapeptide epitope shares sequence homology with a peptide on a 65 kDa HSP in mycobacteria. They further showed that this small peptide epitope induced proliferation of their arthritogenic T lymphocyte lines. Interestingly, however, immunization with the 65 kDa HSP or the epitope did not induce arthritis but, in fact, induced non-responsiveness to arthritis induction (van Eden *et al.*, 1988, Billingham *et al.*, 1990a); this is also the case with SCW-induced arthritis where pre-immunization with HSP induces a state of non-responsiveness (van den Broek *et al.*, 1989). It appears, therefore, that some other endogenous antigen is the target for the arthritogenic T lymphocytes induced by a variety of adjuvants and other materials; these remain to be identified, however.

2.2.2   mAb Therapy of the Rat Polyarthritis Models

In view of the fact that a similar polyarthritis can be induced in the rat by all the above materials, at least when analysed histopathologically, it is convenient to discuss the antiarthritic effects of mAbs to cell surface antigens on T cells and antigen-presenting cells collectively, rather than deal separately with each mAb in each of the individual models. By and large the effect of the mAbs is broadly similar in each model, and it is only when tolerance is addressed that real differences emerge (see below). Historically, the first report of mAb effects in rat polyarthritis was that of Larsson and his colleagues (1985), who reported on the properties of anti-pan T and anti-CD8 (cytotoxic/suppressor) mAbs to T lymphocytes in classical adjuvant arthritis. Since then, between 10 and 20 papers have reported results with mAbs against models of polyarthritis in the rat.

2.2.3   mAbs Directed to T Lymphocytes

Undoubtedly the most effective mAbs at inhibiting the development of the rat polyarthritis models are those directed against the CD4 cell surface molecule-bearing subset, also known as helper T lymphocytes. Billingham and his colleagues (1990b) have studied these mAbs in both classical adjuvant arthritis and that induced by CP20961 and also the type II collagen-induced model of polyarthritis; in addition, these mAbs have been investigated against SCW-induced arthritis by van den Broek *et al.* (1992). Both groups used the anti-CD4 mAbs W3/25 (IgG1) and/or OX35 (IgG2a), originally obtained from the Oxford collection of murine mAbs directed against rat cell surface lymphocyte antigens.

The effect of the anti-CD4 mAb, OX35, against the development of classical mycobacterium-induced arthritis is shown in Fig. 4.2. OX35 was given intraperitoneally at three levels, i.e. in a dose–response manner, just before administration of the mycobacterial arthritogen (day 0) and at days 3 and 6 afterwards. At the level of 3 mg per rat, essentially no symptoms of arthritis developed in the treated rats, although, at the lower levels, some arthritis developed, particularly at 0.75 mg of mAb per rat. A dose of 3 mg of OX35 was sufficient to completely remove circulating CD4+ cells from the peripheral circulation, and these did not return to normal levels until some 10 days after the last OX35 treatment. Even with the return of CD4+ cells, no arthritis was ever seen to develop despite the persistence of arthritogenic mycobacteria in the rats (Billingham *et al.*, 1990b). Very similar results were obtained with W3/25, an IgG1

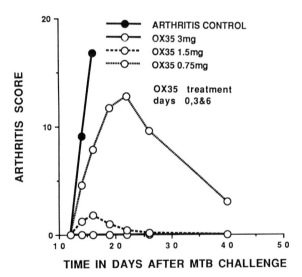

Figure 4.2 Dose–response of the anti-CD4 mAb, OX35, against classical adjuvant arthritis induced by mycobacteria in oil (*M. tuberculosis*, MTB). The anti-CD4 mAb produced a dose-related inhibition of arthritis development in much the same manner as standard antiarthritic drugs. The arthritis was scored as described in Billingham *et al.* (1990a). Note the onset of natural remission after day 23 in the low-dose OX35 group. This and all the experiments described below were performed in the Lewis rat.

isotype, although this mAb was marginally less potent than OX35 (Billingham *et al.*, unpublished observations); again the most profound effects on arthritis development were obtained with fully CD4+ cell-depleting levels of the mAb.

Using a very similar protocol of anti-CD4 mAb treatment to that used by Billingham *et al.* (1990b), van den Broek and her colleagues (1992) were successful in preventing the development of SCW-induced arthritis in Lewis rats. This model is initiated following intraperitoneal administration of a peptidoglycan extract of SCW in phosphate-buffered saline. A dose of 4 mg of W3/25 given to rats at the time of SCW immunization and 3 days later essentially prevented the appearance of arthritic symptoms in their rats, when compared with control rats and others given similar amounts of an isotype control mAb of irrelevant specificity. This level of W3/25 reduced the CD4+ lymphocyte population within the spleen to less than 2% of the normal value, again demonstrating the need for marked depletion of cells to achieve a profound antiarthritic effect. CD4+ lymphocyte levels returned to normal at day 19 of the experiment, i.e. similar to the experience of Billingham *et al.* (1990b), and again there was no appearance of arthritic symptoms despite the continuing presence of SCW. For both mycobacteria- and SCW-induced arthritis models, inhibition of arthritis development by anti-CD4 therapy appeared to be associated with induction of tolerance/non-responsiveness to the inducing arthritogen.

Figure 4.3 shows the effect of mAb OX35 on the development of arthritis induced by the synthetic non-antigenic adjuvant, CP20961 (5 mg of this adjuvant dissolved in paraffin oil produces an arthritis equivalent to that seen with 250 μg of heat-killed mycobacteria). The result was essentially the same as that seen with the mycobacterial model, with the anti-CD4 mAb producing a dose-related inhibition of arthritis development which was similarly dependent on the level of CD4+ cell depletion. This adjuvant, however, does not persist within the rat, so that when the CD4+ cells returned to normal levels, there would be little opportunity for arthritis to develop, even more so as CP20961 is non-antigenic. This experiment could not show that tolerance to CP20961-induced arthritis had been induced by anti-CD4 therapy; this would require rechallenge with CP20961, the initiating arthritogen (see below in Section 3, on tolerance induction).

Finally, with reference to anti-CD4 mAbs, the poly-arthritis induced by type II collagen in the rat can be totally inhibited by such therapy (Billingham *et al.*, 1990b). In this instance, arthritis was induced by injecting 2 mg of bovine type II collagen in incomplete Freund's adjuvant into the base of the tail. A dose of 3 mg of OX35 given on days 0, 3 and 6 prevented the disease from developing as shown in Fig. 4.4; interestingly the rats with collagen-induced arthritis rapidly underwent natural remission around day 26, a phenomenon also seen with both classical adjuvant arthritis and that induced by CP20961 in the Lewis rat used (Billingham *et al.*, 1990b).

The only other circumstance in which anti-CD4 therapy has been investigated is with the adoptive

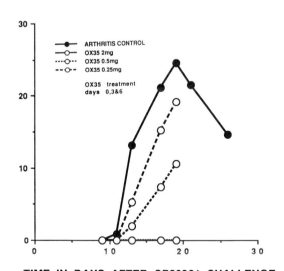

Figure 4.3 Dose–response of the anti-CD4 mAb, OX35, against adjuvant arthritis induced by a lipoidal amine CP20961 (Avridene). Note again the onset of natural remission in the control group which is characteristic of this strain of Lewis rat.

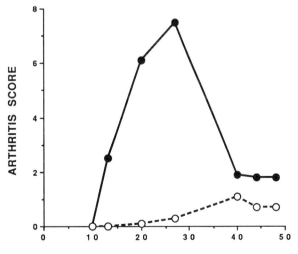

Figure 4.4 Effect of the anti-CD4 mAb, OX35, against type II collagen-induced arthritis in the Lewis rat. This arthritis is essentially confined to the hind feet. Note that natural remission also occurs with this model of arthritis. •, Arthritis control; ○, OX35 3 mg. OX35 treatment was given on days 0, 3 and 6.

transfer of arthritis using arthritogenic T lymphocytes from either mycobacteria- or CP20961-primed rats (Taurog *et al.*, (1983) for methodology). OX35 given on the day of transfer and 3 and 6 days later completely prevented the development of this adoptively transferred disease (Fig. 4.5); again this level of antibody treatment totally depleted the circulating CD4+ cell population (Billingham *et al.*, 1990b). No arthritis developed in these rats when CD4+ cells returned to normal levels, unlike the situation below when the established arthritis was treated with anti-CD4.

The effect of anti-CD4 on established rat polyarthritis, regardless of the initiating arthritogen, has not been so profound as that seen when the mAbs are given prophylactically. van den Broek *et al.* (1992) noted an effect with W3/25 given to rats with established SCW-induced arthritis, and Billingham *et al.* (1990b) found that OX35 lowered the arthritis score in rats with adoptively transferred arthritis as shown in Fig. 4.5. In the case of adoptively transferred disease, the arthritis rebounded at the end of treatment and was associated with the reappearance of CD4+ cells in the circulation; it would appear that once arthritis has developed, a memory system is set up which utilizes CD4+ helper T lymphocytes for maintenance of the arthritis. Alternatively, the administration of anti-CD4 at an early stage of the established arthritis may have compromised the development of natural remission, as this may also reside in a CD4+ cell population (see below in Section 4).

In stark contrast with the effectiveness of anti-CD4 mAbs in the treatment of various rat polyarthritis

models, anti-CD8 mAbs directed to the cytotoxic/suppressor subset have been totally without effect (Larsson *et al.*, 1985; Billingham *et al.*, 1990b). Both these groups used the anti-CD8 mAb, OX8, at various dose levels and differing time periods during development of adjuvant arthritis, and, despite the fact that peripheral blood, spleen, lymph nodes and arthritic lesion sites were depleted of CD8+ lymphocytes, there was no effect on the disease process. Clearly CD8+ T cells are not involved in the development of this model of arthritis. Anti-pan T mAbs such as W3/13 (Larsson *et al.*, 1985) and OX52 (Billingham *et al.*, 1990b), which target all T lymphocytes, were found to delay the onset of adjuvant arthritis when given over the period 0–10 days after adjuvant challenge, but the arthritis subsequently escaped with the arthritic scores approaching untreated control values. In one experiment, Larsson *et al.* (1985) treated their rats with W3/13 every 5 days until day 30 after adjuvant challenge and in this instance just one of the five rats so treated developed a mild arthritis. Thus anti-pan T mAbs may be able to achieve the same degree of effectiveness as anti-CD4, but this requires further substantiation.

Before leaving the subject of mAbs against T lymphocytes, mention should be made of a mAb against T lymphoblasts; this is the work of Schluesener and his colleagues (1986). They developed an antibody to a cell surface antigen which is expressed on a minority of rat T cells late on in the process of lymphocyte activation. This antibody pta-3 recognizes an antigen thought to be equivalent to the Ta1 antigen which is found on the surface of a minor subset of activated T cells in patients with multiple sclerosis (Hafler *et al.*, 1986). Normally, less than 1% of peripheral blood T cells, lymph node cells and thymocytes are pta-3 positive, but this increases to 10–15% after antigen or mitogen stimulation. A dose of 600 μg of pta-3 given to Lewis rats on days 1, 7 and 10 after mycobacterial adjuvant administration essentially inhibited the development of adjuvant arthritis, without having any obvious effect on other T cell subset numbers such as CD4. This antibody regimen was also effective against EAE, and a single treatment at day 11 also prevented the development of neurological symptoms (Schluesener *et al.*, 1986). The authors considered that their more selective approach to immunotherapy, by targeting activation antigens, would be more applicable than one against constitutively expressed cell surface antigens. This sentiment is also expressed by those who favour targeting the IL-2R.

2.2.4   mAbs against the TCR

Attention was focused on the rat TCR shortly after Hunig and his colleagues (1989) developed a mAb to a constant determinant on the antigen receptor for T lymphocyte activation. This antibody, R73, reacts with the $\alpha\beta$ TCR and has been investigated for an antiarthritic effect in several rat polyarthritis models. Adjuvant

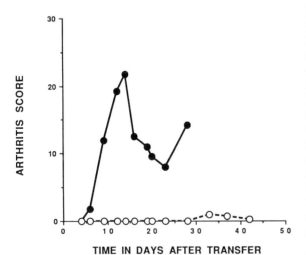

Figure 4.5 Effect of the anti-CD4 mAb, OX35, against adoptively transferred arthritis using arthritogenic T lymphocytes. Prophylactic and therapeutic treatment were both effective, but rebound occurred following treatment of the established arthritis. •, Transfer control (2 mg OX35 on days 13, 15, 17 and 19); ○, 2 mg OX35 on days 0, 3 and 6.

arthritis has been studied by Yoshino *et al.* (1990a,b), type II collagen-induced arthritis by Goldschmidt and Holmdahl (1991) and Yoshino *et al.* (1991b) and finally the model of SCW-induced arthritis by Yoshino *et al.* (1991a). The development of all these models of polyarthritis can be inhibited by prophylactic treatment with R73, and the established diseases of both adjuvant arthritis and type II collagen arthritis can be diminished.

Initial experiments by Yoshino *et al.* (1990a) with adjuvant arthritis demonstrated that 2 mg of R73 given on days 15, 18 and 21 after *M. tuberculosis* administration could profoundly reduce the ongoing arthritis. This was associated with a marked reduction in circulating R73+ lymphocytes to around 10–15% of their pretreatment levels. Newborn rats given the same amount of R73 twice weekly from birth and then challenged with *M. tuberculosis* developed no signs of arthritis, and the $\alpha\beta$ TCR-bearing T cells were even more depleted, although again not entirely. $\alpha\beta$ TCR-bearing T cells reappeared within a few days of cessation of therapeutic treatment with R73 and this was associated with a rebound of arthritic symptoms until the rats underwent natural remission. Further experiments by this group (Yoshino *et al.*, 1990b) showed that as little as 16 μg of R73 given on days 15, 18 and 21 after *M. tuberculosis* modestly inhibited the ongoing arthritis and that 80 μg of the mAb was essentially as good as 2 mg for both cell depletion and arthritis inhibition when given over the same period. Leaving treatment until days 21, 24 and 27, i.e. when arthritis had reached its peak, also reduced the severity of arthritis in comparison with controls and prevented the damage to bone and cartilage seen histologically. Later administration of the mAb was without visible effect against the arthritis both clinically and histologically, but by this time the rats were clearly entering natural remission and were unlikely to be influenced by the antibody. Where therapy was stopped before full development of natural remission, the arthritis rebounded in a similar fashion to that seen upon withdrawal of anti-CD4 therapy, suggesting that anti-CD4 and anti-$\alpha\beta$ TCR mAbs target the same T cell population. In both situations, reappearance of arthritic symptoms was associated with a return of T cells bearing the respective cell surface antigens.

Following a move from Emmrich's laboratory in Erlangen, Germany to Adelaide in Australia, Shin Yoshino went on to demonstrate that R73 could effectively inhibit the development of SCW-induced arthritis (Yoshino *et al.*, 1991a) and also that induced by type II collagen (Yoshino *et al.*, 1991b). For SCW-induced arthritis, the initial acute swelling that occurs over the first few days, which is not T cell-dependent, was unaffected by R73, but the ensuing chronic arthritis characterized by synovitis, periostitis and bone and cartilage erosion was completely inhibited by 100 μg of the mAb given on days 1, 2, 3 and every 3 days thereafter to day 27. As with adjuvant arthritis, therapy with R73 caused a marked depletion of $\alpha\beta$ TCR+ T cells in the peripheral blood.

Using essentially the same protocol of R73 treatment, i.e. 100 μg/rat at the time of immunization and then every 3 days until day 27, Yoshino *et al.* (1991b) completely prevented the appearance of type II collagen-induced arthritis in DA rats; this was accompanied by a depletion of $\alpha\beta$ TCR+ T cells similar to that seen with their SCW model and also an inhibition of delayed-type hypersensitivity to type II collagen. Anti-collagen antibody levels were only modestly inhibited, however. Once arthritis had developed, treatment with the mAb, on days 17, 20, 23 and 26, whilst suppressing further development of the arthritis, had no effect on the anti-collagen antibody titre. These results closely agree with those of Goldschmidt and Holmdahl (1991) who used the same mAb against type II collagen arthritis, again in DA rats. Their protocol involved giving 500 μg per rat of R73 rat on days 0, 1, 6, 7, 12, 13, 18 and 19 after collagen administration. This prevented arthritis development and modestly inhibited anti-collagen antibody production as Yoshino and his colleagues had found. Delaying mAb therapy until just before the arthritis developed, or even until fully developed, was still associated with a profound inhibition of the disease, although again anti-collagen antibody titres were not affected.

The major difference between the two studies was that Goldschmidt and Holmdahl (1991) reported that arthritis developed after they stopped treatment with R73 and that this could be severe. This delayed appearance of arthritis, after prophylactic R73 therapy, was not due to newly emerging T cells from the thymus, as adult thymectomy did not affect the onset of this delayed arthritis. However, in a therapeutic regimen, where therapy began at day 15 and was continued to day 34, some recovery from disease was noted in certain rats. The authors suggested, therefore, that inhibition of their collagen-induced arthritis was associated with functional blockage of the TCR rather than depletion of the $\alpha\beta$ TCR+ T cells, despite the fact that considerable depletion did occur. They found that significant numbers of T cells remained that carried anti-TCR antibodies on their surface and, further, cited the adult thymectomy experiment where arthritis developed after anti-TCR therapy in the absence of newly emerging T cells from the thymus. Presumably some of the $\alpha\beta$ TCR+ T cells "recovered" from R73 treatment and were able to elicit arthritis at the later stage. Yoshino and his colleagues (1991b) did not observe this rebound effect so perhaps their DA rat strain differed in some interesting manner from that used by Goldschmidt and Holmdahl (1991).

These results with anti-TCR mAb therapy clearly demonstrated that T lymphocytes are involved in induction and perpetuation of these polyarthritis models in the rat, up to the point where natural remission occurs.

2.2.5 mAbs against the IL-2R

As with the use of anti-IL-2R antibodies against type II collagen-induced arthritis in the mouse, the value of such therapy in the rat models is that it targets a relatively small population of T cells with consequently less potential for profound immunosuppression than anti-CD4 or anti-TCR mAbs. Unfortunately, where anti-IL-2R mAbs have been used to modulate the development of, for example, adjuvant arthritis, they have been unsuccessful. Neither Stunkel *et al.* (1988) nor Fergusson *et al.* (1988) were able to prevent the development of adjuvant arthritis in the rat following injection of mycobacterial adjuvant in oil. Both groups used ART-18, a mAb that binds to IL-2R (Osawa and Diamanstein, 1983), at levels up to 5 mg/kg for the period 0–10 days after adjuvant injection. However, a total inhibition of the arthritis induced by adoptive transfer of adjuvant arthritis with activated T lymphocytes was reported by the above authors, when ART-18 was given over the first 10 days after transfer of the cells. Fergusson *et al.* (1988) were also able to prevent development of adoptively transferred arthritis by treating the lymphocytes with ART-18 just before transfer. It is unclear why ART-18 was effective against the adoptively transferred arthritis, but could not deal with the active form of the disease. Our own experience is that essentially all the T cells used during adoptive transfer express IL-2R, so it is not surprising that anti-IL-2R mAbs modulate disease development when administered shortly after the cells have been transferred or just before transfer.

The failure to affect the direct form of adjuvant arthritis may be explained by the timing of mAb administration. Another possibility is that after several injections of a murine immunoglobulin, a vigorous host response could have negated the effectiveness of these mAbs in the rat. In relation to the former explanation, neither the work of the two groups above nor our earlier work (Billingham *et al.*, 1989, 1990b) involved giving the anti-IL-2R mAbs for a period longer than 10 days after mycobacterial challenge. It was probably assumed that important proliferative events associated with arthritogenic antigens, involving interaction between IL-2 and its receptor, would have occurred before this time. Our experiments with two other anti-IL-2R mAbs, OX39 and C5A (Billingham *et al.*, 1989, 1990b), were never carried out beyond day 6 after adjuvant injection, and were equally unsuccessful. However, these antibodies are bivalent, with both antigen-binding regions directed to epitope on the IL-2R. Some experiments undertaken by ourselves with a bifunctional mAb, with one binding region aimed at the IL-2R and the other at the vinca alkaloids, i.e. a monovalent anti-IL-2R mAb, indicate that later timing of the administration of bivalent mAbs should be explored (see below).

Earlier work at the Lilly laboratories had been directed successfully to the development of bifunctional mAbs for anti-tumour therapy, i.e. vinca alkaloids to tumours carrying the CEA (Corvalan and Smith, 1987). This technology was subsequently transferred to targetting the IL-2R with vinca alkaloids, for treatment of autoimmune diseases, with the development of a bifunctional mAb, 45-47-12. This mAb was tried initially against the adoptive transfer of adjuvant arthritis as this was known to be sensitive to anti-IL-2R therapy. Figure 4.6 demonstrates the potent inhibitory effect that this mAb has by itself against the development of adoptively transferred arthritis. Given every 2 days from the time of cell transfer to day 8, as little as 50 μg of 45-47-12 had a significant effect on the arthritis; the no-effect level of the mAb against arthritis was 5 μg. Addition of a small amount of vinblastine to this no-effect level of 45-47-12 produced a further reduction of arthritis development as seen in Fig. 4.7, but could not totally prevent it in the manner achieved with higher levels of anti-IL-2R mAbs (Fig. 4.6). Prolonging treatment with the 45-47-12–vinblastine complex to day 15 was also unable to completely suppress arthritis development. Why this is so is unclear, but it is possible that a host anti-mouse immunoglobulin response negates the activity of such low levels of mAb. Figure 4.7 also shows that the adoptively transferred arthritis enters natural remission around day 14, and it is clear that anti-IL-2R mAb therapy does not affect this process, indicating that the cell subtype responsible for remission is not IL-2R positive.

When used to try to prevent the development of the direct model of adjuvant arthritis, subsequent to injection of mycobacteria in oil, some surprising results were obtained; these are shown in Fig. 4.8. Antibody

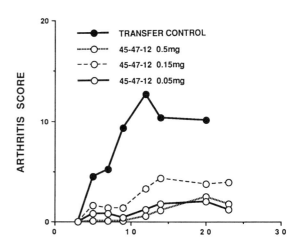

TIME IN DAYS AFTER TRANSFER

Figure 4.6 Inhibition of adoptively transferred adjuvant arthritis with the bifunctional (anti-IL-2R/anti-vinblastine) mAb 45-47-12 (given on days 0, 2, 4, 6 and 8). The no effect level was found to be at 5 μg of mAb on the days indicated.

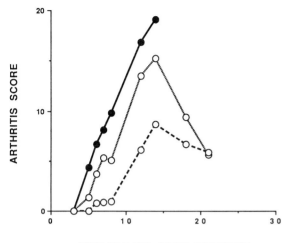

Figure 4.7 Addition of vinblastine to the bifunctional mAb, 45-47-12, enhances its antiarthritic activity. Note that this did not affect natural remission mechanisms. mAb 45-47-12 was given on days 0, 2, 4, 6 and 8. •, Transfer control; ·····○·····, 5 μg of mAb 45-47-12; --○--, 5 μg of mAb 45-47-12 + 3.75 μg of vinblastine.

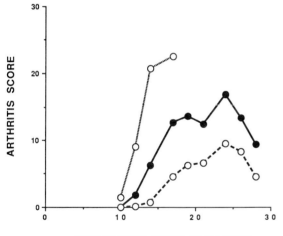

Figure 4.8 Effect of the bifunctional mAb, 45-47-12, on adjuvant arthritis induced by mycobacteria. A single dose of this mAb was able to both enhance and inhibit arthritis development depending on the time of administration. •, Arthritis control; ·····○·····, 100 μg of mAb 45-47-12 on day 0; --○--, 100 μg of mAb 45-47-12 on day 10.

45-47-12 by itself, i.e. without the vinblastine, was found to dramatically enhance the development of arthritis if given at the time of adjuvant injection, although the mechanism of this enhancement is quite unclear. This enhancement was also seen if the mAb was given on any day up to day 3, but after this time the enhancing effect was lost and after day 10 the antibody

actually had an inhibitory effect against arthritis development. As mentioned earlier, anti-IL-2R therapy has been unsuccessful against adjuvant arthritis. Perhaps the initial experiments had missed the window when such therapy could have worked, i.e. after day 10; alternatively this monovalent anti-IL-2R mAb may have unique effects against adjuvant arthritis. There is still much to do therefore with anti-IL-2R mAbs before these issues are resolved, and some further work with the mAb 45-47-12–vinblastine complex against the direct model of adjuvant arthritis needs to be undertaken. It is nonetheless clear that anti-IL-2R therapy is effective against this model of polyarthritis and that IL-2R can be successfully targetted with cytotoxic drugs using bifunctional mAbs. No studies have been reported with the other models of rat polyarthritis, probably because of the initial lack of success against adjuvant disease and the difficulty of adoptively transferring type II collagen- and SCW-induced arthritis with T lymphocytes.

2.2.6 mAbs against MHC class II (anti-Ia)

There is only one study that reports on the effect of anti-Ia mAbs in rat polyarthritis models. Billingham and his colleagues (1990b) demonstrated that OX6 was capable of totally inhibiting the development of classical adjuvant arthritis as shown in Fig. 4.9. OX6 was given on days 0, 3, 6, 9 and 12 after adjuvant injection in a dose–response manner; 1 mg/rat had a modest inhibitory effect but 4 mg/rat essentially abolished arthritis development. Earlier experiments had demonstrated that it was necessary to give OX6 over the 12-day period to see complete inhibition of arthritis and, in this respect, anti-Ia differs from anti-CD4 which is effective when

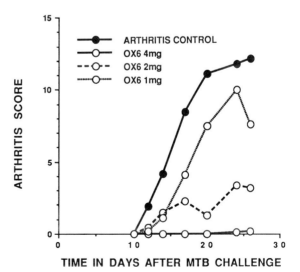

Figure 4.9 Dose–response of the anti-Ia (MHC class II) mAb, OX6, against the development of adjuvant arthritis induced by mycobacteria. OX6 treatment was given on days 0, 3, 6, 9 and 12.

given for just the first 3 days. These experiments demonstrated clearly, however, that interaction between antigen-presenting cells bearing MHC class II and CD4+ helper T lymphocytes is necessary for the development of adjuvant arthritis and most probably for the other polyarthritis models; in this respect they are similar to the mouse type II collagen-induced model.

2.2.7 mAbs against Adhesion Molecules

From a consideration of the interactions depicted in Fig. 4.1, for the induction of an MHC class II-restricted T lymphocyte response to a foreign or autoantigen, it would be expected that targetting the adhesion molecules necessary for successful interaction and lymphocyte involvement should influence the development of arthritis. To date, only Iigo et al. (1991) have addressed this aspect, despite the fact that anti-LFA-1 mAbs can produce the same degree of tolerance to foreign antigen as anti-CD4 (Benjamin et al., 1988). Of course, the availability of suitable mAbs will influence the progress of such studies!

Iigo and his colleagues (1991) developed a mAb to rat ICAM-1 called 1A29 and subsequently investigated its effect on adjuvant arthritis in the rat. They noted that the arthritis could be divided into an induction phase dependent on the interaction between T-helper lymphocytes and antigen-presenting cells and an effector phase when activated cells pass across the endothelium into sites of inflammatory reactivity. At a level of 5 mg/kg, mAb 1A29 given three times a week from day 0 to day 26 profoundly inhibited the development of adjuvant arthritis. The authors also found that giving this level of mAb 1A29 to donor rats used for the adoptive transfer of arthritis, i.e. on days 0, 2, 4, 7 and 9 before cell harvest on day 10, abolished the ability of lymphocytes from these rats to transfer disease to naive hosts. It was clear from these results that mAb 1A29 was interfering with the induction of arthritis during the critical phase of antigen presentation to T lymphocytes; this was confirmed by the observation that cultured lymph node T lymphocytes from 1A29-treated rats did not proliferate in response to exogenous mycobacterial antigen in comparison with saline-treated controls. Interestingly, administration of 1A29 to recipients of arthritogenic T lymphocytes (1 mg/kg, three times a week from day 0 to day 23) also inhibited the development of this adoptively transferred arthritis, indicating that this anti-ICAM-1 mAb influences the passage of inflammatory cells across the endothelium at sites of arthritis, although the authors did not comment on whether T cells or other inflammatory cells such as macrophages were the prime target in such circumstances. Iigo et al. (1991) correctly concluded that ICAM-1-dependent pathways are critically involved in the induction and maintenance of chronic inflammatory disease, particularly as this adhesion molecule is upregulated by inflammatory cytokines (Dustin et al., 1986) and is markedly expressed on

synovial cells, macrophages and endothelial cells in inflamed rheumatoid synovium (Hale et al., 1989).

From Fig. 4.1, it is clear that other adhesion molecules could be targetted for an effect on the induction of arthritis models in the rat, but to date they have not been investigated. The evidence that Springer (1990) has drawn together alluding to their importance in T cell recognition of antigen suggests that selective inhibition of the function of these molecules, e.g. LFA-1–3 (LFA-2 = CD2) and ICAM-2, would modulate development of arthritis.

3. Tolerance Induction with mAbs

The initial indication that certain mAbs may have induced a state of tolerance to arthritis came from studies of the effectiveness of anti-CD4 mAbs against adjuvant arthritis (Billingham et al., 1990b). High levels of treatment with the anti-CD4 mAb, OX35, completely blocked the development of arthritic symptoms (see Fig. 4.2) and caused a major depletion of CD4+ cells in the circulation, spleen and lymph node (van den Broek et al., 1992). Repopulation of these sites and the circulation with CD4+ cells, presumably from the bone marrow, was not associated with the development of arthritis, however, despite the continued presence of potentially arthritogenic mycobacterial cell walls and breakdown products with adjuvant properties, i.e. peptidoglycans and MDP. It appeared as though a state of tolerance or non-responsiveness had been induced to the arthritogenic properties of the mycobacteria by anti-CD4 mAb treatment.

To test this possibility further, rats rendered tolerant to arthritis induction by high levels of the anti-CD4 mAb, OX35, were rechallenged with a second fully arthritogenic level of mycobacteria in oil when CD4+ cells, which had been depleted by the first course of therapy, had returned to normal levels, i.e. after day 20 (see Fig. 4.10). It is clear that the rechallenge with mycobacteria failed to induce any arthritic symptoms, although there was a vigorous cytokine response to the rechallenge at day 27, in terms of release of IL-1 and IL-6, as indicated by the rise in the acute-phase protein α1GP (Billingham et al., 1990b). Under these circumstances of anti-CD4 mAb therapy, the rats were indeed tolerant, or non-responsive, to arthritis induced by mycobacteria, but not by a mechanism that compromised cytokine pathways in general. More likely, a form of antigen-specific tolerance, or non-responsiveness, had been induced, perhaps analogous to that described by Benjamin and Waldmann (1986), where tolerance to foreign antigens, including the anti-CD4 mAb itself, can be induced if they are administered under the cover of anti-CD4 therapy. Such tolerance appears to be maintained by continual exposure to the foreign antigen and, furthermore, can also be induced by anti-LFA-1, another

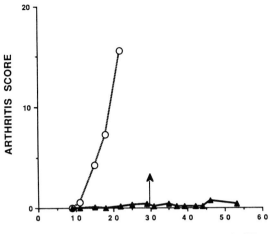

Figure 4.10 Induction of tolerance to adjuvant arthritis induced by mycobacteria with the anti-CD4 mAb, OX35. Early treatment with this mAb prevented development of arthritis and rendered the rats resistant to further attempts to induce arthritis with mycobacteria. ○, Arthritis control; ▲, 3 mg OX35 given on days 0, 3 and 6. The arrow indicates rechallenge with mycobacteria.

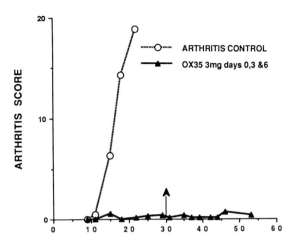

Figure 4.11 Induction of tolerance to adjuvant arthritis induced by the lipoidal amine CP20961. Early prevention of the arthritis with anti-CD4 rendered the rats resistant to further challenge with CP20961 (indicated by arrow).

adhesion molecule critical to the initial handling and presentation of antigen for T lymphocyte activation (Benjamin *et al.*, 1988). In such circumstances, the persistence of the mycobacteria or some other self-antigen could provide the continual antigenic stimulus for the maintenance of tolerance to arthritis induction.

Following from the observations with arthritis induced by mycobacteria, additional experiments were subsequently undertaken at the Lilly laboratories to see if this phenomenon of tolerance to arthritis induction with anti-CD4 mAb therapy extended to other rat polyarthritis models, e.g. those induced by the non-antigenic lipoidal amine, CP20961, and type II collagen. In collaboration with Maries van den Broek and her colleagues (1992), the model of SCW-induced arthritis was also investigated for tolerance induction.

Figure 4.11 shows the situation for arthritis induced by the non-antigenic adjuvant, CP20961. The protocol was identical with that for the mycobacterial arthritis depicted in Fig. 4.9, and essentially the same result was obtained. High-level treatment of the CP20961-induced arthritis with OX35 at the time of induction prevented the appearance of symptoms, and rechallenge with a second fully arthritogenic level of the adjuvant at day 27, when CD4+ cells had returned to normal levels, again failed to induce arthritis. As with rechallenge with mycobacteria, the cytokine axis was not compromised by anti-CD4 therapy, and a vigorous acute-phase protein response occurred with the CP20961 rechallenge, essentially duplicating the situation depicted in Fig. 4.10 for mycobacterial rechallenge.

The next question was whether the tolerance produced by anti-CD4 therapy to mycobacterially induced arthritis, i.e. classical adjuvant arthritis, extended to the non-antigenic adjuvant CP20961, as this might answer some questions about the role of mycobacterial antigens in the pathogenesis of adjuvant arthritis. Fig 4.12 illustrates the situation where rats that have been rendered tolerant to classical adjuvant-induced (mycobacterial) arthritis are rechallenged with CP20961. In this instance, the

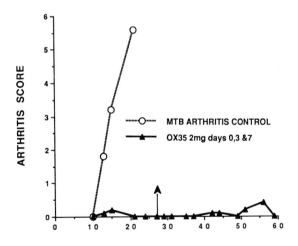

Figure 4.12 Tolerance to adjuvant arthritis induced by mycobacteria, following anti-CD4 treatment, also confers tolerance to adjuvant arthritis induced by the lipoidal amine CP20961. The arrow indicates rechallenge with CP20961.

mycobacterial adjuvant induced a relatively mild disease which was totally blocked by anti-CD4 therapy. However, rechallenge with CP20961 of the rats that had been treated with OX35 did not result in the appearance of arthritis, indicating that induction of tolerance to mycobacterial arthritis also rendered the rats tolerant to CP20961, a totally non-antigenic adjuvant. Performing the experiment the other way round, i.e. challenging rats made tolerant to CP20961 arthritis with mycobacteria, also resulted in a failure to induce significant arthritis, as seen in Fig. 4.13. It became clear, therefore, that both antigenic (mycobacterial) and non-antigenic (CP20961) adjuvants could induce tolerance to arthritis induction either to themselves or to each other, so the role of anti-genic determinants on mycobacteria in the pathogenesis of arthritis comes into question. Being non-antigenic itself, CP20961 would have presumably boosted reactivity to some self-antigen, either endogenous and self or some exogenous antigen, viral or bacterial, which is ubiquitously present and which in turn leads to arthritis development. The non-antigenic adjuvant moiety of mycobacteria, MDP, could also have boosted the same reactivity as CP20961, so it is possible that mycobacterial epitopes present on the cell walls are irre-levant to the development of classical adjuvant arthritis. These results do not preclude a cross-reactivity between some as yet unrecognized determinant on mycobacteria which shares homology with an unknown self-antigen in the rat, but they suggest that the search for the putative arthritogenic self-antigen should be widened.

van den Broek and her colleagues (1992) have asked the same questions of the SCW-induced model of poly-arthritis in the rat, with very similar results. In this instance they used the anti-CD4 mAb, W3/25, to prevent development of SCW-induced arthritis, as described above (in Section 2.2.3). Anti-CD4 therapy completely prevented the development of SCW-induced arthritis, along with an almost total depletion of CD4+ cells, and upon rechallenge with a fully arthritogenic level of SCW at day 83 after the initial challenge, when CD4+ cells were repleted, again no symptoms of arthritis developed. The anti-CD4 mAb had rendered the rats tolerant to SCW-induced arthritis. Most interestingly, when such tolerized rats were rechallenged with an arthritogenic level of mycobacteria in oil, they were also found to be tolerant to this arthritogen (van den Broek et al., 1992). Both Billingham et al. (1990), and van den Broek et al. (1992) found, however, that the tolerance could be overcome by adoptive transfer of large numbers of arthritogenic T lymphocytes. It appears, therefore, that mycobacterial and streptococcal cell walls can induce tolerance to the arthritis that each can initiate, as can CP20961, at least in cases so far investigated, all of which suggests that these arthritogens may activate arthritis by a similar pathway. The actual antigenic stimulus, however, remains elusive and requires a more diligent search.

The above results suggested a common pathway of activation of polyarthritic disease in the rat, but further experimentation with the type II collagen-induced model provided evidence that science should never be viewed as that simple! As discussed above, see Fig. 4.4, anti-CD4 therapy can completely block the development of type II collagen-induced arthritis in the rat. Consequently, rats that had been successfully treated with anti-CD4 to prevent arthritis were rechallenged with a second arthritogenic level of type II collagen. To our surprise, not only had we failed to tolerize these rats to type II collagen-induced arthritis, but they developed a rapid, aggressive form of the disease (Fig. 4.14) upon rechallenge with collagen, somewhat reminiscent of the findings of Goldschmidt and Holmdahl (1991) when they used the anti-TCR antibody, R73, prophylactically in this model. Subsequently, we found that rats rendered tolerant to mycobacterial adjuvant disease by anti-CD4 therapy developed a severe and accelerated arthritis when challenged with type II collagen and, similarly, rats prevented from developing type II collagen arthritis by anti-CD4 therapy were highly susceptible to arthritis development when rechallenged with mycobacteria (Fig. 4.15).

The clear conclusion from these studies is that type II collagen initiates arthritis by a separate route to that of the Gram-positive bacteria (mycobacteria, streptococci, etc.) and non-antigenic adjuvants such as CP20961. They also substantiate the contention of other authors who regard type II collagen-induced arthritis and the adjuvant arthritides of the rat as separate disease entities (e.g. Kaibara et al., 1984; Cremer et al., 1990). Interestingly, the ability of type II collagen to overcome

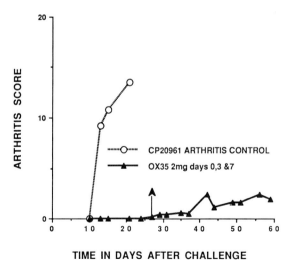

Figure 4.13 Tolerance to adjuvant arthritis induced by the lipoidal amine CP20961, following anti-CD4 treatment, confers tolerance to the arthritis induced by mycobacteria. The arrow indicates rechallenge with mycobacteria.

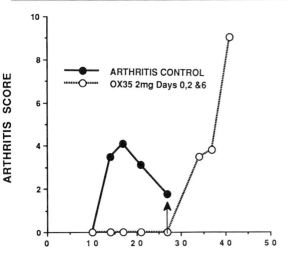

Figure 4.14 Anti-CD4 therapy prevents the development of type II collagen-induced arthritis, but does not induce tolerance to this antigen. This contrasts markedly with the results seen with adjuvant arthritis above. The arrow indicates rechallenge with collagen.

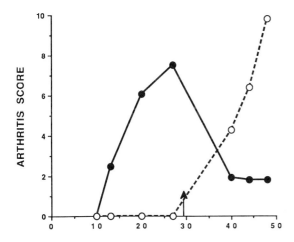

Figure 4.15 Inhibition of the development of type II collagen-induced arthritis with anti-CD4 therapy does not confer tolerance to adjuvant arthritis induced with mycobacteria. This experiment and the ones illustrated in Figures 4.10–4.14 demonstrate that collagen-induced arthritis and the adjuvant arthritides are separate entities. •, Arthritis control; ○, 3 mg OX35 on days 0, 3 and 6. The arrow indicates rechallenge with mycobacteria.

the anti-CD4-induced tolerance to the other arthritogens adds further weight, paradoxically, to the existence of a common pathway to arthritis development which is activated by the adjuvant arthritogens.

Before leaving the subject of tolerance, it needs to be mentioned that CSA appears unable to induce a state of tolerance to arthritis development, despite its ability to inhibit the development of arthritic symptoms in all of the models of polyarthritis in the rat and its profound therapeutic effect in established forms of the models. Withdrawal of prophylactic therapy is frequently associated with the subsequent development of arthritis, particularly in the case of persistent arthritogens such as mycobacteria; in this respect it contrasts totally with the effect of anti-CD4 therapy. When used therapeutically, with marked beneficial effect, withdrawal of CSA is often followed by a severe rebound of arthritic symptoms. The mechanisms behind this phenomenon, however, are best discussed in the context of natural suppression and remission of these rat polyarthritis models (see below).

4. Remission Mechanisms of Rat Polyarthritis

Most strains of rat are capable of developing at least one of the models of polyarthritis induced by the arthritogenic materials described above. A very few are resistant to all, and some strains, such as the inbred Lewis rat, are highly susceptible to all the polyarthritis models. An interesting observation is that, regardless of arthritogen, strain of rat or inherent susceptibility, the arthritic symptoms tend to be short-lived. This is illustrated in Figs 4.2, 4.4 and 4.5, which respectively demonstrate the phenomenon of natural remission in the Lewis rat for classical adjuvant arthritis, the model of type II collagen-induced arthritis and adoptive transfer of adjuvant arthritis. I have experience of strains of rat that enter natural remission by day 22 after challenge with arthritogen, others that tend to peter out around day 35 and the odd one that persists for 3–4 months before entering remission (Billingham, 1990). At present, the mechanisms of natural remission remain to be fully elucidated, but several authors have alluded to the role of subsets of suppressor cells which can abrogate the disease process (Tsukano et al., 1984; Myers et al., 1989; Nanishi and Battisto, 1991).

In some early experiments we noticed that treatment of established adjuvant arthritis with CSA was very effective in inhibiting the disease symptoms, but was always associated with a rebound of active arthritis when therapy was stopped; this rebound was not seen, however, with an anti-inflammatory drug such as indomethacin. Prud'homme and his colleagues (1991) reviewed the immunosuppressive properties of CSA, noting that, whilst it is a potent immunosuppressive agent under certain circumstances, it can paradoxically augment some delayed-type hypersensitivity reactions, aggravate autoimmune disease and even induce specific forms of autoimmunity. They further commented that CSA inhibits production of IL-2 and other cytokines at the transcriptional level, but does not usually prevent antigen-specific priming of T cells, so T cells may be poised to respond as soon as the drug is withdrawn. Their conclusions could provide an explanation for the rebound of arthritis described above, and the priming of T cells for development of adjuvant arthritis before drug withdrawal is dramatically illustrated in Fig. 4.16. In this instance, CSA was given to rats for 40 days, during which time control rats developed arthritis and underwent natural remission. CSA was then withdrawn, whereupon the rats rapidly developed arthritis, which ultimately entered remission just like the control rats. These results were in total contrast with the effect of anti-CD4 mAb therapy of adjuvant disease, where tolerance to adjuvant arthritis is induced by a short course of treatment.

This suggested that CSA was influencing the development and/or function of a suppressor cell population during the evolution of adjuvant arthritis, the normal role of which would be to curtail excessive autoaggressive reactivity. To address this possibility, rats that had developed adjuvant arthritis and undergone natural remission were given a short course of CSA therapy to see if the arthritis could be re-activated. Figure 4.17 shows that adjuvant arthritis can be rekindled by CSA immediately after natural remission and even a few months later. It appears that CSA nullifies the influence of a suppressor population, possibly by inhibiting production of a suppressor cytokine at the transcriptional level; arthritogenic T-helper cells then gain the ascendancy until the suppressor population regains control again.

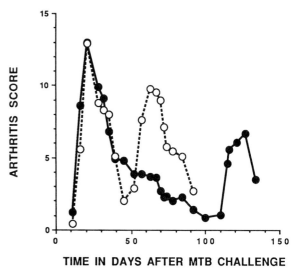

TIME IN DAYS AFTER MTB CHALLENGE

Figure 4.17 Re-activation of adjuvant arthritis by CSA after natural remission has occurred. A short pulse of therapy can re-activate the disease after a few months of remission. This only occurs, however, when the arthritogen persists; it was not seen with the lipoidal amine or after adoptive transfer of arthritis with T lymphocytes. •, CSA (10 mg/kg) on days 100–110; ○, CSA (10 mg/kg) on days 39–49.

Nanishi and Battisto (1991) have, in fact, described a factor from T-suppressor cells which can downregulate the ability of arthritogenic T lymphocytes to adoptively transfer arthritis; the phenotype of their suppressor cell was CD8.

The question then arose as to the identity of the suppressor population responsible for the natural remission we observed. Earlier studies (Billingham *et al.*, 1990b) demonstrated that anti-CD4 therapy of established adjuvant disease could reduce established disease activity, (Figs 4.2, 4.4 and 4.5) and that this rebounded when therapy stopped, as also described by Yoshino *et al.* (1990a) for their anti-TCR mAb in adjuvant arthritis. Rebound of arthritis after withdrawal of CSA is shown again in Fig. 4.18, in comparison with the anti-CD4 mAb, OX35. This is suggestive of a T lymphocyte subset involvement in suppression, possibly CD4+, $\alpha\beta$TCR+ and IL-2R−, but the evidence is insufficient at this stage to support such a conclusion. We subsequently found that this suppression of arthritis could be adoptively transferred to naive hosts with T lymphocytes obtained from rats in remission from adjuvant arthritis.

Others have subscribed to T lymphocyte-mediated suppression of arthritis and other models of autoimmunity in rodents. Myers *et al.* (1989) described some experiments in mice in which they isolated a suppressor population from donors injected with type II collagen. Injection of these cells into naive mice, 3 days before induction of type II collagen-induced arthritis, considerably inhibited the development of arthritis. Interestingly,

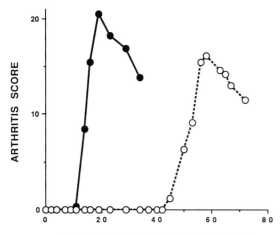

TIME IN DAYS AFTER MTB CHALLENGE

Figure 4.16 CSA is unable to induce tolerance to adjuvant arthritis. Therapy prevents development of arthritis, but, on withdrawal, arthritis develops and then undergoes natural remission in a similar fashion to the control rats. The rapid onset at the end of therapy indicates that the priming for arthritis occurred in the presence of CSA. •, Arthritis control; ○, 10 mg of CSA/kg on days 0–40.

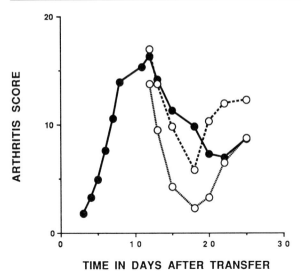

Figure 4.18 Effect of the anti-CD4 mAb, OX35, and CSA on the established phase of adoptively transferred adjuvant arthritis. Inhibition of arthritis with both therapies was associated with a rebound of symptoms when treatment was withdrawn. Both may be influencing the same cell population. •, Transfer control; ·····○·····, CSA (10 mg/kg) on days 12–19; --○--, OX35 (3 mg) on days 12–19.

treatment of the donor mice with CSA prevented the induction of the suppressor population. Phenotypic analysis demonstrated that this suppressor population was CD4+, and that CD8+ lymphocytes were not involved in the process. The CD4+ suppressor subset was characterized further as being positive for the Pgp-1 surface marker, which is present on a small population of memory cells, leading Myers *et al.* (1989) to suggest that a CD4+ memory cell downregulates autoimmunity. The situation may be more complex in the rat, as Larsson *et al.* (1989) have provided evidence for a CD8+ T cell involvement in the resistance to adjuvant arthritis produced by pre-immunization with very small amounts of mycobacteria; however, this may be a separate phenomenon from natural remission and the suppression described by Myers *et al.* (1989) and Swanborg and his colleagues below.

For EAE in the rat, Karpus and Swanborg (1989) have described a CD4+ T suppressor cell that induces the remission of this autoimmune disease, suggesting also that it mediates this suppression by differential inhibition of lymphokine production. This population of T suppressor cells could block the production of IFNγ from effector T lymphocytes in culture, but not IL-2. Later work on the potential mechanism of this suppression by the CD4+ population suggests that both TGFβ (Karpus and Swanborg, 1991) and IL-4 (Karpus *et al.*, 1992) may be involved.

It appears, therefore, that separate subsets of T lymphocytes battle for supremacy during the animal

models of arthritis described above, yet scientists by and large have been preoccupied with only one aspect. Clearly, there are powerful mechanisms in existence in animal models of autoimmunity for limiting the destruction that may be induced. However, this aspect has had nowhere near the attention of the effector side of the equation. Encouraging the natural mediation of suppression and downregulation may be less compromising to host defence mechanisms than the more generally immunosuppressive approaches currently being pursued with monoclonal antibodies.

5. Concluding Comments

In relation to the cellular interactions involved in MHC class II-restricted antigen presentation to helper T cells (Fig. 4.1), it is clear that mAbs directed to all those so far investigated can abrogate the development of arthritis in rats and mice, regardless of the initiating arthritogen. For anti-CD4 in the rat, this also leads to the development of tolerance to the initiating arthritogen, apart from type II collagen, and has demonstrated that the arthritogenic properties of Gram-positive bacteria, such as mycobacteria and streptococci, probably initiate arthritis by the same mechanism. This mechanism appears also to be shared by non-antigenic adjuvants, e.g. CP20961, as tolerance to this arthritogen confers tolerance to the Gram-positive bacterial arthritogens, and thus brings into question the relevance of bacterial antigens in the actual pathogenesis of the adjuvant arthritides. Some other endogenous antigen may well be responsible.

Comparison with the effects of CSA in the same model systems has shown that the mAbs are far superior in their overall properties, but this is in relation to induction of arthritis. In established arthritis, the mAbs are effective, but rebound frequently occurs when therapy is withdrawn, as is also the case with CSA. Use of both mAbs and CSA has additionally focused attention on the potential for control of arthritis by natural suppressor mechanisms, as is seen so frequently in the rat models of polyarthritis. This neglected aspect clearly requires more exploitation than it is currently receiving, as it may well be a safer alternative to the immunosuppressive mAbs at present being tried in human RA.

Attempts are being made to focus on the subsets of effector lymphocytes that are responsible for the development and maintenance of arthritis, by targetting activation antigens on lymphocytes, but we are a long way from selecting targets associated with the initiating arthritogens; in fact, this may never be achieved.

As was pointed out in the Introduction, other targets exist such as the macrophage and the effector mesenchymal cells of the actual connective tissue matrix destruction. Questions have been posed by Firestein and Zvaifler (1990) about the role of lymphocytes in the maintenance of chronicity of matrix destruction, as their products are much less apparent than the macrophage and mesenchymal cytokines. Finally, the results of Shiozawa and his colleagues (1992) demonstrating destruction of cartilage and bone in the absence of lymphocytes point to progress from the present approach which concentrates heavily on the T lymphocyte. The animal models may be misleading in relation to the chronicity of human RA, as the most studied tend to be short lived, e.g. the rat, with very little chronic destruction of matrix. Models have, however, been very useful for dissecting the intricate control of arthritis initiation, and the currently available mAbs have been invaluable for this purpose. No doubt new and more selective antibodies will help to carry our understanding of arthritic disease much further.

6.   Acknowledgements

I would like to thank Caroline Hicks who performed the studies illustrated in this text and who has "green fingers" in the adoptive transfer of arthritis and remission with T lymphocytes in the rat, also my collaborators, Bill Smith, Ann Kingston and Steve Carney for reagents and suggestions for some of the experiments described, and, finally, Eli Lilly and Company for providing an environment where basic research is encouraged as an integral part of the process towards the discovery of novel therapies.

7.   References

Acha-Orbea, H., Mitchell, D.A., Timmermann, L., Wraith, D.C., Tausch, G.S., Waldor, M.K., Zamvil, S.S., McDevitt, H.O. and Steinman, L. (1988). Limited heterogeneity of T-cell receptors from lymphocytes mediating autoimmune encephalomyelitis allows specific immune intervention. Cell 54, 263–273.

Adelman, N.E., Watling, D.L. and McDevitt, H.O. (1983). Treatment of (NZB × NZW)F1 disease with anti-Ia monoclonal antibodies. J. Exp. Med. 158, 1350–1355.

Andersson, M., Kramer, M.A., Terato, K., Burkhardt, H. and Holmdahl. R (1991). Analysis of type II collagen reactive T cells in the mouse. II. Different localization of immunodominant T cell epitopes on heterologous and autologous type II collagen. Scand. J. Immunol. 33, 505–510.

Banerjee, S., Haqqi, T.M., Luthra, H.S., Stuart, J.M. and David, C.S. (1988a). Possible role of V beta T cell receptor genes in susceptibility to collagen-induced arthritis in mice. J. Exp. Med. 167, 832–839.

Banerjee, S., Wei, B-Y., Hillman, K., Luthra, H.S. and David C.S. (1988b). Immunosuppression of collagen-induced arthritis in mice with an anti-IL2 receptor antibody. J. Immunol. 141, 1150–1154.

Benjamin, R.J. and Waldmann, H. (1986). Induction of tolerance by monoclonal antibody therapy. Nature (London) 320, 449–451.

Benjamin, R.J., Qin, X.I., Wise, W.P., Cobbold, S.P. and Waldmann, H. (1988). Mechanisms of monoclonal antibody-facilitated tolerance induction: a possible role for the CD4 (L3T4) and CD11a (LFA-1) molecules in self–non-self discrimination. Eur. J. Immunol. 18, 1079–1088.

Billingham, M.E.J. (1990). In "Anti-Rheumatic Drugs" (ed. M. Orme), pp 1–48. Pergamon Press, New York.

Billingham, M.E.J., Robinson, B.V. and Gaugas, J.M. (1970). Two anti-inflammatory components in anti-lymphocyte serum. Nature (London) 227, 276–277.

Billingham, M.E.J., Fairchild, S., Griffin, E., Drayer, L. and Hicks, C.A. (1989). In "The Therapeutic Control of the Inflammatory Response". (ed. A.J. Lewis, N.S. Doherty and N.R. Ackerman, pp 242–253, Elsevier, New York.

Billingham, M.E.J., Carney, S.L., Butler, R. and Colston, M.J. (1990a). A mycobacterial 65-kD heat shock protein induces antigen-specific suppression of adjuvant arthritis, but is not arthritogenic itself. J. Exp. Med. 171, 339–344.

Billingham, M.E.J., Hicks, C.A. and Carney, S.L. (1990b). Monoclonal antibodies and arthritis. Agents Actions 29, 77–87.

van den Broek, M.F., van den Berg, W.B. and van de Putte, L.B.A. (1986). Monoclonal anti-Ia antibodies suppress the flare up reaction of antigen induced arthritis in mice. Clin. Exp. Immunol. 66, 320–330.

van den Broek, M.F., Hogervorst, E.J.M., van Bruggen, M.C.J., van Eden, W., van der Zee, R. and van den Berg, W. (1989). Protection against streptococcal cell wall-induced arthritis by pretreatment with the 65-kD mycobacterial heat shock protein. J. Exp. Med. 170, 449–466.

van den Broek, M.F., van de Langerigt, L.G.M., van Bruggen, M.C.J., Billingham, M.E.J. and van den Berg, W.B. (1992). Treatment of rats with monoclonal anti-CD4 induces long-term resistance to streptococcal cell wall-induced arthritis. Eur. J. Immunol. 22, 57–61.

Burns, F.R., Li, X.B., Shen, N., Offner, H., Chou, Y.K., Vandenbark, A.A. and Heber-Katz, E. (1989). Both rat and mouse T cell receptors specific for the encephalitogenic determinant of myelin basic protein use similar $V\alpha$ and $V\beta$ chain genes even though the major histocompatibility complex and encephalitogenic determinants being recognized are different. J. Exp. Med. 169, 27–39.

Chang, Y.H., Pearson, C.M. and Abe, C. (1980). Adjuvant polyarthritis, IV. Induction by a synthetic adjuvant: immunologic, histopathologic and other studies. Arth. Rheum. 23, 62–71.

Chiocchia, G., Boissier, M.-C. and Fournier, C. (1991). Therapy against murine collagen-induced arthritis with T cell receptor $V\beta$-specific antibodies. Eur. J. Immunol. 21, 2899–2905.

Cooper, S.M., Sriram, S. and Ranges, G.E. (1988). Suppression of murine collagen-induced arthritis with monoclonal anti-Ia antibodies and augmentation with INF-γ. J. Immunol. 141, 1958–1962.

Courtenay, J.S., Dallman, M.J., Dayan, A.D., Martin, A. and Mosedale, B. (1980) Immunisation against heterologous type II collagen induces arthritis in mice. Nature (London) 238, 666–668.

Corvalan, J.R.F. and Smith, W. (1987). Construction and characterization of a hybrid–hybrid monoclonal antibody recognising both carcinoembryonic antigen (CEA) and vinca alkaloids. Cancer Immunol. Immunother. 24, 127–132.

Cremer, M.A., Townes, A.S. and Kang, A.H. (1990). Adjuvant-induced arthritis in rats. Evidence that autoimmunity to homologous collagens types I, II, IX and XI is not involved in the pathogenesis of arthritis. Clin. Exp. Immunol. 82, 307–312.

Currey, H.L.F. and Ziff, M. (1968). Suppression of adjuvant disease in the rat with heterologous anti-lymphocyte serum. J. Exp. Med. 127, 185–203.

Dustin, L.M., Rothlein, R., Bhan, A.K., Dinarello, C.A. and Springer, T.A. (1986). Induction by IL1 and interferonγ: tissue distribution, biochemistry and function of a natural adherence molecule (ICAM-1). J. Immunol. 137, 245–254.

van Eden, W., Thole, J.E.R., van der Zee, R., Noordzij, A., van Embden, J.D.A., Hensen, E.J. and Cohen, I.R. (1988). Cloning of the mycobacterial epitope recognized by T-lymphocytes in adjuvant arthritis. Nature (London) 331, 171–173.

Eisenberg, S.P., Evans, R.J., Arend, W.P., Verderber, E., Brewer, M.T., Hannum, C.H. and Thompson, R.C. (1990). Primary structure and functional expression from complementary DNA of a human interleukin-1 receptor antagonist. Nature (London) 343, 341–346.

Fergusson, K.M., Osawa, H., Diamanstein, T., Oronsky, A.L. and Kerwar, S.S. (1988). Treatment with an anti-interleukin 2 receptor antibody protects rats from passive but not adjuvant arthritis. Int. J. Immunother. IV, 29–33.

Firestein, G.S. and Zvaifler, N.J. (1990). How important are T-cells in chronic rheumatoid arthritis. Arth. Rheum. 33, 768–773.

Goldschmidt, T.J. and Holmdahl, R. (1991). Anti-T cell receptor antibody treatment of rats with established autologous collagen-induced arthritis; suppression of arthritis without reduction of anti-type II collagen autoantibody levels. Eur. J. Immunol. 21, 1327–1330.

Goldschmidt, T.J., Jannson, L. and Holmdahl, R. (1990). In vivo elimination of T cells expressing specific T-cell receptor V_β chains in mice susceptible to collagen-induced arthritis. Immunology 69, 508–514.

Granstein, R.D., Goulston, C. and Gaulton, G.N. (1986). Prolongation of murine skin allograft survival by immunologic manipulation with anti-interleukin 2 receptor antibody. J. Immunol. 136, 898–902.

Hafler, D.A., Fox, D.A., Benjamin, D. and Weiner, H.L. (1986). Antigen reactive memory T cells are defined by Ta1. J. Immunol. 137, 414–418.

Hale, L.P., Martin, M.E., McCollum, D.E., Nunley, J.A., Springer, T.A., Singer, K.H. and Haynes, B.F. (1989). Immunohistologic analysis of the distribution of cell adhesion molecules within the inflammatory synovial microenvironment. Arth. Rheum. 32, 22–30.

Hancock, W.W., Muller, W.A. and Cotran, R.S. (1987a). Interleukin 2 receptors are expressed by alveolar macrophages during pulmonary sarcoidosis, and are inducible by lymphokine treatment of normal lung macrophages, blood monocytes and monocyte cell lines. J. Immunol. 138, 185–191.

Hancock, W.W., Lord, R.H., Colby, A.J., Diamanstein, T., Rickles, R.J., Dijkstra, C., Hogg, N. and Tilney, N.L. (1987b). Identification of IL-2r+ T cells and macrophages within rejecting cardiac allografts, and comparison of the effects of treatment with anti-IL-2r monoclonal antibody or cyclosporin. J. Immunol. 138, 164–170.

Holoshitz, J., Naparstek, Y., Ben-Nun, A. and Cohen, I.R. (1983). Lines of T-lymphocytes induce or vaccinate against autoimmune arthritis. Science 219, 56–58.

Hom, J.T., Butler, L.D., Riedl, P.E. and Bendele, A.M. (1988). The progression of the inflammation in established collagen-induced arthritis can be altered by treatments with immunological or pharmacological agents which inhibit T cell activities. Eur. J. Immunol. 18, 881–888.

Horneff, G., Burmester, G.R., Emmrich, F. and Kalden, J.R. (1991). Treatment of rheumatoid arthritis with an anti-CD4 monoclonal antibody. Arth. Rheum. 34, 129–140.

Hunig, T., Wallny, H-J., Hartley, J.K., Lawetsky, A. and Tiefenthaler, G. (1989). A monoclonal antibody to a constant determinant of the rat T cell antigen receptor that induces T cell activation. Differential reactivity with subsets of immature and mature T lymphocytes. J. Exp. Med. 169, 73–86.

Hunneyball, I.M., Billingham, M.E.J. and Rainsford K.D. (1989). In "New Developments in Antirheumatic Therapy" (ed K.D. Rainsford), pp 93–132. Kluwer, Dordrecht, The Netherlands.

Iigo, Y., Takashi, T., Tamatani, T., Miyasaka, M., Higashida, T., Yagita, H., Okumura, K. and Tsukada, W. (1991). ICAM-1-dependent pathway is critically involved in the pathogenesis of adjuvant arthritis in rats. J. Immunol. 147, 4167–4171.

Kaibara, N., Hotokebuchi, T., Takagishi, K., Katsuki, I., Morinaga, M., Arita, C. and Jingushi, S. (1984). Pathogenetic difference between collagen arthritis and adjuvant arthritis. J. Exp. Med. 159, 1388–1396.

Karpus, W.J. and Swanborg, R.H. (1989). CD4+ suppressor cells differentially affect the production of INF-γ by effector cells of experimental autoimmune encephalomyelitis. J. Immunol. 143, 3492–3497.

Karpus, W.J. and Swanborg, R.H. (1991). CD4+ suppressor cells inhibit the function of effector cells of experimental autoimmune encephalomyelitis through a mechanism involving transforming growth factor-β. J. Immunol. 146, 1163–1168.

Karpus, W.J., Gould, K.E. and Swanborg, R.H. (1992). CD4+ suppressor cells of autoimmune encephalomyelitis respond to T cell receptor-associated determinants on effector cells by interleukin-4 secretion. Eur. J. Immunol. 22, 1757–1763.

Kirkman, R.L., Barrett, L.V., Gaulton, G.N., Kelley, V.E., Ythier, A. and Strom, T.B. (1985). Administration of an anti-interleukin-2 receptor antibody prolongs cardiac allograft survival in mice. J. Exp. Med. 162, 358–362.

Kohashi, O., Tanaka, A., Kotani, S., Shiba, T., Kusumoto, S., Yokogawa, K., Kawata, S. and Ozawa, A. (1980). Arthritis inducing ability of a synthetic adjuvant, N-acetyl muramyl dipeptides, and bacterial disaccharide peptides related to different oil vehicles and their composition. Infect. Immun. 29, 70–75.

Kohashi, O., Aihara, K., Ozawa, A., Kotani, S. and Azuma, I. (1982). New model of a synthetic adjuvant, N-acetylmuramyl-L-alanyl-D-isoglutamine-induced arthritis: clinical and histologic studies in athymic nude and euthymic rats. Lab. Invest. 47, 27–36.

Larsson, P., Holmdahl, R., Bencker, L. and Klareskog, L. (1985). In vivo treatment with W3/13 (anti-pan T) but not OX8 (anti-suppressor/cytotoxic T) monoclonal antibodies impedes the development of adjuvant arthritis. Immunology 56, 383–391.

Larsson, P., Holmdahl, R. and Klareskog, L. (1989). *In vivo* treatment with anti-CD8 and anti-CD5 monoclonal antibodies alters induced tolerance to adjuvant arthritis. J. Cell. Biochem. 40, 49–56.

Malek, T.R. and Korty, P.E. (1986). The murine interleukin-2 receptor. IV. Biochemical characterisation. J. Immunol. 136, 4092–4098.

Mori, L., Loetscher, H., Kakimoto, K., Bleuthmann, H. and Steinmetz, M. (1992). Expression of a transgenic T cell receptor β chain enhances collagen induced arthritis. J. Exp. Med. 176, 381–388.

Myers, L.K., Stuart, J.M. and Kang, A.H. (1989). A CD4 cell is capable of transferring suppression of collagen-induced arthritis. J. Immunol. 143, 3976–3980.

Nanishi, F. and Battisto, J.R. (1991). Down-regulation of adoptive adjuvant-induced arthritis by suppressor factor(s). Arth. Rheum. 34. 180–186.

Newbould, B.B. (1963). Chemotherapy of arthritis induced in rats by injection of mycobacterial adjuvant. Br. J. Pharmacol. 21, 127–136.

Osawa, H. and Diamanstein, T. (1983). The characteristics of a monoclonal antibody that binds specifically to rat T lymphoblasts and inhibits IL–2 receptor functions. J. Immunol. 130, 51–55.

Pearson, C.M. (1956). Development of arthritis, periarthritis and periostitis in rats given adjuvants. Proc. Soc. Exp. Biol. 91, 95–101.

Prud'homme G.J., Parfrey, N.A. and Vanier, L.E. (1991). Cyclosporin-induced autoimmunity and immune hyperreactivity. Autoimmunity 9, 345–356.

Ranges, G.E., Sriram, S. and Cooper, S.M. (1985). Prevention of type II collagen induced arthritis by *in vivo* treatment with anti-L3T4. J. Exp. Med. 162, 1105–1110.

Riechmann, L., Clark, M., Waldmann, H. and Winter, G. (1988). Reshaping human antibodies for therapy. Nature (London) 332, 323–327.

Robb, R.J.A., Munck, A. and Smith, K.A. (1981). T-cell growth factor receptors: quantitation, specificity and biological relevance. J. Exp. Med. 154, 1455–1474.

Schluesener, H., Brunner, C., Vass, K. and Lassmann, H. (1986). Therapy of rat autoimmune disease by a monoclonal antibody specific for T lymphoblasts. J. Immunol. 137, 3814–3820.

Shiozawa, S., Tanaka, Y., Fujita, T. and Tokuhisa, T. (1992). Destructive arthritis without lymphocyte infiltration in H2-c-fos transgenic mice. J. Immunol. 148, 3100–3104.

Springer, T.A. (1990). Adhesion receptors of the immune system. Nature (London) 346, 425–434.

Sriram, S. and Steinman, L. (1983). Anti-Ia antibody suppresses active encephalomyelitis: treatment model for diseases linked to Ir genes. J. Exp. Med. 158, 1362–1367.

Steinman, L., Rosenbaum, J.T., Sriram, S. and McDevitt, H.O. (1981). *In vivo* effects of antibodies to immune response gene products: prevention of experimental allergic encephalomyelitis. Proc. Natl Acad. Sci. USA 78, 7111–7114.

Stoerk, H.C., Bielinski, T.C. and Budzilovich, T. (1954). Chronic polyarthritis in rats injected with spleen in adjuvants. Am. J. Pathol. 30, 616–621.

Stunkel, K.G., Theisen, P., Mouzaki, A., Diamanstein, T. and Schlumberger, H.D. (1988). Monitoring of interleukin-2 receptor (IL2r) expression *in vivo* and studies on an IL-2R-directed immunosuppressive therapy of active and adoptive adjuvant-induced arthritis in rats. Immunology 64, 683–689.

Taurog, J.D., Sandberg, G.P. and Mahowald, M.L. (1983). The cellular basis of adjuvant arthritis. II. Characterisation of the cells mediating passive transfer. Cell. Immunol. 80, 198–204.

Tsukano, M., Nawa, Y. and Kotani, M. (1984). Characterisation of low dose induced suppressor cells in adjuvant arthritis in rats. Clin. Exp. Immunol. 53, 60–66.

Waldor, M., Sriram, S., McDevitt, H.O. and Steinman, L. (1983). *In vivo* therapy with monoclonal anti-Ia antibody suppresses the immune response to acetyl choline receptor. Proc. Natl Acad. Sci. USA 80, 2713–2717.

Watson, W.C. and Townes, A.S. (1985). Genetic susceptibility to murine collagen II autoimmune arthritis. Proposed relationship to the IgG2 autoantibody subclass response, complement C5, major histocompatibility (MHC) and non-MHC loci. J. Exp. Med. 162, 1878–1891.

Wooley, P.H., Luthra, H.S., Stuart, J.M. and David, C.S. (1981). Type II collagen-induced arthritis in mice. I. Major histocompatibility complex (I region) linkage and antibody correlates. J. Exp. Med. 688–700.

Wooley, P.H., Dillon, A.M., Luthra, H.S., Stuart, J.M. and David, C.S. (1983). Genetic control of Type II collagen-induced arthritis in mice: factors influencing disease susceptibility and evidence for multiple MHC-associated gene control. Trans. Proc. 15, 180–188.

Wooley, P.H., Luthra, H.S., Griffiths, M.M., Stuart, J.M., Huse, A. and David, C.S. (1985a). Type II collagen-induced arthritis in mice. IV. Variations in immunogenetic regulation provide evidence for multiple arthritogenic epitopes on the collagen molecule. J. Immunol. 135, 2443–2451.

Wooley, P.H., Luthra, H.S., Lafuse, W.P., Huse, A. Stuart, J.M. and David, C.S. (1985b). Type II collagen-induced arthritis in mice. III. Suppression of arthritis by using monoclonal and polyclonal anti-Ia antisera. J. Immunol. 134, 2366–2374.

Yoshino, S., Kinne, R., Hunig, T. and Emmrich, F. (1990a). The suppressive effect of an antibody to the αβ cell receptor in rat adjuvant arthritis: studies on optimal treatment protocols. Autoimmunity 7, 255–266.

Yoshino, S., Schlipkoter, E., Kinne, R., Hunig, T. and Emmrich, F. (1990b). Suppression and prevention of adjuvant arthritis in rats by a monoclonal antibody to the αβ T cell receptor. Eur. J. Immunol. 20, 2805–2808.

Yoshino, S., Cleland, L.G., Mayrhofer, G., Brown, R.R. and Schwab, J.H. (1991a). Prevention of chronic erosive streptococcal cell wall-induced arthritis in rats by treatment with a monoclonal antibody against the T cell antigen receptor αβ. J. Immunol. 146, 4187–4189.

Yoshino, S., Cleland, L.G. and Mayrhofer, G. (1991b). Treatment of collagen-induced arthritis in rats with a monoclonal antibody against the αβ T cell antigen receptor. Arth. Rheum. 34, 1039–1047.

5. Anti-CD4 and Other Antibodies to Cell Surface Antigens for Therapy

Frank Emmrich, Hendrik Schulze-Koops and Gerd Burmester

1. Introduction

The technique of monoclonal antibody production has had a significant impact for the rapid development of new research tools. An ever increasing number of cell surface molecules can now be characterized by means of specific mAbs. They are designated as CD (cluster of differentiation) with a distinct number referring to a standardized nomenclature based on the similarity of antigen distribution in various cell populations and cell lines

Immunopharmacology of Joints and Connective Tissue
ISBN 0–12–206345–7

(Spiegelhalter and Gilks, 1987). After characterization of the molecules, functional analyses have also been performed and have provided us with a wealth of information on the role of cell surface molecules in cell–cell interaction and signal transduction. Soon after the corresponding mAbs became available in larger amounts about 10 years ago, several laboratories began investigating their *in vivo* effects and potential therapeutic use in experimental animal models of autoimmune diseases, organ transplantation and cancer.

Particularly interesting results were generated by exploring the effects of mAbs to T cells, thereby extending the knowledge already accumulated using polyclonal anti-lymphocyte or anti-thymocyte globulin. Beyond this, it became possible to specifically address T cell subpopulations such as helper/inducer and cytotoxic T cells, characterized by the nearly exclusive expression of either CD4 or CD8 surface antigens. These studies have revealed the central role of helper/inducer T cells in the majority of experimental autoimmune diseases which could be prevented by early treatment with anti-CD4 mAbs. Moreover, already established experimental autoimmune diseases, such as EAE (Brinkman *et al.*, 1985), diabetes mellitus in NOD-mice (Shizuru *et al.*, 1988), the SLE-like disease in NZB/NZW F1 mice (Wofsy and Seaman 1987) and rat adjuvant arthritis (Billingham *et al.*, 1989), were susceptible to treatment. These findings have stimulated pilot trials in human diseases beginning with RA in 1987 (Herzog *et al.*, 1987).

Many observations suggest that activated T lymphocytes contribute significantly to the disease process in RA. Early during the onset of the disease, infiltrating T cells appear in the synovial membrane and constitute characteristic elements of joint inflammation. They express activation markers, and those that are responsive to IL-2 frequently show clonality (Korthäuer *et al.*, 1992). The extremely low frequency of T cells intimately involved in pathogenesis by their antigen specificity may have prevented the identification of putative autoantigens in the disease. Association of the disease with MHC class II gene products has been taken as an additional argument for the contribution of helper T lymphocytes, which are only able to recognize antigen in conjunction with MHC class II molecules. As the putative autoantigen(s) have not yet been defined, strategies using antigen or antigenic peptides for tolerance induction are not applicable at present, although some have been developed in animal models. However, lymphocyte depletion achieved by drainage of the thoracic duct (Paulus *et al.*, 1977), leucapheresis (Karsh *et al.*, 1981; Wilder and Decker, 1983) or total lymph node irradiation (Kotzin *et al.*, 1981) markedly reduced disease activity, thereby providing further support for the implication of T lymphocytes. Promising clinical improvements seen with the more specific reagents to CD4+ T cells confirmed the early observations and have initiated a series of additional clinical studies.

The use of mAbs as therapeutic agents has been studied most extensively in the area of cancer treatment and organ transplantation. These studies will not be the main focus of this review but have contributed significantly to the understanding of the mechanisms of antibody therapy and possible adverse reactions to antibody application. The anti-CD3 mAb, OKT3, directed against all mature T cells, has been used for prophylaxis and treatment of rejection crises (Todd and Brogden, 1989) in thousands of patients undergoing renal transplantation and these experiences are the reference for some aspects of mAb therapy in humans.

Most remarkable was the observation that induction of long-lasting tolerance could be achieved by treatment with anti-T cell mAbs including anti-CD4 in transplantation models (Waldmann *et al.*, 1989). Even tolerance to certain soluble protein antigens could be demonstrated if the protein was administered under the "umbrella" of a short-term anti-CD4 treatment (Benjamin and Waldmann, 1986). These observations have generated hope that "reprogramming" (Cobbold *et al.*, 1990) of the immune system should be possible even in adult individuals, which may have a tremendous therapeutic impact for both organ transplantation and autoimmune diseases. Besides CD3, CD4 and CD8, mAbs to other cell surface molecules have also been investigated in clinical pilot trials (Table 5.1).

In the following sections, we will discuss experiences with, and the rationale behind the use of, antibodies as therapeutic agents for treatment of autoimmune diseases in humans. The main focus will be RA and the use of anti-CD4 mAbs.

2.   Target Molecules of Antibody Therapy in Autoimmune Diseases

CD4+ helper/inducer T cells are key elements in the development of aberrant immune responses mediated predominantly by either antibodies or autoreactive cells. Therefore, interference with antigen recognition and/or T cell activation and long-term suppression of those T cells involved in the pathogenesis of a particular autoimmune disease are the major goals of therapeutic intervention. It is not surprising that the majority of cell surface molecules that have been proposed as targets for antibody therapy are found on activated CD4+ T cells. To become activated, CD4+ T cells have to recognize processed antigen associated with class II MHC-gene products on the surface of antigen-presenting cells (Babbitt *et al.*, 1985; Buus *et al.*, 1986). This interaction involves the TCR which consists of two polypeptide chains (α and β) with N-terminal variable regions for antigen recognition (Saito *et al.*, 1987). Associated with this "recognition unit" is the CD3 complex responsible for signal transduction after ligand binding. However,

Table 5.1   Characteristics of cell surface molecules used as targets for therapeutic mAbs in human autoimmune diseases and in organ transplantation

Target molecule	Biochemistry	Main cellular reactivity	Disease	Reference
CD2	m, gp50	T cells	Multiple sclerosis	Hafler et al. (1988)
CD3	m, gp26(γ); m gp20(δ); m, p20(ε); hod p16(ζ)	T cells	Allograft rejection	reviewed by: Todd and Brogden (1989), Chatenoud and Bach (1991), Norman and Leone (1991)
			Myocarditis	Gilbert et al. (1988)
CD4	m, gp60	T cell subset, monocytes, macrophages	See Table 5.3	
CD5	m, gp67	T cells, B cell subsets	Rheumatoid arthritis[a]	Strand et al. (1990, 1991)
CD6	m, gp100	T cells, B cell subsets	Allograft rejection	Kirkman et al. (1983)
CD7	gp40	T cells	Rheumatoid arthritis	Kirkham et al. (1988)
CD11a	hed, gp180/95	Leucocytes	Allograft rejection	Fischer et al. (1986, 1991)
CD25	m, gp55	Activated T cells, activated B cells, activated monocytes	Allograft rejection	e.g. Soulillou et al. (1987), Diamantstein et al. (1989), Waldmann et al. (1990), Wijdenes et al. (1990), Kirkman et al. (1991)
			Rheumatoid arthritis	Kyle et al. (1989)
CDw52	gp21–28	Leucocytes	Vasculitis[b]	Mathieson et al. (1990)
TCR $\alpha\beta$	hed	T cells	Liver transplantation	Wonigeit et al. (1989)

m, monomer; hod, homodimer; hed, heterodimer; gp, glycoprotein; p, phospoprotein.
[a] Antibody coupled to ricin A-chain; [b] Used before application of anti-CD4.

before T cell activation programmes resulting in cytokine production or cell division can be fully implemented, second signals are required which are normally provided by accessory cells. Adjunctive T cell molecules such as CD28 may transmit the additional signals required for an optimal T cell response (Jenkins et al., 1991). Unfortunately, although the ligand for CD28 has been identified (Linsley et al., 1991; Koulova et al., 1991), the natural ligands for most surface molecules are unknown. Some of them have the potential of generating interfering signals for T cell activation when ligated by specific antibodies.

The main goal of anti-T cell mAb therapy is the calming of unwarranted T cell responses which may be achieved by either deletion or functional inactivation. If possible, the treatment should challenge only those cells that are intimately involved in the disease process. They may be deleted by (i) direct killing or (ii) preparation for destruction by other cells. Functional inactivation may be achieved by (i) receptor blockade or (ii) generation of negative signals to cell activation. Modulation of the idiotype network or interactive units of T cell subsets, i.e. more complex interactions within the immune system, may be a third mode of action. Another possibility is interference with cell adhesion and redistribution of cells between body compartments. In many cases, we find combinations of several mechanisms which makes precise evaluation of their individual contributions difficult.

In the following, we will briefly comment on those surface molecules that are being used as targets for antibody therapy. Clinical studies using anti-CD4 mAbs and treatment trials of arthritis with antibodies to other cell surface molecules will be outlined in the following sections.

2.1 T CELL RECEPTOR (TCR)

mAbs to the TCR α and β chains can be categorized into those recognizing (i) common determinants, (ii) determinants restricted to certain TCR gene families or (iii) clonotype-restricted determinants. To be effective, the latter two types of reagent require preferential usage of certain TCRs by pathogenic T cells and can be predicted to provide a highly specific type of T cell suppression. This has been demonstrated in EAE in both mice and rats. In B10PL mice, 80% of the encephalitogenic T cells utilize the Vβ8.2 TCR-V gene (Urban et al., 1988), and, in the Lewis rat, 100% of the encephalitogenic T cells recognizing the myelin basic protein, peptide 72–86, express an homologous Vβ gene (Chluba et al., 1989) . Taking advantage of the limited heterogeneity of the TCR used by encephalitogenic T cells, it has been possible to prevent and treat EAE by using mAbs against Vβ8 (Acha-Orbea et al., 1988; Urban et al., 1988). Until now, no mAbs to clonotypic TCR or to TCR families with restricted usage have been applied therapeutically in humans. However, an antibody to a determinant commonly expressed by all TCR α/β chains was investigated in the treatment of acute graft-versus-host disease as well as rejection crises in kidney and liver transplantation (Beelen et al., 1988; Wonigeit et al., 1989; Pfeffer et al., 1990). It demonstrated effectiveness with only mild side effects compared with OKT3.

2.2 CD3

Associated with the α and β chains of the TCR is a number of non-polymorphic polypeptides called γ, δ, ε, ζ and η which comprise the CD3 complex (reviewed by Clevers et al., 1988). Only one mAb to mouse CD3 has been described recently and this was used for therapeutic studies (Hirsch et al., 1988), contrasting with the situation in humans for which there are numerous different anti-CD3 mAbs, mostly directed to CD3ε, such as the prototype antibody OKT3 (Transy et al., 1989). In general anti-CD3 mAbs are not cytotoxic and appear to act by steric blockade of antigen recognition via the TCR when used in organ transplantation. There is one case report on the use of anti-CD3 mAbs in a human autoimmune disease (Gilbert et al., 1988). Anti-CD3 mAbs are able to short-cut the natural pathway of signals from TCR to CD3 followed by induction of cytokine secretion and proliferation if cross-linked on the cell membrane by contact with Fc-receptor positive accessory cells (Tax et al., 1983). Most of the side effects described in the use of anti-CD3 in vivo are probably due to T cell activation, illustrating the potential danger of overstimulation of autoimmune T cells.

2.3 MHC CLASS II MOLECULES

Gene products of MHC class II are able to present antigenic peptides after cleavage (processing) of the intact protein to the T cell (Babbitt et al., 1985; Rudensky et al., 1991). They are expressed on antigen-presenting cells which comprise monocytes, macrophages, B lymphocytes and dendritic cells, but also, at least in humans, on activated T cells.

There is a genetic risk for RA conferred by the HLA allele DR4 and the linked D locus specificity Dw4 and Dw14 (Winchester, 1981; Nepom et al., 1989), and it has been demonstrated that certain amino acid positions, especially in the third hypervariable region of the DR β1 chain, are important for disease susceptibility. Possibly, as yet unknown peptides of the pathogenic antigen(s) are presented in association with this molecule to T cells. Therefore, prevention of appropriate presentation by using blocking antibodies to the critical MHC molecules involved has been suggested as a therapeutic concept (Steinman et al., 1986, 1988). Therapy with anti-MHC class II mAbs rests on the promise that such antibodies will selectively suppress the response to antigens under the control of the relevant MHC class II molecule without causing complete immunosuppression. The

blocking mAb should be specific for a single chain of the MHC class II molecule, so that, in heterozygotes, there would be two unblocked heterodimers to permit a normal response to foreign antigens. Such a concept has been validated by preventing EAE in mice or by reducing the frequency of relapses in the established disease (Steinman et al., 1986). Various other experimentally investigated autoimmune diseases have been attenuated by this kind of immunotherapy. It was also effective in suppressing the occurrence of collagen-induced arthritis in mice (Wooley et al., 1985).

2.4 CD4

The CD4 molecule is a plasma membrane glycoprotein of 55 kDa which is expressed on helper/inducer T lymphocytes (Reinherz and Schlossman, 1980; Maddon et al., 1985). CD4 has four extracellular immunoglobulin-like domains and a cytoplasmic tail highly conserved across mammalian species (Maddon et al., 1987). Recently, the three-dimensional structure was described for the first two domains resembling the β strand sandwich structure of immunoglobulin molecules (Wang et al., 1990; Ruy et al., 1990). The natural ligands for CD4 are MHC class II molecules on antigen-presenting cells which are also ligated by the TCR (reviewed by Swain (1983) and Emmrich (1988)). This may explain why CD4+ T cells recognize antigen only in association with MHC II molecules, a phenomenon known as MHC restriction. It was shown that close physical contact between CD4 and TCR–CD3 mediated by MHC class II molecules as a physiological "clamp" initiates a strong activation signal for the T cell (Emmrich et al., 1987, 1988). A possible mediator is the protein tyrosine kinase p56^{lck}, found in association with the cytoplasmic part of CD4 (Rudd et al., 1988; Veillette et al., 1988). Separate ligation of CD4 by an anti-CD4 mAb may (i) prevent the physical association with TCR–CD3 which is required for activation or may (ii) pre-activate the p56^{lck} thus generating a refractory state with regard to subsequent triggering via TCR–CD3 (Tsygangov et al., 1993). Besides its function as an accessory molecule for T cell recognition and activation, the CD4 molecule seems to be a low-affinity adhesion molecule, as demonstrated by binding experiments with CD4-transfected fibroblasts (Doyle and Strominger, 1987).

Soluble anti-CD4 mAbs are able to inhibit physiological stimulation of resting T cells by nominal antigen in vitro with regard to their proliferative response (Biddison et al., 1982; Wilde et al., 1983) as well as to lymphokine secretion (Wilde et al., 1983). It does not matter whether soluble or cellular antigens are used; particularly sensitive to inhibition by anti-CD4 is the autologous mixed lymphocyte culture of CD29+ T cells (Takeuchi et al., 1987).

mAbs to CD4 have been used in mice and rats to prevent onset of collagen type II-induced arthritis (Ranges et al., 1985) or rat adjuvant arthritis (Billingham et al., 1989) when given before or shortly after induction of the disease. It is still possible early in disease manifestation of adjuvant arthritis to achieve an immediate and significant improvement upon anti-CD4 treatment. Susceptibility to treatment even after onset of disease has been demonstrated in murine lupus erythematosus (Wofsy and Seaman, 1987) and a series of pilot studies was initiated in human autoimmune diseases, including RA, which will be outlined in the following section.

2.5 CD25

One of the earliest events following T cell activation is induction of the high-affinity receptor, IL-2R. It consists of two independently expressed chains, a p55 α chain (Tac antigen) (Uchiyama et al., 1981) and a p70/75 β chain (Tsudo et al., 1986). Both chains are able to bind IL-2 on its own, although only with low (α chain) or intermediate (β chain) affinity (Lowenthal and Greene, 1987). Once an α/β heterodimer is formed, it represents the high-affinity receptor for IL-2, able to induce T cell proliferation upon IL-2 binding (Tsudo et al., 1987).

As IL-2R is almost exclusively expressed in activated T cells (Robb et al., 1984), mAbs against IL-2R provide the opportunity to specifically address activated T cells which may be eliminated (Tanaka et al., 1989). Anti-IL-2R mAbs have been used for prevention and treatment of allograft rejection crises in animal models (Kirkman et al., 1985a,b, 1987; Shapiro et al., 1987) and are currently being investigated in clinical studies. It should be noted that only adoptively transferred rat adjuvant arthritis and not the actively induced disease is susceptible to mAb treatment (Stunkel et al., 1988).

2.6 CD5 AND CD7

The CD5 molecule can interfere with the T cell activation process. It has been shown that perturbation of the CD5 molecule by some anti-CD5 mAbs may enhance T cell activation (Fiebig et al., 1989). Anti-CD5 mAbs have been coupled to the ricin A-chain for clinical use (Strand et al., 1990, 1991). The function of CD7 is largely unknown. Although many anti-CD7 mAbs are inactive in vitro, it has been reported that a certain anti-CD7 antibody (7G5) effectively inhibits primary mixed lymphocyte cultures in vitro (Lazarovits et al., 1987). Others have described efficacy in preventing rhesus monkeys from rejecting skin allografts (Tax et al., 1984) or humans from renal allograft rejection (Raftery et al., 1985).

2.7 OTHERS

Only limited therapeutic experience is available regarding mAbs to other T cell surface molecules. Interesting for several reasons is LFA-1 which is found on human leucocytes as a heterodimeric molecule consisting of CD11a

and CD18 (Uciechowski and Schmidt 1989). It is involved in cellular adhesion which is an important prerequisite for homing, migration and cell–cell interactions initiating certain T cell functions. Migration of leucocytes to the site of inflammation starts with cellular adhesion to endothelial cells. A severe combined immunodeficiency may result from a genetic defect of CD18 (Kishimoto et al., 1987). mAbs to LFA-1 in an animal model inhibited granulocyte infiltration into an inflammatory site (Barton et al., 1989) which may add to the expected inhibition of T cell function when applied therapeutically.

Another molecule that is important for intracellular adhesion is CD2. Antibodies to CD2 may interfere with ligand binding of LFA-3 (CD58) to CD2 and have been shown to block in vitro stimulation in mixed lymphocyte cultures (Hafler et al., 1988). In a preliminary study, an anti-CD2 mAb was used in four cases of multiple sclerosis but no effect on the disease could be recorded after a short course of treatment (Hafler et al., 1988).

An interesting antibody is Campath 1 and its "humanized" derivative Campath 1H, both directed to CDw52, which is expressed on leucocytes, predominantly T cells and monocytes (Hale et al., 1989; Hadam, 1989). Campath 1 is cytolytic and able to activate human complement (Hale and Waldmann, 1988).

Finally, it should be mentioned that a mAb to CD6 (T12) has been successfully applied in patients after renal transplantation in an attempt to reverse allograft rejection crises (Kirkman et al., 1983).

3. Anti-CD4 Therapy

3.1 IMMEDIATE EFFECTS OF ANTI-CD4 mAb ADMINISTRATION

In this section we will try to generalize on some observations made with anti-CD4 mAb administration. The data were generated primarily in RA patients (Fig. 5.1), but they are very likely to be independent of this particular disease.

3.1.1 Body Distribution and Imaging

Little is known about body distribution of anti-T cell mAbs in humans. However, it is a common experience that injected immunoglobulin accumulates unspecifically at the site of inflammation probably because of leaky endothelium (Kushner and Sommerville, 1971). This has been demonstrated by isotype-matched and ^{99m}Tc-labelled mAbs in rat adjuvant arthritis (Kinne et al., 1992) and may be very important for discussion of mechanisms, as nature provides us with an antibody targeting which we do not have to implement. Besides unspecific accumulation, Kinne et al. (1992) demonstrated a specific enrichment of anti-CD4 mAbs in organs

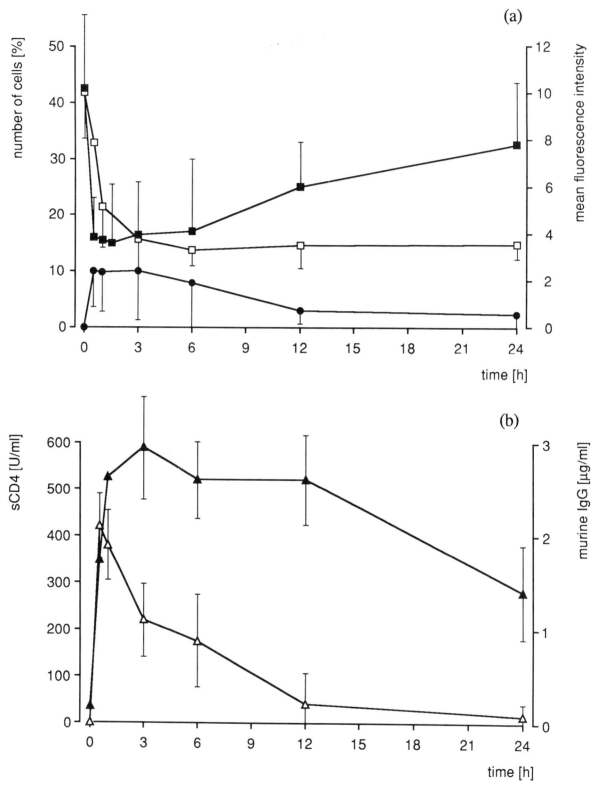

Figure 5.1 (a) Depletion of CD4+ cells (■), modulation of CD4 (□) and kinetics of anti-CD4-coated cells (•) and (b) release of soluble CD4 (▲) and clearance of the anti-CD4 mAbs (△) are shown for the first 24 h after infusion of 20 mg of MAX.16H5 for 30 min beginning at 0 h. Nine patients with severe RA were investigated (Horneff *et al.*, 1991a).

containing a high number of CD4+ cells (e.g. spleen, lymph nodes).

In humans, a higher target-to-background ratio was found with ^{99m}Tc anti-CD4 (MAX.16H5) than with non-specific immunoglobulins in arthritic joints (Kinne et al., 1993). This seems to indicate that imaging of tissues rich in CD4+ cells might be an interesting diagnostic approach (Becker et al., 1990).

3.1.2 Kinetics of Circulating mAbs

The serum level of circulating anti-CD4 mAbs after injection is a function of the applied dose as well as of duration of infusion. After infusion of 20 mg anti-CD4 mAb MAX.16H5 (IgG1) over 30 min a peak level of 2.4 mg/l ($n = 6$ patients) was detected, with the first measurement 30 min after the end of infusion (Horneff et al., 1991a). The level of free antibody rapidly declined with a half-life of about 3 h, and, 12 h after the infusion, murine mAbs were no longer detectable (Fig. 5.1b). Using the same dose of a different antibody (MT-151, IgG2a), the peak level in RA patients after a 30 min infusion was measured 1 h after the infusion at 1.5 ± 1.0 mg/l, and the antibody became undetectable after 7 h (Reiter et al., 1991a). Interestingly, a considerable variation in plasma mAb levels between individual patients was described in this study. Another murine IgG2a mAb to CD4 (BL4) was employed in renal transplantation, reaching peak levels after infusion of 10 or 20 mg, comparable with previous studies (500–900 μg/l and 400–2200 μg/l respectively) although clearance, as assessed after 24 h, was markedly delayed (100–400 μg/l and 100–700 μg/l respectively) (Morel et al., 1990). These data taken together show that the half-life of murine anti-CD4 mAb varies considerably depending on the individual antibody but not on the isotype.

Not many data are available about the kinetics of chimerized anti-CD4 antibodies consisting of mouse variable region linked to a human constant part. They do, however, seem to be consistent with the observations made with anti-cancer antibodies of a 4 to 6-fold longer half-life of chimeric antibodies than their murine counterparts (LoBuglio et al., 1989).

3.1.3 Coating of Cells

The percentage of circulating lymphocytes coated with anti-CD4 after infusion of the antibody in vivo was determined cytofluorimetrically by FITC-labelled anti-mouse Ig (Fig. 5.1a). The data obtained with different antibodies were quite similar and revealed that a maximum of antibody-coated cells (1–33% mean 14% with BL4 (Morel et al., 1990), $11 \pm 7\%$ with MAX.16H5 (Horneff et al., 1991a)) was reached at the end of the infusion and declined to 0–5% of circulating lymphocytes 12 h thereafter. Owing to a rapid disappearance of CD4+ cells immediately after the infusion of anti-CD4 (see Section 3.1.5), over an estimated period of 3 h, saturation of circulating CD4+ cells with the anti-CD4 was seen in one study (Horneff et al., 1991a), e.g. the number of circulating antibody-coated cells was similar to the number of remaining CD4+ cells, while no saturation was found in another study (Morel et al., 1990).

3.1.4 Soluble CD4

Shortly after infusion of 20 mg MT-151 over 30 min, soluble CD4 became detectable in the sera of patients (Reiter et al., 1991a). The peak level (approximately 100 ng/ml) was reached 3 h after antibody infusion and the level declined to pretreatment values by 20 h. Similar results were observed with MAX.16H5 (Fig. 5.1b) (Horneff et al., 1992). Absorption with immobilized anti-mouse IgG completely removed soluble CD4 from sera, thus indicating that soluble CD4 was complexed with the anti-CD4 antibody (Reiter et al., 1991a).

3.1.5 Cell Depletion

The most impressive immediate effect observed to various degrees with many murine anti-CD4 mAbs was the rapid clearance of CD4+ lymphocytes from the circulation (Fig. 5.1a). With most mAbs, the number of CD4+ lymphocytes reached pretreatment levels within 24 h after an initial fall to 17% (MT-151; Reiter et al., 1991a), 30% (MT-412; van der Lubbe et al., 1991a) and 50% (BL4; Morel et al., 1990) within the first hour of infusion.

In contrast, mAb MAX.16H5 had a much more pronounced depletory effect on CD4+ lymphocytes (Horneff et al., 1991a). After a 30 min infusion with this antibody, up to 90% of the CD4+ cells disappeared from the circulation within 1 h. Subsequently, throughout the next 24 h the number of CD4+ cells increased gradually up to a mean of 50% of the pretreatment level with a marked interindividual variation. Each daily infusion throughout the following 7 days yielded similar kinetics of depletion and reappearance of CD4+ cells. After a 7-day treatment course by daily infusions of 20 mg MAX.16H5, the CD4+ cell count was reduced to about 50% of the pretreatment level, staying at this level for at least 2 months. Prolongation of the infusion time further enhanced the extent and duration of CD4+ cell depletion.

Chimerization of mAb MT-412 resulted in prolonged depletion of CD4+ lymphocytes compared with the murine origin which might be due to the 4 to 6-fold prolonged half-life of the chimeric antibody compared with its murine equivalent. After an initial decrease within 1 h of mAb infusion, the number of CD4+ cells remained below 50% of the pretreatment level for at least 6 weeks (van der Lubbe et al., 1991b; Moreland et al., 1991; Choy et al., 1991). Remarkably, the chimerized antibody SK3 used for treatment of patients with mycosis fungoides did not cause any depletion of CD4+ cells (Knox et al., 1991). In conclusion, the extent and duration of CD4+ cell depletion varies noticeably among the anti-CD4 antibodies used for treatment.

Because of CD4+ cell depletion, the total number of T cells, as assessed by anti-CD3 staining, decreased in parallel with the decline in CD4+ cells. As the absolute number of CD8+ cells was not affected in most recipients, anti-CD4 infusion resulted in a reversed CD4/CD8 ratio, which remained below 1 in one patient for at least 24 months without any obvious clinical signs of severe immunosuppression (Horneff et al., 1992). Two single case reports described a temporary decrease of CD8+ cells to 60% of the baseline level within the first hours of infusion (Reiter et al., 1991a; Hiepe et al., 1991). Whereas the number of B cells and natural killer cells remained unaffected, one study reports on a transient depletion of monocytes (Horneff et al., 1991a).

3.1.6 CD4 Modulation

Antibody binding to cell surface antigens may induce disappearance of the corresponding surface molecule – a phenomenon called modulation. It is well known as a regular feature of anti-CD3 antibody. In contrast, modulation of the CD4 molecule induced by murine anti-CD4 mAb in vivo has only been observed upon administration of MAX.16H5 (Fig. 5.1a). The surface density of CD4 declined over a period of 24 h to 33 ± 8% of the original value and, after a 7-day treatment cycle with daily antibody infusion, reached a minimum of 30 ± 5% at day 8, increasing again to 72 ± 16% at day 14 and 90 ± 16% at day 28 (Horneff et al., 1991a). The permanent reduction in CD4 density continuing for more than 14 days after the first treatment is in contrast with the kinetics after depletion of CD4+ cells, which began reappearing shortly after the infusion was stopped. No co-modulation could be found for CD2, CD3, CD8, CD25, CDw29, CD45R, CD45RO and HLA-DR. In vivo modulation was always more pronounced than in vitro modulation by MAX.16H5 with cells of the same patient. The in vitro experiments also revealed that the requirements for CD4 modulation resemble the requirements for CD3 modulation induced by anti-CD3 antibody, e.g. presence of viable monocytes and the use of whole antibody molecules (Horneff et al., 1993a).

Only preliminary data are available on chimeric anti-CD4 mAbs showing, if any, only a mild CD4 modulation (Knox et al., 1991; Reiter et al., 1991b).

3.1.7 Complement Activation

Binding of complement components after anti-CD4 antibody infusion to lymphocytes was investigated with mAbs MT-151 and MAX.16H5 (Reiter et al., 1991a; Horneff et al., 1992). Cytofluorimetric analyses with specific rabbit antisera revealed deposition of C1s, C3d, C4d, C4-binding protein and C5 on circulating T cells. In contrast, C9 was hardly detected. The peak concentration of fixed complement was reached 3 h after mAb infusion.

3.2 TREATMENT OF RHEUMATOID ARTHRITIS

3.2.1 Study Populations and Treatment Modalities

The patient populations treated so far have consisted of individuals with severe and active disease. Most patients had been treated previously with several DMARD regimens without success and had been considered refractory to conventional therapy. In the majority of studies, patients received only NSAIDs and no or a maximum of 10 mg of prednisone. The individual dosage regimens are outlined in Table 5.2. In general, daily dosages of 10–100 mg were administered, resulting in total dosages of 70–700 mg per treatment cycle. Individual treatment courses consisted of 5–7 days, even though single injections at certain time points have been carried out as well. Currently, several trials are being performed in search of the optimum dosing regimens.

3.2.2 Laboratory Changes

Even though directed against the same cell surface molecule, analysis of the data reported so far has revealed some striking differences in the immunological and clinical effects of the various reagents used. Thus, for instance, one major difference between antibody MAX.16H5 and the antibodies MT-151, VIT4 and the chimeric reagent MT-412 is the apparent profound influence on laboratory parameters. These include the significant reductions in the erythrocyte sedimentation rate (ESR), α_2-globulin fraction and rheumatoid factors induced by MAX.16H5. These findings are paralleled by marked decreases in parameters indicative of monocyte–macrophage activation, such as serum neopterin or IL-6 levels or the in vitro production of IL-1 and TNF-α (Horneff et al., 1993b). Moreover, the enhanced lymphocyte responsiveness after treatment observed in some individuals treated with MAX.16H5 appears to be unique to this antibody.

In a study carried out by Horneff et al. (1991a) using antibody MAX.16H5, there was a significant and usually parallel reduction in acute-phase reactants as determined by the ESR, CRP and the α_2-globulin fraction within the first week of therapy documented in most patients. Decreased ESR values persisted for more than 4 months in some patients. The majority of patients also exhibited a decrease in total IgG and rheumatoid factors ($P < 0.02$); one patient became rheumatoid factor negative (Waaler Rose test) upon treatment.

In most studies performed so far, there was a decrease in T cell function in vitro after treatment, which reverted to normal levels upon normalization of blood T cell numbers. Unexpectedly, however, using antibody MAX.16H5, two groups of patients could be distinguished according to the stimulation values. Although in all patients a nearly complete unresponsiveness occurred

Table 5.2 Summary of clinical and immunological data derived from anti-CD4 trials in RA

Antibody	Isotype	No. of patients reported	Total dosage (mg)	Modulation of CD4 antigen	CD4+ T cells (% of pretreatment values) Maximum depletion	End of treatment	ESR, CRP or rheumatoid factor	Articular index improved (Ritchie) (no. of individuals affected)	Adverse effects (no. of individuals affected)	HAMA (incidence)	References
MT-151/VIT4	IgG2a	8	70	No	19	120	No change	8/8	Low-grade fever (1)	6/8	Herzog et al. (1989)
MAX.16H5	IgG1	10	105–210	Strong	9	40	Reduced	7/9	Fever, nausea (4), allergy (1)	6/10	Horneff et al. (1991a,b)
MT-151	IgG2a	10	140	Marginal	18	97	No change	6/10 (>25%)	Allergy (1)	6/10	Reiter et al. (1991a)
B-F5	IgG1	10	100/150/200	n.a.	n.a.	92	Reduced	10/10	Fever (1)	2/10	Wendling et al. (1991)
B-F5	IgG1	10	200/300	n.a.	n.a.	n.a.	No change	6/10 (>25%)	Fever, shivers (2)	9/10	Didry et al. (1991)
cMT-412	c-human IgG1	33	70/350/700	Strong	25	43	No change	n.a., $P < 0.005$	Flu-like (21), haemodyn. (2)	HACA, low	van der Lubbe et al. (1991b)
cMT-412	c-human IgG1	25	10–700	n.a.	18	13 (3 × 300 mg)	No change	8/15 (>50%)	Flu-like symptoms	HACA, low	Moreland et al. (1991)

n.a., data not available; ESR, erythrocyte sedimentation rate; CRP, C-reactive protein; HAMA, human anti-mouse antibodies; HACA, human anti-chimeric antibodies.

upon maximum depletion of CD4+ T cells usually 1 h after administration, there was a persistently decreased mitogen and antigen stimulation in only a few patients. In contrast, in a second group, there was a striking increase in T cell responsiveness to both mitogens and antigens to above pretreatment levels. This was particularly evident in antigen-induced proliferation where a complete unresponsiveness reverted to high stimulation values. Interestingly, these data did not correlate with the various CD4/CD8 ratios nor with the total amounts of CD4+ T cells.

The antibody characteristics that drive these different laboratory changes are not easily recognized. MAX.16H5 is the only murine reagent leading to a profound *in vivo* modulation of the CD4 antigen (Horneff *et al.*, 1993a). Alternatively, different effects may be due to the immunoglobulin isotype of MAX.16H5 which is IgG1, in contrast with IgG2a, in the case of MT-151. Interestingly, the other monoclonal reagent inducing significant decreases in inflammatory parameters is reagent B-F5 which is also of the IgG1 isotype (Wendling *et al.*, 1991). However, while treatment with MAX.16H5 resulted in a marked and frequently long-lasting depletion, B-F5 antibody therapy did not lead to a persistent decrease in circulating T cell numbers. It is notable that, although most findings with the same reagent in two different trials (Table 5.3) were remarkably similar, the data obtained with the B-F5 reagent differed considerably between centres (Wendling *et al.*, 1991; Didry *et al.*, 1991).

There were different kinetics for the mAb, MAX.16H5, and the corresponding CD4+ cells upon prolonging the infusion period to 6 h. The integrals of the two kinetic curves were different, with a smaller total amount of detectable serum anti-CD4 in the 6 h application mode. This treatment resulted in a very strong depletion of CD4+ cells which was already evident after 30% of the reagent had been administered. In a typical patient, after 12 h, the CD4+ cells were reduced to 17% and after 24 h to 42% of the corresponding pretreatment values. At the end of the 7-day treatment cycle, the CD4/CD8 ratio was persistently decreased to levels of 0.33 for up to 24 months after this second therapy (Horneff *et al.*, 1992).

3.2.3 Clinical Evaluation

Despite the profound differences in laboratory findings, the clinical efficacy of all anti-CD4 reagents used so far appear quite similar. Thus, in all studies, significant clinical improvements were demonstrated in 60–75% of patients lasting for an average period of 3 months after a single treatment course (Table 5.2). This is particularly remarkable, as the patients treated so far usually represented the far end spectrum of intractable individuals in whom conventional treatment regimens had failed.

In detail, clinical parameters at the beginning and after the first or second treatment cycle demonstrated that the

Table 5.3   Human diseases treated with anti-CD4 mAb

Antibody	Disease	No. of patients	Reference
MT-151, VIT4	Rheumatoid arthritis	5/8[a]	Herzog et al. (1987, 1989)
MT-151		10	Reiter et al. (1991a)
MAX.16H5		10	Horneff et al. (1991a)
B-F5		10	Wendling et al. (1991)
B-F5		10	Didry et al. (1991)[b]
cMT-412		25	Moreland et al. (1991)[b]
cMT-412		33	van der Lubbe et al. (1991b)[b]
19THY5D7	Multiple sclerosis	4	Hafler et al. (1988)
MAX.16H5	Allograft rejection crisis	5	Reinke et al. (1991)
BL4		12	Morel et al. (1990)
Chimeric SK3	Mycosis fungoides	7	Knox et al. (1991)
MAX.16H5	CIBD	3	Emmrich et al. (1991)
MAX.16H5	SLE	1	Hiepe et al. (1991)
cMT-412	Psoriasis vulgaris	1	Prinz et al. (1991)
BB14		3	Nicolas et al. (1991)
MT-412	Relapsing polychondritis	1	van der Lubbe et al. (1991a)
cMT-412		1	Choy et al. (1991)
13B8.2	AIDS	7	Dhiver et al. (1989)
YNB46.1.8SG2B1.19	Vasculitis	1[c]	Mathieson et al. (1990)

CIBD, chronic inflammatory bowel disease.
[a] Reports on the same patients, including one patient with psoriatic arthritis.
[b] Meeting abstract.
[c] Used after application of Campath 1H.

most significant change was a decrease in the number of swollen joints in all patients with a marked reduction of synovitis (day 8 $P < 0.04$, day 28 $P < 0.01$) (Horneff et al., 1991a). The Ritchie index decreased in 7/9 patients (day 8 $P = 0.058$, day 28 $P < 0.02$) and grip strength increased (day 8 $P = 0.06$, day 28 $P < 0.04$). Morning stiffness decreased in 6/9 patients. In general, clinical improvement was already evident at the end of the 7-day treatment period and lasted up to 6 months. In one patient with rheumatoid vasculitis, the leg ulcer due to this extra-articular manifestation healed completely after 1 week of therapy. Repeated treatment cycles resulted in a far better and more sustained improvement in one patient (Fig. 5.2) and in a similar improvement in two individuals with a prolonged duration (3/4 weeks versus more than 3/2 months). In one patient, similar, but only minor, clinical benefits occurred within 6 weeks after both treatment cycles.

Little is known about the kinetics of lymphocyte migration from blood and lymphatic compartments into synovial sites and how anti-CD4 monoclonal antibody therapy affects intra-articular tissue sites. However, the data obtained so far indicate that, despite an immediate entry of the reagent, as demonstrated by immunoscintigraphy (Becker et al., 1990) or coating of intra-articular CD4+ T cells (Herzog et al., 1989), it takes a considerable time to alter the cellular composition of the lymphocyte population in the synovial fluid or the synovial tissue (Horneff et al., 1992). Therefore, it is unlikely that the effects of anti-CD4 therapy are due to an immediate depletion of intra-articular CD4+ T cells.

3.3   TREATMENT TRIALS OF OTHER DISEASES

Anti-CD4 antibodies have not only been used in patients with RA but also in various other autoimmune diseases, the histological and immunological findings from the majority of which indicate a contribution of activated T cells to their pathogenesis (Table 5.3).

3.3.1   Systemic Lupus Erythematosus (SLE)

SLE is a systemic autoimmune disease, characterized serologically by high titres of IgG ANAb, e.g. anti-DNA (dsDNA, ssDNA, z-DNA), anti-histone and anti-non-histone antibodies. Clinically, SLE is characterized by a systemic vasculitis involving multiple organs. Many would agree that T and B lymphocyte dysregulation contributes to the pathogenesis of the disease (Gleichmann et al., 1982; Theofilopoulos et al., 1985). Stimulated by the beneficial effects of anti-T cell mAb treatment in a mouse model (MRL/lpr mice) of SLE (Wofsy et al., 1984), Wofsy and Seaman (1985) succeeded in treating spontaneously developing SLE in NZB/NZW F1 mice with an anti-CD4 mAb. Weekly injections of anti-CD4 beginning at an age of 4 months dramatically reduced autoantibody concentrations, retarded renal disease and prolonged life (Wofsy and Seaman, 1985; Wofsy et al., 1988).

Recently, a case report on treatment of a patient with SLE has been published (Hiepe et al., 1991). The 21-year-old patient with a 6-year history of severe SLE had frequent exacerbations of disease despite aggressive

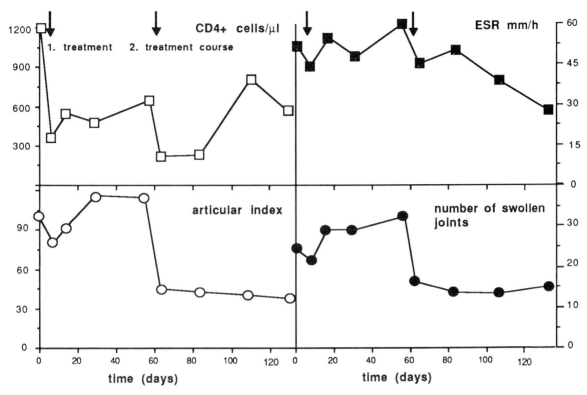

Figure 5.2 Clinical course of one patient with RA undergoing repeated cycles of anti-CD4 treatment. While there was no response to therapy after the first cycle despite depletion of CD4+ T cells, the second treatment course resulted in a marked reduction of the Ritchie articular index and the number of swollen joints, along with a decrease in ESR.

immunosuppressive treatment with azathioprine, cyclophosphamide and high doses of corticosteroids, as well as total lymphoid irradiation. Anti-dsDNA antibody corresponded well with disease activity. When the patient developed an exacerbation of disease (nephrotic syndrome, pericarditis, anaemia, anti-dsDNA titre 1:64), he was given daily infusions of 0.3 mg/kg body weight mAb MAX.16H5 for 7 consecutive days. A prednisolone dose of 50 mg/day was maintained.

The clinical effect of anti-CD4 antibody treatment was rapid: by the end of the 7-day treatment cycle, proteinuria was reduced to almost 50% of pretreatment values and continuously declined for the following 2 weeks. In parallel, serum albumin increased. Most interestingly, the anti-DNA titres decreased from 1:64 to 1:8 on day 7. However, 4 weeks after treatment, the patient developed a flare-up, as indicated by clinical signs as well as by increasing autoantibody levels. As a consequence, the patient was given a methylprednisolone bolus for 5 days, and complete remission was initiated lasting, to date, more than 20 months. Corresponding to the clinical signs, the anti-DNA titre became negative and a marked reduction in *in vitro* production of IgG and anti-DNA antibody was observed.

3.3.2 Chronic Inflammatory Bowel Disease

In Crohn's disease and ulcerative colitis, the therapeutic effects of corticosteroids and immunosuppressive agents, as well as histological and immunological findings, indicate a hyperreactive immune system (Selby *et al.*, 1983) in the gut with B and T cell infiltrates in the mucosa (MacDermott and Stenson, 1988; Qin *et al.*, 1988). Three patients with active steroid-resistant or steroid-dependent disease were treated (Emmrich *et al.*, 1991) with the same antibody, MAX.16H5, and the same treatment protocol as mentioned above. All patients included in the study had a long-lasting history of disease with multiple relapses despite aggressive immunosuppressive therapy.

One patient with Crohn's disease rapidly improved after treatment. Moreover, ESR and CRP as indicators of active systemic disease declined. Like the patient with SLE (Hiepe *et al.*, 1991), a mild relapse occurring 4 weeks after anti-CD4 treatment responded to a higher dose of prednisolone.

The other two patients both suffered from ulcerative colitis. While the first patient had a relapse after a 4-week period of clinical improvement following the anti-CD4 treatment, the second patient has now been in complete clinical, endoscopic and biochemical remission for more than 22 months.

3.3.3   Generalized Severe Psoriasis

Generalized pustular psoriasis is a rarely occurring severe progression of psoriasis vulgaris. The initial phase of this severe disease is dominated by epidermal infiltration of activated CD4+ T lymphocytes (Baker *et al.*, 1984; Valdimarson *et al.*, 1986). Two recent studies have reported on treatment of severe generalized psoriasis with anti-CD4 antibodies (Prinz *et al.*, 1991; Nicolas *et al.*, 1991).

In the first report (Prinz *et al.*, 1991), a 63-year-old male patient, who had developed severe generalized pustular psoriasis, despite the administration of oral steroids, was given the chimerized anti-CD4 antibody cMT-412 in alternating doses of 10 and 20 mg on days 1, 2, 3, 6 and 7. The clinical effect was rapid: 2 days after initiation of treatment, the pustules had dried off and by day 11 erythroderma, desquamation and extensive peripheral lymphoedema had disappeared. Clinical improvement was parallelled by a reduction in CRP to normal levels. A mild relapse after day 14 was effectively treated with another infusion of 20 mg antibody. Moreover, conventional therapy proved to be effective again in treating single guttate lesions, developing 4 weeks after treatment. The second study (Nicolas *et al.*, 1991) describes treatment of three patients with severe, generalized psoriasis. The monoclonal anti-CD4 antibody BB14 (IgG1) was given daily for 8 consecutive days over a 2 h infusion period in different dosages. The first patient (8×0.2 mg/kg body weight BB14) had a rapid onset of clinical improvement by day 4, and most pronounced on day 30, but deteriorated progressively thereafter. In contrast, no relapses were noted in the other two patients receiving a higher dose of the antibody (3×0.8 mg/kg body weight, 5×0.4 mg/kg body weight). These patients experienced maximum clinical improvement 3–4 weeks after treatment. It should be mentioned that two observations of effective treatment by anti-CD4 mAbs in psoriasis had already been published (Prinz *et al.* (1991) and Nicolas *et al.* (1991)) as short descriptions. One AIDS patient with psoriasis improved under anti-CD4 therapy (mAb 13B8.2; Dhiver *et al.*, 1989), and improvement of psoriasis was also described in a case of psoriatic arthritis treated with mAb MT-151 (Herzog *et al.*, 1987).

3.3.4   Relapsing Polychondritis

Two patients with a progressing form of relapsing poly-chondritis have been treated with anti-CD4 mAbs. The first report (van der Lubbe *et al.*, 1991a) was on a 45-year-old woman who, despite aggressive immunosup-pressive therapy in the past, presented with saddle nose deformity, deterioration of flow-volume curves in pul-monary function tests and inflammation in the trachea

and main bronchi as revealed by bronchoscopy. A dose of 25 mg of murine MT-412 was given daily for 7 con-secutive days while prednisolone (30 mg/day) was main-tained during treatment. The clinical effect was a disease regression (clinically, pulmonary function tests) and the prednisolone dose could be reduced to 15 mg/day. A relapse 6 months after initial treatment was successfully re-treated with the same antibody infusion protocol. By the regimen described, the disease progression could be effectively blocked for more than 1 year.

The second report (Choy *et al.*, 1991) described a 27-year-old male who presented with steroid-dependent progressive disease refractory to methotrexate. He was given 50 mg cMT-412 fortnightly for 6 weeks. As described in Section 3.1, the CD4 lymphocyte depletion was markedly prolonged compared with the effect of the murine MT-412, measured by van der Lubbe *et al.* (1991a) in the first study on relapsing polychondritis. The steroid dose of the patient could be successfully reduced to 7.5 mg/day after treatment. However, the clinical follow-up has not been described for longer than 2 weeks, during which the patient did well.

3.3.5   Mycosis Fungoides

Mycosis fungoides is a T cell lymphoma, characterized by infiltrates in the skin which are composed primarily of a monoclonal proliferation of CD4+ cells (Wood *et al.*, 1986) eventually penetrating other organs. Despite con-ventional treatment (chemotherapy, radiation therapy, PUVA), the disease may progress and, once lymph nodes, bone marrow and visceral organs are involved, will have a poor prognosis of less than 2 years (Kaye *et al.*, 1989; Young, 1989).

Seven patients with mycosis fungoides, which was progressive despite conventional treatment, were treated twice a week for 3 weeks intravenously with different dosages ranging from 10 to 80 mg per infusion of a chi-meric IgG1$\varkappa$ anti-CD4 mAb (Knox *et al.*, 1991). The authors observed some clinical efficacy, e.g. reduction of both erythema and induration of skin lesions, as well as reduction of erythroderma and improvement of adenopathy in all patients with a rapid onset. However, the improvement was of relatively short duration, lasting from 9 days to 12 weeks with a mean duration of approxi-mately 2 weeks. Interestingly, one patient with joint involvement of the lymphoma developed a complete res-olution of gross and microscopic CD4+ synovial infiltrate 3 weeks after the completion of therapy. The best responses were seen in the patients treated with 80 mg antibody per dose.

3.3.6   Graft Rejection

In contrast to autoimmune diseases, in organ trans-plantation the immune system is challenged by a known cellular antigen at definite time points, which allows treatment in the inductive phase of the ongoing immune response. In animal models, induction of transplantation tolerance by anti-T cell mAb has been successfully demonstrated (Waldmann *et al.*, 1989). However, to date, no study has been reported in humans, in which anti-CD4 mAb was given before transplantation. In two studies, the patients received anti-CD4 mAbs at different time points after transplantation. Twelve patients were treated daily with 10 mg (5) or 15 mg (7) of the murine mAb BL4 for 12 consecutive days, starting at day 1 after transplantation (Morel *et al.*, 1990). Associated immunosuppressive treatment consisted of azathioprine and prednisolone. The authors conclude that, in their study, the number of documented rejection episodes was comparable with that of patients treated with anti-lymphocyte globulin. In the second study (Reinke *et al.*, 1991), five patients with acute rejections of long-term renal allografts were treated with the anti-CD4 mAb, MAX.16H5. Late rejections are usually more resistant to steroids and OKT3 treatment, resulting in an allograft loss rate of 35% compared with less than 10% in early post-transplantation rejection episodes (Venkateswara *et al.*, 1989; Reinke *et al.*, 1991). The patients received 0.6 mg of the antibody/kg body weight over 3 consecutive days. After completion of treatment, the histological signs of severe acute rejection disappeared in all patients along with a reduction in interstitial infiltrates. In all patients, serum creatinine declined rapidly within 5 days. Two patients deteriorated by week 3 to 4 and one rejection occurred by week 10. However, creatinine values could be stabilized in two of the three patients with a methylprednisolone bolus treatment. The third patient received an additional anti-CD4 treatment and has been stable for more than 10 weeks at the time of report.

3.3.7 Multiple Sclerosis

One of the earliest treatments with anti-CD4 mAbs was performed in patients with multiple sclerosis (Hafler *et al.*, 1988). By using the mouse IgG2a anti-CD4 mAb 19THY5D7 four patients received a 5-day course of daily infusions of 0.2 mg/kg body weight per day. After treatment, immunosuppressive effects, as measured by reduced PWM-induced immunoglobulin synthesis were observed. However, as the study population was part of a phase I study, no clinical effects have been reported.

3.3.8 AIDS

CD4 is the target molecule for the HIV gp120 envelope protein, thereby representing the major, if not the only, receptor for HIV (Maddon *et al.*, 1984). Thus, anti-CD4 mAbs could have some benefits in HIV infection by (i) blocking HIV binding to CD4+ cells, (ii) delivering negative signals to T cells, thereby preventing T cell activation and viral replication, (iii) depletion of CD4+ T cells from the circulation and (iv) inducing anti-idiotype antibodies, which in turn may enhance the anti-gp120 immune response provided that the anti-idiotype

represents the internal image of the antigen (Dhiver *et al.*, 1989).

In vitro, anti-CD4 mAbs efficiently inhibited HIV infection of T cells when added immediately after incubation of the cells with HIV 1 (Rieber *et al.*, 1990).

In vivo, seven patients, classified as CDC group IV (seropositive, less than 100 CD4+ T cells/μl, at least one opportunistic infection) were treated with various doses of the murine anti-CD4 mAb 13B8.2 (IgG1) for 10 consecutive days (Dhiver *et al.*, 1989). Two of the seven patients responded to therapy, e.g. they became negative for the virus protein p24 and reverse transcriptase assays. However, the response was transient and by day 45, the viral antigen was detected again. Interestingly, both responders developed a transient increase in the number of CD4+ cells upon anti-CD4 mAb treatment. Interestingly, during the course of therapy and for 4–7 months after the last mAb infusion, no opportunistic infections were observed.

3.3.9 Systemic Vasculitis

One patient with a long-lasting history of severe vasculitis was successfully treated with a combination of the humanized anti-CDw52 antibody (Campath 1H) and a rat anti-CD4 mAb (YNB46.1.8 SG 2B1.19) given consecutively (Mathieson *et al.*, 1990). The previous treatment of the patient included prednisolone, dapsone, azathioprine, cyclophosphamide and plasmapheresis. Despite this aggressive treatment, the patient presented again with an exacerbation of disease, and subsequently received an 8-day course of Campath 1H, which resulted in a dramatic improvement but only for 10 days. Therefore, two more courses of Campath 1H were carried out with the same results. Finally, the patient received a 3-day course of Campath 1H, followed by a 12-day course of anti-CD4. This sequential use of both antibodies was followed by a complete remission, lasting for 12 months, at the time of this report. Despite profound CD4 depletion and depressed CD4/CD8 ratio, the patient did well and did not develop opportunistic infections. The working hypothesis for this combined treatment will be outlined in Section 3.4.

3.4 POSSIBLE MODE OF ACTION

Effective treatment in animal models as well as in human diseases by anti-CD4 mAbs needs explanation of the mechanism(s) in operation. In this section, we will discuss several possibilities that may explain (i) the immediate effects observed during and shortly after application of the antibody and (ii) the more prolonged effects lasting longer than 1 month. With regard to the immediate effects, we will differentiate between inhibition of CD4 T cell functions as a consequence of direct antibody binding to the cells and the more complex results of redistribution of antibody-coated cells to other body compartments.

3.4.1   Immediate Effects on Cell Function

3.4.1.1   Complement-Mediated Killing or ADCC

Figure 5.3 schematically depicts several possible consequences of anti-CD4 binding. Most suggestive at the
beginning of anti-T cell mAb therapy was the idea that
T cells were killed either directly by complement-
mediated mechanisms or by ADCC involving Fc-
receptor-bearing cytotoxic cells. mAbs to CD52, which
are able to lyse human lymphocytes by using human
complement, have demonstrated that cytolytic antibodies can be developed that are particularly valuable for
purging T cells from donor marrow in clinical bone-
marrow transplantation (Hale and Waldmann, 1988).
Hierarchies of antibody isotypes have been established
which demonstrated that mouse IgG2a was the best isotype for lysis and C1q binding and mouse IgG1 was the
worst (Neuberger and Rajewsky, 1981). However, the
target surface antigen seems to play a critical role, as the
majority of mAbs to other T cell surface antigens are not
cytolytic. There is no report on an anti-human CD4 antibody which is able to kill directly, in a complement-
mediated manner or by ADCC. However, as complement split products are found on CD4+ cells (see
Section 3.1.7) after treatment, it cannot be excluded that
the lifetime of these cells will be reduced.

3.4.1.2   Modulation

Reduction of CD4 density could be imagined to impair
T cell recognition and activation. Variable results were
observed with CD4 depending on the antibody used
(Horneff *et al.*, 1993a). Even the best modulating mAb
reduced the CD4 density by only 60–70%. Similarly to
the anti-CD3-mediated modulation, there was a requirement for Fc-receptor-bearing accessory cells. *In vitro*
experiments and some observations with CD4-
modulated cells after antibody treatment gave no evidence for impaired T cell function solely induced by
modulation. Interestingly, CD4-modulated T cells seem
to respond even better to mitogenic signals and to anti-
CD3 stimulation (Schrezenmeier and Fleischer, 1988;
Horneff *et al.*, 1993a). There is no strong argument that
limited CD4 modulation *per se* impairs T cell activation.

3.4.1.3   Soluble CD4

If soluble CD4 were to bind to MHC class II molecules,
it would be considered as an immunosuppressive agent.
The release of soluble CD4 immediately after anti-CD4
injection has been described by several groups, with
varied duration of the plasma level of soluble CD4+
(Reiter *et al.*, 1991a; Horneff *et al.*, 1992). However, it
is known from studies with recombinant soluble CD4 in
primates that this compound is not immunosuppressive

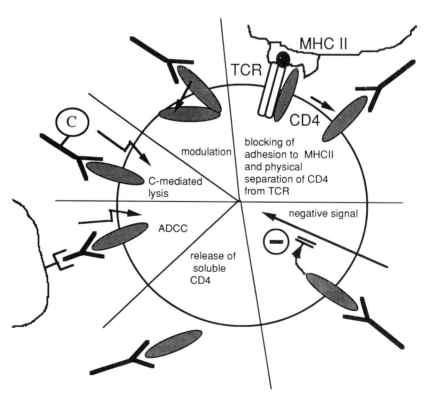

**Figure 5.3 Possible inhibitory effects which could act immediately after anti-CD4 binding. Confirmed by *in vitro*
experiments is the inhibition of T cell activation by separate ligation and the transmission of negative signals
upon antibody binding.**

(Watanabe *et al.*, 1989). Similar results were obtained by *in vitro* experiments (Liu and Liu, 1988). This result is probably due to a low avidity of soluble CD4 for MHC class II molecules, insufficient to compete effectively with the physiological antigen recognition by T cells.

3.4.1.4 Blocking of Antigen Recognition and Separate Ligation of CD4

In Section 2 of this chapter, we described CD4 as a ligand for MHC class II molecules, which are also targets for the TCR. Interference with this associative recognition by anti-CD4 can be accomplished in different ways: it may (i) reduce cell adhesion, (ii) block the physiological antigen recognition and (iii) lead to a separate ligation of CD4 and TCR–CD3. Separate ligation of CD4, however, reduces TCR–CD3-mediated signals (Emmrich *et al.*, 1987; Tsygankov *et al.*, 1993).

3.4.1.5 Negative Signal

Interestingly, anti-CD4 mAbs inhibit lectin-stimulated T cell functions also in the presence of MHC class II-negative accessory cells (Bekoff *et al.*, 1985). This can be demonstrated even with rather artificial ligands such as PMA and Ca^{2+} ionophore, which are very unlikely to involve the TCR–CD3 complex. Therefore, it appears as if a direct negative signal can be transmitted by anti-CD4 independent of TCR–CD3 ligation. Pretreatment with anti-CD4 significantly reduces intracellular Ca^{2+} mobilization and the proliferative response to subsequent stimulation by cross-linking anti-CD3 (Tsygankov *et al.*, 1993). Recently, a direct antiproliferative effect by anti-CD4 has been described, but this seems to be restricted to certain T cell clones (Blue *et al.*, 1988). The significance of negative signals for any effect seen under anti-CD4 treatment remains unclear.

3.4.2 Immediate Effects on Cell Distribution

Several anti-T cell mAbs are able to deplete T cells. It should be kept in mind that "depletion" in animal experiments normally means depletion from lymphoid tissues whereas in human studies, with few exceptions, only depletion from the circulation can be assessed. The latter involves only a small portion of the total lymphocyte pool. Consequently, redistribution of T cells between organ compartments may take place even in the absence of significant depletion from the circulation. Little is known about the compartments to which T cells are shifted once they are coated by a depleting antibody. However, it is easy to imagine that reduction in cell number in the lymphatic organs together with "blinding" of T cell recognition and inhibition of activation may have dramatic consequences for the immune system. At least in neonatal mice, anti-CD4 mAbs reach the thymus and may interfere with selection mechanisms (MacDonald *et al.*, 1988).

It would be interesting to know more about the mechanism(s) altering the migration behaviour of antibody-coated cells. As reported recently, anti-CD4 inhibits low-affinity and antigen-independent adhesion of CD4 T cells to MHC class II-bearing cells such as B cells (Doyle and Strominger, 1987). The expression of potential adhesion molecules seems not to be influenced by anti-CD4 binding to resting T cells. However, the enhanced adhesiveness of CD4 T cells induced by TCR-mediated signals can be inhibited by anti-CD4 (Mazerolles *et al.*, 1991). Another observation with certain anti-CD4 antibodies like MAX.16H5 is a tendency to aggregate T cells. Whether or not these *in vitro* phenomena contribute to depletion and redistribution remains to be determined.

It should also be kept in mind that multiple epitopes have been described for CD4 (Jonker *et al.*, 1985). Different biological functions described for distinct anti-CD4 mAbs cannot always be explained by different isotypes.

3.4.3 Long-term Effects on T Cells

It was a very encouraging observation in two naturally occurring autoimmune diseases, diabetes mellitus in NOD-mice and the SLE-like disease in NZB/NZW F1 mice, that prolonged anti-CD4 therapy could prevent or attenuate the disease and that treatment could eventually be stopped without disease recurrence (Shizuru *et al.*, 1988; Wofsy and Seaman, 1987). A few observations of long-lasting remissions in severe human autoimmune diseases have been reported even after short courses of anti-CD4 treatment. We have commented on these observations in Section 3.3. Such long-term improvement maintained after complete degradation of the injected antibody require additional explanations.

A very interesting concept was suggested by Waldmann *et al.* (1989) based on their experiments with tolerance induction by giving anti-CD4 shortly before antigenic challenge (Benjamin and Waldmann, 1986). A long-term unresponsiveness could be produced towards the isotype of the anti-CD4 mAb (Benjamin *et al.*, 1986; Gutstein *et al.*, 1986) and likewise to xenogeneic immunoglobulin (Benjamin and Waldmann, 1986). Cell depletion was not required, as non-depleting F(ab')2 fragments of anti-CD4 were comparable with regard to their effectiveness (Gutstein and Wofsy, 1986; Benjamin *et al.*, 1988). This form of tolerance was induced in T helper cells and not in B cells, and no suppressor cells were detected on adoptive transfer (Benjamin *et al.*, 1988). However, not only anti-CD4 but also a non-depleting mAb to another adhesion molecule (LFA-1) facilitated tolerance induction (Benjamin *et al.*, 1988). Similar strategies have been successfully applied for the induction of transplantation tolerance to skin grafts and were shown to induce stable chimerism after bone-marrow transplantation (Quin *et al.*, 1989).

A hypothesis was developed to explain these fascinating observations (Waldmann *et al.*, 1989; Cobbold *et al.*, 1990) which is based on (i) the critical role of co-stimulatory signals required to provide an "ON" signal upon TCR triggering and (ii) the assumption that tolerance induction is facilitated in the absence of appropriate co-stimulatory signals. The hypothesis makes use of the two-signal concept of Bretscher and Cohn (1970) and is compatible with observations in T cell clones (Jenkins et al., 1987) but, in addition, takes into account disruption of more complex cellular interactions. Co-stimulatory signals may be provided not only by cytokines but also by cell interactions via surface receptors. It is suggested that these co-stimulatory signals accumulate gradually until a threshold is reached for switching on the cellular activation programmes. It is well established that T cell clones become unresponsive to further antigenic challenge if the antigen is presented by fixed accessory cells unable to provide appropriate co-stimulatory signals (Jenkins et al., 1987). mAbs against adhesion molecules or receptors for co-stimulatory signals may act in a similar manner in vivo by disrupting collaborative cellular units either physically by cell depletion or merely in a functional way. Under these conditions with a drastically reduced number of responsible helper T cells, the antibodies disappear by degradation, and T cells are released, in a gradual process, from blockade. Surrounded by non-responding cells, i.e. "silence" with regard to co-stimulatory signals, they will encounter the putative autoantigen and thereby tolerance will be induced or reinforced. The situation seems to be similar to that in animals after depletion of lymphocytes by thoracic-duct drainage or irradiation, or in neonatal mice where tolerance is easy to establish.

A selective T cell blockade induced by anti-CD4 treatment has been described recently for the induction of transplantation tolerance to pancreatic islets of Langerhans in mice. In this study, clonal anergy without cell deletion was induced in Vβ11+ T cells reactive to the donor's MHC class II molecules (I-EK) as demonstrated by unresponsiveness to Vβ11-specific mAbs (Alters et al., 1991). With regard to autoimmune diseases, the question remains whether clonal anergy can also be implemented in memory cells or whether it is restricted to the application of anti-CD4 in the inductive phase of an immune response.

3.4.4 Other Possible Effects of Anti-CD4 Treatment

Little is known about possible effects of anti-CD4 treatment with other cells, although CD4 is found, at least in the human system, also on monocytes–macrophages (Wood et al. 1983), skin Langerhans cells (Wood et al., 1983), eosinophils (Lucey et al., 1989) and endothelial cells of the hepatic sinusoids (Scoazec and Feldmann, 1990). A 1.8 kB RNA transcript of CD4 has also been found in brain (Littman, 1987). A moderate reduction in circulating monocytes is demonstrated with some anti-CD4 mAbs (Horneff et al., 1991a), and IL-1 peaks lasting for 3–6 h after treatment were observed in some

patients (Horneff et al., 1991c). Preliminary data indicate no direct signalling via CD4 in monocytes but the possibility to engage Fc-receptors when anti-CD4 mAbs are cross-linked by secondary antibody (Guse et al., 1992). The functional consequences are unknown.

Anti-CD4 may also disturb binding of ligands other than MHC molecules. Recently, a cytokine, the lymphocyte chemoattractant factor, was reported to bind CD4 and also to transmit signals to the cell (Rand et al., 1991). It may be too early to speculate, but interference with cytokine binding by anti-CD4 mAbs could perhaps contribute to the redistribution of CD4 cells.

3.4.5 Future Prospects

Undoubtedly, the observation of long-term improvement with anti-CD4 mAbs in a few cases of severe autoimmune diseases and the results obtained with antibody-mediated tolerance induction in experimental animal models require more extended mechanistic studies. It is the general experience from these studies that anti-CD4 treatment is most effective during the early phase of an autoimmune disease, as demonstrated by total prevention of clinical manifestation when applied at the time or shortly after disease induction (Billingham et al., 1989). It is seen with other anti-T cell antibodies as well that delayed onset of treatment in rat adjuvant arthritis is accompanied by a gradual decline in therapeutic benefits (Yoshino et al., 1990) and a relapse after cessation of treatment. Therefore, anti-CD4 treatment in juvenile RA might be a promising approach. On the other hand, therapy starting a few months after disease onset might be too late and we have to consider other strategies. The main goal would be tolerance induction in memory T cells. Alternatively, it has been proposed to shift the whole immune system back to a quasi-neonate state where tolerance induction is much more easy to establish by means of a massive "debulking" of T cells (Waldmann et al., 1989). Thereby, a platform may be established on to which tolerance induction by non-depleting antibodies would be facilitated. Such a combined treatment using anti-CDw52 followed by anti-CD4 appeared to be successful in a patient with severe vasculitis (Mathieson et al., 1991).

It may also be worth considering the combined use of various mAbs. Combining two different mAbs to distinct rat CD4 epitopes, permitted a drastic reduction in the antibody dose (Qin et al., 1987), and only the combined use of anti-CD4, anti-CD8 and anti-LFA-1 together with low-dose irradiation made it possible to induce transplantation tolerance of skin grafts across complete H-2 differences (Waldmann et al., 1989). Until now, no reports are available documenting the use of antibody combinations in arthritis. Our own preliminary experiences with an anti-TCR mAb together with anti-CD4 in rat adjuvant arthritis suggest a synergistic effect (unpublished data). Combinations with conventional drug therapy aimed at supporting T cell blockade and, more importantly, at suppression of co-stimulatory signals provided by accessory cells will be another developmental pathway to be followed. At a time when animal experiments tend to become more and more restricted by regulatory issues it should be mentioned that the value of these therapeutic strategies is impossible to investigate without extended experimental proof.

4. Experiences with Other Antibodies in Rheumatoid Arthritis

4.1 CD5

Parallel to the anti-CD4 trials described above, phase I and subsequently phase II trials have been conducted using an anti-CD5 reagent coupled to the ricin A-chain by genetic engineering and designated CD5 Plus (Strand *et al.*, 1990). A considerable number of patients with RA (about 100) and recently also individuals with SLE (four patients) have been included in these trials (Hiepe *et al.* personal communication; Chatenoud *et al.* 1992; Moreland *et al.*, 1993, Strand *et al.*, 1993; Olsen *et al.*, 1993; Wacholtz *et al.*, 1992). The dosages administered to the patients treated are similar to those used in the anti-CD4 trials, with a mean tolerable dose of CD5 Plus of 0.20 mg/kg per day. Dose limitations were primarily due to constitutional symptoms including fever, chills and nausea with vomiting. In addition, approximately 50% of patients experienced rashes; myalgias and arthralgias occurred in 20%. However, no infectious episodes were caused by the treatment.

Immunological findings included a decrease in CD3+ T cell counts from 1200 cells/μl to a minimum of 570 cells/μl after 2 months, with a gradual increase to 730 after 3 months (0.33 mg/kg per day for 5 days; Cannon *et al.* (1991). Thus, the depletion efficacy does not appear to be higher than for the anti-CD4 reagents. There was a moderate reduction in *in vitro* T cell function after treatment. It is of special interest that the *in vitro* production of IgM rheumatoid factors increased at the time of maximum depletion of CD3+ T cells (Olsen *et al.*, 1991). There were no significant changes in routine laboratory parameters (serum immunoglobulins, rheumatoid factors or other autoantibody levels).

The clinical evaluation demonstrated a significant improvement in 75% (57/76) of patients by day 29 (>20% in 4/6 Paulus criteria) (Strand *et al.*, 1991). In a follow-up study 6 months after the first or the second treatment episode, 32 patients remained evaluable. Of these, 17 had a 50% improvement by the Paulus criteria. Thus, the authors concluded that one or two treatment courses resulted in significant objective improvements in patients with active RA who had failed at least one DMARD treatment. In a subset of patients, this improvement was sustained for more than 6 months. The amounts of human antibody generated against CD5 Plus appear to be remarkably high with titres of as much as >1:1 000 000 after a second treatment course. However, even very high titres of anti-CD5 Plus did not lead to a reduction in depletion efficacy compared with the first treatment episode. The same is true for those patients who had been treated with anti-CD4 reagents and developed human anti-mouse antibodies. Also in these instances re-treatment resulted in the same degree of CD4 cell depletion (Horneff *et al.*, 1991a; Reiter *et al.*, 1991a).

4.2 CD25 AND CD7

Small cohorts of patients have been treated using the murine anti-CD7 mAb RFT2 (IgG2a-isotype) or the chimeric version of the latter reagent (Kirkham *et al.* (1988); B. Kirkham (personal communication)). While the response using the murine reagent was very modest showing improvements in 2/6 patients, the clinical response to the chimerized reagents was more pronounced (Kirkham *et al.*, 1992).

Kyle and co-workers used Campath 6, a rat IgG2b mAb to IL-2R, in three patients with active RA (Kyle *et al.*, 1989). In this study, two patients were described as having an excellent clinical response with long-lasting significant changes in pain scores, morning stiffness and the Ritchie articular index. One other individual had an initial response, but a relapse after 1 month. Two patients had a febrile reaction during the first infusion, but there were no other side effects. Interestingly, CRP levels rose in these two individuals, but later markedly decreased to undetectable levels after 1 month.

5. Side Effects of Antibody Therapy

The longest experience with mAb treatment in man has been gained in patients with malignancies for which treatment is aimed at destruction of malignant cells (Koprowski *et al.*, 1979; Nadler *et al.*, 1980). Such mAbs are directed to so-called tumour-associated antigens and exert cytotoxic activity either directly (Masucci *et al.*, 1988; Vadhan-Raj *et al.*, 1988; Lubeck *et al.*, 1988) or via coupling with toxic compounds such as chemotherapeutics and radioisotopes (Kalofonos *et al.*, 1988; von Wussow *et al.*, 1988). Cancer treatment has always been impeded by the general difficulties in generating useful antibodies against weak antigens (Pirowski *et al.*, 1990). Moreover, virtually all patients developed a host immune response against the xenogeneic proteins (Shawler *et al.*, 1985; Schroff *et al.*, 1985; Courtenoy-Luck *et al.*, 1986; Dillman, 1989). A detailed description of side effects observed after mAb therapy in cancer patients has been published elsewhere (van der Linden *et al.*, 1988; Dillman, 1989; Frödin *et al.*, 1990) and this section will primarily focus on side effects associated with mAb therapy in patients with autoimmune diseases as well as in allograft rejection.

Side effects of mAb therapy in autoimmune disorders and organ transplantation may be classified into three distinct types related to the underlying mechanism. The first type of side effect is an immediate generalized reaction, usually seen within minutes of the first injection of antibody and presenting as a "flu-like syndrome". It is most prominent in patients receiving the anti-CD3 murine mAb, OKT3, and appears to be a consequence of mAb-mediated cell activation resulting in cytokine release. The second type of side effect results from the recipient's immune response to the therapeutic mAb and develops within the second week of therapy. It bears the danger of anaphylactic reactions, although the degree of the host response upon sensitization varies markedly depending on the antibody used. As a third type of possible side effects, overimmunosuppression of the recipient's immune system must be considered, especially when mAb therapy is combined with other immunosuppressive treatments.

5.1   IMMEDIATE REACTIONS FOLLOWING mAb INFUSION

Since the first clinical trials with OKT3, a poor tolerance has been reported with this particular mAb (Cosimi *et al.*, 1981a,b, 1987; Ortho Multicenter Transplant Study Group, 1985; Goldstein *et al.*, 1986; Norman *et al.*, 1988a; Thistlethwaite *et al.*, 1988). Patients receiving the initial 5 mg dose of OKT3 spontaneously developed high fever, chills, nausea, vomiting, diarrhoea, headache and/or anorexia. Usually, these symptoms are mild. However, they can be severe and require intensive care. The onset of the "first-dose-reaction" is at 45–60 min after the injection of the antibody, and symptoms spontaneously disappear after 2–3 days. Remarkably, the symptoms occur only during administration of the first two or three doses of OKT3. More severe but infrequent symptoms seen after OKT3 injection are pulmonary oedema due to a capillary leak in the presence of pre-existing fluid overload (Rowe *et al.*, 1987), aseptic meningitis (Emmons *et al.*, 1986; Thomas *et al.*, 1987; Martin *et al.*, 1988), marked hypotension (Hosenpud *et al.*, 1989) and seizures (Norman and Leone, 1991).

The precise pathophysiology of the described symptoms remains elusive. However, there is some evidence, that the mediators of the symptoms are cytokines, released by OKT3-induced T cell activation (Ellenhorn *et al.*, 1990) and/or lysis of opsonized T cells by mononuclear cells (Cosimi, 1987): (i) the first OKT3 infusions are followed by a sharp increase in cytokines (TNF-α, IL-6, IFNγ) with a peak level 1 h (TNFα) and 4 h (IL-6 and IFNγ) after infusion (Abramowicz *et al.*, 1989; Chatenoud *et al.*, 1989; Chatenoud and Bach, 1991; Norman and Leone, 1991; Gaston *et al.*, 1991). An increase in IL-2 was only observed in the absence of prior steroid treatment, and not all investigators have found an increase in this cytokine; (ii) the symptoms are not related to hypersensitivity, e.g. no increase in anti-OKT3 IgE was found (Chatenoud and Bach, 1991); (iii) similar acute manifestations can be induced by injecting pure recombinant cytokine molecules (IL-1, IL-2, TNF-α, IFNγ) (Remick *et al.*, 1987; Rosenberg *et al.*, 1987; Billiau, 1987); (iv) a refractory state is reached after repeated injections (e.g. usually after the fourth dose of OKT3) with regard to both cytokine release and clinical reactions (Ortho Multicenter Transplant Study Group, 1985; Cosimi, 1987; Abramowicz *et al.*, 1989; Chatenoud *et al.*, 1989); (v) the clinical symptoms can almost totally be abrogated by the use of an anti-human TNF mAb, given 1 h before OKT3 (Chatenoud and Bach, 1991). This antibody not only neutralizes TNF_1 but also results in modulation of the levels of other cytokines produced; (vi) *in vitro*, OKT3 is a powerful mitogen for triggering T cell proliferation (van Wauwe *et al.*, 1980).

Anti-CD4 mAbs are remarkably better tolerated than OKT3. Among 152 reported patients with various diseases who had received an anti-CD4 mAb (see Sections 3.2 and 3.3), no serious side-effects (either immediate or long-lasting) have been observed. A very few patients developed a flu-like syndrome with low-grade fever and chills (Herzog *et al.*, 1989; Horneff *et al.*, 1991a; Wendling *et al.*, 1991; Nicolas *et al.*, 1991; van der Lubbe *et al.*, 1991b; Didry *et al.*, 1991; Moreland *et al.*, 1991). The symptoms resolved spontaneously within 24 h and, in some studies, were parallelled by increased levels of cytokines such as TNF-α, IFNγ and IL-2 or IL-6 (Horneff *et al.*, 1991c; van der Lubbe *et al.*, 1991b). Although one has to consider that some patients were treated with histamine receptor blockers (which do not influence the OKT3-associated first-dose reaction), the clinical symptoms following anti-CD4 infusion were by no means comparable with the OKT3-induced symptoms with respect to their frequency, intensity and severity. Some recent reports indicate that the chimeric mAb cMT-412 is more frequently accompanied by a flu-like syndrome (Moreland *et al.*, 1991; van der Lubbe *et al.*, 1991b).

Antibodies against the IL-2R were usually well tolerated (Soulillou *et al.*, 1987; Diamantstein *et al.*, 1989; Kyle *et al.*, 1989; Waldmann *et al.*, 1990; Wijdenes *et al.*, 1990; Kirkman *et al.*, 1991). In one study with 27 patients receiving anti-IL-2R mAb 33B3.1 (rat IgG2a) for prevention of kidney allograft rejection, mild fever was reported in most patients during the first 48 h of therapy (Soulillou *et al.*, 1987). In a study with a different mAb (anti-Tac, murine IgG2a), three patients out of 40 developed flushes or chills, two patients suffered from pruritus, and eight patients developed fever during the whole treatment course, which, however, could not clearly be attributed to antibody therapy (Kirkman *et al.*, 1991). With another anti-IL-2R mAb (Campath 6, rat IgG2b), two of three patients had fever during the first infusion (Kyle *et al.*, 1989), whereas none of 32 patients treated for steroid-resistant acute graft-versus-host disease had any side effects in a study using the mouse IgG1 mAb, B-B10 (Wijdenes *et al.*, 1990). No side effects were reported in 23 patients receiving the anti-blast antibody CBL1 (Culler *et al.*, 1985; Takahashi *et al.*, 1983).

5.2 ANTI-mAb IMMUNE RESPONSE

When OKT3 was first administered to patients, it was much to the surprise of the investigators that the antibody was highly immunogenic, resembling the predecessors of mAb therapy, e.g. polyclonal anti-lymphocyte sera. Similar to murine antibodies used in cancer patients (Shawler *et al.*, 1985; Schroff *et al.*, 1985; Courtenoy-Luck *et al.*, 1986; Dillman, 1989), almost every individual developed an immune response against the antibody when treated with OKT3 alone (Cosimi *et al.*, 1981a; Chatenoud *et al.*, 1982; Ortho Multicenter Transplant Study Group, 1985; Goldstein *et al.*, 1986). Anti-OKT3 antibodies were first detected during or after the second week of treatment. In the majority of patients, titres did not exceed 1 : 100 with peak levels of 1 : 1000–1 : 100 000 in a few cases.

The human anti-mouse response tended to be primarily of the IgG isotype and was less frequently IgM (Chatenoud *et al.*, 1982, 1983, 1986a; Ortho-Multicenter Study Group, 1985). Importantly, the predominant component of the immune response was an anti-idiotypic antibody (Jaffers *et al.*, 1986; Chatenoud *et al.*, 1986a,b) with neutralizing capacity for OKT3, thus leading to an accelerated clearance of the mAb. OKT3 clearance was followed by an increasing number of CD3+ cells, which parallelled the onset of overt clinical and histological rejection episodes (Chatenoud *et al.*, 1983).

The anti-isotypic antibody did not interfere with OKT3-mediated immunosuppressive effects, although they bound to OKT3 (Baudrihaye *et al.*, 1984; Chatenoud *et al.*, 1986a). It was shown *in vitro* that binding of anti-isotypic antibody to OKT3-coated T cells induced an even more effective antigenic modulation of the CD3–TCR complex which may increase efficacy of treatment (Chatenoud and Bach, 1984). IgM antibodies against OKT3 usually express low affinity to the antibody thereby lacking an effective OKT3 neutralization (Chatenoud *et al.*, 1986a).

The human anti-mouse response to OKT3 was clonally restricted (Chatenoud *et al.*, 1986b). However, this seems not to be a unique feature of the OKT3-induced immune response and was also seen in monkeys treated with anti-CD4 and in rodents treated with anti-CD8 mAbs (Benjamin *et al.*, 1986; Villemain *et al.*, 1986).

A further mAb injection into patients who had developed an immune response to OKT3 boosted their anti-mouse response. Half of the patients not responding to the first treatment cycle developed anti-mouse antibodies after the second course of treatment (Norman *et al.*, 1988b). However, the second exposure to OKT3, appeared to stimulate predominantly non-blocking antibodies i.e. non-idiotypic antibodies or IgM (Norman *et al.*, 1988b).

Human anti-mouse antibodies are also induced by anti-CD4 therapy with different mAbs (Hafler *et al.*, 1988; Dhiver *et al.*, 1989; Herzog *et al.*, 1989; Morel *et al.*, 1990; Horneff *et al.*, 1991a; Knox *et al.*, 1991; Reiter *et al.*, 1991a; Wendling *et al.*, 1991); The frequency of patients developing anti-mouse antibodies upon anti-CD4 treatment varies considerably, presumably depending on the amount of mAb given, the state of immunocompetence of the recipient, and the immunogenicity of the individual mAb. The levels of anti-CD4-induced human anti-mouse antibodies were significantly lower than the OKT3-induced titres. It should be kept in mind that up to 5% of healthy blood donors ($n = 170$) apparently have low titres of preformed circulating anti-mouse antibodies (Reiter *et al.*, 1991a). The low amount of anti-mouse antibodies arising after anti-CD4 therapy may be explained by a significant immunosuppression caused by anti-CD4 therapy preventing a vigorous anti-mouse response. In addition, most patients had received concomitant immunosuppressive drug therapy. This hypothesis is supported by the observation in a mouse model that application of low-dose anti-CD4 antibody did elicit an immune response, and high doses did not (Gutstein and Wofsy, 1986). Concordantly, decreasing the amount of injected OKT3 also leads to a higher sensitization rate (Chatenoud and Bach 1991).

Anti-mouse antibodies usually become detectable 2–3 weeks after initiation of treatment but may appear earlier in rare cases (Dhiver *et al.*, 1989; Didry *et al.*, 1991). They normally remain detectable for 10–12 weeks after a single treatment cycle and are primarily of the IgG isotype. A second course of treatment enhances the anti-mouse response in a quite similar way to the OKT3-induced response. With MAX.16H5, about 25% of the anti-mouse response is directed against the idiotype (Horneff *et al.*, 1991a) and anti-mouse antibodies that could block *in vitro* binding of anti-CD4 are found after treatment with MT-151 (Reiter *et al.*, 1991a) and BL4 (Morel *et al.*, 1990). Probably the affinity of the particular anti-CD4 mAb will determine whether these anti-idiotypic antibodies effectively compete with the CD4 molecule. Although the experience is still limited to four patients who received a second treatment cycle, no interference of the human anti-mouse response with the clinical efficacy of MAX.16H5 has been observed (Horneff *et al.*, 1991b).

One patient who developed an anaphylactic reaction during a second treatment course developed IgE anti-mouse antibodies (Reiter *et al.*, 1991a). In another patient with skin urticaria after the first injection, no anti-mouse IgE, IgM or IgG could be detected (Horneff *et al.*, 1991b) which, however, in the case of IgE may have been due to the lower sensitivity of the assay system.

In treatment protocols with other mAbs, human anti-mouse antibodies could be detected with variable frequency. Four of four patients treated with anti-CD7 antibodies were described as developing an anti-mouse response (Kirkham *et al.*, 1988), and, in 14 of 19 patients treated with an anti-blast mAb, anti-mouse antibodies could be detected within 2 weeks of initiation of treatment (Takahashi *et al.*, 1983). However, higher antibody levels were found in three patients only without abrogating treatment efficacy. An anti-T12 mAb used for treatment of allograft rejection in renal transplant patients induced an immune response in 14 of 19 patients with equal distribution of IgG and IgM isotypes which were exclusively directed against non-idiotypic determinants (Kirkman *et al.*, 1983). Again, one has to consider the concomitant immunosuppressive therapy in these patients when interpreting the data. After anti-IL-2R mAb infusions, about 85% of the patients developed an anti-mouse response with a high proportion of neutralizing anti-idiotypic antibodies (Soulillou *et al.*, 1987; Diamantstein *et al.*, 1989;. Waldmann *et al.*, 1990; Wijdenes *et al.*, 1990; Kirkman *et al.*, 1991). However, patients treated for adult T cell leukaemia (ATL) with anti-IL-2R mAbs did not produce any human anti-mouse antibodies presumably because of their underlying disease resulting in a concomitant immunodeficiency.

An important, but mainly logistic, side effect of circulating human anti-mouse antibodies is their interference with *in vitro* assays, for example ELISA, operating with anti-murine sera, thus leading to false positive serum levels of the proteins investigated, e.g. for carcino-embryonic antigen (Hansen *et al.*, 1989) or thyroid-stimulating hormone (Zweig *et al.*, 1987).

Numerous efforts have been undertaken to reduce the incidence of sensitization towards therapeutic mAbs. By combining antibody therapy with conventional immunosuppressive drugs, the sensitization rate could be successfully reduced to an incidence of only 10–20% with concomitant treatment by OKT3 together with cyclosporin A. In addition, the frequency of non-blocking antibodies was increased by this regimen (Norman *et al.*, 1988; Schroeder *et al.*, 1990; Hricik *et al.*, 1990).

5.3   SIDE EFFECTS DUE TO OVERIMMUNOSUPPRESSION

One of the major goals of T cell-directed mAb therapy is specific targeting of the immunosuppressive effect to certain cell subsets, leaving other parts of the immune system unaffected to control infections and malignancies. However, unless specific targeting can be achieved to

only T cells that initiate and maintain the disease, one has to consider unwanted "over"immunosuppression.

Patients that have received an organ graft are generally on a profound immunosuppressive therapy. Infections and malignancies during the post-transplant course caused by the potent conventional immunosuppressive regimens are not uncommon (Penn, 1983; Chatenoud and Bach, 1991). However, no increased incidence of lymphomas has been reported in OKT3-treated patients compared with a control group receiving conventional immunosuppressive therapy after kidney and liver transplantation (Abramowicz *et al.*, 1991; Chatenoud and Bach, 1991; Cosimi and Rubin, 1991; Norman and Leone, 1991). In contrast, an increase in lymphoproliferative disorders has been described in cardiac-grafted patients (Swinnen *et al.*, 1990) who received a cumulative dose of OKT3 of more than 75 mg, in addition to a full dose of cyclosporin A starting at the time of transplantation. This finding has initiated an extended and controversial discussion (Emery and Lake, 1991; Brouwer *et al.*, 1991).

Patients with a history of herpes simplex virus infections frequently re-activate these infections upon OKT3 therapy unless acyclovir is used for prophylaxis (Singh, 1988). CMV antibody titres in CMV-positive patients were increased by OKT3. However, CMV-negative individuals receiving a CMV-positive transplant have no increased risk of developing a CMV infection upon OKT3 treatment (Chou and Norman, 1985; Chou *et al.*, 1987). In general, it appears that the risk of acquiring infections is increased in patients receiving OKT3 compared with the healthy control population, but not increased in comparison with control groups receiving other potent immunosuppressive regimens.

Only one report (Moreland *et al.* 1993) of opportunistic infection but no malignancy have been published for any patient treated with anti-CD4 mAbs until now. In contrast, one patient with a known herpes zoster infection did not show any activation of this disease (Herzog *et al.*, 1989) and, interestingly, of seven patients with AIDS, none developed increased opportunistic infection during the treatment course and 4–7 months thereafter (Dhiver *et al.*, 1989).

Moreover, one patient who developed a long-lasting CD4+ cell depletion (200–500 cells/μl for more than 2 years) with an inversed CD4/CD8 ratio (0.2–0.4) after two 1-week cycles of anti-CD4 mAb therapy (MAX.16H5) and a subsequent continuous treatment with chlorambucil did not suffer from increased infection nor did he develop signs of malignancies during the entire follow-up period (Horneff *et al.*, 1992).

In vitro as well as *in vivo* experiments with T cells after anti-CD4 treatment revealed no major damage to T lymphocyte function. After CD4 modulation, *in vivo* T cells responded even better to anti-CD3-induced triggering of the TCR–CD3 complex by increasing the intracellular Ca^{2+} concentrations (Horneff *et al.*, 1993a). These findings indicate that even low numbers of circulating CD4+ T cells, as seen after anti-CD4 treatment, are sufficient to maintain a functional cellular immune system.

Similarly to anti-CD4 antibody, no increased rates of infection or malignancies have been reported for treatment trials with mAbs to IL-2R, CD7, T12 and blast cells. However, only limited numbers of patients have been treated, and more experience is required.

6. Engineered Antibodies

In 1975, Köhler and Milstein published their famous experiment on the generation of murine mAbs with selected specificity generated by fusing a mouse myeloma cell with a normal B cell (Köhler and Milstein, 1975). In this setting, the normal B cell contributes the specific antibody while the myeloma cell contributes its capability of continuous growth. The most appropriate antibody-producing "hybridoma" has to be selected by screening. Hybridoma cells form stable cell lines with an almost unlimited capacity to multiply, and many of them synthesize large amounts of mAb normally in the range of 1–100 μg/ml of culture supernatant. They are permanent cellular sources of homogeneous antibodies which can be produced in the peritoneal cavity of mice as ascites or in large-scale suspension cultures using fermenters or bioreactors with immobilized cells and perfusion systems. The technologies are constantly being improved. However, together with some recent developments in mAb technology requests have emerged for more refined molecules.

In Fig. 5.4 a range of principal inventions is depicted which illustrate the potential of antibody engineering. Bispecific antibody can be generated by somatic cell genetics, i.e. fusion of hybridomas which codominantly express antibody genes of two different specificities but have to be purified from a variety of different H- and L-chain combinations. They have been used for redirecting potential effector cells to their targets (Staerz and Bevan, 1986). Univalent antibodies often show a greatly improved complement-mediated lysis (Glennie and Stevenson, 1982) and may be produced by either enzymatic cleavage of one Fab arm or, like bispecific antibodies, from hybrid–hybridomas with subsequent purification.

To avoid unwarranted immune responses to mouse immunoglobulin determinants, several fusion partners of human origin were developed for the production of human mAbs. Unfortunately, most hybridomas obtained by this means are not very stable and produce only low amounts of antibody. Human mAbs to cell surface determinants cannot be obtained in this way because B cells specific for human cell surface antigens should have been eliminated during ontogeny of the immune system and are not available in normal lymphocyte populations.

Nowadays, the newly developed molecular genetic tools have provided us with the opportunity to construct human antibodies equipped with recognition sites obtained from selected mouse mAbs. The first step towards "humanization" of mouse mAbs was the linking of rodent variable regions and human constant regions, thus generating "chimeric" antibodies (Neuberger et al., 1985). However, framework determinants within the foreign V-region still retain a considerable immunogenicity as demonstrated in an elegant study by Brüggemann et al. (1989). No attenuation of the anti-V response against the chimeric antibody was observed in comparison with a fully xenogeneic antibody carrying the same V-region.

Therefore, a more sophisticated method of additional replacement of the V-region framework had to be developed. It relies on grafting the antigen-binding site – the so-called complementarity-determining regions – from rodent to human antibody (Riechmann et al., 1988). Such "reshaping" leading to fully humanized antibodies often requires molecular modelling and stepwise fitting of the key contact between antigen-binding loop and framework in order to restore the affinity of the wild-type rodent mAb. As demonstrated with a fully humanized antibody (Campath 1H) no anti-mouse response could be detected (Hale et al., 1988).

It is also possible to alter the biological function of mAbs, which mostly resides in the Fc portion, by generating immunoglobulin class switch variants or by recombining the same variable region with another constant region. It has been demonstrated already that the human IgG1 isotype was highly effective in several in vitro assays with chimeric antibodies bearing the same anti-CD4 recognition site (Dalesandro et al., 1991). Binding sites for Fc-receptors and for the first component (C1q) of complement reside in the constant region and may be altered like other biological functions by cutting and pasting of restriction fragments or by site-directed mutagenesis. In turn, the effector functions of Fc fragments can be transferred to other proteins, as demonstrated by linking CD4 to Fc fragments (CD4 immunoadhesion), thus creating an artificial ligand for the viral glycoprotein gp120 (Byrn et al., 1990).

Smaller fragments lacking the Fc portion, i.e. F(ab)2, Fab or Fv fragments, and derivatives thereof, mediate function primarily via antigen binding. They may penetrate tissue faster (Sutherland et al., 1987) and are also cleared faster which will be advantageous if these compounds are used for imaging or as drug carriers. Some further engineering may be required to avoid dissociation of unstable Fv fragments which can be overcome by a flexible linker peptide (Bird et al., 1988) or by introducing disulphide bonds between the domains. The use of single-domain antibodies (Ward et al., 1989) or the "minimal recognition unit" possibly on the background of another protein molecule will mainly depend on the possibility of retaining an appropriate affinity and, in the

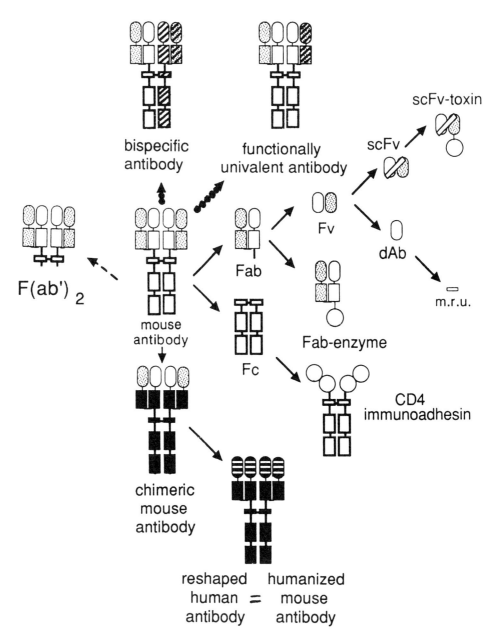

Figure 5.4 Illustrated are engineered antibodies and fragments. Each box represents a domain. Fab fragments and single-chain Fv fragments (scFv) have been used to target enzymes and toxins. Size reduction of the variable region can be achieved by using VH domains (dAb) or even single minimal recognition units (m.r.u.) which retain antigen-binding activities. In immunoadhesins, a specific ligand (CD4) is attached to an Fc fragment. The terms "reshaped human antibody" and "fully humanized mouse antibody" are used synonymously. Bispecific antibodies consist of two different but functional sets of H and L chains while functionally univalent antibodies bear one irrelevant L chain. The constructs are generated by genetic engineering (——), somatic cell genetics followed by antibody purification (••••) or by enzyme cleavage (---) (modified from Winter G. and Milstein C. (1991)). (Reprinted by permission from Nature vol. 349, p. 295. Copyright (C) 1991 Macmillan Magazines Ltd.)

case of Fv fragments, on the reduction of their hydrophobicity.

Another possibility of introducing novel biological functions is linking totally different molecules such as enzymes to Fab fragments (Neuberger *et al.*, 1984).

It is difficult to say whether any of these inventions will be of particular benefit for the anti-CD4 treatment as long as the rationale of immediate and long-term effects is not completely understood. Chimeric antibodies have demonstrated clinical efficacy (Moreland *et al.*, 1991; van der Lubbe *et al.*, 1991b) but a considerable anti-V framework response may require further humanization and reshaping of the antibody. However, all biological functions mediated by the Fc region of individual anti-CD4 mAbs are likely to be lost and may be difficult to restore by additional genetic manipulations.

7. Conclusion

Beneficial prophylactic and therapeutic effects of mAbs to T cell surface molecules, in particular on CD4+ (helper/inducer) T cells, have been demonstrated in animal models of autoimmune disorders including inflammatory joint diseases. Studies in humans were encouraged by these observations, which have led to an ever-increasing number of clinical trials in RA and other human autoimmune diseases implicating T cells. Of particular interest were results with anti-CD4 antibodies which have demonstrated that in RA (i) CD4+ T cells do contribute to the disease process in many cases even in a late and chronic stage and (ii) the immune system of the adult can be modulated towards clinical improvement. Most patients treated had severe diseases that were intractable to all other conventional therapies, thereby providing unfavourable conditions for immunomodulation which is not able to reverse already established destruction of joint tissue. Nevertheless, the transient but significant improvement, lasting at least several weeks and up to a few months in the majority of patients treated, is a promising result. However, the number of patients investigated over the past 3 years is still small, and the study designs are not always comparable. It is important to note that adverse effects of anti-CD4 treatment and also of treatment with other anti-T cell antibodies are not very frequent and only mild. Thus far, no increased susceptibility to infectious diseases or lymphoproliferative disorders has been reported.

The immunological mechanisms upon which anti-CD4 therapy is based are still not fully understood. Immediate effects are probably due to blocking of antigen recognition and/or a negative signal transmitted to the cell by ligation of anti-CD4 mAbs separate from TCR. In contrast, depletion of CD4 cells from the circulation or cell killing and also release of soluble CD4 molecules and modulation of the CD4 molecule from cell membranes does not seem to contribute very much to therapeutic effects, although it is difficult to exclude the idea that combinations of certain mechanisms studied separately may have a synergistic effect. In animal models, the antibody isotype is very critical, which has not been observed by comparing IgG2a and IgG1 mouse anti-human-CD4 antibodies with regard to their clinical efficacy. Many observations point to the importance of different CD4 epitopes which may explain why some antibodies differ in their biological activities. The capability of one antibody (MAX.16H5) to reduce rheumatoid factor concentration and other laboratory parameters of inflammation is not parallelled by other anti-CD4 monoclonals. Thus far, there are no test systems available for determining the most effective anti-CD4 before its use in humans.

Besides mouse mAbs, chimeric antibodies expressing only immunoglobulin V-regions and fully "humanized" mAbs have also been developed, and preliminary data on the use of a chimeric anti-CD4 antibody in RA are available. At present, it is still too early to decide whether they will provide clear advantages over their murine counterparts.

Undoubtedly, additional carefully controlled double-blind studies are required to investigate the clinical use of anti-CD4 and other T cell antibodies in autoimmune diseases. There is only preliminary information available on repeated courses of treatment, and longer treatment periods, or more frequent single administrations, combinatorial therapies of different antibodies with or without further combination with conventional drug therapy should also be considered. More experience is needed in monitoring parameters and markers helpful for identifying potential therapy responders before treatment.

However, clinical studies and more refined antibodies are not the only developments that should be pursued. We should not forget to intensify exploration of the basic mechanisms which will require animal experiments to optimize immunomodulatory protocols. Although not yet observed in the treatment of RA with the current protocols, the hope remains (supported by experimental studies and a few observations in other human autoimmune diseases) that we might be able in the future to induce long-lasting improvement or even remissions by a relatively short-term treatment with anti-T cell antibodies.

8. References

Abramowicz, D., Schandene, L., Goldman, M., Crusiaux, A., Vereerstraeten, P., DePauw, L., Wybran, J., Kinnaert, P., Dupont, E. and Toussaint, C. (1989). Release of tumor necrosis factor, interleukin-2, and gamma-interferon in serum after injection of OKT3 monoclonal antibody in kidney transplant recipients. Transplantation 47, 606–608.

Abramowicz, D., Goldman, M., DePauw, L., Deutrelepont, J.-M., Kinnaert, P., Vanherweghem, J.-L. and Vereerstraeten, P. (1991). Post-transplantation lymphoproliferative disorder and OKT3. N. Engl. J. Med. 324, 1438–1439.

Acha-Orbea, H., Mitchell, D.J., Timmerman, L., Wraith, D.C., Tausch, G.S., Waldor, M.K., Zamvil, S.S., McDevitt, H.O. and Steinman, L. (1988). Limited heterogeneity of T cell receptors from lymphocytes mediating autoimmune encephalomyelitis allows specific immune intervention. Cell 54, 263–273.

Alters, S.A., Shizuru, J.A., Ackerman, J., Grossman, D., Seydel, K.B. and Fathman, C.G. (1991). Anti-CD4 mediates clonal anergy during transplantation tolerance induction. J. Exp. Med. 173, 491–494.

Babbitt, B.P., Allen, P.M., Matsueda, G., Haber, E. and Unanue, E.R. (1985). Binding of immunogenic peptides to Ia histocompatibility molecules. Nature (London) 317, 359–361.

Baker, A.S., Swain, A.F., Fry, L. and Valdimarsson, H. (1984). Epidermal T lymphoctye and HLA-DR expression in psoriasis. Br. J. Dermatol. 110, 555–564.

Barton, R.W., Rothlein, R., Ksiazek, J. and Kennedy, C. (1989). The effect of anti-intercellular adhesion molecule-1 on phorbol-ester-induced rabbit lung inflammation. J. Immunol. 143, 1278–1282.

Baudrihaye, M.F., Chatenoud, L., Kreis, H., Goldstein, G. and Bach, J.-F. (1984). Unusually restricted anti-isotype human immune response to OKT3 monoclonal antibody. Eur. J. Immunol. 14, 686–691.

Becker, W., Emmrich, F., Horneff, G., Burmester, G.R., Seiler, F., Schwarz, A., Kalden, J.R. and Wolf, F. (1990). Imaging autoimmune rheumatoid arthritis specifically with technetium 99m CD4-specific (T-helper lymphocytes) antibodies. Eur. J. Nucl. Med. 7, 156–159.

Beelen, D.W., Graeven, U., Schulz, G., Grosse-Wilde, H., Doxiadis, I., Schaefer, U.W., Quabeck, K., Sayer, H. and Schmidt, C.G. (1988). Treatment of acute graft-versus-host disease after HLA-partially matched marrow transplantation with a monoclonal antibody (BMA031) against the T cell receptor. First results of a phase-I/II trial. Onkologie 11, 56–58.

Bekoff, M., Kakiuchi, T. and Grey, M.H. (1985). Accessory cell junction in the Con A response: role of Ia-positive and Ia-negative accessory cells. J. Immunol. 134, 1373–1343.

Benjamin, R.J. and Waldmann, H. (1986). Induction of tolerance by monoclonal antibody therapy. Nature (London) 320, 449–451.

Benjamin, R.J., Cobbold, S.P., Clark, M.R. and Waldmann, H. (1986). Tolerance to rat monoclonal antibodies. Implications for serotherapy. J. Exp. Med. 163, 1539–1552.

Benjamin, R.J., Qin, S.X., Wise, M.P., Cobbold, S.P. and Waldmann, H. (1988). Monoclonal antibodies for tolerance induction: a possible role for CD4 (L3T4) and CD11a (LFA-1) molecules in self–non-self discrimination. Eur. J. Immunol. 18, 1079–1088.

Biddison, W.E., Rao, P.E., Talle, M.A., Goldstein, G. and Shaw, S. (1982). Possible involvement of the OKT4 molecule in T cell recognition of class II HLA antigens. Evidence from studies of cytotoxic T lymphocytes specific for SB antigens. J. Exp. Med. 156, 1065–1076.

Billiau, A. (1987). Interferons and inflammation. J. Interferon Res. 7, 559–567.

Billingham, M.E.J., Fairchild, S., Griffin, E., Drayer, L. and Hicks, C. (1989). In "Therapeutic Approaches to Inflammatory Diseases" (ed A.J. Lewis, N.S. Doherty and N.R. Ackerman), pp 242–253. Elsevier Science Publishing Co., Inc., Amsterdam.

Bird, R.E., Hardman, K.D., Jacobson, J.W., Johnson, S., Kaufman, B.M., Lee, S.M., Lee, T., Pope, S.H., Riordan, G.S. and Whitlow, M. (1988). Single-chain antigen-binding proteins. Science 242, 423–426.

Blue, M.-L., Hafler, D.A., Daley, J.F., Levine, H. and Craig, K.A. (1988). Regulation of T cell clone via CD4 and CD8 molecules. J. Immunol. 140, 376–383.

Bretscher, P. and Cohn, M. (1970). A theory of self–non-self discrimination. Science 169, 1042–1049.

Brinkman, C.J.J., Ter Laak, H.J. and Hommes, O.R. (1985). Modulation of experimental allergic encephalomyelitis in Lewis rats by monoclonal anti-T cell antibodies. J. Neuroimmunol. 7, 237–238.

Brouwer, R.M.L., Balk, A.H.M.M. and Weimar, W. (1991). Post-transplantation lymphoproliferative disorder and OKT3. N. Engl. J. Med. 324, 1437.

Brüggemann, M., Winter, G., Waldmann, H. and Neuberger, M.S. (1989). The immunogenicity of chimeric antibodies. J. Exp. Med. 170, 2153–2157.

Buus, A., Sette, A., Colon, S.M., Jenis, D.M. and Grey, H.M. (1986). Isolation and characterization of antigen–Ia complexes involved in T cell recognition. Cell 47, 1071–1077.

Byrn, R.A., Mordenti, J., Lucas, C., Smith, D., Marsters, S.A., Johnson, J.S., Cossum, P., Chamow, S.M., Wurm, F.M., Gregory, T., Groopman, J.E. and Capon, D.J. (1990). Biological properties of a CD4 immunoadhesin. Nature (London) 344, 667–670.

Cannon, G.W., Marble, D.A., Griffiths, M.M., Shulman, S.F. and Strand, V. (1991). Immunologic assessment during treatment of rheumatoid arthritis with anti-CD5 immunoconjugate. Arth. Rheum. 34, S 157.

Chatenoud, L. and Bach, J.-F. (1984). Antigenic modulation. A major mechanism of antibody action. Immunol. Today 5, 20.

Chatenoud, L. and Bach, J.-F. (1991). In "The British Council, Immunotherapy with Monoclonal Antibodies", Speakers' note 9132, Cambridge, 7–13 April 1991.

Chatenoud, L., Baudrihaye, M.F., Kreis, H., Goldstein, G., Schindler, J. and Bach, J.-F. (1982). Human in vivo antigenic modulation induced by the anti-T cell OKT3 monoclonal antibody. Eur. J. Immunol. 12, 979–982.

Chatenoud, L., Baudrihaye, M.F., Chkoff, N., Kreis, H. and Bach, J.-F. (1983). Immunologic follow-up of renal allograft recipients treated prophylactically by OKT3 alone. Transplant. Proc. 15, 643–645.

Chatenoud, L., Baudrihaye, M.F., Chkoff, N., Kreis, H., Goldstein, G. and Bach, J.-F. (1986a). Restriction of the human in vivo immune response against the mouse monoclonal antibody OKT3. J. Immunol. 137, 830–838.

Chatenoud, L., Jonker, M., Villemain, F., Goldstein, G. and Bach, J.-F. (1986b). The human immune response to the OKT3 monoclonal antibody is oligoclonal. Science 232, 1406–1408.

Chatenoud, L., Gerran, C., Reuter, A., Legendre, C., Gevaert, Y., Kreis, H., Franchimont, P. and Bach, J.-F. (1989). Systemic reaction to the anti-T cell monoclonal antibody OKT3 in relation to serum levels of tumor necrosis factor and interferon-γ. N. Engl. J. Med. 320, 1420–1421.

Chatenoud, L., Goldberg, D., Viard, J.-P., Dain, M.-P.,

Bach, J.F. and Menkes, C.-J. (1992) A pilot study using an anti-CD4 monoclonal antibody therapy in rheumatoid arthritis. Arthritis Rheum. (Suppl) 35, S. 106.

Chluba, J., Steeg, C., Becker, A., Wererle, H. and Epplen, J.T. (1989). T cell receptor chain usage in myelin basic protein-specific rat T lymphocytes. Eur. J. Immunol. 19, 279–284.

Chou, S. and Norman, D.J. (1985). Effect of OKT3 antibody therapy on cytomegalovirus reactivation in renal transplant recipients. Transplant. Proc. 17, 2755–2756.

Chou, S., Kim, D.Y. and Norman, D.J. (1987). Transmission of cytomegalovirus by pretransplant leukocyte transfusions in renal transplant candidates. J. Infect. Dis. 155, 565–567.

Choy, E.H.S., Chikanza, J.C., Kingsley, G.H. and Panayi, G.S. (1991). Chimaeric anti-CD4 monoclonal antibody for relapsing polychondritis. Lancet 338, 450.

Clevers, H., Alarcon, B., Wileman, T. and Terhorst, C. (1988). The T cell receptor/CD3 complex: a dynamic protein ensemble. Annu. Rev. Immunol 6. 629–662.

Cobbold, S., Qin, S. and Waldmann, H. (1990). Reprogramming the immune system for tolerance with monoclonal antibodies. Semin. Immunol. 2, 377–387.

Cosimi, A.B. (1987). OKT3: first-dose safety and success. Nephron 46, 12–18.

Cosimi, A.B. and Rubin, R.H. (1991). Post-transplantation lymphoproliferative disorder and OKT3. N. Engl. J. Med. 324, 1438.

Cosimi, A.B., Colvin, R.B., Burton, R.C., Rubin, R.H., Goldstein, G., Kung, P.C., Hansen, P., Delmonico, F.L. and Russell P.S. (1981a). Use of monoclonal antibodies to T cell subsets for immunologic monitoring and treatment in recipients of renal allografts. N. Engl. J. Med. 305, 308–314.

Cosimi, A.B., Burton, R.C., Colvin, R.B., Goldstein, G., Delmonico, F.L. LaQuaglia, M.P., Tolkoff-Rubing, R.H., Herrin, J.T. and Russell, P. (1981b). Treatment of acute renal allograft rejection with OKT3 monoclonal antibody. Transplantation 32, 535–539.

Courtenoy-Luck, N.S., Epenetos, A.A., Moore, R., Larche, M., Pectasides, D., Dhokio, B. and Ritter, M.A. (1986). Development of primary and secondary immune responses to mouse monoclonal antibodies used in the diagnosis and therapy of malignant neoplasms. Cancer Res. 46, 6489–6493.

Culler, F.L., O'Connor, R., Kaufmann, S., Jones, K.L and Roth, J.C. (1985). Immunospecific therapy for type I diabetes mellitus. N. Engl. J. Med. 311, 1701–1702.

Dalesandro, M.N., Pak, K.Y., Tam, S., Wilson, E., Reiter, C., Knight, D., Looney, J., Ghrayeb, J., Rieber, E.P., Riethmüller, G. and Daddona, P. (1991). In vitro efficacy of a mouse/human chimeric CD4 antibody: functional contributions of isotype and Fc. J. Cell. Biochem. (Suppl. 15E) 179, O 403.

Dhiver, C., Olive, D., Rousseau, S., Tamalet, C., Lopez, M., Galindo, J.-R., Mourens, M., Hirn, M., Gastaut, J.-A. and Mawas, C. (1989). Pilot phase I study using zidovudine in association with a 10-day course of anti-CD4 monoclonal antibody in seven AIDS patients. AIDS 3, 835–842.

Diamantstein, T., Kupiec-Weglinski, J.W., Strom, T.B. and Tilney, N.L. (1989). Current stage of interleukin 2 receptor targeted therapy. Exp. Clin. Endocrinol. 93, 114–124.

Didry, C., Portalés, P., Adary, M., Brochier, J., Combe, B., Clot, J. and Sany, J. (1991). Treatment of rheumatoid arthritis (RA) with monoclonal anti-CD4 antibodies. Clinical results. Arth. Rheum. 34, S92 (A162).

Dillman, R.O. (1989). Monoclonal antibodies for treating cancer. Ann. Int. Med. 111, 592–603.

Doyle, C. and Strominger, J.L. (1987). Interaction between CD4 and class II MHC molecules mediates cell adhesion. Nature (London) 330, 256–259.

Ellenhorn, J.D.I., Woodle, E.S., Chobreal, I., Thistlethwaite, J.R. and Bluestone, J.A. (1990). Activation of human T cells in vivo following treatment of transplant recipients with OKT3. Transplantation 50, 608–612.

Emery, R.W. and Lake, K.D. (1991). Post-transplantation lymphoproliferative disorder and OKT3. N. Engl. J. Med. 324, 1437.

Emmons, C., Smith, J. and Flanigan, M. (1986). Cerebrospinal fluid inflammation during OKT3 therapy. Lancet ii, 510–511.

Emmrich, F. (1988). Activation of T cells by crosslinking the T cell receptor complex with the differentiation antigens CD4 and CD8. Implications for the generation of MHC-restriction and for repertoire selection in the thymus. Immunol. Today 9, 296–300.

Emmrich, F., Kanz, L. and Eichmann, K. (1987). Cross-linking of the T cell receptor complex with the subset-specific differentiation antigen stimulates interleukin 2 receptor expression in human CD4 and CD8 T cells. Eur. J. Immunol. 17, 529–534.

Emmrich, F., Rieber, P., Kurrle, R. and Eichmann, K. (1988). Selective stimulation of human T lymphocyte subsets by heteroconjugates of antibodies to the T cell receptor and to subset-specific differentiation antigens. Eur. J. Immunol. 18, 645–648.

Emmrich, J., Seyfarth, M., Fleig, W.E. and Emmrich, F. (1991). Treatment of inflammatory bowel disease with anti-CD4 monoclonal antibody. Lancet 338, 570–571.

Fiebig, H., Behn, I., Hommel, U., Kupper, H. and Eichler, W. (1989). In "Leucocyte Typing IV" (ed. W. Knapp, B. Dörken, W.R. Gilks, E.P. Rieber, R.E. Schmidt, H. Stein and A.E.G.Kr. von dem Borne), pp 332–335. Oxford University Press, Oxford.

Fischer, A., Griscelli, C., Blanche, S., LeDeist, F., Veber, F., Lopez, M., Delaage, M., Olive, D., Mawas, C. and Janossy, G. (1986). Prevention of graft failure by an anti HLFA-1 monoclonal antibody in HLA-mismatched bone marrow transplantation. Lancet 2, 1058–1061.

Fischer, A., Friedrich, W., Fasth, A., Blance, S., LeDeist, F., Girault, D., Veber, F., Vossen, J., Lopez, M., Griscelli, C. and Hirn, M. (1991). Reduction of graft failure by a monoclonal antibody (anti-LFA-1 CD11a) after HLA nonidentical bone marrow transplantation in children with immunodeficiencies, osteopetrosis, and Fanconi's anemia: A European group for immunodeficiency/European group of bone marrow transplantation report. Blood 77, 249–256.

Frödin, J.-E., Lefvert, A.-K. and Mellstedt, H. (1990). Pharmacokinetics of the mouse monoclonal antibody 17-1A in cancer patients receiving various treatment schedules. Cancer Res. 50, 4866–4871.

Gaston, R.S., Deierhoi, M.H., Patterson, T., Prasthofer, E., Julian, B.A., Barber, W.H., Laskow, D.A., Diethelm, A.G. and Curtis, J.J. (1991). OKT3 first-dose reaction: Association with T cell subsets and cytokine release. Kidney Int. 39, 141–148.

Gilbert, E.M., O'Connell, J.B., Hammond, M.E., Renlund, D.G., Watson, F.S. and Bristow, M.R. (1988). Treatment of myocarditis with OKT3 monoclonal antibody. Lancet i, 759.

Gleichmann, E., van Elven, E.H. and van der Veen, J.P.W. (1982). A systemic lupus erythematosus (SLE)-like disease in mice induced by abnormal T-B cell cooperation. Preferential formation of autoantibodies characteristic of SLE. Eur. J. Immunol. 12, 152–159.

Glennie, M.J. and Stevenson, G.T. (1982). Univalent antibodies kill tumour cells in vitro and in vivo. Nature (London) 295, 712–714.

Goldstein, G., Fuccello, A.G., Norman, D.J., Shiled, C.F. III, Colvin, R.B. and Cosimi, A.B. (1986). OKT3 monoclonal antibody plasma levels during therapy and the subsequent development of host antibodies to OKT3. Transplantation 42, 507–511.

Guse, A.H., Roth, E., Bröker, B.M. and Emmrich, F. (1992). Complex inositol polyphosphate response induced by co-crosslinking of CD4 and Fc receptors in the human monocytoid cell line U937. J. Immunol. 149, 2452–2458.

Gutstein, N.C. and Wofsy, D. (1986). Administration of F(ab)$_2$ fragments of monoclonal antibody to L3T4 inhibits humoral immunity in mice without depleting L3T4 cells. J. Immunol. 137, 3414–3419.

Gutstein, N.L., Seaman, W.E., Scott, J.H. and Wofsy, D. (1986). Induction of tolerance by administration of monoclonal antibody to L3T4. J. Immunol. 137, 1127–1132.

Hadam, M.R. (1989). In "Leucocyte Typing IV" (ed W. Knapp, B. Dörken, W.R. Gilks, E.P. Rieber, R.E. Schmidt, II. Stein and A.E.G.Kr. von dem Borne), pp 670–673. Oxford University Press, Oxford.

Hafler, D.A., Ritz, J., Schlossman, S.F. and Weiner, H.L. (1988). Anti-CD4 anti-CD2 monoclonal antibody infusions in subjects with multiple sclerosis. Immunosuppressive effects and human anti-mouse responses. J. Immunol. 141, 131–138.

Hale, G. and Waldmann, H. (1988). Campath 1 for prevention of GvHD and graft rejection. Summary of results from a multicentre study. Bone Marrow Transplant. 1, 11.

Hale, G., Dyer, M.J.S., Clark, M.R., Phillips, J.M., Marcus, R., Reichmann, L., Winter, G. and Waldmann, H. (1988). Remission induction in non-Hodgkin's lymphoma with the reshaped human monoclonal antibody CAMPATH-1H. Lancet ii, 1394–1399.

Hale, G., Xia, M. and Waldmann, H. (1989). In "Leucocyte Typing IV" (ed W. Knapp, B. Dörken, W.R. Gilks, E.P. Rieber, R.E. Schmidt, H. Stein and A.E.G.Kr. von dem Borne), pp 673–674. Oxford University Press, Oxford.

Hansen, H.J., LaFontaine, G., Newman, E.S., Schwartz, M.K., Malkin, A., Mojzisik, K., Martin, E.W. and Goldenberg, D.M. (1989). Solving the problem of antibody interference in commercial "sandwich"-type immunoassay of carcinoembryonic antigen. Clin. Chem. 35, 146–151.

Herzog, C., Walker, C., Pichler, W., Aeschlimann, A., Wassmer, P., Stockinger, H., Knapp, W., Rieber, W. and Müller, W. (1987). Monoclonal anti-CD4 in arthritis. Lancet 333, 1461–1462.

Herzog, C., Walker, C., Müller, W., Rieber, P., Reiter, C., Riethmüller, G., Wassmer, P., Stockinger, H., Madic, O. and Pichler, W.J. (1989). Anti-CD4 antibody treatment of patients with rheumatoid arthritis: I. Effect on clinical course and circulating T cells. J. Autoimmun. 2, 627–642.

Hiepe, F., Volk, H.-D., Apostoloff, E., von Baehr, R. and Emmrich, F. (1991). Treatment of severe systemic lupus erythematosus with anti-CD4 monoclonal antibody. Lancet 338, 1529–1530.

Hirsch, R., Eckhaus, M., Auchinloss, H.J., Sachs, D.H. and Bluestone, J.A. (1988). Effects of in vivo administration of anti-T3 monoclonal antibody on T cell function in mice. I Immunosuppression of transplantation response. J. Immunol. 140, 3766.

Horneff, G., Burmester, G.R., Emmrich, F. and Kalden, J.R. (1991a). Treatment of rheumatoid arthritis with an anti-CD4 monoclonal antibody. Arth. Rheum. 34, 129–140.

Horneff, G., Winkler, T., Kalden, J.R., Emmrich, F. and Burmester, G.R. (1991b). Human anti-mouse antibody response induced by anti-CD4 monoclonal antibody therapy in patients with rheumatoid arthritis. Clin. Immunol. Immunopathol. 59, 89–103.

Horneff, G., Krause, A., Emmrich, F., Kalden, J.R. and Burmester, G.R. (1991c). Elevated levels of circulating tumor necrosis factor-α, interferon-γ and interleukin-2 in systemic reactions induced by anti-CD4 therapy in patients with rheumatoid arthritis. Cytokine 3, 1–2.

Horneff, G., Emmrich, F., Reiter, C., Kalden, J.R. and Burmester, G.R. (1992). Persistent depletion of CD4+ T cells and inversion of the CD4/CD8 T cell ratio induced by anti-CD4 therapy. J. Rheumatol. 19, 1845–1850.

Horneff, G., Guse, A.H., Schulze-Koops, H., Kalden, J.R. and Burmester, G.R. (1993a). Human CD4-modulation in vivo induced by antibody-treatment. Clin. Immunol. Immunopathol. 66, 80–90.

Horneff, G., Sack, U., Kalden, J.R., Emmrich, F. and Burmester, G.R. (1993b). Reduction of monocyte-macrophage activation markers upon anti-CD4 treatment. Decreased levels of IL-1, IL-6, neopterin and soluble CD14 in patients with rheumatoid arthritis. Clin. Exp. Immunol. 91, 207–213.

Hosenpud, J.D., Norman D.J. and Pantley, G.A. (1989). OKT3 induced hypotension in cardiac allograft recipients treated for resistant rejection. J. Heart Transplant. 8, 159–166.

Hricik, D.E., Mayes, J.T. and Schulak, J.A. (1990). Inhibition of anti-OKT3 antibody generation by cyclosporine. Results of a prospective randomized trial. Transplantation 50, 237–240.

Jaffers, G.J., Fuller, T.C., Cosimi, A.B., Russell, P.S., Winn, H.J. and Colvin, R.B. (1986). Monoclonal antibody therapy: anti-idiotypic and non-anti-idiotypic antibodies to OKT3 arising despite intense immunosuppression. Transplantation 41, 572–578.

Jenkins, M.K., Pardoll, D.M., Mizuguchi, I., Quill, H. and Schwartz, R.H. (1987). T-cell unresponsiveness in vivo and in vitro: fine specificity of induction and molecular characterization of the unresponsive state. Immunol. Rev. 95, 113–135.

Jenkins, K.M., Taylor, P.S., Norton, S.D. and Urdahl, K.B. (1991). CD28 delivers a costimulatory signal involved in antigen-specific IL-2 production by human T cells. J. Immunol. 147, 2461–2466.

Jonker, M., Slingerlan, W., Niphuis, H., Solub, E.S., Thornton, G.B., Smit, L. and Goudsmit, J. (1989). In "Leucocyte Typing IV" (ed W. Knapp et al.), pp 319–322. Oxford University Press, Oxford.

Kalofonos, H.P., Stewart, S. and Epenetos, A.A. (1988). Antibody-guided diagnosis and therapy of malignant lesions. Int. J. Cancer 2S, 74–80.

Karsh, J., Klippel, J.H., Plotz, P.H., Decker, J.L., Wright, D.G. and Flye, M.W. (1981). Lymphapheresis in rheumatoid arthritis. Arth. Rheum. 24, 867–873.

Kaye, F.J., Bunn, P.A., Steinberg, S.M., Stocker, J.L., Ihde, D.C., Fischmann, A.B., Glatstein, E.J., Schechter, G.P., Phelps, R.M., Foss, F.M., Parlette, H.L., Anderson, M.J. and Sausville, E.A. (1989). A randomized trial comparing combination electron-beam radiation and chemotherapy with topical therapy in the initial treatment of mycosis fungoides. N. Engl. J. Med. 321, 1784–1790.

Kinne, R.W., Becker, W., Schwab, J., Simon, G., Schwarz, A., Wolf, F., Kalden, J.R., Burmester, G. and Emmrich, F. (1992). In "Advances in Rheumatology and Inflammation" vol. 2 (eds J. Fritsch and R. Mueller-Peddinghaus) pp 161–174, Basle, Euler Verlag, (in press).

Kinne, R.W., Becker, W., Simon, G., Paganelli, G., Palombo-Kinne, E., Wolski, A., Block, S., Schwarz, A., Wolf, F. and Emmrich, F. (1993). Joint uptake and body distribution of a Technetium-99m-labeled anti-rat CD4 monoclonal antibody in rat adjuvant arthritis. J. Nucl. Med. 34, 92–98.

Kirkham, B., Chikanza, I., Pitzalis, C., Kingsley, G.H., Grahame, R., Gibson, T. and Panayi, G.S. (1988). Response to monoclonal CD7 antibody in rheumatoid arthritis. Lancet i, 589.

Kirkham, B.W., Thien, F., Pelton, B.K., Pitzalis, C., Amlot, P., Denman, A.M. and Panayi, G.S. (1992) Chimeric CD7 monoclonal antibody therapy in rheumatoid arthritis. J. Rheumatol. 19, 1348–1352.

Kirkman, R.L., Araujo, J.L., Busch, G.J., Carpenter, C.B., Milford, E.L., Reinherz, E.L., Schlossman, S.F., Strom, T.B. and Tilney, N.L. (1983). Treatment of acute renal allograft rejection with monoclonal anti-T12 antibody. Transplantation 36, 620–626.

Kirkman, R.L., Barrett, L.V., Gaulton, N.G., Kelley, V.E., Kontun, W.A., Schoen, F.J., Ythier, A.A. and Strom, T.B. (1985a). The effect of anti-interleukin 2 receptor monoclonal antibody on allograft rejection. Transplantation 40, 719–721.

Kirkman, R.L., Barrett, L.V., Gaulton, G.N., Kelley, V.W., Ythier, A.A. and Strom, T.B. (1985b). Administration of anti-interleukin 2 receptor monoclonal antibody prolongs cardiac allograft survival in mice. J. Exp. Med. 162, 358–362.

Kirkman, R.L., Barrett, L.V., Koltun, W.A. and Diamantstein, T. (1987). Prolongation of murine cardiac allograft survival by the anti-interleukin 2 receptor monoclonal antibody AMT 13. Transplant. Proc. 19, 618–621.

Kirkman, R.L., Shapiro, M.E., Carpenter, C.B., McKay, D.B., Milford, E.L., Ramos, E.L., Tilney, N.L., Waldmann, T.A., Zimmerman, C.E. and Strom, T.B. (1991). A randomized prospective trial of anti-TAC monoclonal antibody in human renal transplantation. Transplantation 51, 107–113.

Kishimoto, T.K., Hollander, T., Roberts, T.M., Anderson, D.C. and Springer, T.A. (1987). Heterogenous mutations in the beta subunit common to the LFA-1, Mac-1, and p 150, 95 glycoproteins cause leukocyte adhesion deficiency. Cell 50, 193–202.

Knox, S.J., Levy, R., Hodgkinson, S., Bell, R., Brown, S., Wood, G.S., Hoppe, R., Abel, E.A., Steinman, L., Berger, R.G., Gaiser, C., Young, G., Bindl, J., Hanham, A. and Reichert, T. (1991). Observations on the effect of chimeric anti-CD4 monoclonal antibody in patients with mycosis fungoides. Blood 77, 20–30.

Koprowski H., Steplewski, Z., Mitchell, K., Herlyn, M., Herlyn, D. and Fuhrer, P. (1979). Colorectal carcinoma antigens detected by hybridoma antibodies. Somat. Cell Genet. 5, 957–971.

Korthäuer, U., Hennerkes, B., Menninger, H., Mages, H.-W., Zacher, J., Potocnik, A.J., Emmrich, F. and Kroczek, R.A. (1992). Oligoclonal T cells in rheumatoid arthritis: Identification strategy and molecular characterization of a clonal T cell receptor. Scand. J. Immunol. 36, 855–863.

Kotzin, B.L., Strober, S., Engleman, E.G., Calin, A., Hoppe, R.T., Kansas, G.S., Terrel, C.P. and Kaplan, H.S. (1981). Treatment of intractable rheumatoid arthritis with total lymphoid irradiation. N. Engl. J. Med. 305, 969–976.

Koulova, L., Clark, E.A., Shu, G. and Dupont, B. (1991). The CD28 ligand B7/BB1 provides costimulatory signal for allo-activation of CD4+ T cells. J. Exp. Med. 173, 759–762.

Köhler, G. and Milstein, C. (1975). Continuous cultures of fused cells secreting antibody of redefined specificity. Nature (London) 256, 495–497.

Kushner, I. and Sommerville, J.A. (1971). Permeability of human synovial membrane to plasma proteins. Arth. Rheum. 14, 560–570.

Kyle, V., Coughlan, R.J., Tighe, H., Waldmann, H. and Hazleman, B.L. (1989). Beneficial effect of monoclonal antibody to interleukin 2 receptor on activated T cells in rheumatoid arthritis. Ann. Rheum. Dis. 48, 428–429.

Lazarovits, A.I., Colvin, R.B., Camerini, D., Karsh, J. and Kurnick, J.T. (1987). In "Leucocyte Typing III" (ed A.J. McMichael, P.C.L. Beverley, S. Cobbold, M.J. Crumpton, W. Gilks, F.M. Gotch, N. Hogg, M. Horton, N. Ling, I.C.M. MacLennan, D.Y. Mason, C. Milstein, D. Spiegelhalter and H. Waldmann), pp 219–223. Oxford University Press, Oxford.

Linsley, P.S., Brady, W., Grosmaire, L., Aruffo, A., Damle, N.K. and Ledbetter, J.A. (1991). Binding of the B cell activation antigen B7 to CD28 costimulates T cell proliferation and interleukin 2 mRNA accumulation. J. Exp. Med. 173, 721–730.

Littman, D.R. (1987). The structure of the CD4 and CD8 genes. Annu. Rev. Immunol. 5, 561–584.

Liu, M.A. and Liu, T. (1988). Effect of recombinant soluble CD4 on human peripheral blood lymphocytes responses in vitro. J. Clin. Invest. 82, 2176–2180.

LoBuglio, A.F., Wheeler, R.H., Trang, J., Hanes, A., Rogers, K., Harvey, E.B., Sun, L., Ghrayeb, J. and Khazaeli, M.B. (1989). Mouse/human chimeric monoclonal antibody in man: Kinetics and immune response. Proc. Natl Acad. Sci. USA 86, 4220–4224.

Lowenthal, J.L. and Greene, W.C. (1987). Contrasting interleukin-2 binding properties of the alpha (p55) and beta (p70) protein subunits of the human high-affinity interleukin-2 receptor. J. Exp. Med. 166, 1156–1161.

Lubeck, M.D., Kimoto, Y., Steplewski, Z. and Koprowski, H. (1988). Killing of human tumor cell lines by human monocytes and murine monoclonal antibodies. Cell. Immunol. 111, 107–117.

Lucey, D.R., Dorsky, D.I., Nicholson-Weller, A. and Weller, P.F. (1989). Human eosinophils express CD4 protein and bind human immunodeficiency virus 1 gp120. J. Exp. Med. 169, 327–332.

McDermott, R.P. and Stenson, W.F. (1988). Alterations of the immune system in ulcerative colitis and Crohn's disease. Adv. Immunol. 42, 285–328.

MacDonald, H.R., Hengartner, H. and Pedrazzini, T. (1988). Intrathymic deletion of self-reactive cells prevented by neonatal anti-CD4 antibody treatment. Nature (London) 335, 174–176.

Maddon, P.J., Dalgleish, A.G., McDougal, J.S., Clapham, P.R., Weiss, R.A. and Axel, R. (1984). The T4 gene encodes the AIDS virus receptor and is expressed in the immune system and brain. Cell 47, 333–348.

Maddon, P.J., Littman, D.R., Godfrey, M., Maddon, D.E., Chess, L. and Axel, R. (1985). The isolation and nucleotide sequence of cDNA encoding the T cell surface protein T4: A new member of the immunoglobulin gene family. Cell 42, 93–104.

Maddon, P.J., Molineaux, S.M., Maddon, D.E., Zimmerman, K.A., Godfrey, M., Alt, F.W., Chess, L. and Axel, R. (1987). Structure and expression of the human and mouse T4 genes. Proc. Natl Acad. Sci. USA 84, 9155–9159.

Martin, M.A., Massanari, R.M., Nghiem, D.D., Smith, J.L. and Cory, R.J. (1988). Nosocomial aseptic meningitis associated with administration of OKT3. JAMA 259, 2002–2005.

Masucci, G., Lindemalm, C., Fröding, J.-E., Hagström, B. and Mellstedt, H. (1988). Effect of human blood mononuclear cell populations in antibody dependent cellular cytotoxicity (ADCC) using two murine (CO17-1A and Br55-2) and one chimeric (17-1A) monoclonal antibodies against a human colorectal carcinoma cell line (SW948). Hybridoma 7, 429–440.

Mathieson, P.W., Cobbold, S.P., Hale, G., Clark, M.R., Oliveira, D.B.G., Lockwood, C.M. and Waldmann, H. (1990). Monoclonal antibody therapy in systemic vasculitis. N. Engl. J. Med. 323, 250–254.

Mazerolles, F., Hauss, P., Barbat, C., Figdor, C.G. and Fischer, A. (1991). Regulation of LFA-1-mediated T cell adhesion by CD4. Eur. J. Immunol. 21, 887–894.

Morel, P., Vincent, C., Cordier, G., Panaye, G., Carosella, E. and Revillard, J.-P. (1990). Anti-CD4 monoclonal antibody administration in renal transplanted patients. Clin. Immunol. Immunopathol. 56, 311–322.

Moreland, L.W., Bucy, R.P., Pratt, P.W., Khazaeli, M.B., LoBuglio, A.F., Ghrayeb, J., Daddona, P., Sanders, M.E., Kilgariff, C., Riethmüller, G. and Koopman, W.J. (1991). Use of a chimeric anti-CD4 monoclonal antibody in refractory rheumatoid arthritis. Arth. Rheum. 34, S49 (97).

Moreland, L.W., Bucy, R.P., Tilden, A., Pratt, P.W., LoBuglio, A.F., Khazaeli, M., Everson, M.P., Daddona, P., Ghrayeb, J., Kilgarriff, C., Sanders, M.E. and Koopman, W.J. (1993) Use of a chimeric monoclonal anti-CD4 antibody in patients with refractory rheumatoid arthritis. Arthritis Rheum. 36, 307–318.

Nader, I.M., Stashenko, P., Hardy, R., Kaplan, W.D., Button, L.N., Kufe, D.W., Antman, K.H. and Schlossman, S.F. (1980). Serotherapy of a patient with a monoclonal antibody directed against a human lymphoma-associated antigen. Cancer Res. 40, 3147–3154.

Nepom, G.T., Seyfried, C., Holbeck, S., Byers, P., Wilske, K., Palmer, J., Robinson, D. and Nepom, B. (1989). In "Immunobiology of HLA. Vol. II" (ed B. Dupont), pp 404–406. Springer Verlag, New York.

Neuberger, M.S. and Rajewsky, K. (1981). Activation of mouse complement by mouse monoclonal antibodies. Eur. J. Immunol. 11, 1012–1018.

Neuberger, M.S., Williams, G.T. and Fox, R.O. (1984). Recombinant antibodies possessing novel effector functions. Nature (London) 312, 604–608.

Neuberger, M.S., Williams, G.T., Mitchell, E.B., Jouhal, S.S., Flanagan, J.G. and Rabbits, T.H. (1985). A hapten-specific chimeric IgE antibody with human physiological effector function. Nature (London) 314, 268–270.

Nicolas, J.F., Chamchick, N., Thivolet, J., Wijdenes, J., Morel, P. and Revillard, J.P. (1991). CD4 antibody treatment of severe psoriasis. Lancet 338, 321.

Norman, D.J. and Leone, M.R. (1991). The role of OKT3 in clinical transplantation. Pediatr. Nephrol. 5, 130–136.

Norman, D.J., Shield, C.F., Barry, J., Bennett, W.M., Henell, K., Kimball, J., Gunnell, B. and Hubert, B. (1988a). Early use of OKT3 monoclonal antibody in renal transplantation to prevent rejection. Am. J. Kidney Dis. 11, 107–110.

Norman, D.J., Shield, C.F. III, Henell, K.R., Kimball, J., Barry, J.M., Bennett, W.M. and Leone, M.R. (1988b). Effectiveness of a second course of OKT3 monoclonal anti-T cell antibody for treatment of renal allograft rejection. Transplantation 46, 523–529.

Olsen, N.J., Teal, G.P. and Strand, V. (1993). In vivo T cell depletion in rheumatoid arthritis is associated with increased in vitro IgM-rheumatoid factor synthesis. Clin. Immunol. Immunopathol. 67, 124–129.

Ortho Multicenter Transplant Study Group (1985). A randomized clinical trial of OKT3 monoclonal antibody for acute rejection of cadaveric renal transplants. N. Engl. J. Med. 313, 337–342.

Paulus, H.E., Machleder, H.I., Levine, S., Yu, D.T.Y. and MacDonald, N.S. (1977). Lymphocyte involvement in rheumatoid arthritis: studies during thoracic duct drainage. Arth. Rheum. 20, 1249–1262.

Penn, I. (1983). Lymphomas complicating organ transplantation. Transplant. Proc. 15S, 2790–2797.

Pfeffer, P.F., Jakobsen, A., Albrechtsen, D., Sodal, G., Brekke, I., Bentdal, O. Leivestad, T., Fauchald, P. and Flatmark, A. (1990). BMA 031 effectively reverses steroid resistant rejection in renal transplants. Transplant. Proc. 23, 1099–1100.

Pirofski, L., Casadevall, A., Rodriguez, L., Luckier, L.S. and Scharff, M.D. (1990). Current state of the hybridoma technology. J. Clin. Immunol. 10 (6 Suppl.) 5S–12S, discussion 12S–14S.

Prinz, J., Braun-Falco, O., Meurer, M., Daddona, P., Reiter, C., Rieber, P. and Riethmüller, G. (1991). Chimaeric CD4 monoclonal antibody in treatment of generalised pustular psoriasis. Lancet 338, 320–321.

Qin, O.Y.Q., El-Youssef, M., Yen-Lieberman, B., Sapatnekar, W., Youngman, K.R., Dusugami, K. and Focchi, C. (1988). Expression of HLA DR antigens in inflammatory bowel disease mucosa: role of intestinal lamina propria mononuclear cell-derived interferon gamma. Dig. Dis. Sci. 33, 1528–1536.

Qin, S.X., Cobbold, S., Tighe, H., Benjamin, R. and Waldmann, H. (1987). CD4 monoclonal antibody pairs for immunosuppression and tolerance induction. Eur. J. Immunol. 17, 1159–1165.

Qin, S.X., Cobbold, S.P., Benjamin, R. and Waldmann, H. (1989). Induction of classical transplantation tolerance in the adult. J. Exp. Med. 169, 779–794.

Raftery, M.J., Lang, C.J., Ivory, K., Tidman, N., Sweny, P., Fernando, O.N., Moorhead, J.F. and Janossy, G. (1985). Successful transplantation despite a positive fluorescence-activated cell sorter crossmatch following plasma exchange of donor-specific anti-HL. Transplantation 41, 131–133.

Rand, T.H., Cruikshank, W.W., Center, D.M. and Weller, P.F. (1991). CD4-mediated stimulation of human eosinophils: Lymphocyte chemoattractant factor and other

CD4-binding ligands elicit eosinophil migration. J. Exp. Med. 173, 1521–1528.

Ranges, G.E., Sriram, S. and Cooper, S.M. (1985). Prevention of type II collagen-induced arthritis by *in vivo* treatment with anti-L3T4. J. Exp. Med. 162, 1105–1110.

Reinherz, E.L. and Schlossman, S.F. (1980). The differentiation and function of human T lymphocytes. Cell 19, 821–827;

Reinke, P., Miller, H., Fietze, E., Herberger, D., Volk, H.-D., Neuhaus, K., Herberger, J., von Baehr, R. and Emmrich, F. (1991). Anti-CD4 therapy of acute rejection in long-term renal allograft recipients. Lancet ii, 338, 702–703.

Reiter, C., Kakavand, B., Rieber, E.P., Schattenkirchner, M., Riethmüller, G. and Krüger, K. (1991a). Treatment of rheumatoid arthritis with monoclonal CD4 antibody M-T151. Arth. Rheum. 34, 525–536.

Reiter, C., van der Lubbe, P.A., Breedveld, F.C., Daddona, P., Kürger, K., Kakavand, B. and Riethmüller, G. (1991b). Chimeric monoclonal CD4 antibody cM-T412 induces a long lasting CD4 cell depletion in rheumatoid arthritis (RA) patients. Arth. Rheum. 34 S 91 A154.

Remick, D.G., Kunkel, R.G., Larrick, J.W. and Kunkel, S.L. (1987). Acute *in vivo* effects of human recombinant tumor necrosis factor. Lab. Invest. 56, 583–590.

Rieber, E.P., Reiter, C., Gürtler, L., Deinhardt, F. and, Riethmüller, G. (1990). Monoclonal CD4 antibodies after accidental HIV infection. Lancet 336, 1007–1008.

Riechmann, L., Clark, M., Waldmann, H. and Winter, G. (1988). Reshaping human antibodies for therapy. Nature (London) 332, 323–327.

Robb, R.J., Greene, W.C. and Rusk, C. (1984). Low and high affinity cellular receptors for interleukin 2. J. Exp. Med. 160, 1126–1130.

Rosenberg, S.A., Lotze, M.T., Mutt, L.M., Chang, A.E., Avis, F.P., Leitman, S., Lineham, W.M., Robertson, C.N., Lee, R.E. and Rubin, J.T. (1987). A progress report on the treatment of 157 patients with advanced cancer using lymphokine-activated killer cells and interleukin-2 or high dose interleukin-2 alone. N. Engl. J. Med. 316, 889–897.

Rowe, P.A., Rocker, G.M., Morgan, A.G. and Shale, D.J. (1987). OKT3 and pulmonary capillary permeability. Br. Med. J. 295, 1099–1100.

Rudd, C.E., Trevillyan, J.M., Dasgupta, J.V., Wong, L.L. and Schlossman, S.F. (1988). The CD4 receptor is complexed in detergent lysates to a protein-tyrosine kinase (pp58) from human T lymphocytes. Proc. Natl Acad. Sci. USA 85, 5190–5194.

Rudensky, A.Y., Preston-Hurlburt, P., Hong, S.C., Barlow, A. and Janeway, C.A. Jr. (1991). Sequence analysis of peptides bound to MHC class II molecules. Nature (London) 353, 622–627.

Ruy, S.-E., Kwong, P.D., Truneh, A., Porter, T., Arthos, J., Rosenberg, M., Dai, X., Yuong, N., Axel, R., Sweet, R. and Hendrickson, W. (1990). Crystal structure of an HIV-binding recombinant fragment of human CD4. Nature (London) 348, 419–426.

Saito, T., Weiss, A., Miller, J., Norcross, M.A. and Germain, R.N. (1987). Specific antigen-Ia activation of transfected human T cells expressing murine Ti $\alpha\beta$-human T3 receptor complexes. Nature (London) 325, 125–130.

Schrezenmeier, H. and Fleischer, B. (1988). A regulatory role for the CD4 and CD8 molecules in T cell activation. J. Immunol. 141, 398–403.

Schroeder, T.J., First, M.R., Mansour, M.E., Hurtubise, P.E., Hariharan, S., Ryckman, F.C., Munda, R., Melvin D.B., Penn, I., Ballistreri, W.F. and Alexander, J.W. (1990). Antimurine antibody formation following OKT3 therapy. Transplantation 49, 48–51.

Schroff, R.W., Foon, K.A., Beatty, S.M., Oldham, R.K. and Morgan, A.C. Jr. (1985). Human anti-murine immuno-globulin responses in patients receiving monoclonal antibody therapy. Cancer Res. 45, 879–885.

Scoazec, J.Y. and Feldmann, G. (1990). Both macrophages and endothelial cells of the human hepatic sinusoid express the CD4 molecules: possible implications for HIV infection. Hepatology 12, 505–510.

Selby, W.J., Janossy, G., Mason, D.Y. and Jewell, D.P. (1983). Expression of HLA-DR antigens by colonic epithelium in inflammatory bowel disease. Clin. Exp. Immunol. 53, 614–618.

Shapiro, M.E., Kirkman, R.L., Reed, M.H., Puskas, J.D.M., Mazouijan, G., Letvin, N.L., Carpenter, C.B., Milford, E.L., Milford, T.A., Waldman, T.A., Strom, T.B. and Schlossman, S.F. (1987). Monoclonal anti-IL-2 receptor antibody in primate renal transplantation. Transplant. Proc. 19, 594–597.

Shawler, D.L., Bartholomew, R.M., Smith, L.M. and Dillman, R.O. (1985). Human immune response to multiple injections of murine monoclonal IgG. J. Immunol. 135, 1530–1535.

Shizuru, J.A., Taylor-Edwards, C., Banks, B.A., Gregory, A.K. and Fathmann, G.C. (1988). Immunotherapy of the nono-bese diabetic mouse: treatment with an antibody to helper T cells. Science 240, 659–662.

Singh, N. (1988). Impact of OKT3 therapy on cytomegalovirus and herpes simplex virus infections after liver transplantation. Transplant. Proc. 20, 661–662.

Soulillou, J.P., LeMauff, B., Olive, D., Delaage, M., Peyronnet, P., Hourmant, M., Mawas, C., Hirn, M. and Yacques, Y. (1987). Prevention of rejection of kidney trans-plants by monoclonal antibody directed against interleukin 2. Lancet i, 1339–1342.

Spiegelhalter, D.J. and Gilks, W.R. (1987). In "Leucocyte Typing III" (ed A.J. McMichael *et al.*), pp 14–24. Oxford University Press, Oxford.

Staerz, V.D. and Bevan, M.J. (1986). Hybrid hybridoma producing a bispecific monoclonal antibody that can focus effector T cell activity. Proc. Natl Acad. Sci. USA 83, 1453–1457.

Steinman, L., Waldor, M.K., Zamvel, S.S., Lim, M., Herzen-berg, L., Herzenberg, L., McDevitt, H.O., Mitchell, D. and Sriram, S. (1986). Therapy of autoimmune disease with anti-body to immune response gene products or to T cell surface markers. Ann. N.Y. Acad. Sci. 475, 274–283.

Steinman, L., Zamvil, S.S., O'Hearn, M., Schwartz, G., Sriram, S., Mitchell, D. and Waldor, M.K. (1988). In "Immune Intervention, Vol. 2" (ed J. Brochier, J. Clot and J. Sany), pp 109–128. Academic Press, London.

Strand, V., Fishwild, D. and the XOMA Rheumatoid Arthritis Investigators Group (1990). Treatment of rheumatoid arthritis with an anti-CD5 immunoconjugate: clinical and immunologic findings and preliminary results of re-treatment. Arth. Rheum. 33, S25.

Strand, V., Lipsky, P.E., Cannon, G.W., Calabrese, L.H., Wiesenhutter, C., Cohen, S.B., Olsen, N.J., Lee, M.L., Lorenz, T.J., Nelson, B. and the CD5 plus rheumatoid arthritis investigators group. Arthritis Rheum. 36, 620–630.

Stunkel, K.G., Theisen, P., Mouzaki, A., Diamantstein, T. and Schlumberger, H.D. (1988). Monitoring of interleukin-2 receptor (Il-2R) expression *in vivo* and studies on an Il-2R-directed immunosuppressive therapy of active and adoptive adjuvant-induced arthritis in rats. Immunology 64, 683–689.

Sutherland, R., Buchegger, F., Schreyer, M., Vacca, A. and Mach, J.P. (1987). Penetration and binding of radiolabeled anti-carcino-embryonic antigen monoclonal antibodies and their antigen binding fragments in human colon. Cancer Res. 47, 1627–1633.

Swain, S.L. (1983). T cell subsets and the recognition of MHC class. Immunol. Rev. 74, 129–142.

Swinnen, L.J., Costanzo-Nordin, M.R., Fischer, S.G., O'Sullivan, E.J., Johnson, M.R., Herouxi, A.L., Dizihes, G.J., Pifarre, R. and Fisher, R.I. (1990). Increased incidence of lymphoproliferative disorder after immunosuppression with monoclonal antibody OKT3 in cardiac-transplant recipients. N. Engl. J. Med. 323, 1723–1728.

Takahashi, H., Terasaki, P.I., Kinukawa, T., Chia, D., Miura, K., Okazaki, H., Iwaki, Y., Taguchi, Y., Hardiwidjaja, S., Ishizaki, M. and Billing, R. (1983). Reversal of transplant rejection by monoclonal antiblast antibody. Lancet ii, 1155–1157.

Takeuchi, T., Schlossman, S.F. and Morimoto, C. (1987). The T4 molecule differentially regulating the activation of subpopulations of T4+ cells. J. Immunol. 139, 665–671.

Tanaka, K.W., Hancock, W.W., Osawa, H., Stunkel, K.G., Alverghini, T.V., Diamantstein, T., Tilney, N.L. and Kupiec-Weglinski, J.W. (1989). Mechanism of action of anti-Il-2R monoclonal antibodies. ART-18 prolongs cardiac allograft survival in rats by elimination of Il-2R+ mononuclear cells. J. Immunol. 143, 2873–2879.

Tax, W.J.M., Willems, H.W., Reekers, P.P.M., Capel, P.J.A. and Koene, R.A.P. (1983). Polymorphism in mitogenic effect of IgG1 monoclonal antibodies against T3 antigen on human T cells. Nature (London) 304, 445–447.

Tax, W.J.M., Tidman, N., Janossy, G., Trejdosiewicz, L., Willems, R., Ledeuwenberg, J. Dewitte, T.J.M., Capel, P.J.A. and Koene, R.A.P. (1984). Monoclonal antibody (WT 1) directed against a T cell surface glycoprotein: characteristics and immunosuppressive activity. Clin. Exp. Immunol. 55, 427–436.

Theofilopoulos, A.N., Prod'homme, G.J. and Dixon, F.J. (1985). Autoimmune aspects of systemic lupus erythematosus. Concepts Immunopathol. 1, 190–218.

Thistlethwaite, J.R., Stuart, J.K., Mayes, J.T., Gaber, A.O., Woodle, S., Buckingham, M.R. and Stuart, F.P. (1988). Complications and monitoring of OKT3 therapy. Am. J. Kidney Dis. 11, 112–119.

Thomas, D.M, Nicholls, A.J., Feest, T.G. and Ried, H. (1987). OKT3 and cerebral oedema. Br. Med. J. 295, 1486.

Todd, P.A. and Brogden, R.N. (1989). Muromonab CD3. A review of its pharmacology and therapeutical potential. Drugs 37, 871–899.

Transy, C., Moingeon, P.E., Marshall, B., Stebbins, C. and Reinherz, E.L. (1989). In "Leucocyte Typing IV" (ed W. Knapp *et al.*), pp 293–295. Oxford University Press, Oxford.

Tsudo, M., Kozak, R.W., Goldman, C.K. and Waldmann, T.A. (1986). Demonstration of a new (non-Tac) peptide that binds interleukin-2: a potential participant in a multichain interleukin-2 receptor complex. Proc. Natl Acad. Sci. USA 83, 9694–9698.

Tsudo, M., Kozak, R.W., Goldman, C.K. and Waldmann, T.A. (1987). Contribution of a p75 interleukin-2 binding peptide to a high-affinity interleukin-2 receptor complex. Proc. Natl Acad. Sci. USA 84, 4215–4218.

Tsygankov, A.Yu., Bröker, B.N., Guse, A.H., Meinke, U., Roth, E., Rossmann, C. and Emmrich, F. (1993). Preincubation with anti-CD4 influences activation of human T cells by subsequent co-crosslinking with CD3. J. Leukocyte Biol. (in press)

Uchiyama, T., Broder, S. and Waldmann, T.A. (1981). A monoclonal antibody (anti-Tac) reactive with activated and functionally mature human T cells. J. Immunol. 126, 1393–1397.

Uciechowski, P. and Schmidt, R.E. (1989). In "Leucocyte Typing IV" (ed W. Knapp, B. Dörken, W.R. Gilks, E.P. Rieber, R.E. Schmidt, H. Stein and A.E.G.Kr. von dem Borne), pp 543–554. Oxford University Press, Oxford.

Urban, J.L., Jumar, V., Kono, D.H., Gomez, C., Horvath, S.J., Clayton, J., Ando, D.G., Sercarz, E.E. and Hood, L. (1988). Restricted use of T cell receptor V genes in murine autoimmune encephalomyelitis raises possibilities for antibody therapy. Cell 54, 577–592.

Vadhan-Raj, S., Cordon-Cardo, C., Carswell, E., Mintzer, D., Dantis, L., Duteau, C., Templeton, M.A., Oettgen, H.F., Old, L.J. and Houghton, A.N. (1988). Phase I trial of a mouse monoclonal antibody against G_{d3} ganglioside in patients with melanoma: induction of inflammatory responses at tumor sites. J. Clin. Oncol. 6, 1636–1648.

Valdimarsson, H., Baker, B.S., Jonsodottir, I. and Fry, L. (1986). Psoriasis: a disease of abnormal keratinocyte proliferation induced by T lymphocytes. Immunol. Today 7, 256–259.

van der Linden, E.F.H., van Kroonenburgh, M.J.P.G. and Pauwels, E.K.J. (1988). Side-effects of monoclonal antibody infusions for the diagnosis and treatment of cancer. Int. J. Biol. Markers 3, 147–153.

van der Lubbe, P.A., Miltenburg, A.M. and Breedveld, F.C. (1991a). Anti-CD4 monoclonal antibody for relapsing polychondritis. Lancet 337, 1349.

van der Lubbe, P.A., Reiter, C., Riethmüller, G., Sandes, M.E. and Breedveld, F.C. (1991b). Treatment of rheumatoid arthritis (RA) with chimeric CD4 monoclonal antibody. Arth. Rheum. 34, S89 (A143).

Van Wauwe, J.P., DeMay, J.R and Goossens, J.G. (1980). OKT3: a monoclonal anti-human T lymphocyte antibody with potent mitogenic properties. J. Immunol. 124, 2708–2713.

Veillette, A., Bookman, M.A., Horak, E.M. and Bolen, J.B. (1988). The CD4 and CD8 T cell surface antigens are associated with the internal membrane tyrosine-protein kinase p 56^{lck}. Cell 55, 301–308.

Venkateswara, R.K., Kaiske, B.L. and Bloom, P.M. (1989). Acute graft rejection in the late survivors of renal transplantation. Transplantation 47, 290–292.

Villemain, F., Jonker, M., Bach, J.-F. and Chatenoud, L. (1986). Fine specificity of antibodies produced in rhesus monkeys following *in vivo* treatment with anti-T cell murine monoclonal antibodies. Eur. J. Immunol. 16, 945–949.

von Wussow, P., Spitler, L., Block, B. and Deicher, H. (1988). Immunotherapy in patients with advanced malignant melanoma using a monoclonal antimelanoma antibody Ricin A immunotoxin. Eur. J. Cancer Clin. Oncol. 24, S69–S73.

Wacholtz, M., and Lipsky, P.E. (1992). Treatment of lupus nephritis with CD5 plus, an immunoconjugate of anti-CD5 monoclonal antibody and ricin A chain. Arthritis Rheum. 35, 837–839.

Waldmann, H. (1989). Manipulation of T cell responses with monoclonal antibodies. Ann. Rev. Immunol. 7, 407–444.

Waldmann, H., Cobbold, S.P., Qin, S., Benjamin, R.J. and Wise, M. (1989). Tolerance induction in the adult using monoclonal antibodies to CD4, CD8, and CD11a (LFA-1). Cold Spring Harb. Symp. Quant. Biol. 54, 885–892.

Waldmann, T.A., Grant, A., Tendler, C., Greenberg, S., Goldman, C., Bamford, R., Junghans, R.P. and Nelson, D. (1990). Lymphokine receptor-directed therapy: A model of immune intervention. J. Clin. Immunol. 10S, 19–29.

Wang, J.H., Yan, Y.W., Garrett, T.P., Liu, J.H., Rodgers, D.W., Garlick, R.L., Tarr, G.E., Husain, Y., Reinherz, E.L. and Harrison, S.C. (1990). Atomic structure of a fragment of human CD4 containing two immunoglobulin-like domains. Nature (London) 348, 411–418.

Ward, E.E., Guessow, D., Griffiths, A.D., Jones, P.T. and Winter, G. (1989). Binding activities of a repertoire of single immunoglobulin variable domains secreted from *Escherichia coli*. Nature (London) 341, 544–546.

Watanabe, M., Reimann, K.A., DeLong, P.A., Liu, T., Fisher, R.A. and Letvin, N.L. (1989). Effects of recombinant soluble CD4 in rhesus monkeys with simian immunodeficiency virus of macaques. Nature (London) 337, 267–270.

Wendling, D., Wijdenes, J., Radacot, E. and Morel-Fourrier, B. (1991). Therapeutic use of monoclonal anti-CD4 antibody in rheumatoid arthritis. J. Rheumatol. 18, 325–327.

Wijdenes, J., Beliard, R., Muot, S., Herve, P. and Peters, A. (1990). A semi-pharmaceutical approach for the preparation of an anti-Il2 receptor monoclonal antibody in the treatment of acute GvHD in a multicentric study. Dev. Biol. Standard. 71, 103–111.

Wilde, D.B., Marrack, P., Kappler, J., Dialynas, D.P. and Fitch, F.W. (1983). Evidence implicating L3T4 in class II MHC antigen reactivity: monoclonal antibody GK1.5 (anti-L3T4a) blocks class II MHC antigen-specific proliferation, release of lymphokines, and binding by clones of murine helper T lymphocyte lines. J. Immunol. 131, 2178–2183.

Wilder, R.L. and Decker, J.L. (1983). T-inducer lymphocytes, leukapheresis and the pathogenesis of rheumatoid arthritis. Clin. Exp. Rheumatol. 1, 89–91.

Winchester, R.G. (1981). Genetic aspects of rheumatoid arthritis. Springer Semin. Immunopathol. 4, 89–102.

Wofsy, D. and Seaman, W.E. (1985). Successful treatment of autoimmunity in NZB/NZW F1 mice with monoclonal antibody to L3T4. J. Exp. Med. 161, 378–391.

Wofsy, D. and Seaman, W.E. (1987). Reversal of advanced murine lupus in NZB/NZW F1 mice by treatment with monoclonal antibody to L3T4. J. Immunol. 138, 3247–3253.

Wofsy, D., Ledbetter, J.A., Hendler, P.L. and Seaman, W.E. (1984). Treatment of murine lupus with monoclonal anti-T cell antibody. J. Immunol. 134, 852–857.

Wofsy, D., Chiang, N.Y., Greenspan, J.S. and Ermak, T.H. (1988). Treatment of murine lupus with monoclonal antibody to L3T4. I. Effects on the distribution and function of lymphocyte subsets and on the histopathology of autoimmune disease. J. Autoimmun. 1, 415–431.

Wonigeit, K., Nashan, B., Schwinzer, R., Schlitt, H.J., Kurrle, R., Racenberg, J., Seiler, F., Ringe, B. and Pichlmayr, R. (1989). Use of a monoclonal antibody against the T cell receptor for prophylactic immunosuppressive treatment after liver transplantation. Transplant. Proc. 21, 2258–2259.

Wood, G.S., Warner, N.L. and Warnke, R.A. (1983). Anti-Leu-3/T4 antibodies react with cells of monocytes/macrophages and Langerhans lineage. J. Immunol. 131, 212–216.

Wood, G.S., Abel, E.A., Hoppe, R.T. and Warnke, R.A. (1986). Leu-8 and Leu-9 antigen phenotypes: Immunologic criteria for the distinction of mycosis fungoides from cutaneous inflammation. J. Am. Acad. Dermatol. 14, 1006–1013.

Wooley, P.M., Luthra, H.S., Lafuse, W.P., Huse, A., Stuart, J. and David, C.S. (1985). Type-II collagen-induced arthritis in mice. III. Suppression of arthritis by using monoclonal and polyclonal anti-Ia antisera. J. Immunol. 134, 2361–2371.

Yoshino, S., Kinne, R., Hünig, T. and Emmrich, F. (1990). The suppressive effect of an antibody to the αβ T cell receptor in rat adjuvant arthritis. Studies on optimal treatment protocols. Autoimmunity 7, 255–266.

Young, R.C. (1989). Mycosis fungoides: The therapeutic search continues. N. Engl. J. Med. 321, 1822–1824.

Zweig, M.H., Csako, G., Benson, C.C., Weintraub, B.D. and Kahn, B.B. (1987). Interference by anti-immunoglobulin G antibodies in immunoradiometric assays of thyreotropin involving mouse monoclonal antibodies. Clin. Chem. 33, 840–844.

6.   Are Imbalances in Cytokine Function of Importance in the Pathogenesis of Rheumatoid Arthritis?

M. Feldmann, F.M. Brennan, E.R. Abney, A. Hales, Y. Chernajovsky, P. Katsikis, A. Corcoran, C. Haworth, A. Cope, D. Gibbons, C.Q. Chu, M. Field, B. Deleuran, R.O. Williams and R.N. Maini

1. Introduction

Cytokines are major mediators of immune and inflammatory function. Hence they are likely to be intimately involved in autoimmune disease. Investigating cytokine expression during this process should provide information about the pathogenesis of the disease, and possibly provide clues for therapeutic approaches.

Over the past 7 years we have studied the role of cytokines in the pathogenesis of RA. There is access to the actual disease site, and in diseases like RA with pronounced local manifestations, the most interesting events must be local. In another autoimmune disease, Graves' thyroiditis, we have been able to show that, in the maintenance phase of the disease, there is interaction between autoantigen-reactive T cells and tissue APCs. In this case, thyrocytes were induced to express MHC class II and adhesion molecules, and produce cytokines (Londei *et al.*, 1985; Grubeck-Loebenstein *et al.*, 1989). In RA, activated T cells specific for collagen type II were found in three consecutive operative specimens from a patient over a 3-year period (Londei *et al.*, 1989). The persistence of these cells, specific for an antigen that is restricted in its distribution to the joint, argues strongly that these T cells are involved in the pathogenesis. Similar cells were not detectable in blood taken at the same time. This argues that T cell–APC interactions are probably also important in RA, as they are in thyroiditis (Bottazzo *et al.*, 1983; Feldmann, 1989), and that the overall scheme (Fig. 6.1) is likely also to be relevant in RA.

In the past few years, progress in the cytokine field has been very rapid. The cloning of cDNAs for numerous cytokines and the cloning of many cytokine receptor chains has meant that the majority of molecules interacting in the cytokine system are known, and most importantly can be readily assayed – at the protein

Immunopharmacology of Joints and Connective Tissue
ISBN 0–12–206345–7

CONCEPT OF AUTOIMMUNITY

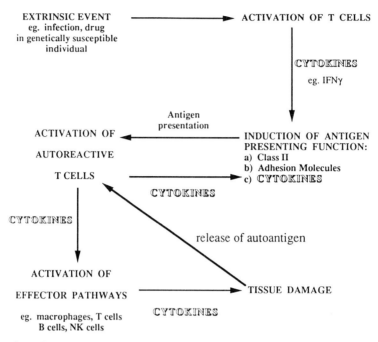

Figure 6.1 Concept of autoimmunity. Aetiology and pathogenesis of autoimmunity: interactions of T cells, APCs and cytokines.

(e.g. by ELISA) and mRNA level (Northern, slot blotting or polymerase chain reaction), and functionally by their action in bioassays. Despite the fact that bioassays are usually not molecule-specific, they are still of importance, as cytokines detected by mRNA and ELISA need not be bioactive, and only bioactive cytokines transmit signals.

In most biological systems, the fine regulation needed to maintain health dictates that there are ways of inhibiting or interfering with intercellular signalling; thus the cholinesterase enzyme exists in close proximity to acetylcholine receptors, and degrades the free transmitter, acetylcholine. The ways in which cytokine signals are limited were not fully appreciated until the recent discovery of cytokine inhibitors. This added to the previously known pulsatile production of cytokines, and the limited and regulatable expression of cytokine receptors which provides a very flexible system of regulating cytokine function. In view of the potent and wide ranging effects of cytokines, this is essential.

The aim of this chapter is to review current knowledge of the cytokine pathways in RA together with the expression and regulation of cytokine receptors and inhibitors in order to yield a credible portrait of how cytokines may be involved in disease.

2.   *Cytokines and Pathogenesis*

2.1   HOW CAN CYTOKINE FUNCTION BE DOCUMENTED?

As cytokines are local mediators, often produced by one cell to act on its near neighbours, it is difficult (if not impossible) to sample their intercellular concentrations and measure their actions. The inability to detect cytokines in a cell supernatant does not exclude their presence in quantities sufficient to trigger the adjacent cells. The high affinity of cytokine receptors implies that abundance in supernatants would only occur after most local receptors are saturated. Furthermore, for an increasing range of cytokines (e.g. TNF, TGF-β, M-CSF), it is clear that there is a membrane-bound form which could not be detected by assays of supernatants (Kriegler *et al.*, 1988).

It is also a problem to establish which type of assay to use. The cloning and expression of the genes controlling cytokine production has led to the development of many new assays: mRNA assays using cDNA probes and binding assays using rabbit and monoclonal antibodies. These supplement the bioassays, which remain vital to ensure that the cytokines detected are in fact functional and not degraded or neutralized molecules. The use of recombinant cytokines has demonstrated that the original bioassays for cytokines were not molecule-specific. Thus cell lines used to assay IL-2 usually detect IL-4 also, and possibly IL-7 which is also a powerful T cell growth factor (Londei *et al.*, 1990), and the murine thymocyte assay detects human IL-1, IL-6 and IL-7 (Chantry *et al.*, 1989a). Neutralizing antibodies raised against recombinant proteins can (and must) be used to make the bioassays specific (e.g. Grubeck-Loebenstein *et al.*, 1989).

Another problem is the interpretation of the data, and the appropriate controls to use for pathological tissues. The synovial tissue of the normal joint is almost acellular, apart from the two-cell-thick lining layer. As the majority of the cells infiltrating an RA joint are derived from the blood, we have used mitogen-activated blood cells for comparison, although the cellular composition is obviously somewhat different. Other inflammatory diseases of the joint have also been studied, but these may have similarities in their pathogenesis, and as such are not appropriate as "controls". In a potentially heterogeneous disease, it is also of importance to assay reasonable numbers of samples, as there may be an influence of the treatment or stage of disease on cytokine production.

The advent of pure recombinant cytokines has made simple experiments possible, by adding cytokines to pure cell populations and assaying the effects. However, this does not resemble what happens *in vivo*, where cell populations are heterogeneous, and cells, once activated, do not release single cytokines but a wide spectrum of molecules. Thus *in vivo* any given cell will be exposed concurrently to a multitude of cytokines and a gradient of concentrations. It is also now known that important synergies occur between cytokines; for example, IFNγ and TNF-α synergize in cytotoxicity or MHC class II expression (Pujol-Borrell *et al.*, 1987), and IL-2 and IL-4 synergize in T cell activation (Carding and Bottomly, 1988). However, in humans, IL-2 and IL-4 are antagonistic for the generation of LAK cells and on B cells (e.g. Kawakami *et al.*, 1989). The consequences of such synergies (and antagonisms) between cytokines renders studies of single cytokines in a disease context virtually meaningless in terms of immunopathology.

In addition, adsorption of cytokines to carrier proteins, degradation by enzymes and competition by inhibitors makes accurate quantification of cytokines using a single technique impossible.

2.2 CYTOKINE PRODUCTION IN THE RHEUMATOID JOINT

In view of the problems outlined above, we initially concentrated on documenting the spectrum of cytokines produced by cells isolated from the rheumatoid joint,

and not in synovial fluid. This is because synovial fluid is a viscous "soup" of enzymes, proteins and hyaluronic acid at very high concentration, and this heterogeneous mixture could lead to problems in many of the assays, especially bioassay. Furthermore, it is in the synovial membrane that the important pathology is present, and it is clear that many cytokines that may be active in the membrane may not escape in detectable quantities into the synovial fluid.

However, many of the clinical samples obtained for these studies contained relatively small numbers of cells (often less than 5×10^6/sample), so it was necessary to make use of assays in which the amount of information obtained from a single sample was optimized. We therefore used RNA slot blotting followed by hybridization to cDNA probes as a convenient and simple screening procedure. This only requires small numbers of cells ($1-2 \times 10^6$), and allows the filter to be stripped and reprobed for other cytokines yielding a large amount of information from a single sample (5–10 cytokines). This approach was combined with the use of appropriate bioassays on cell supernatants (rendered specific by the use of neutralizing antibodies) and ELISAs to demonstrate the presence of the corresponding protein. Table 6.1 summarizes the data obtained from these studies (e.g. Buchan *et al.*, 1988a; Hirano *et al.*, 1988; Feldmann *et al.*, 1991).

From these results it is apparent that, although the levels of mRNA and protein for some cytokines such as

Table 6.1 Summary of cytokines produced spontaneously by RA synovial cells

Cytokine	mRNA	Protein
IL-1α	Yes	Yes
IL-1β	Yes	Yes
TNF-α	Yes	Yes
Lymphotoxin	Yes	(+/−)[a]
IL-2	Yes	(+/−)[a]
IL-3	No	No
IL-4	?	No
IFNγ	Yes	(+/−)[a]
IL-6	Yes	Yes
GM-CSF	Yes	Yes
IL-8/NAP-1	Yes	Yes
RANTES	Yes	?
G-CSF	Yes	?
M-CSF	No	?
TGF-β	Yes	Yes
EGF	Yes	Yes
TGF-α	No	No
PDGF-A	Yes	Yes
PDGF-B	Yes	Yes

[a] +/− = demonstration of protein has proved difficult. Abbreviations: RANTES, regulated on activation, normal T expressed and secreted; PDGF, platelet-derived growth factor.

IL-1 and TNF-α are often concordant, for some mediators (chiefly the products of T cells), this is not the case (Brennan *et al.*, 1989a). Possible mechanisms to overcome the lack of readily detectable protein for cytokines such as IL-2, IL-4, lymphotoxin and IFNγ include adsorption to receptors, degradation by enzymes, inhibition by antagonists and translational regulation of the induced cytokine mRNA by other cytokines, such as TGF-β, which has been shown to act in this manner (Chantry *et al.*, 1989b). The lack of appreciable protein is of particular interest with IFNγ, as its presence in RA joints has been strongly suspected on the basis of the marked MHC class II expression and macrophage activation. For IFNγ there is evidence for downregulation of its production, as, upon culture, mRNA levels tend to increase (Buchan *et al.*, 1988a). It is also of interest with lymphotoxin, where high mRNA levels can be detected but the protein levels are in complete contrast (see Table 6.2).

From this preliminary survey, it was found that the usually most abundant form of IL-1 (IL-1β) was relatively less abundant in the RA joint. IL-1α mRNA was in most patients somewhat more abundant than IL-1β. Assaying supernatants of joint cells for IL-1α and IL-1β protein revealed that there was an approximately equivalent amount of each secreted (Buchan *et al.*, 1988b). Furthermore, *in vitro* both IL-1α (Fig. 6.2) and IL-1β mRNA was produced spontaneously in joint cell cultures. This suggested to us that the cytokine regulation in the RA joint was different from a normal immune response.

In RA joints, the most abundant cytokines detected are IL-6, TNF-α, IL-1, IL-8, TGF-β and GM-CSF (Hirano *et al.*, 1988; Brennan *et al.*, 1989b, 1990a,b; Haworth *et al.*, 1991). However, no definitive correlation can be made between abundance and importance, as discussed in the preceding section.

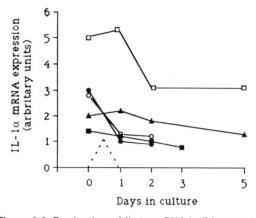

Figure 6.2 Production of IL-1α mRNA in RA synovial joint mononuclear cell cultures. RNA from RA MNC (solid line) cultured for 5 days was extracted at times indicated, blotted on to nitrocellulose, and probed with IL-1α. Normal peripheral blood MNC were stimulated with PHA/PMA for 48 h. RNA was extracted at times indicated (dotted line), and probed with IL-1α as described. Data from Buchan *et al.* (1988).

2.3   CYTOKINE REGULATION IN THE RHEUMATOID JOINT

The presence of high levels of cytokines expressed consistently in RA samples suggests that these cytokines are continuously produced *in vivo*, unlike the pulsatile cytokine production induced by stimuli *in vitro*. To evaluate whether this is the case, synovial cells were cultured in the absence of extrinsic stimulation. High levels of IL-1, IL-6, TNF-α and other cytokines were generated, and remained at high levels for the 5–6-day culture period. The initial cultures were performed in RPMI 1640 supplemented with fetal calf serum. As the latter

Table 6.2   Discordance between lymphotoxin and IFNγ mRNA and protein production in RA synovial cultures

| | Lymphotoxin (pg/ml) | | | | | | IFNγ (pg/ml) | | | | | |
| | mRNA | | | Protein | | | mRNA | | | Protein | | |
Days in culture	1	3	6	1	3	6	1	3	6	1	3	6
RA culture 1	4116	4674	3878	<50	<50	<50	722	7642	3611	<50	<50	<50
RA culture 2	2018	1205	nd	<50	<50	<50	435	9102	nd	<50	<50	<50
RA culture 3	4320	4518	5015	<50	<50	<50	3197	10330	9097	<50	<50	<50

RA synovial cells were placed in culture without exogenous stimulus for periods of up to 6 days. mRNA was extracted and assessed for lymphotoxin and IFNγ gene expression. mRNA levels are expressed as arbitrary units of integration as determined by densitometry. Protein was determined by a specific immunoassay (detection limit 50 pg/ml). nd = not determined because of insufficient tissue in sample.

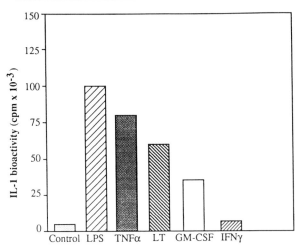

Figure 6.3 Induction of IL-1 protein by cytokines. Cells were cultured in the presence of LPS (1 µg/ml), TNF-α (2500 units/ml), lymphotoxin (LT) (2500 units/ml), and GM-CSF (2500 units/ml). Supernatants were collected and assayed for IL-1 bioactivity by the mouse thymocyte comitogenic assay. Data from Portillo et al. (1988).

et al., 1986; Saklatvala *et al.*, 1985; Thomas *et al.*, 1987), we concentrated initially on the regulation of IL-1 production.

We have investigated which signals are capable of inducing IL-1 production (Portillo *et al.*, 1989). Of these, TNF-α and lymphotoxin were particularly potent in inducing IL-1 mRNA and protein (Fig. 6.3). GM-CSF is also active in inducing IL-1 (Chantry *et al.*, 1990). Elsewhere we have documented that cryoprecipitated immune complexes free of LPS can induce IL-1 production and that cytokines such as IFNγ and TNF augment this (Chantry *et al.*, 1989c). These were thought to be of possible importance in RA. The strategy chosen for determining which of these many signals may be of major importance, for example in regulating IL-1 production in the joint cell cultures, involved using neutralizing antibodies at the beginning of the culture period, to remove the activity of a single cytokine, and evaluating the effects on various immune functions during the subsequent culture period. As TNF-α and lymphotoxin were found to be among the strongest inducers of IL-1 (after LPS), neutralizing antisera to these two cytokines were initially used *in vitro* (Brennan *et al.*, 1989b). The results were quite striking. In RA joint cell cultures, anti-TNF-α (but not anti-lymphotoxin) abrogated the production of IL-1 bioactivity, assayed after 3–6 days in culture (Fig. 6.4), and reduced mRNA levels even earlier.

These results have been controlled in many ways: normal rabbit immunoglobulin and anti-lymphotoxin sera did not influence IL-1 levels, viability of the cells was unaffected, and the thymocyte assay used detected IL-1 (and not IL-6) as judged by neutralizing antibodies to IL-1 and IL-6. To ensure that this result was representative of the disease process, seven RA patients have been investigated so far, and in all, anti-TNF-α inhibited IL-1 production, ranging from 50 to 99%. Anti-lymphotoxin had an inhibitory effect on IL-1 production in only one patient (of seven) indicating that low levels of

may contain antigenic material recognized by T cells and APCs in the RA joint cell mixture, analogous experiments have been performed with human serum and serum-free media; all yielded prolonged cytokine production from RA cells.

The results obtained (Table 6.1) indicate that the signals (cellular and molecular) responsible for the maintenance of cytokine production were present in the joint cell cultures, and therefore these cultures provide an experimental system for studying cytokine regulation in the RA joint. Because there was evidence that IL-1 is of importance in joint pathology, for example its ability to induce the destruction of cartilage and bone (Pettipher

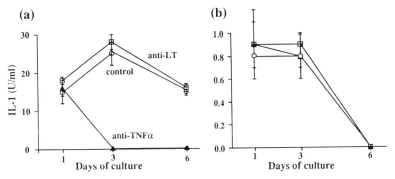

Figure 6.4 Inhibition of IL-1 protein by anti-TNF-α in RA but not OA synovial cultures. RA (a) or OA (b) synovial membrane cells were incubated in culture with polyclonal antibodies to TNF-α (▲), polyclonal antibodies to lymphotoxin (□) or equivalent amount of control rabbit IgG (○). IL-1 levels were measured in the supernatants after 1, 3 and 6 days culture by the mouse comitogenic thymocyte assay. Data from Brennan et al. (1989b).

lymphotoxin (<50 pg/ml) were present and contributing to the production of IL-1 in that instance (Brennan *et al.*, 1989b).

The experiment illustrated in Fig. 6.4(a) was repeated using joint tissues from osteoarthritic joints. Here the results were quite different. In six of seven samples, anti-TNF had no effect on the IL-1 levels (Fig. 6.4b), but in one sample, anti-TNF reduced IL-1 production. The exception was the OA patient whose joint cells made relatively high levels of IL-1 comparable with the RA patients. In both RA and OA, there are abundant macrophages, and TNF-α production is comparable in both; however, in OA, TNF-α does not induce IL-1 production. Comparable data have been subsequently obtained for RA samples using monoclonal antibodies to TNF-α. The degree of reduction in IL-1 activity depended on the neutralizing capacity of the monoclonal anti-TNF-α.

This preliminary attempt to unravel the complexities of the cytokine interactions in RA tissues has shown that neutralizing antibodies provide a viable strategy, and has also shown that there may be dominant signals regulating certain functions, e.g. TNF-α regulating IL-1 production (Brennan *et al.*, 1989b), GM-CSF production (Haworth *et al.*, 1991) and MHC class II expression (unpublished). In view of the presence of bioactive TNF-α, and its above effects and on cell adhesion, lymphocyte activation and the destruction of cartilage and bone, we have developed the working hypothesis that TNF-α is of pivotal importance in the rheumatoid process and thus would be a suitable therapeutic target (Feldmann, 1991; Feldmann *et al.*, 1990; Brennan *et al.*, 1992a). Attempts to delve further into this hypothesis especially *in vivo* will be described below.

2.4   Cytokine Localization

As cytokines act primarily as local mediators, their effects are likely to be influenced by the microenvironment of the producing cell. It was therefore important to localize mediators within the joint and investigate whether they could also be detected in circulating blood cells.

Two techniques are appropriate for the localization of cytokines: *in situ* hybridization using cDNA or RNA probes, and immunostaining with anti-cytokine antibodies. We have concentrated on the latter technique as, in our hands, this appears to allow the producing cell type to be more readily identified. The results obtained from these studies are in agreement with those obtained using dissociated cells, in that those cytokines that are abundant in cell culture supernatants are detectable by immunostaining. In addition, this approach has allowed the identification of the major sites of synthesis of cytokines such as IL-6 and TNF in the rheumatoid joint (Field *et al.*, 1991; Chu *et al.*, 1991).

The major source of cytokines was found to be the synovial lining layer; for example, IL-1, IL-6 and TNF-α were most abundant there. However, these were also found in the deeper layers, nodules and the interstitium. Abundant cytokine production has also been found at the CPJ junction.

There are two morphological types of cartilage/pannus junction, the "discrete CPJ" and the "diffuse CPJ" (Allard *et al.*, 1987). The discrete CPJ is an active erosive state, and the dominant cell type appears to be macrophage–monocyte. There are few T cells compared with other areas of synovium, and fibroblastic cells are common. The diffuse CPJ appears to be a healing site, and the dominant cell type is fibroblastic. It was of interest to compare the cytokine profiles of these two types of CPJ. The discrete CPJ contained abundant TNF-α, IL-1α, IL-6 and TGF-β. IL-1β was surprisingly not detectable with the reagents used, which were effective at staining adjacent synovium. In the diffuse CPJ, only TGF-β was detectable. Staining for TNF-Rs revealed that abundant p55 and p75 TNF-R were detectable in both (Deleuran *et al.*, 1992a), as was IL-1 type I (p50) receptor (Deleuran *et al.*, 1992b).

Double staining was used to identify which cells produced most of a particular cytokine. Thus for IL-1, IL-6 and TNF-α it was the macrophage–monocyte series. Other workers have produced analogous results, e.g. Firestein *et al.* (1990) and Wood *et al.* (1991), with ready detection of IL-1, TNF and IL-6.

2.5   Cytokine Receptor Expression

With the recent characterization of a large number of cytokine receptors (e.g. Sims *et al.*, 1988; Gray *et al.*, 1990), it is now possible to investigate the expression of cytokine receptors in RA joint tissues. The IL-2R p55 protein was identified in 1983 and its expression in RA tissues was the first receptor to be investigated. It is present on a variable percentage of T cells, from a usual 1–2% to an occasional 12% in our experience.

More recently, the receptors for the cytokines most abundantly expressed in the RA joint have been identified and their cDNAs cloned. Thus the expression of IL-6, IL-1 type I and both TNF receptors (p55 and p75) are now amenable to study by the simplest procedure, using monoclonal antibodies, by both binding to isolated cells and immunostaining on sections of RA joints. Because of our interest in TNF-α in RA tissues, and the evidence presented above that its overexpression may be of major importance in the pathogenesis of RA, we have explored TNF-α receptor expression in RA tissues using monoclonal antibodies to the p55 and p75 TNF-Rs.

By flow cytometry, expression of TNF-R was observed on both monocytic (p55 and p75) and lymphocytic cells (p75) isolated from the RA synovial joint. Expression of both receptors was increased compared with cells isolated from OA synovial joints (Fig. 6.5). Furthermore, both receptors were increased on synovial joint cells isolated

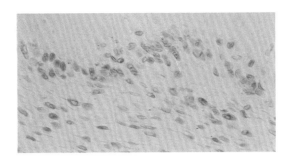

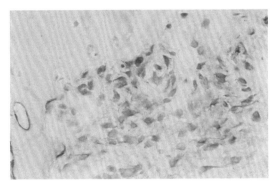

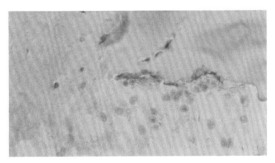

Plate 1 (see Chapter 6) Localization of TNF-Rs at the CPJ in RA. Immunostaining with anti-p55 TNF-R monoclonal antibody (top) and anti-p75 TNF-R monoclonal antibody (middle) shows that cells at the interface of the CPJ express both receptors. Normal mouse IgG1 (bottom) failed to stain these cells. Data from Deleuran *et al.* (1992a).

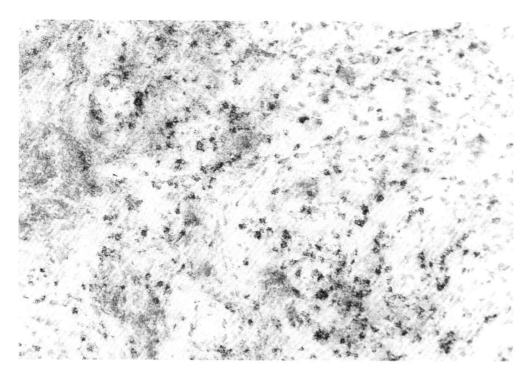

Plate 2 (see Chapter 8) Combined immunophenotyping/*in situ* hybridization for CD14 + macrophages and IL-1β mRNA in rheumatoid synovium. CD14 + macrophages are indicated by red staining and IL-1β mRNA-positive cells by overlying dense silver granules. The figure shows combined localization in perifollicular areas. Taken from Wood *et al*. (1992).

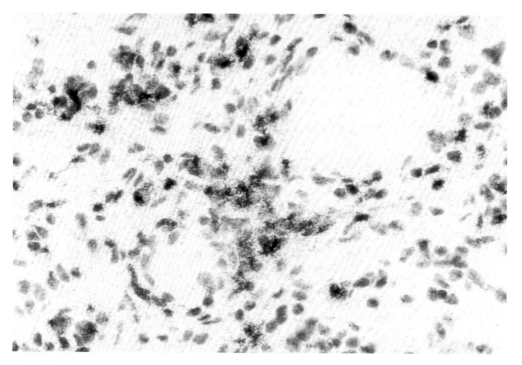

Plate 3 (see Chapter 8) *In situ* hybridization for IL-6 mRNA in rheumatoid synovium. IL-1 + cells are indicated by overlying dense silver granules and are shown in a "transitional" area of rheumatoid synovium. Taken from Wood *et al*. (1992).

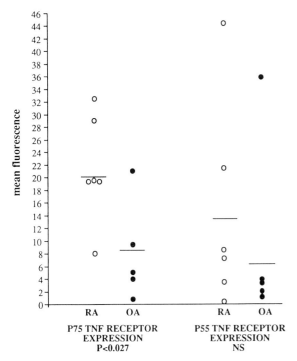

Figure 6.5 TNF receptor expression on mononuclear cells isolated from RA and OA synovial membrane. RA (○) and OA (•) synovial joint cells were immunostained with monoclonal anti-p55 (HTR-9) and anti-p75 (UTR-1) TNF-R and analysed by flow cytometry. Results are expressed as mean fluorescence after subtraction of background binding. Data from Brennan *et al.* (1992b).

from RA joints compared with matched peripheral blood samples (Brennan *et al.*, 1992b).

Immunocytochemistry showed that the expression of both TNF-Rs was elevated in the RA joint (Deleuran *et al.*, 1992a). Most striking was the expression at the synovial lining layer, which is the major site of TNF-α production. In view of the fact that joint damage occurs primarily at the CPJ, it was noteworthy that there was coexpression of both TNF-Rs (p55 and p75) (Plate 1) and TNF-α at the CPJ (Deleuran *et al.*, 1992a). This would be compatible with the concept that TNF-α has an important role in the destructive process in the RA joint.

2.6 CYTOKINE INHIBITORS

Two types of cytokine inhibitors have been described. There is an IL-1Ra, which is related to IL-1β and IL-1α, and binds to the two IL-1Rs without triggering them. It is thus a receptor antagonist (reviewed by Arend (1991)). However, its physiological function *in vivo* is unclear, as assays for this entity are still at an early stage and little is known of its concentrations in tissues and body fluids in different circumstances. As it takes a 100-fold molar excess to inhibit IL-1 activity, it is unlikely that its role

is to totally block IL-1 action, but rather to limit its duration or range of action. There is production of IL-1Ra in rheumatoid joints, detected by immunostaining (Deleuran *et al.*, 1992b) and *in situ* hybridization (Firestein *et al.*, 1991). However, as rheumatoid tissue releases bioactive IL-1, there is currently no evidence that endogenous IL-1Ra has a major regulatory role in the disease process. Exogenous IL-1R may be effective if sufficient quantities can be delivered.

The major group of cytokine inhibitors reported are soluble receptors derived from the extracellular domain of many cytokine receptors. This was first reported for the IL-2R p55 (Tac) chain, and soluble IL-2R is elevated in RA and correlates with disease activity (Symons *et al.*, 1988). Subsequently, many others, e.g. soluble forms of IL-4, IL-6, IL-7, IFNγ and both TNF-Rs, have been described (reviewed by Feldmann (1991)).

In view of our working hypothesis that TNF-α is of pivotal importance in RA, we have analysed the production of TNF inhibitors in some detail. OA joint cell cultures, which did not downregulate their IL-1 production with anti-TNF sera (Brennan *et al.*, 1989b), were found to lack bioactive TNF-α (Brennan *et al.*, 1992c). Additional recombinant TNF-α added to OA culture supernatants was neutralized. Radiolabelled OA joint cells synthesized a protein capable of binding to TNF-α. These observations are all consistent with the presence of TNF inhibitors in OA tissues. Direct ELISA for the p55 and p75 soluble TNF-Rs readily detected both (Brennan *et al.*, 1992c).

As there was bioactive TNF-α in RA culture supernatants and less bioactive TNF-α in OA culture supernatants, the possibility that the RA process is partly due to a relative lack of soluble TNF-R was investigated. Comparing levels of bioactive TNF-α in RA and OA showed that, whereas all RA samples had bioactive TNF-α, the average level of bioactivity was 54%, and many OA samples had no bioactivity, and the average TNF bioactivity was 40% (Brennan *et al.*, 1993). However, when soluble TNF-R levels were compared, these were higher in synovial fluid or synovial cell supernatant from RA than OA patients (Cope *et al.*, 1992; Brennan *et al.*, 1992b), so the RA process does not occur as a result of an absolute lack of this receptor. The soluble TNF-R is upregulated, but still not sufficiently to abrogate the elevated levels of active TNF-α produced. The OA samples were derived from patients with sufficient joint destruction to require joint replacement, and hence it is not surprising that the OA samples also had bioactive TNF-α.

Assays of soluble TNF-R in serum and synovial fluid in arthritic diseases have confirmed that production of this receptor is upregulated. It is elevated in RA serum (compared with normals and OA), more so in the more active cases, and, in matched synovial/serum samples, the former were 3 to 4-fold higher, suggesting that there is local production. To verify that the soluble TNF-R measured had TNF-α-inhibitory activity, its capacity to protect TNF-α assay lines from TNF-α lysis was verified. This protection was neutralized by antibodies to TNF-R (Cope *et al.*, 1992).

Thus our current concept is that TNF-α bioactivity is of major importance in the pathogenesis of RA. Despite upregulation of soluble TNF-R, the inhibitor of TNF-α, TNF-α production outstrips that of the inhibitor, and it is the imbalance between the two that is of major importance, and permits TNF-α to exert its effects. The upregulation of membrane TNF-R probably facilitates signal transduction.

3. Conclusions

3.1 CAN CYTOKINE INTERACTIONS DETECTED *IN VITRO* BE SHOWN TO OCCUR ALSO *IN VIVO*?

Collagen-induced arthritis in the DBA/1 mouse resembles RA in its histopathology and erosion of cartilage and bone. This model was chosen to ascertain whether TNF-α is of pivotal importance in arthritis *in vivo*. The effects of neutralizing TNF-α was evaluated *in vivo* using TN3.19.2, a hamster anti-murine TNF-α monoclonal antibody donated by Dr R. Schreiber.

Weekly antibody injections from the time collagen was injected reduced the inflammation. More dramatic was the effect on joint destruction and ankylosis, which was markedly diminished. This shows that blocking TNF-α can prevent aspects of the arthritis process (Williams *et al.*, 1992).

To evaluate whether blocking TNF-α would have a therapeutic effect on established arthritis, monoclonal or rabbit anti-TNF-α serum was injected just after the onset of arthritis (Table 6.3). Both regimens prevented progression of the arthritis, both the inflammation and the joint destruction (Williams *et al.* (1992) and unpublished data). These results support the hypothesis that TNF-α is of pivotal importance in RA, and demonstrate the therapeutic potential of anti-TNF-α therapy.

Transgenic mice have been useful in evaluating the effects of abnormal gene expression. Attempts were made to evaluate the effects of augmented TNF-α gene expression in these mice. Kollias and colleagues (Keffer *et al.*, 1991) replaced the 3′ untranslated region of the human TNF-α gene, which is of importance in reducing the half-life of TNF-α mRNA (Caput *et al.*, 1986), by the 3′ untranslated region of β-globin, which has a long half-life mRNA. The transgenic mice, with disregulated TNF-α mRNA expression, developed arthritis at about 4 weeks of age, which was totally abrogated by injection of monoclonal anti-human TNF-α antibody.

Thus, both antigen-induced and transgenic murine

Table 6.3   Anti-TNF treatment of established collagen-induced arthritis

	Clinical score	Maximum paw-swelling (%)
TN3-19.12	3.4 ± 0.6[*]	35 ± 10[*]
L2	6.7 ± 0.8	52 ± 19
PBS	5.6 ± 1.0	48 ± 13
Rb anti-TNF	1.9 ± 0.5[†]	21 ± 13[†]
NRS	5.0 ± 0.9	41 ± 10
PBS	6.3 ± 0.8	38 ± 11

Mice were treated with monoclonal (12 mg/kg) or polyclonal (rabbit) anti-TNF (80 mg/kg) sera for 2 weeks, starting immediately after the onset of clinical arthritis. Injections were given intraperitoneally (i.p.) twice per week. TN3-19.12, hamster monoclonal, anti-TNF; L2, hamster IgG1 antibody; Rb anti-TNF, rabbit anti-TNF. [*]$P < 0.05$ TN3-19.12 vs L2, [†]$P < 0.05$ Rb anti-TNF vs NRS.

models of arthritis support the concept that TNF-α is of pivotal importance in the pathogenesis of arthritis.

3.2 WHY IS TNF-α PRODUCTION NOT BALANCED BY TNF INHIBITORS IN RA?

It is well known that human TNF-α acts on murine cells, as murine cells are routinely used to assay human TNF-α. However, the cloning studies of the murine TNF-Rs revealed that human TNF-α binds to murine p55, and not p75 (Barrett *et al.*, 1991).

Thus mouse soluble p75 TNF inhibitor should not inhibit human TNF-α, and possibly murine p55 inhibitor does not inhibit human TNF-α efficiently. Thus the human TNF-α-induced transgenic model of arthritis also probably occurs as the result of an imbalance between TNF-α and TNF inhibitor production, as the amount of TNF-α detected is not large (Keffer *et al.*, 1991).

It is not known why there is an imbalance between TNF-α and TNF-R production. One hypothesis is that, despite upregulation of TNF-R on the membrane, and augmented cleavage of membrane receptor to form the soluble TNF-R, the maximal rate of TNF-R production is less than that of TNF-α produced by the numerous macrophages recruited to the synovium. This may especially be the case if the major source of soluble TNF-R is different from that of TNF-α. As very little is known about the mechanism (presumed enzymic) of cleavage of TNF-R, the effect of therapy on the cleavage of TNF-R is unknown, but could be of importance: TIMP, an inhibitor of the proteolytic enzymes, stromelysin and collagenase, may also inhibit the receptor cleavage enzyme and so could inhibit the production of soluble TNF-R. Much work needs to be performed to define what drives TNF-α production in RA, and to define the mechanism of regulation of soluble TNF-R production.

4. Acknowledgements

This work would not have been possible without many generous donations of reagents. In particular, we wish to thank Dr H.M. Shepard (Genentech), Dr C. Henney and S. Gillis (Immunex), Dr M. Schreier (Sandoz), Dr S. Clark (Genetics Institute), Dr P. Lomedico (Roche) and Dr. R.D. Schreiber (Washington University) for their support. This work was funded by the ARC, MRC, Nuffield Foundation, Wellcome Trust and Xenova.

5. References

Allard, S.A., Muirden, K.D., Camplejohn, K.L. and Maini, R.N. (1987). Chondrocyte-derived cells and matrix at the rheumatoid cartilage-pannus junction identified with monoclonal antibodies. Rheumatol. Int. 7, 153–159.

Arend, W.P. (1991). Interleukin 1 receptor antagonist. J. Clin. Invest. 88, 1445–1451.

Barrett, K., Taylor-Fishwick, D.A., Cope, A.P., Kissonerghis, A.M., Gray, P.W., Feldmann, M. and Foxwell, B.M.J. (1991). Cloning, expression and cross-linking analysis of the murine p55 tumor necrosis factor receptor. Eur. J. Immunol. 21, 1649–1656.

Bottazzo, G.F., Pujol-Borell, R., Hanafusa, T. and Feldmann, M. (1983). Hypothesis: Role of aberrant HLA-DR expression and antigen presentation in the induction of endocrine autoimmunity. Lancet ii, 1115–1118.

Brennan, F.M., Chantry, D., Jackson, A.M., Maini, R.N. and Feldmann, M. (1989a). Cytokine production in culture by cells isolated from the synovial membrane. J. Autoimmunity, 2 (Suppl) 177–186.

Brennan, F.M., Chantry, D., Jackson, A., Maini, R.N. and Feldmann, M. (1989b). Inhibitory effect of TNF-α antibodies on synovial cell interleukin-1 production in rheumatoid arthritis. Lancet ii, 244–247.

Brennan, F.M., Zachariae, C.O.C., Chantry, D., Larsen, C.G., Turner, M., Maini, R.N., Matsushima, K. and Feldmann, M. (1990a). Detection of interleukin-8 (IL-8) biological activity in synovial fluids from patients with rheumatoid arthritis and production of IL-8 mRNA by isolated synovial cells. Eur. J. Immunol. 20, 2141–2144.

Brennan, F.M., Chantry, D., Turner, M., Foxwell, B., Maini, R.N. and Feldmann, M. (1990b). Detection of transforming growth factor-β in rheumatoid arthritis synovial tissue: lack of effect on spontaneous cytokine production in joint cell cultures. Clin. Exp. Immunol. 81, 278–285.

Brennan, F.M., Maini, R.N. and Feldmann, M. (1992a). TNF-α – a pivotal role in rheumatoid arthritis. Br. J. Rheumatol. 31, 293–298.

Brennan, F.M., Gibbons, D.L., Mitchell, T., Cope, A.P., Maini, R.N. and Feldmann, M. (1992b). Enhanced expression of TNF receptor mRNA and protein in mononuclear cells isolated from rheumatoid arthritis synovial joints. Eur. J. Immunol. 22, 1907–1912.

Brennan, F.M., Katsikis, P., Gibbons, A.P., Aderka, D., Wallach, D., Maini, R.N. and Feldmann, M. (1993). TNF-binding proteins are produced spontaneously by RA and OA synovial joint cell cultures: inhibition of TNF bioactivity (in preparation).

Buchan, G., Barrett, K., Fujita, T., Maini, R.N. and Feldmann, M. (1988a). Detection of activated T-cell products in the rheumatoid joint using cDNA probes to interleukin-2 (IL-2) receptor and IFN-γ. Clin. Exp. Immunol. 71, 295–301.

Buchan, G., Barrett, K., Turner, M., Chantry, D., Maini, R.N. and Feldmann, M. (1988b). Interleukin-1 and tumour necrosis factor mRNA expression in rheumatoid arthritis: prolonged production of IL-1α. Clin. Exp. Immunol. 73, 449–455.

Caput, D., Beutler, B., Hantog, K, Brown Shimer, S. and Cerami, A. (1986). Identification of a common nucleotide sequence in the $3'$ untranslated region of mRNA molecules specifying inflammatory mediators. Proc. Natl Acad. Sci. USA 83, 1670–1674.

Carding, S.R. and Bottomly, K. (1988). IL-4 (B cell stimulatory factor 1) exhibits thymocyte growth factor activity in the presence of IL-2. J. Immunol. 140, 1519–1526.

Chantry, D., Turner, M. and Feldmann, M. (1989a). Interleukin 7 (murine pre-B cell growth factor/lymphopoietin 1) stimulates thymocyte growth: regulation by transforming growth factor beta. Eur. J. Immunol. 19, 783–786.

Chantry, D., Turner, M., Abney, E. and Feldmann, M. (1989b). Modulation of cytokine production by transforming growth factor beta. J. Immunol. 142, 4295–4300.

Chantry, D., Winearls, C.G., Maini, R.N. and Feldmann, M. (1989c). Mechanism of immune complex mediated damage: induction of interleukin 1 by immune complexes and synergy with interferon γ and tumour necrosis factor α. Eur. J. Immunol. 19, 189–192.

Chantry, D., Turner, M., Brennan, F.M. and Feldmann, M. (1990). GM-CSF induces both HLA-class expression and cytokine expression by human monocytes. Cytokine 2, 60–67.

Chu, C.Q., Field, M., Feldmann, M. and Maini, R.N. (1991). Localization of tumour necrosis factor in the synovial tissues and at the cartilage-pannus junction in patients with rheumatoid arthritis. Arth. Rheum. 34, 1125–1132.

Cope, A., Aderka, D., Doherty, M., Engelmann, H., Gibbons, D., Jones, A C., Brennan, F.M., Maini, R.N., Wallach, D. and Feldmann, M. (1992). Increased levels of soluble tumour necrosis factor receptors in the sera and synovial fluid of patients with rheumatic diseases. Arth. Rheum. 35, 1160–1169.

Deleuran, B., Chu, C.Q., Field, M., Brennan, F.M., Mitchell, T., Brockhaus, M., Feldmann, M. and Maini, R.N. (1992a). Localization of TNF receptors in the synovial tissue and cartilage/pannus junction in rheumatoid arthritis: implications for local actions of TNFα. Arthr. Rheum. 35, 1170–1178.

Deleuran, B., Chu, C.Q., Field, M., Brennan, F.M., Katsikis, P., Feldmann, M. and Maini, R.N. (1992b). Localization of interleukin 1α (IL-1α), type 1 IL-1 receptor and interleukin 1 receptor antagonist protein in the synovial membrane and cartilage-pannus junction in rheumatoid arthritis. Br. J. Rheum. 31, 801–809.

Feldmann, M. (1989). Molecular mechanisms involved in human autoimmune diseases: relevance of chronic antigen presentation, class II expression and cytokine production. Immunol. Suppl. 2, 66–71.

Feldmann, M. (1991). Review: Cytokine networks: Do we understand them well enough to facilitate clinical benefits? Eur. Cytokine Net. 2, 5–9.

Feldmann, M., Brennan, F.M., Chantry, D., Haworth, C., Turner, M., Abney, E., Buchan, G., Barrett, K., Barkley, D., Chu, A., Field, M. and Maini, R.N. (1990). Cytokine production in the rheumatoid joint: implications for treatment. Ann. Rheum. Dis. 51, 480–486.

Feldmann, M., Brennan, F.M., Chantry, D., Haworth, C., Turner, M., Katsikis, P., Londei, M., Abney, E., Buchan, G., Barrett, K., Corcoran, A., Kissonerghis, M., Zheng, R.. Grubeck-Loebenstein, B., Barkley, D., Chu, A., Field, M. and Maini, R.N. (1991). Cytokine assays: Role in evaluation of the pathogenesis of autoimmunity. Immunol. Rev. 119, 105–123.

Field, M., Chu, C.Q., Feldmann, M. and Maini, R.N. (1991). Interleukin-6 localisation in the synovial membrane in rheumatoid arthritis. Rheumat. Int. 11, 45–50.

Firestein, G.S., Alvaro-Garcia, J.M. and Maki, R. (1990). Quantitative analysis of cytokine gene expression in rheumatoid arthritis. J. Immunol. 144, 3347–3353.

Firestein, G.S., Berger, N.E., Chapman, D.L., Tracey, D.E., Chosay, J.G. and Zvaifler, N.J. (1991). IL-1 receptor antagonist protein (IRAP) production and gene expression by RA and OA synovium. Clin. Res. 39, 291A.

Gray, P.W., Barrett, K., Chantry, D., Turner, M. and Feldmann, M. (1990). Cloning of human tumour necrosis factor (TNF) receptor cDNA and expression of recombinant soluble TNF-binding protein. Proc. Natl Acad. Sci. USA 87, 7380–7384.

Grubeck-Loebenstein, B., Buchan, G., Chantry, D., Kassal, H., Londei, M., Pirich, K., Barrett, K., Turner, M., Waldhausl, W. and Feldmann, M. (1989). Analysis of intrathyroidal cytokine production in thyroid autoimmune disease: thyroid follicular cells produce IL-1a and interleukin-6. Clin. Exp. Immunol. 77, 324–330.

Haworth, C., Brennan, F.M., Chantry, D., Turner, M., Maini, R.N. and Feldmann, M. (1991). Expression of granulocyte-macrophage colony stimulating factor (GM-CSF) in rheumatoid arthritis: regulation by tumour necrosis factor a. Eur. J. Immunol. 21, 2575–2579.

Hirano, T., Matsuda, T., Turner, M., Miyasaka, N., Buchan, G., Tang, B., Sato, K., Shimizu, M., Maini, R., Feldmann, M. and Kishimoto, T. (1988). Excessive production of interleukin 6/B cell stimulatory factor-2 in rheumatoid arthritis. Eur. J. Immunol. 18, 1797–1801.

Kawakami, Y., Custer, M.C., Rosenberg, S.A. and Lotze, M.T. (1989). IL-4 regulates IL-2 induction of lymphokine activated killer activity from human lymphocytes. J. Immunol. 142, 3452–3461.

Keffer, J., Probert, L., Cazlaris, H., Georgopoulos, S., Kaslaris, E., Kioussis, D. and Kollias, G. (1991). Transgenic mice expressing human tumour necrosis factor: a predictive genetic model of arthritis. EMBO J. 10, 4025–4031.

Kriegler, M., Perez, C., De Fay, K., Albert, I. and Lu, S.D. (1988). A novel form of TNF/cachectin is a cell surface cytotoxic transmembrane protein: ramifications for the complex physiology of TNF. Cell 53, 45–53.

Londei, M., Bottazzo, G.F. and Feldmann, M. (1985). Human T-cell clones from autoimmune thyroid glands: specific recognition of autologous thyroid cells. Science 228, 85–89.

Londei, M., Savill, C., Verhoef, A., Brennan, F., Leech, Z.A., Duance, V., Maini, R.N. and Feldmann, M. (1989). Persistence of collagen type II specific T cell clones in the synovial membrane of a patient with RA. Proc. Natl Acad. Sci. USA 86, 636–640.

Londei, M., Verhoef, A., Hawrylowics, C., Groves, J., De Berardinis, P. and Feldmann, M. (1990). Interleukin 7 is a growth factor for mature human T cells. Eur. J. Immunol. 20, 425–428.

Pettipher, E.J., Higgs, G.A. and Henderson, B. (1986). Interleukin 1 induces leucocyte infiltration and cartilage degradation in the synovial joint. Proc. Natl Acad. Sci. USA 83, 8749–8753.

Portillo, G., Turner, M., Chantry, D. and Feldmann, M. (1989). Effect of cytokines on HLA-DR and IL-1 production by a monocytic tumour, THP-1. Immunology 66, 170–175.

Pujol-Borrell, R., Todd, I., Doshi, M., Bottazo, G.F., Sutton, R., Gray, D., Adolf, G.R. and Feldmann, M. (1987). HLA class II induction in human islet cells by interferon-γ plus tumour necrosis factor or lymphotoxin. Nature (London) 326, 304–306.

Saklatvala, J., Sarsfield, S.J. and Townsend, Y. (1985). Pig interleukin-1. Purification of two immunologically different leukocyte proteins that cause cartilage resorption lymphocyte activation and fever. J. Exp. Med. 162, 1208–1222.

Sims, J., March, C.J., Cosman, D., Widmer, M.R.M., Macdonald, H.R., Masmahai, C.J., Grubin, C.K., Wignall, J.M., Jackson, J.K., Call, S.M., Friend, D., Aepert, C.R., Gillis, S., Urdal, D.L. and Dower, S.K. (1988). cDNA expression cloning of the IL-1 receptor – a member of the immune globulin super family. Science 241, 585–589.

Symons, J.A., Wood, N.C., Di Giovine, F.S. and Duff, G.W. (1988). Soluble IL-2, receptor in rheumatoid arthritis. Correlation with disease activity, IL-1 and IL-2 inhibition. J. Immunol. 141, 2612–2618.

Thomas, B.M., Mundy, G.R. and Chambers, T.J. (1987). Tumour necrosis factor α and β induce osteoblastic cells to stimulate osteoclast bone resorption. J. Immunol. 138, 775–779.

Williams, R.O., Feldmann, M. and Maini, R.N. (1992). Anti-TNF ameliorates joint disease in murine collagen-induced arthritis. Proc. Natl Acad. Sci. USA 89, 9784–9788.

Wood, N.C., Symons, J.A., Dickens, E. and Duff, G.W. (1991). *In situ* hybridization of IL-6 in rheumatoid arthritis. Clin. Exp. Immunol. 87, 183–189.

7. Naturally Occurring Inhibitors of Cytokines

William P. Arend and Jean-Michel Dayer

1. Introduction

Human autoimmune or inflammatory disease may be triggered by endogenous or exogenous stimuli. These diseases may result from overactivation of normal cells, selection of an abnormal clone of cells or a defect in host defence mechanisms. Cytokines from both immune and non-immune cells play major roles in these disease

Immunopharmacology of Joints and Connective Tissue
ISBN 0-12-206345-7

Table 7.1   Levels of interference with cytokine effects

1. *Cytokine production*
   Receptor triggering (e.g. HDL–LPS complexes; interference with integrins)
   Signal transduction
   Transcription rate (e.g. glucocorticoids)
   Translation, mRNA stability
   Inhibition of cytokine release (e.g. Ca^{2+} level, myristoylation)
2. *Latent versus active cytokines*
   Inhibitors of proteases cleaving the inactive precursor
   Binding to matrix (e.g. fibronectin, collagen, proteoglycan, TGF-β, FGF)
3. *Binding proteins (BP)*
   Neutralization of ligand
   Naturally occurring autoantibodies
   Carrier molecules (e.g. α_2-macroglobulin) which modify biopharmacology
   Formation of inactive ligand/BP complexes (e.g. shedding of receptor fragments, soluble TNF-R)
4. *Receptor antagonists*
   Interaction with receptor ligand binding (e.g. IL-1Ra)
5. *Downregulation of ligand receptors*
   e.g. number and/or affinity of the receptors
6. *Inactivation of the ligand*
   Alteration by mutation
   Proteases, pH, temperature, oxidation, clearing factors
7. *Inhibition of post-receptor events*
8. *Cytokines with conflicting biological activities*
   (e.g. IFNγ and TGF-β in collagen synthesis; IFNγ and IL-4/IL-10 in cytokine production)

Abbreviations: FGF, fibroblast growth factor; TNF-R, TNF receptor.

processes. Cytokines are involved in initiation of the immune response, induction of acute inflammatory events and transition to or persistence of chronic inflammation. However, they exist in a network with overlapping and redundant effects; cells also exhibit concomitant production of specific and non-specific cytokine inhibitors.

This chapter will summarize the numerous ways by which the cytokine network may be modulated or inhibited by naturally occurring processes. If a given cytokine fails to exert its usual biological effects, this may be due to events occurring from the stage of activation of cytokine-producing cells to the level of cytokine activation of target cells (Table 7.1). Cytokine production can be affected at several levels: prevention of interaction between lymphocytes and monocytes; cytokines can oppose the action of each other; cytokines in solution can be bound by antibodies, soluble receptors or other proteins; and specific antagonists may block receptor binding of cytokines. New therapeutic approaches to human diseases are directed at interfering with the cytokine network at these multiple levels.

2. *Inhibitors of Cytokine Production*

Cytokine production may be inhibited at the level of induction following ligand binding to cell surface receptors. The ligand can be either a soluble factor or a membrane-bound glycoprotein involved in direct cell contact. One of the most potent triggers of monocyte–macrophages is endotoxin or LPS. The cell surface glycoprotein CD14 is known to play a major role as a receptor for LPS–protein complexes (Wright *et al.*, 1990), interference with CD14 function inhibits LPS activity.

Direct contact of monocyte–macrophages with activated lymphocytes stimulates the production of IL-1, TNF-α and IL-6 to a marked extent (Vey *et al.*, 1992). It is possible that soluble fragments of integrin receptors may interfere with this monocyte response (Isler *et al.*, 1993). As TNF-α and IL-1 may be associated with a variety of diseases in man, it is important to understand the mechanisms that might block production or biological activities of these cytokines (Seckinger and Dayer, 1992). The following are examples of inhibition of TNF-α and IL-1 production or action.

2.1 INHIBITION OF TNF-α SYNTHESIS, PROCESSING AND RELEASE

In high concentrations (100 nM), PGE_2 suppresses accumulation of LPS-induced TNF-α mRNA by exerting effects at both transcriptional and post-transcriptional levels. TNF-α activates the cyclooxygenase pathway, and the resultant PGE_2 in turn downregulates TNF-α production. Other agents that cause an increase in cAMP activity may also reduce TNF-α production. In contrast, the lipoxygenase pathway appears to stimulate TNF-α production. Corticosteroids markedly suppress the endotoxin-induced increase in TNF-α mRNA through both transcriptional and post-transcriptional mechanisms. Lastly, inhibition of the protease that cleaves the 26 kDa precursor propeptide of TNF-α into the fully active form represents another potential mechanism for regulating TNF-α effects (Beutler *et al.*, 1992).

2.2 INHIBITION OF TNF-α BIOLOGICAL ACTIVITY AT THE TARGET CELL LEVEL

Reversible phosphorylation of intracellular proteins controlled by various kinases may be one of the mechanisms by which TNF-α acts on target cells (Seckinger and Dayer, 1992). Dephosphorylation of these proteins by the activation of specific phosphatases renders the cells resistant to the effects of TNF-α. The TNF-α transduction mechanism may involve receptor coupling to GTP-binding proteins (G-proteins), leading to an increase or decrease in cytoplasmic cAMP through modulation of adenylate cyclase activity. A pivotal role for a pertussis toxin-sensitive G-protein has been established in some biological responses to TNF-α. In addition, as PLA2 is activated through a G-protein, it may be essential to block this enzyme in order to regulate TNF-α cytotoxicity.

TNF-α destroys cells by at least two distinct mechanisms. One of them is dependent on *de novo* protein synthesis, but the second one is independent of this step. Both dexamethasone and indomethacin block TNF-α-induced cytotoxicity, suggesting that PLA2 may play a key role in cytotoxicity. In addition, the cytocidal action of TNF-α has been shown to involve lysosomal enzymes; inhibition of their activities might therefore block TNF-α cytotoxicity. Finally, scavengers of toxic oxygen metabolites (reactive oxygen species) reduce the cytotoxicity of TNF-α. Enzymes such as catalase, glutathione peroxidase and superoxide dismutase may therefore be essential in preventing the cytotoxic effects of TNF-α. All these mechanisms have recently been reviewed (Baglioni, 1992; Wong *et al.*, 1992).

2.3 REGULATION OF TNF-α AND IL-1 RECEPTORS

TNF-α receptors are downregulated by IL-1 and mitogens in some cells, probably mediated by PKA. This is not due to enhanced internalization of the TNF-α receptor, nor to its shedding, but to an influence on ligand-binding affinity. In contrast, stimulation of PKA results in the enhancement of TNF-α receptor expression (Pfizenmaier *et al.*, 1992). The possibilities of up- and down-regulation of TNF-α receptor expression are listed in Table 7.2.

Table 7.2 Factors inducing up- and down-regulation of TNF-α receptors

Upregulation	Downregulation
IFNγ, IFNα, IFNβ	LPS
IL-4, IL-6, IL-2	PMA (PKC)
Monocyte differentiation	IL-1
Dibutyryl cAMP (PKA)	

IL-1 receptor expression is also upregulated or downregulated on different cells. IL-1 receptor levels on T cells are decreased by IL-1 or TGF-β, but increased by IL-4. In addition, IL-1 receptor expression is enhanced by culture of fibroblasts with PDGF and of keratinocytes with IFNγ.

2.4 INHIBITION OF IL-1 AT THE LEVELS OF INDUCTION AND PRODUCTION

As LPS strongly induces IL-1 production, agents that temper LPS effects could be considered potential inhibitors of IL-1 production. Some of these agents act in combination with the LPS molecule, blocking the LPS-triggering signal at the membrane level (Baumberger *et al.*, 1991). Inhibition of the proteolytic cleavage of IL-1β may be another mechanism to prevent production of 17 kDa extracellular IL-1β (Mizutani *et al.*, 1991; Thornberry *et al.*, 1992). An increase in cellular cAMP or a decrease in the available Ca^{2+} ions may also reduce the production of IL-1 by stimulated monocytes. In contrast, interference with protein kinases does not decrease IL-1 production but only its secretion (Bakouche *et al.*, 1992). Specific pharmacological approaches at these levels will certainly be important in the future.

Other cytokines such as IL-4, IL-6, IL-10 and IFNα may decrease the production of IL-1 in some *in vitro* systems under particular conditions. However, these cytokines do not affect IL-1 exclusively; they also reduce TNF-α and other monocyte–macrophage products (reviewed in Arend and Dayer, 1993).

3. *Opposing Effects of Cytokines*

The concept of cytokine inhibition encompasses the entire cytokine network. To almost any cytokine with an agonist activity there is another cytokine with an antagonistic activity, although primarily shown *in vitro* (Table 7.3). One of the most challenging and disputed concepts is the balance between the Th2/Th1 lymphocytes and their respective production of lymphokines (Table 7.4). Th2 lymphocytes can control Th1 lymphocytes and vice versa. Thus, Th2 cells inhibit via IL-4 and

Table 7.3   Examples of the cytokine-induced decrease in cytokine production

Activator	Events	Inhibitor
IL-1	Production of IL-2	TGF-β
TGF-β	Collagen synthesis	IFNγ
IL-1, TNF-α	Protease synthesis	IFNγ
IL-1	PMN adhesion	IL-8
IL-1, TNF-α	Production of IL-1/TNF-α	IL-4, IL-6, IL-10, TGF-β
IFNγ	Production of IFNγ	IL-10
IL-1, TNF-α	Protease production	IL-4, IL-10
IFNγ	IgE production	IL-4

Table 7.4   Cytokines secreted by T lymphocytes

Cytokine	Cytotoxic T lymphocytes (CD8)	T helper lymphocytes (Th1/CD4)	T helper lymphocytes (Th2/CD4)
IFNγ	+ +	+ +	–
IL-2	±	+ +	–
TNF-β	+	+ +	–
GM-CSF	+ +	+ +	+
TNF-α	+	+ +	+
IL-3	+	+ +	+ +
IL-4	–	–	+ +
IL-5	–	–	+ +
IL-6	–	+ / --	+ +
IL-10	?	–	+ +

IL-10 the production of cytokines by Th1 and NK cells (Quesniaux, 1992). By releasing IFNγ, Th1 cells block the proliferation and differentiation of basophils/mast cells or eosinophils controlled by the Th2 production of IL-2, IL-4, IL-5 and IL-10 (Thompson-Snipes et al., 1991).

In tissue destruction, the relationship between IL-4 and IFNγ and their effects on the production of cytokines and metalloproteinases by human macrophages is of particular interest (Lacraz et al., 1992). IL-4 decreases IL-1 and TNF-α production, whereas IFNγ increases this response in macrophages. On the same target cell, both IL-4 and IFNγ decrease metalloproteinase production (e.g. 92 kDa collagenase and stromelysin). Another remarkable example of opposite effects regards synthesis of collagen and fibronectin by fibroblasts; this response is induced by TGF-β but opposed by IFNγ and TNF-α. Lastly, both IL-4 and IL-10 block monocyte production of a variety of cytokines, whereas IL-4 enhances LPS-induced IL-1Ra production by these cells.

4.   Antibodies to Cytokines

4.1   INTRODUCTION

Autoantibodies to cytokines represent another potential mechanism for altering the *in vivo* effects of specific cytokines. Naturally occurring antibodies to IL-1α, IL-6, IFN and TNF in human circulation have been described. In addition, cytokine-reactive antibodies may result after therapeutic administration of some recombinant human cytokines. Only the naturally occurring autoantibodies will be discussed in this chapter.

It remains unclear whether these autoantibodies act to inhibit or enhance the effects of cytokines *in vivo* (Fig. 7.1) (Bendtzen et al., 1990). An antibody that bound to the active site of a cytokine, and with an affinity high enough to prevent transfer of the cytokine to a membrane receptor, would theoretically inhibit the effects of that cytokine *in vivo*. In contrast, a lower-affinity antibody might enhance cytokine effects by acting as a carrier *in vivo*. In this situation the antibody would pick up the cytokine from the site of synthesis, possibly carry it to another location and then transfer the cytokine to high-affinity cell surface receptors. In addition, antibodies may prolong the lifespan of cytokines by preventing both urinary excretion and proteolytic degradation.

4.2   AUTOANTIBODIES TO IL-1α

Autoantibodies specific for IL-1α have been found in the sera of both normals and patients with a variety of autoimmune diseases. A pool of normal human sera was found to competitively inhibit the binding of ^{125}I-IL-1α to specific receptors on EL-4 murine thymoma cells (Svenson et al., 1989). The responsible activity in the normal sera was shown to be IgG antibodies by three criteria: size of 100–200 kDa by gel filtration chromatography, binding to immobilized staphylococcal-protein A, and precipitation of ^{125}I-IL-1α-antibody complexes by rabbit anti-human IgG antibodies.

Subsequent studies have further characterized these antibodies to IL-1α found in normal sera (Svenson et al., 1990). These antibodies were of IgG1, IgG2 and IgG4 subclasses and did not demonstrate any cross-reactivity with IL-1β, IL-2, IL-6 or TNF-α. Interestingly, up to 50% of these antibodies were IgG4, a subclass of IgG that fixes complement poorly. The specific anti-IL-1α antibodies were found in 25% of normal male sera and 22% of normal female sera. Most importantly, this IgG was demonstrated to bind IL-1α through the Fab portion of the molecule. Either one or two Fab fragments were bound to a single molecule of IL-1α. The intact antibodies bound IL-1α with a high affinity, exhibiting a mean K_d of 11 pM with IgG from female sera and 5.5 pM with IgG from male sera by Scatchard analysis. These

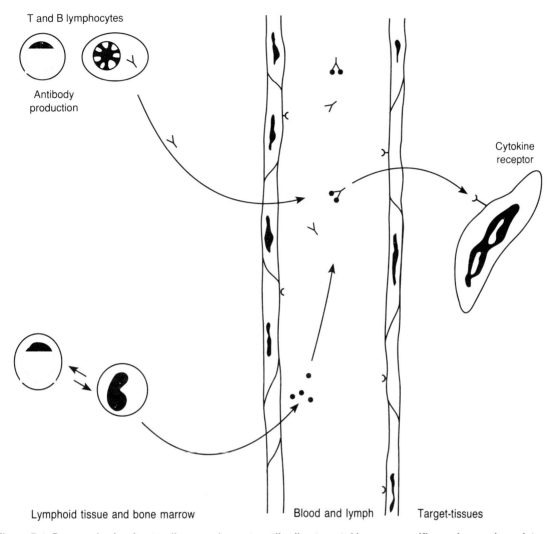

T and B lymphocytes

Antibody
production

Cytokine
receptor

Lymphoid tissue and bone marrow | Blood and lymph | Target-tissues

Figure 7.1 Proposed role of naturally occurring autoantibodies to cytokines as specific carriers and regulators of cytokines. Taken, with permission, from Bendtzen et al. (1990).

antibodies were capable of cross-linking IL-1α molecules to form a lattice-work as ^{125}I-IL-1α added to normal sera formed immune complexes as large as 700 kDa.

Autoantibodies to IL-1α were demonstrated to interfere with the detection of IL-1α by ELISA (Mae et al., 1991). Again, these antibodies were shown to be IgG and bound IL-1α with an affinity of 470 pM by Scatchard analysis and 100 pM by the Sips plot. This affinity is sufficiently high to compete with binding of IL-1α to cell surface receptors. In this study, as in the earlier studies, no antibodies to IL-1β were detected.

Anti-IL-1α antibodies also have been described in the sera of seven of 41 RA patients (Suzuki et al., 1989). These antibodies were proven to be IgG and they inhibited IL-1-induced proliferation of murine thymocytes, IL-1 upregulation of adhesion molecule expression on endothelial cells, and binding of ^{125}I-IL-1α to

receptors on synovial cells (Suzuki et al., 1990). The antibodies from rheumatoid sera bound IL-1α with a K_d of 55 pM, and, like the antibodies found in normal sera, did not bind IL-1β or TNF-α. However, these investigators found autoantibodies to IL-1α in <5% of normal sera. The differences between these results and those of earlier studies by others may be due to methodological variations in detection of the anti-IL-1α antibodies.

Anti-IL-1α antibodies have been detected in other diseases including 66% of patients with Schnitzler's syndrome (urticaria and macroglobulinaemia) (Saurat et al., 1991). Again, these antibodies were found disproportionately in the IgG4 subclass but IgA anti-IL-1α antibodies were also detected. It was demonstrated in rat studies that the IgG anti-IL-1α antibodies prolonged the presence of ^{125}I-IL-1α in circulation, probably by retarding glomerular filtration. However, not all of the

IgG antibodies blocked receptor binding of IL-1α. Thus, autoantibodies to IL-1α might potentiate the effects of IL-1α *in vivo* in these patients by prolonging circulation and allowing further opportunity for target cell stimulation.

Two more sensitive competitive assays for autoantibodies to IL-1α have recently been described: a radioimmunoassay and an indirect ELISA (Hansen *et al.*, 1993). Using these assays, antibodies to IL-1α were found in the sera of 28% of normals, 75% of Grave's disease and 44% of pernicious anaemia. The titre of these antibodies was no higher in the diseased sera than in normal sera. Again, no antibodies to IL-1β were found in normal or diseased sera. In addition to inhibiting the binding of soluble IL-1α to receptors on human T cells, thymocytes and fibroblasts, IgG antibodies also inhibited the activity of membrane-bound IL-1α (Svenson *et al.*, 1993). In addition, these antibodies failed to inhibit receptor binding of the specific IL-1Ra molecule.

4.3   AUTOANTIBODIES TO IL-6

Antibodies specific for IL-6 have also been found in 10% of normal sera (Hansen *et al.*, 1991). These antibodies interfered with the detection by ELISA of exogenously added IL-6. It is of interest that five of seven normal sera examined contained antibodies to both IL-1α and IL-6. The anti-IL-6 antibodies were also found predominantly in the IgG4 subclass and inhibited receptor binding of IL-6 (Bendtzen *et al.*, 1992). Again, it remains unclear whether these antibodies act as carriers for IL-6 *in vivo* or block receptor binding.

4.4   AUTOANTIBODIES TO IFN

Natural antibodies to IFNγ were found in very low titre in virtually all of 180 normal sera examined (Caruso *et al.*, 1990). These antibodies were present in much higher titres in the sera of virus-infected patients. The anti-IFNγ antibodies were solely IgG and failed to inhibit the antiviral activity of IFNγ. However, these antibodies may inhibit the effects of IFNγ on immune cells. In another study, normal sera possessed antibodies against IFNα and β as well as γ, and neutralized antiviral activities of the different interferons (Ross *et al.*, 1990). In addition, these antibodies were of both the IgG and IgM classes. The possible importance of anti-IFN antibodies *in vivo* remains to be examined.

4.5   AUTOANTIBODIES TO TNF-α

Lastly, antibodies reactive with TNF-α detected by immunoblotting were found in 40% of normal sera (Fomsgaard *et al.*, 1989). These antibodies were more prevalent in patients with Gram-negative sepsis (66%), cystic fibrosis with chronic lung infection (72%) and rheumatic diseases (61%). The TNF-α-reactive antibodies

were of both the IgM and IgG classes. It has not been reported whether they block the receptor binding of TNF-α.

4.6   SUMMARY AND CONCLUSIONS

Recently published studies have described the presence of naturally occurring antibodies to various cytokines in normal sera: to IL-1α in up to 30%, to IL-6 in 10%, to IFNγ in all and to TNF-α in 40%. The antibodies to IL-1α have been characterized most completely. These anti-cytokine antibodies block receptor binding *in vitro* but may function primarily as a carrier or transport mechanism *in vivo*. The relevance of other anti-cytokine antibodies remains to be determined.

5.   *Protein Binding of Cytokines*

5.1   INTRODUCTION

It had long been noted by many investigators that high-molecular-mass forms of some cytokines were present in plasma or other body fluids. These observations implied that cytokines may bind to larger-sized proteins. Some of this discrepancy in cytokine size was undoubtedly due to the presence of autoantibodies, particularly specific for IL-1α (see above). However, two other proteins, uromodulin and α2-macroglobulin, may bind various cytokines. Although the *in vivo* biological relevance of protein binding of cytokines remains unclear, it is possible that this interaction interferes with the biological activity of some cytokines but not of others.

5.2   CYTOKINE BINDING TO UROMODULIN

Uromodulin, known also as Tamm–Horsfall glycoprotein, is an 85 kDa molecule found primarily in pregnancy urine. This protein had previously been known to inhibit antigen-induced proliferation of human lymphocytes. Semi-purified uromodulin was shown to inhibit IL-1-induced proliferation of murine thymocytes, but actually to enhance the effects of IL-2 in this assay (Brown *et al.*, 1986). This effect of uromodulin was due to a high-affinity direct binding of both IL-1α and IL-1β (Matsuda *et al.*, 1986). This interaction was dependent upon intact glycosylation of the uromodulin molecule (Muchmore and Decker, 1987). It is of interest that uromodulin inhibited the effects of IL-1 in any T cell assay examined. In contrast, uromodulin was co-stimulatory with IL-1 in induction of PGE2 synthesis by fibroblasts. This apparent paradox may be due to the variable direct effects of uromodulin itself in these cell assays.

Molecular cloning of uromodulin led to a further characterization of its interactions with cytokines

(Hession *et al.*, 1987). In addition to both forms of IL-1, uromodulin also directly bound TNF-α. Immunohistological localization studies indicated that IL-1 and TNF could bind to uromodulin in sections of human kidneys. This observation suggested that uromodulin may bind these cytokines in renal tissue *in vivo*, possibly influencing either circulating levels or the local effects of IL-1 and TNF-α.

5.3   CYTOKINE BINDING TO α_2M

α_2-Macroglobulin is a major serum protein that binds a variety of substances including enzymes, mitogens, LPS, histones and a number of ions. An important biological function of α_2M appears to be in the clearance of potentially noxious materials from the circulation. The interaction between α_2M and proteolytic enzymes conformationally alters native α_2M from an electrophoretically slow to a fast form. This structural change exposes a hydrophobic region on α_2M that binds to specific surface receptors on macrophages, fibroblasts and hepatocytes. The binding of α_2M–protein complexes to these cells leads to phagocytosis and degradation. It is unlikely that this process induces any significant biological responses in the phagocytosing cell.

The fast form of α_2M is capable of binding numerous cytokines including NGF, PDGF, TFG-β, TNF-α, IL-1, IL-2 and IL-6 (James, 1990). The consequences of this interaction are potentially great, as summarized in Table 7.5. However, a great deal of variability exists between results from different laboratories in the effects of α_2M on cytokine function. Certainly, α_2M may alter detection of cytokines in serum or plasma by ELISA. The binding of cytokines by α_2M, however, may be primarily an *in vitro* phenomenon and of little relevance *in vivo* (Peterson and Moestrup, 1990).

Recent studies have clarified further details of IL-1β binding to α_2M. Cleavage of the internal thiol ester bond in both C3 and α_2M leads to IL-1β binding (Borth *et al.*, 1990b). In disease situations characterized by the presence of α_2M–proteinase complexes and activated C3, as in the rheumatoid joint, binding of IL-1 may

occur. IL-1β binds to fast α_2M by both covalent and non-covalent bonds (Borth *et al.*, 1990a). Penicillamine inhibits the non-covalent binding of IL-1β by α_2M (Teodorescu *et al.*, 1991). However, neither form of binding appears to inhibit appreciably the biological activity of the bound IL-1β. A similar situation exists for IL-6 where binding to α_2M rendered the cytokine resistant to proteolysis but did not inhibit receptor binding or biological activity (Matsuda *et al.*, 1989). Thus, α_2M binding of IL-1β and IL-6 may prolong the half-life of these cytokines in the body and possibly deliver them to various tissues.

A different situation exists for TGF-β where binding to fast α_2M blocks any interaction of TGF-β with specific cell surface receptors. In recent studies the α_2M–TGF-β complexes were rapidly removed from circulation by binding to receptors on hepatocytes specific for conformationally altered α_2M (LaMarre *et al.*, 1991). This is the first demonstration that α_2M binding of a cytokine leads to hepatic clearance. The ultimate fate of this α_2M–TGF-β complex was not explored in this study but the cytokine was probably degraded by proteolysis.

5.4   SUMMARY AND CONCLUSIONS

Cytokines may interact with uromodulin or α_2M in the body, in addition to binding to specific antibodies. The consequences of this interaction may not be the same for all cytokines. This protein binding may interfere with accurate measurements of particular cytokines in various body fluids by ELISA. Protein binding of cytokines may affect their fate in the body, i.e. uromodulin may confine cytokines to the kidney or urine and α_2M may retain cytokines in the circulation or extravascular space. α_2M binding of TGF-β leads to rapid hepatic clearance but it is not known whether other α_2M–cytokine complexes undergo the same fate. IL-1β and IL-6 bound to α_2M largely retain biological activity whereas this is not true for TGF-β. In any case, rather than acting as immunomodulatory agents, uromodulin and α_2M may function primarily in the transport or clearance of cytokines *in vivo*.

Table 7.5   Possible consequences of cytokine binding of α_2M

A.	Assays	
	1. Immunoassays	α_2M may mask antigenic epitopes
	2. Bioassays	α_2M may influence the generation, cell binding or stability of cytokines
B.	Therapy	
	1. Biodistribution	May be affected by concentration of α_2M
	2. Bioavailability	α_2M may inhibit receptor binding of cytokines
	3. Stability	α_2M binding of cytokines may inhibit proteolytic degradation
	4. Clearance	May be enhanced by fast α_2M binding to specific receptors on macrophages, hepatocytes and fibroblasts

Adapted from James (1990)

6. Soluble Cytokine Receptors

Another potential mechanism for inhibition of cytokine effects is through the presence of soluble cytokine receptors. When present in the fluid phase, these soluble receptors could potentially bind cytokines and prevent their interaction with cell surface receptors. However, this binding may not necessarily inhibit cytokine effects. If the affinity of binding of a cytokine to its soluble receptor is less than the affinity of that cytokine for binding to a cell surface receptor, the soluble receptor may function as a transport mechanism and give up the cytokine to the cell. This appears to be the case for IL-4, as discussed below. In contrast, binding of IL-6 to its soluble receptor leads to cell activation, as this complex interacts with the cell surface accessory molecule gp130 and transduces a cellular response. However, soluble receptors for IL-1 and TNF-α block these cytokines from activating cells *in vitro* and at present are being evaluated as potential therapeutic agents in human diseases (Dayer and Fenner, 1992).

6.1 SOLUBLE TNF-α RECEPTORS

Originally discovered in the urine of febrile patients (Seckinger *et al.*, 1988), TNF-α-inhibitory activities have since been found in other biological fluids, e.g. the plasma of cancer patients and, to a lesser extent, the urine of healthy volunteers (Engelmann *et al.*, 1989; Olsson *et al.*, 1989; Gatanaga *et al.*, 1990; Aderka *et al.*, 1991). Purification of the TNF-α-inhibitory material to homogeneity yielded a protein with a novel amino acid sequence. This protein binds to the ligand itself to form a stable complex, its affinity being higher for TNF-α than for TNF-β. The TNF-α inhibitor proved to be a soluble fragment of the TNF-α receptor itself (Englemann *et al.*, 1989; Seckinger *et al.*, 1990). It not only blocks collagenase and PGE2 production by synovial cells, but also the neutrophil respiratory burst induced by TNF-α (Ferrante *et al.*, 1991) and B cell functions (Tucci *et al.*, 1992).

As there are two different TNF-α receptors (55 and 75 kDa), there are two different soluble fragments, originating from the two chains. They are also referred to as TNF-binding proteins I and II, or sTNFR-β and sTNFR-α, respectively. The terminology is less confusing when bearing in mind the molecular masses (see review by Dayer and Fenner, 1992) of the receptors: TNF-R55-BP and TNF-R75-BP (BP = binding protein). Proteolytic cleavage of the two TNF-α receptor molecules is probably an important mechanism for controlling the release of the two soluble receptor proteins (Porteu and Nathan, 1990, 1992; Nortier *et al.*, 1991; Porteu *et al.*, 1991). TNF-R55-BP and TNF-R75-BP can be detected in synovial fluids from patients with inflammatory arthritis (Roux-Lombard *et al.*, 1993), in the supernatants of alveolar macrophages and in several biological fluids in

Table 7.6   Evidence for the presence *in vivo* of TNF-R55-BP and TNF-R75-BP

ng amounts (1–3 ng/ml) in serum of healthy individuals
Up to 60–80 ng/ml in serum from patients presenting with:
   high temperature
   infection
   cancer
   inflammatory diseases
Present in synovial fluid and serum of RA patients
Present in BAL (fluids and AM culture supernatant)

inflammatory diseases (Suter *et al.*, 1992; Andus *et al.*, 1992). These naturally occurring soluble TNF-α receptor molecules may function as inhibitors of TNF-α *in vivo* (Table 7.6).

The possible imbalance between ligand (TNF-α) and ligand inhibitor (TNF-R-BP) may be important for the clinical prognosis of severe diseases. High TNF-α concentrations have been demonstrated to correlate with the severity of infectious purpura and meningococcal infection (Girardin *et al.*, 1988). In view of the deleterious effect of TNF-α in septic shock, the relative proportions of TNF-α and its inhibitors may also determine the clinical outcome. Indeed, large amounts of TNF-R55-BP or TNF-R75-BP are produced in conditions where circulating concentrations of TNF-α are increased, and high values correlate with fatal outcome. More important is the finding that patients who did not survive had a higher TNF-α/TNF-R-BP ratio, suggesting an inadequate endogenous inhibitory activity (Girardin *et al.*, 1992).

If the hypothesis regarding the imbalance between ligand and ligand inhibitor is confirmed, administration of exogenous TNF-R-BP, at least in an acute condition, may be beneficial in that it blocks excess TNF-α. A similar imbalance may exist not only in acute but also in chronic inflammatory diseases. Administration of exogenous TNF-R-BP in experimental animal models of disease has yielded beneficial results (Ashkenazi *et al.*, 1991; Piguet *et al.*, 1992; Van Zee *et al.*, 1992).

6.2 SOLUBLE IL-1 RECEPTORS

6.2.1 Introduction

Two different IL-1 receptors exist on both human and murine cells: type I IL-1R is found on T cells, fibroblasts and endothelial cells; and type II IL-1R predominates on B cells, neutrophils and monocytes–macrophages. The cDNAs for both types of IL-1R have been cloned with expression of recombinant receptors. Only the soluble type II IL-1R has been described to occur naturally and consists of the extracellular domain. Soluble type I IL-1R has been created by expressing a truncated cDNA that encodes only the extracellular domain. The soluble type

I IL-1R has been examined in a few *in vitro* systems or animal models of disease.

6.2.2 Soluble Type I IL-1 Receptors

Both the murine (Sims *et al.*, 1988) and human (Sims *et al.*, 1989) type I IL-1R were cloned from T cells and exhibited similar structures. The type I IL-1R is a single chain possessing an extracellular portion of 319 amino acids, a transmembrane region of 20 amino acids (human) and a large cytoplasmic portion of 213 amino acids (human). This receptor is a member of the immunoglobulin superfamily and the extracellular portion is organized into three domains with predicted immunoglobulin-like folding structures. The cytoplasmic portion is highly conserved between the mouse and man with 78% amino acid sequence identity. Interestingly, when transfected into COS cells, the human type I IL-1R cDNA led to the expression of both high- and low-affinity IL-1R, similar to the native membrane-bound receptors on T cells.

The type I IL-1R was solubilized by detergents from plasma membranes of murine EL-4 thymoma cells (Paganelli *et al.*, 1987; Bird *et al.*, 1989). This full-length receptor possessed a molecular mass of 80 kDa. After enzymatic removal of N-linked oligosaccharides, the peptide core was 53–62 kDa. The solubilized type I IL-1R exhibited binding characteristics virtually identical with the membrane-bound receptor with an apparent K_d of 120–360 pM. IL-1α and IL-1β competed equally for binding to both the membrane-bound and solubilized type I IL-1R. These results support the conclusion that the type I IL-1R consists of a single-chain glycoprotein of 80 kDa.

The extracellular binding domain of the murine type I IL-1R was obtained by expressing a partial cDNA, encoding residues 1–316, in HeLa cells (Dower *et al.*, 1989). This truncated soluble IL-1R was secreted into the supernatants and was affinity-purified on an IL-1α column. This molecule possessed a molecular mass of 54–60 kDa, reduced to 34 kDa after *N*-glycanase treatment. The truncated type I IL-1R exhibited binding characteristics similar to those of the native surface receptor. The complex of IL-1α and this soluble receptor contained one molecule of each.

This soluble form of the type I IL-1R inhibited IL-1 induced proliferation of murine B cells (Maliszewski *et al.*, 1990). This observation is particularly intriguing as no IL-1R was detected on either resting or activated B cells by binding of ^{125}I-IL-1β. This finding supports the argument that target cells may respond to very few bound IL-1 molecules, perhaps 1–10 per cell. Administration of the soluble extracellular portion of the murine type I IL-1R led to a prolongation in survival of heterotopic heart allografts in mice (Fanslow *et al.*, 1989). In addition, lymph node hyperplasia in response to a local injection of allogeneic cells was blocked. However, these responses to the soluble IL-1R may have been due

to anti-inflammatory rather than immunosuppressive effects.

6.2.3 Soluble Type II IL-1 Receptors

The type II IL-1R has been cloned from both murine and human B cells (McMahan *et al.*, 1991). This 60 kDa glycoprotein receptor is also a member of the immunoglobulin superfamily and consists of three domains. The extracellular and transmembrane domains were similar in size to those of the type I IL-1R but the cytoplasmic domain for the type II IL-1R was much shorter at 29 residues. The type II IL-1R is also glycosylated, as the predicted size for this protein minus the signal sequence is 44 kDa. Surprisingly, the mRNA for both types of IL-1R were found together in many different cells, although in varying amounts. A variety of B cells, bone marrow cells and keratinocytes all expressed more type I IL-1R mRNA than type II. Because of the very short cytoplasmic domain, the type II IL-1R may not be capable of transducing biological responses.

Binding studies with both natural and recombinant types I and II IL-1R revealed some interesting differences. All three forms of human IL-1 (α, β and Ra) bound equally well to both human and murine type I IL-1R, either natural or recombinant (McMahan *et al.*, 1991). However, IL-1β bound tenfold more avidly to natural or recombinant human type II IL-1R than did IL-1α or IL-1Ra. In addition, IL-IRa bound well to recombinant murine type II IL-1R but poorly to the natural type II receptors. Thus, the murine type II IL-1R is capable of binding human IL-1Ra but apparently is relatively unavailable as expressed in the plasma membrane.

A naturally occurring soluble form of the human type II IL-1R has been found in plasma (Eastgate *et al.*, 1990), in the supernatant of activated mononuclear cells (Symons *et al.*, 1990) and in the supernatant of a human B cell line (Symons and Duff, 1990; Symons *et al.*, 1991). This soluble receptor has a molecular mass of ~43 kDa, reduced to ~30 kDa after *N*-glycanase digestion. These findings are consistent with the soluble type II IL-1R representing the extracellular domain. This naturally occurring soluble IL-1R may be a product of enzyme cleavage. The binding characteristics data for the soluble type II IL-1R varied between two laboratories. In one instance, this soluble human receptor bound only the mature or propeptide forms of IL-1β, and failed to bind either human IL-1α or IL-1Ra (Symons *et al.*, 1991). In another laboratory, the soluble type II IL-1R purified from the same B cell line (Raji) bound both IL-1β and IL-1α, although binding of IL-1β was 16-fold greater than IL-1α (Giri *et al.*, 1990). These latter results are consistent with a more avid binding of IL-1β than IL-1α to membrane-bound human type II IL-1R. Lastly, the soluble type II IL-1R inhibited binding of ^{125}I-IL-1β to Raji B cells and blocked IL-1 induction of PGE$_2$ production by fibroblasts (Giri *et al.*, 1990). Whether this

Table 7.7   Characteristics of soluble IL-1 receptors

Characteristic	Type 1	Type II
Origin	Genetically engineered	Naturally occurring
Cells	T cells, FB, EC	B cells, PMN, MØ
Domain of intact receptor	Extracellular	Extracellular
Size		
Glycosylated	54–60 kDa	43 kDa
Protein core only	43 kDa	30 kDa
Binding of IL-1	$\beta = \alpha = $ Ra	$\beta > \alpha = $ Ra
Effects on IL-1 stimulation	Inhibits	Inhibits

naturally occurring soluble IL-1R functions as an inhibitor or carrier of IL-1β *in vivo* remains to be determined.

6.2.4   Summary and Conclusions

Soluble forms of both types I and II IL-1R, consisting of the extracellular domains, have been described (Table 7.7). Soluble type I IL-1R has been created by genetic engineering and soluble type II IL-1R occurs naturally in human plasma and B cell supernatants. Soluble type I IL-1R blocks binding of both IL-1α and IL-1β to either membrane receptor while soluble type II IL-1R blocks binding of IL-1β more avidly. Administration of soluble type I IL-1R may block some effects of IL-1 *in vivo* and a derivatized version of this molecule is currently undergoing evaluation in treatment of human autoimmune and inflammatory diseases.

6.3   OTHER SOLUBLE CYTOKINE RECEPTORS

In addition to soluble receptors for TNF-α and IL-1, soluble receptors have been described for IL-2, IL-4, IL-6, IL-7 and IFNγ (reviewed by Fernandez-Botran, 1991). These soluble receptors again are truncated forms of the full-length receptor, representing only the extracellular ligand-binding domain. Soluble cytokine receptors can arise by proteolytic cleavage of the membrane receptor or by synthesis from alternatively spliced mRNAs that encode only the extracellular portion of the molecule. Again, some of these soluble receptors may function as cytokine inhibitors and others as carriers *in vivo*.

6.3.1   Soluble IL-2 Receptors

The high-affinity IL-2 receptor consists of two chains: a p75 chain constitutively present on resting T cells, and a p55 chain that must be induced. Activated T cells release the extracellular portion of the p55 chain as a 40–50 kDa soluble IL-2 receptor, probably by enzyme cleavage of the membrane-bound receptor (Rubin *et al.*, 1990b). Soluble IL-2 receptors representing the N-terminal 192 amino acids of the p55 or α chain have also been generated through expression of an artificially truncated cDNA

(Jacques *et al.*, 1990). Both the naturally occurring and recombinant soluble IL-2R α chain bind IL-2 with low affinity.

A soluble version of the p75 or β chain of the IL-2 receptor has also been generated through expression of an artificially truncated cDNA that encodes only the extracellular portion of this chain (Tsudo *et al.*, 1990). In addition, spontaneous release of soluble IL-2 receptor β chains by a T cell line and by PMA-induced PBMCs has been described (Honda *et al.*, 1990). This soluble version of the IL-2 receptor β chain also binds IL-1 less avidly than does the full two chain receptor on the cell surface.

The naturally occurring soluble IL-2 receptor representing the extracellular portion of the p55 or α chain has been described in low concentrations in the serum or urine of normal humans and animals. However, over 10 to 100-fold higher concentrations of soluble IL-2 receptors are present in the serum of patients with autoimmune, inflammatory, malignant and infectious disorders (reviewed by Rubin and Nelson, 1990). These soluble IL-2 receptors are thought to be secondary to general T cell activation. Because of the low affinity of soluble IL-2 receptor α chains for IL-2, it is unlikely that these molecules inhibit or function as a carrier for IL-2 *in vivo*.

The serum levels of soluble IL-2 receptors are particularly elevated in HTLV-1-associated T cell leukaemia, hairy cell leukaemia and non-Hodgkin's disease. Measurement of serum levels of soluble IL-2 receptors may be clinically useful in the diagnosis and treatment of these diseases, as well as in some chronic human autoimmune diseases.

6.3.2   Soluble IL-4 Receptors

Molecular cloning of the murine IL-4 receptors revealed three cDNAs encoding for three different proteins: a 140 kDa membrane-bound form with extracellular, intramembranous and cytoplasmic domains; a second form lacking most of the intracytoplasmic domain; and a third form of only the extracellular domain (Mosley *et al.*, 1989). Thus, the soluble IL-4 receptor may be the first example of an extracellular receptor domain encoded by an alternative cDNA. The soluble form of the IL-4 receptor binds IL-4 with an affinity similar to that of the membrane-bound receptor.

Soluble IL-4 is capable of inhibiting many effects of IL-4 *in vitro*. These include B cell activation (Maliszewski *et al.*, 1990), proliferation of PHA-induced PBMCs, IgE production and IgE receptor expression by PBMCs (Garrone *et al.*, 1991). The pharmacokinetics of soluble IL-4 receptors in mice have been described (Jacobs *et al.*, 1991) and this molecule inhibited alloreactivity *in vivo* (Fanslow *et al.*, 1991). Naturally occurring forms of soluble IL-4 receptors have been described in the serum, urine and ascitic fluid of mice (Fernandez-Botran and Vitetta, 1990). However, recent studies indicate that these molecules may function more as carriers than as inhibitors of IL-4 *in vivo* (Fernandez-Botran and Vitetta, 1991). This is because at $37°C$ the complexes of IL-4 and soluble receptors rapidly dissociate, giving up the IL-4 to membrane-bound receptors.

6.3.3 Other Soluble Receptors

Soluble IL-6 and IFNγ receptors were originally described in normal human urine (Novick *et al.*, 1989). These molecules bind their respective ligands *in vitro* but their abilities to function as inhibitors or carriers *in vivo* have not been examined. Similarly to IL-4, a naturally occurring cDNA clone has been described that encodes for a variant form of the IL-7 receptor lacking an intramembranous portion (Goodwin *et al.*, 1990). Expression of this cDNA led to the production of soluble IL-7 receptors that bound to IL-7 in solution and inhibited interaction of IL-7 with membrane bound receptors *in vitro*.

6.4 SUMMARY AND CONCLUSIONS

Soluble forms of IL-4 and IL-7 receptors may result from alternative cDNAs, whereas soluble IL-2, IL-6, TNF-α and IFNγ receptors appear to be products of enzyme cleavage of membrane-bound receptors. Soluble IL-2 receptors bind IL-2 with low affinity and serum levels may reflect relative T cell activity in human malignant or autoimmune diseases. In contrast, soluble IL-4 receptors bind IL-4 with high avidity but probably function as carriers *in vivo*, as the complex rapidly dissociates at $37°C$.

7. *IL-1 Receptor Antagonist*

7.1 INTRODUCTION

IL-1 is thought to play an important role in mediating tissue damage in RA and in other chronic autoimmune or inflammatory diseases. Because of the ubiquitous presence of IL-1 in various body compartments and tissues, and its pleiotropic effects, it had long been thought by investigators that ways must exist to regulate the *in vivo* effects of IL-1 (Dinarello, 1991). Numerous inhibitors of IL-1 bioactivity had been described in various body fluids or in the supernatants of cultured cells (Larrick, 1989). However, these activities had not been further purified or characterized and their mechanism of action remained unknown.

7.2 DISCOVERY OF IL-1Ra

In the mid 1980s two laboratories described IL-1 inhibitor bioactivities by a 22 kDa protein, which subsequently were shown to be due to a specific receptor antagonist. Balavoine *et al.* (1985, 1986) described this IL-1 inhibitor in the urine of patients with monocytic leukaemia, and Arend *et al.* (1985) described a similar bioactivity in the supernatants of human monocytes cultured on adherent IgG. The semi-purified molecule from human urine was shown to block IL-1α binding to specific receptors on murine EL-4 thymoma cells (Seckinger *et al.*, 1987a). The molecule from human monocytes was subsequently shown to also function as a receptor antagonist (Arend *et al.*, 1989). The IL-1 inhibitor reported from both laboratories was a specific IL-1 receptor antagonist as it did not affect the binding or stimulation seen with numerous other cytokines (Seckinger *et al.*, 1987b; Arend *et al.*, 1989).

7.3 CHARACTERIZATION OF IL-1Ra

The purification of native IL-1Ra from IgG-induced monocyte supernatants, sequencing of the protein, cloning of cDNAs, and expression of recombinant IL-1Ra were first reported in early 1990 (Hannum *et al.*, 1990; Eisenberg *et al.*, 1990). Another laboratory subsequently cloned and expressed the same IL-1Ra molecule from supernatants of the human myelomonocytic cell line U937 after differentiation in PMA and GM-CSF (Carter *et al.*, 1990). A summary of these studies, and of some of the characteristics of IL-1Ra, can be found in three recent reviews (Dinarello and Thompson, 1991; Arend, 1991, 1993).

Some molecular and biochemical characteristics of IL-1Ra are summarized in Table 7.8. This unique new molecule is a member of the IL-1 family by four criteria. IL-1Ra binds specifically to both known types of human IL-1 receptors and competitively inhibits the binding of both IL-1α and IL-1β. Secondly, this molecule fails to induce interiorization of ligand–receptor complexes or to stimulate any detectable intracellular responses (Dripps *et al.*, 1991). Thirdly, in addition to amino acid sequence homology to IL-1α and IL-1β, the gene structures of these three forms of IL-1 are remarkably similar (Eisenberg *et al.*, 1991). Lastly, the genes for IL-1Ra, IL-1α and IL-1β, as well as for types I and II IL-1 receptors, are all clustered on the same region of human chromosome 2 (Steinkasserer *et al.*, 1992; Lennard *et al.*, 1992;

Table 7.8   Molecular and biochemical characteristics of IL-1Ra

(1) Synthesized as a 177-amino acid propeptide with a 25-amino acid leader sequence

(2) Mature protein 152 amino acids with an N-linked glycosylation site

(3) Natural molecule has two primary forms: 22–25 kDa molecules with varying degrees of glycosylation and non-glycosylated 17 kDa form

(4) Amino acid sequence homology 30% with IL-1β and 19% with IL-1α

(5) Exhibits no immunological cross-reactivity with either IL-1α or IL-1β

(6) Produced by monocytes, macrophages, neutrophils, keratinocytes and other epithelial cells

(7) Binds to types I and II IL-1 receptors on target cells with a similar avidity to that of IL-1 but fails to elicit biological responses

Patterson *et al.*, 1993). Although curious, the biological relevance of this chromosomal proximity of the genes for these three ligands and their two receptors remains unknown.

7.4   INDUCERS AND REGULATION OF IL-1Ra PRODUCTION

Many different substances can induce IL-1Ra production in monocytes including adherent or aggregated IgG, bacterial endotoxin, phorbol esters, IL-3, IL-4, GM-GSF and unknown substances in serum. IL-1β and IL-1Ra production is differentially regulated in monocytes (Roux-Lombard *et al.*, 1989; Poutsiaka *et al.*, 1991; Arend *et al.*, 1991). LPS stimulates production of both molecules in near-equal amounts while IgG induces only IL-1Ra protein. In contrast, IL-4 enhances LPS-induced IL-1Ra production by monocytes while inhibiting LPS-induced IL-1β production. Thus, the same cell or group of cells can synthesize both an agonist and an antagonist simultaneously, but the production of each molecule is regulated separately.

The availability of large amounts of recombinant human IL-1Ra has permitted *in vitro* and *in vivo* studies by numerous investigators. In spite of similar affinities of direct binding, 10- to 500-fold excess amounts of IL-1Ra over IL-1 were found to be necessary to effect 50% inhibition of cell responses to IL-1 *in vitro* (Arend *et al.*, 1990). This is because target cells are exquisitely sensitive to very small amounts of IL-1, requiring only a few molecules per cell for full biological responses to occur. Because target cells have 200–2000 IL-1 receptors per cell, excess amounts of IL-1Ra are required to block binding of only a few molecules of IL-1. Because of this extreme sensitivity to IL-1 and the "spare receptor effect", large amounts of IL-1Ra may be necessary to inhibit the action of IL-1 *in vivo*.

IL-1Ra blocks the stimulatory effects of IL-1 on numerous target cells *in vitro* including chondrocytes, bone cells, synovial cells, endothelial cells, thymocytes and pancreatic β cells (summarized by Dinarello and Thompson 1991 and Arend 1993. In all of these studies from different laboratories, no clear-cut agonist effects of this molecule have been described. It is of great interest that IL-1Ra does not inhibit T cell proliferation induced by mitogens, soluble antigens or allogeneic determinants (Nicod *et al.*, 1992). IL-1Ra will block the augmentation of these responses seen with exogenous IL-1 administration, but will not inhibit the baseline T cell responses.

7.5   IL-1Ra PRODUCTION BY OTHER CELLS

In addition to monocytes, recent studies have shown IL-1Ra to be produced by tissue macrophages, neutrophils and keratinocytes (Table 7.9). In contrast with monocytes, alveolar macrophages spontaneously produce large amounts of IL-1Ra (Galve-de Rochemonteix *et al.*, 1990) with a further enhancement in the presence of GM-CSF (Janson *et al.*, 1993). In addition, *in vitro*-derived macrophages also spontaneously produce large amounts of IL-1Ra, particularly after differentiation in GM-CSF (Janson *et al.*, 1991; Galve-de Rochemonteix *et al.*, 1992). In contrast with monocytes, neither LPS nor adherent IgG induced IL-1Ra production in *in vitro*-derived or alveolar macrophages. Lastly, synovial macrophages also produce IL-1Ra (Roux-Lombard *et al.*, 1992). Thus, tissue macrophages may be primed by exposure to GM-CSF or other differentiating agents to produce considerable quantities of IL-1Ra.

In recent studies, neutrophils have been found to produce small amounts of IL-1Ra, approximately 1% per cell of the maximal amounts observed with monocytes or macrophages (Table 7.9) (McColl *et al.*, 1992; M. Malyak and W.P. Arend, unpublished observations).

Table 7.9   IL-1Ra production by different cells

| Cell | Stimulus | IL-1Ra | |
		ng/10^6 cells	% in lysates
Monocyte	None	1.6	61
	Adherent IgG	48.5	14
	GM-CSF	8.2	49
Macrophage (alveolar)	None	24.0	50
	Adherent IgG	24.0	50
	GM-CSF	34.0	46
Neutrophil	None	0.08	64
	GM-CSF	0.35	69
	TNF-α	0.23	64
Keratinocyte	None	38.4	99
	TNF-α	70.4	99

Neutrophil IL-1Ra production is stimulated by GM-CSF, TNF-α, IL-4 and LPS, but not by adherent IgG. Most IL-1Ra produced by neutrophils remains cell-associated. In inflammatory lesions, such as rheumatoid synovial effusions, where massive amounts of neutrophils accumulate, these dying or dead cells may be a major source of IL-1Ra (Roux-Lombard et al., 1992).

Lastly, cultured keratinocytes produce large amounts of IL-1Ra which remain almost entirely intracellular (Table 7.9). Recent studies have established that keratinocytes and other epithelial cells produce a structural variant of the originally described monocyte IL-1Ra (Haskill et al., 1991; Bigler et al., 1992). Keratinocyte IL-1Ra lacks a leader sequence, and thus cannot be secreted. The keratinocyte variant of this molecule is identical with the mature extracellular form of monocyte IL-1Ra but possesses an additional seven N-terminal amino acids. However, both forms of IL-1Ra appear to be equally capable of blocking IL-1 interaction with receptors on T cells (Bigler et al., 1992). Keratinocytes also synthesize large amounts of IL-1α which also remain intracellular (Gruaz-Chatellard et al., 1991). Both IL-1Ra and IL-1α may be released by dying keratinocytes, making the skin potentially a large reservoir of these cytokines.

7.6 USE OF IL-1Ra IN ANIMAL MODELS OF DISEASE OR IN HUMAN DISEASE

A rationale exists for the therapeutic use of IL-1Ra in a variety of human diseases where IL-1 has been implicated as a mediator of tissue destruction or as an important autocrine growth factor. However, IL-1 has been implicated as an inducer of B and T cell proliferation in vitro. Therefore, an important concern about the possible in vivo administration of IL-1Ra was possible side effects on the normal immune response. Recent studies have shown that IL-1Ra does not block humoral or cellular antigen-specific immune responses in vivo in mice (Faherty et al., 1992). This observation makes possible clinical applications of this molecule even more feasible.

7.6.1 Rheumatoid Arthritis

The possible roles of IL-1, TNF and other cytokines in RA have been described in a recent review (Arend and Dayer, 1990) and have been summarized by Feldmann and his co-workers in Chapter 6 of this volume. The possible beneficial consequences of inhibition of IL-1 or TNF-α effects in the rheumatoid joint have been emphasized by many investigators. The net effects of blocking these pro-inflammatory cytokines might be a reduction in tissue destruction and an enhancement in repair.

The administration of IL-1Ra was shown to reduce the inflammation and tissue destruction in two animal models of RA: collagen-induced arthritis in mice and streptococcal cell wall-induced arthritis in rats (Schwab et al., 1991). However, in a third animal model, antigen-induced arthritis in mice, administration of IL-1Ra had no effect on the disease process. This observation emphasizes that the pathophysiological mechanisms of tissue damage may vary between animal models of arthritis and that IL-1 may not be an important mediator in all. Nevertheless, in streptococcal cell wall-induced arthritis in rats, administration of IL-1Ra significantly prevented joint swelling, inhibited pannus development and reduced the destruction of both bone and cartilage.

Studies in humans showed that the synovial fluids of over one-half of patients with active RA possessed markedly elevated levels of IL-1Ra protein (Malyak et al., 1993). The fact that these patients still exhibited active synovitis would suggest that the synovial fluid IL-1Ra may not be sufficiently effective at the tissue level. IL-1Ra and IL-1β proteins and mRNAs have been localized in synovial tissue, primarily in macrophages both in the lining layer and around blood vessels (Firestein et al., 1992; Koch et al., 1992). The possibility exists that the ratio of IL-1Ra to IL-1 may not be high enough in active rheumatoid synovitis to inhibit the inflammatory disease process. The results of a phase I clinical trial of IL-1Ra in RA indicates excellent tolerance with some promising early beneficial effects (Lebsack et al., 1991). In an open-label trial, 15 patients received once daily subcutaneous injections of IL-1Ra for 7 days; decreases were observed in mean tender joint count, erythrocyte sedimentation rate (ESR) and C-reactive protein. This material is at present undergoing evaluation in a large phase II clinical trial in RA.

7.6.2 Other Diseases

IL-1 is spontaneously produced by AML cells in vitro, induces synthesis of colony-stimulating factors and functions as an autocrine growth factor for these cells. The addition of IL-1Ra to AML cells in vitro inhibited cell proliferation in a dose- and time-dependent fashion (Rambaldi et al., 1991). Furthermore, IL-1Ra reduced the spontaneous release of GM-CSF and IL-1β by the AML cells from one-half or more of patients, shutting down the further stimulus for autocrine growth. Similar results have been obtained in studies with cells from CML patients (Estrov et al., 1991). IL-1Ra blocks the formation of haematopoietic colonies from CML cells in vitro, both in the absence and presence of added growth factors. These results have led to clinical trials of IL-1Ra in CML patients.

GVHD is the major complication of allogeneic bone marrow transplantation. Both TNF-α and IL-1 are found in the skin of mice with GVHD. However, the relative importance of these two inflammatory molecules in mediating organ consequences of GVHD remained unclear. The in vivo administration of IL-1Ra reduced the mortality and immunosuppression of murine GVHD without impairing the engraftment of haematopoietic cells (McCarthy *et al.*, 1991). These results indicate that IL-1 is a significant mediator of tissue damage in murine GVHD. IL-1Ra is currently being evaluated in humans with GVHD following bone marrow transplantation.

The i.v. administration of small amounts of endotoxin to human volunteers led to peak plasma levels of IL-1Ra that were one hundredfold greater than those of IL-1β (Granowitz *et al.*, 1991). Both IL-1 and TNF-α have long been thought to be important mediators of shock and death in patients with sepsis syndrome. The exogenous administration of IL-1Ra dramatically reduced mortality from endotoxin shock in rabbits (Ohlsson, *et al.*, 1990; Wakabayashi *et al.*, 1991) and mice (Alexander *et al.*, 1991). In addition, the hypotension and decreased systemic vascular resistance of the septic shock were markedly attenuated without change in circulating levels of IL-1 or TNF-α. These observations suggest that IL-1 is a primary mediator of cardiovascular collapse in sepsis syndrome and that the role of TNF-α may be primarily in stimulating IL-1 production. A phase I/II clinical trial of IL-1Ra in patients with sepsis syndrome showed highly promising results and this material is currently being evaluated in a large phase III trial.

IL-1Ra is also being evaluated in patients with chronic inflammatory bowel disease and asthma. Additional animal models of disease where IL-1Ra has been shown to have beneficial effects include infection-induced premature labour, bleomycin-induced pulmonary fibrosis and reperfusion myocardial injury.

7.7   SUMMARY AND CONCLUSIONS

IL-1Ra is the first described naturally occurring receptor antagonist of a human cytokine or hormone-like molecule. IL-1Ra is a member of the IL-1 family but binds to both types I and II human IL-1 receptors without inducing interiorization or detectable intracellular responses. IL-1Ra is produced by monocytes, macrophages and neutrophils, with an intracellular structural variant found in keratinocytes and other epithelial cells. IL-1Ra and IL-1 are produced by the same cells but are regulated separately and possibly in a differential fashion. The administration of IL-1Ra has been beneficial in animal models of arthritis, GVHD, sepsis syndrome, inflammatory bowel disease and asthma. IL-1Ra is currently being evaluated for the treatment of these and other human diseases.

8. *Miscellaneous IL-1 Inhibitors*

In addition to IL-1Ra, a variety of other IL-1-inhibitory bioactivities have been described in human body fluids or in the supernatants of cultured cells (reviewed by Arend *et al.* (1989) and Larrick (1989)). These IL-1 inhibitors are heterogeneous in size and biological properties. In a few

instances these bioactivities have been further purified and characterized.

8.1   POSSIBLE IL-1Ra

Some additional studies, other than those reviewed in Section 7, may have described the bioactivity of the molecule now known as IL-1Ra. A variety of IL-1-inhibitory bioactivities were noted in these studies: found in the sera of normal donors injected with endotoxin (Dinarello *et al.*, 1981); present in the supernatants of cultured rheumatoid synovial fluid mononuclear cells (Lotz *et al.*, 1986b); secreted from monocytes after EBV infection of PBMCs (Lotz *et al.*, 1986a); identified in the lysates and supernatants of human neutrophils (Tiku *et al.*, 1986); secreted by LPS-stimulated Kupffer cells (Shirahama *et al.*, 1988); found in normal human urine (Svenson and Bendtzen, 1988); secreted by the monocytic leukaemia cell line THP-1 (Gaffney *et al.*, 1989); and produced by cultured human alveolar macrophages (Gosset *et al.*, 1988). Although none of these IL-1-inhibitory bioactivities were further purified, their size and biological characteristics suggest that they may have been due, at least in part, to the presence of IL-1Ra.

8.2   IL-1 INHIBITOR FROM M20 CELLS

A 52 kDa IL-1 inhibitor was described in the supernatants of unstimulated human myelomonocytic M20 cells (Barak *et al.*, 1986). This material abrogated the effects of IL-1 on lymphocytes and fibroblasts but did not alter IL-2 stimulation of thymocyte proliferation. In addition, the M20-derived IL-1 inhibitor was effective *in vivo* in various animal models of IL-1-induced inflammation or disease (Barak *et al.*, 1991). Although this material seemed to work by blocking receptor binding of IL-1, the M20 IL-1 inhibitor was different from IL-1Ra by size and charge. In addition, an antiserum specific for IL-1Ra did not recognize the M20-derived IL-1 inhibitor in a Western blot and did not neutralize the bioactivity of this material.

8.3   LOW MOLECULAR MASS SERUM INHIBITOR OF IL-1

A 5–9 kDa inhibitor of IL-1 bioactivity has been described in the supernatants of unstimulated human PBMCs (Berman *et al.*, 1986). This material blocked IL-1 effects in the murine thymocyte assay but, paradoxically, enhanced the stimulatory effects of IL-1 on fibroblast proliferation (Sandborg *et al.*, 1986), and on Ca^{2+} release from bone (Watrous *et al.*, 1990). This IL-1-inhibitory bioactivity was found at higher levels in the supernatants of cultured PBMCs from patients with scleroderma or AIDS (Berman *et al.*, 1987; Locksley *et al.*, 1988) than from healthy normal controls. In recent studies, this 5–9 kDa IL-1 inhibitor blocked the cytotoxic effects of IL-1β on cultured rat pancreatic islet cells without altering the IL-1β-induced suppression of insulin secretion (Kawahara *et al.*, 1991). This material did not bind to IL-1 receptors and was effective even if added up to 24 h after initiation of culture, suggesting an effect on later stages of IL-1-induced cell stimulation.

8.4 OTHER IL-1 INHIBITORS IN URINE

Although IL-1Ra has been identified in the urine of patients with myelomonocytic leukaemia or fever, other IL-1 inhibitors are present in urine as well. A 20–40 kDa inhibitor of IL-1 but not IL-2 effects on murine thymocytes was described in normal and febrile urine (Liao *et al.*, 1984). This material was purified to two molecular masses of 29 and 32 kDa (Liao *et al.*, 1985) and appeared to alter IL-1 effects on thymocytes after receptor binding and initial cell activation (Brown and Rosenstreich, 1987). Further purification showed that this material was the enzyme DNase I and not a specific IL-1 inhibitor at all (Rosenstreich *et al.*, 1988).

Possibly the same artifactual 30 kDa inhibitor of IL-1 was found in febrile urine by other investigators (Kimball *et al.*, 1984; Kabir and Wigzell, 1989). Similar to the 6–9 kDa IL-1 inhibitor from scleroderma serum, this 30 kDa material blocked the effects of IL-1 in the thymocyte assay but enhanced IL-1-induced fibroblast production of PGE$_2$ (Korn *et al.*, 1987). This material has not been further characterized but possibly could also be DNase I or another enzyme. Endopeptidase 24.11, an enkephalinase that degrades neuropeptides, has been reported to inactivate IL-1 (Pierart *et al.*, 1988).

8.5 IL-1 INHIBITORS PRODUCED BY VIRALLY INFECTED CELLS

A variety of IL-1-inhibitory bioactivities have been described in the supernatants of virally infected lymphocytes or macrophages. These include: 95 kDa material from an EBV-transformed human B cell line (Scala *et al.*, 1984); a 95 kDa inhibitor from cytomegalovirus-infected human monocytes or U937 cells (Rodgers *et al.*, 1985); and 100 kDa material from human monocytes exposed to influenza or respiratory syncytial viruses (Roberts *et al.*, 1986; McCarthy *et al.*, 1989; Salkind *et al.*, 1991). This large-molecular mass IL-1 inhibitor(s) has not been further characterized.

8.6 OTHER IL-1 INHIBITORS

Other IL-1-inhibitory activities have been described over the past 10 years. UV-irradiated epidermal cells release a 40 kDa inhibitor of IL-1 effects on both thymocytes and fibroblasts (Schwarz *et al.*, 1987). A synthetic peptide CKS-17, homologous to a highly conserved region of the immunosuppressive retroviral envelope protein p15E, reduces IL-1-induced IL-2 production by thymocytes probably by inhibiting protein kinase C (Kleinerman *et al.*, 1987; Gottlieb *et al.*, 1989). The neuropeptide α-melanocyte-stimulating hormone inhibits IL-1 and TNF effects *in vitro* and *in vivo*, probably by acting at a post-receptor level (Cannon *et al.*, 1986; Robertson *et al.*, 1988). Pertussin toxin inhibits IL-1-induced production of IL-2 in EL4 murine thymoma cells by acting at a late level in the cell response, after the possible involvement of a G-protein (O'Neill *et al.*, 1992). Lastly, uncharacterized IL-1 inhibitors have been described in extracts of rat submandibular glands (Kemp *et al.*, 1986), supernatants of human gingival organ cultures (Walsh *et al.*, 1986, 1987) and the LPS-stimulated murine macrophage cell line P388D$_1$ (Nishihara *et al.*, 1988).

In addition to the specific IL-1 receptor antagonist, a number of largely uncharacterized IL-1-inhibitory bioactivities have been described. Some of these may represent unrecognized IL-1Ra, others are clearly different, and some apparent IL-1 inhibitors have been shown to be artifactual. The possibility exists that another biologically important IL-1 inhibitor may emerge out of these heterogeneous observations.

9. *Summary and Conclusions*

Cytokines are important mediators of cell–cell interactions both *in vitro* and *in vivo*. The cytokine network exhibits a marked redundancy with different factors possessing the same or overlapping biological effects. The potentially injurious effects of sustained cytokine action suggest that multiple mechanisms must be present in the body to modify or inhibit specific cytokine effects.

This review has focused on mechanisms of cytokine inhibition that occur naturally. However, the full *in vivo* relevance of these potentially regulatory mechanisms has not been established. Most of these possible cytokine inhibitors have been more thoroughly studied *in vitro*. Further work is necessary to indicate whether these mechanisms are operative in modulating the function of various cytokines in normal biological processes as well as in pathophysiological conditions.

At least two naturally occurring types of cytokine inhibitor appear to have potential as therapeutic agents in human diseases: soluble receptors for IL-1 and TNF, and the specific IL-1 receptor antagonist. Both of these approaches have been successful in ameliorating various animal models of disease and at present are being evaluated in a variety of human autoimmune, infectious and inflammatory diseases.

10. References

Aderka D., Engelmann, H., Hornik, V., Skornick, Y., Leno, Y., Wallach, D. and Kushtai, G. (1991). Increased serum levels of soluble receptors for tumor necrosis factor in cancer patients. Cancer Res. 51, 5602–5607.

Alexander, H.R., Doherty, G.M., Buresh, C.M., Venzon, D.J. and Norton, J.A. (1991). A recombinant human receptor antagonist to interleukin 1 improves survival after lethal endotoxemia in mice. J. Exp. Med. 173, 1029–1032.

Andus, T., Gross, V., Holstege, A., Ott, M., Weber, M., David, M., Gallati, H., Gerok, W. and Schölmerich, J. (1992). High concentrations of soluble tumor necrosis factor receptors in ascites. Hepatology 16, 749–755.

Arend, W.P. (1991). Interleukin 1 receptor antagonist. A new member of the interleukin 1 family. J. Clin. Invest. 88, 1445–1451.

Arend, W.P. and Dayer, J.-M. (1990). Cytokines and cytokine inhibitors or antagonists in rheumatoid arthritis. Arth. Rheum. 33, 305–315.

Arend, W.P. and Dayer, J.-M. (1993). "Textbook of Rheumatology" (ed W.N. Kelley, E.D. Harris, Jr., S. Ruddy and C.B. Sledge), 4th edn, pp 227–247. W.B. Saunders Co., London (in press).

Arend W.P., Joslin, F.G. and Massoni, R.J. (1985). Effects of immune complexes on production by human monocytes of interleukin 1 or an interleukin 1 inhibitor. J. Immunol. 134, 3868–3875.

Arend, W.P., Joslin, F.G., Thompson, R.C. and Hannum, C.H. (1989). An IL-1 inhibitor from human monocytes. Production and characterization of biologic properties. J. Immunol. 143, 1851–1858.

Arend, W.P., Welgus, H.G., Thompson, R.C. and Eisenberg, S.P. (1990). Biological properties of recombinant human monocyte-derived interleukin 1 receptor antagonist. J. Clin. Invest. 85, 1694–1697.

Arend, W.P., Smith, M.F. Jr., Janson, R.W. and Joslin, F.G. (1991). IL-1 receptor antagonist and IL-1β production in human monocytes are regulated differently. J. Immunol. 147, 1530–1536.

Ashkenazi, A., Marsters, S.A., Capon, D.J., Chamow, S.M., Figari, I.S., Pennica, D., Goeddel, D.V., Palladino, M.A. and Smith, D.H. (1991). Protection against endotoxic shock by a tumor necrosis factor receptor immunoadhesin. Proc. Natl Acad. Sci. USA 88, 10535–10539.

Baglioni, C. (1992). In "Tumor Necrosis Factors: The Molecules and their Emerging Role in Medicine", pp 425–438. Raven Press, New York.

Bakouche, O., Moreau, J.L. and Lachman, L.B. (1992). Secretion of IL-1: role of protein kinase C. J. Immunol. 1, 84–91.

Balavoine, J.-F., de Rochemonteix, B., Cruchaud, A. and Dayer, J.-M. (1985). In "The Physiologic, Metabolic, and Immunologic Actions of Interleukin-1". pp 429–436. Alan R. Liss, Inc., New York.

Balavoine, J.-F., de Rochemonteix, B., Seckinger, P., Cruchaud, A. and Dayer, J.-M. (1986). Prostaglandin E₂ and collagenase production by fibroblasts and synovial cells is regulated by urine-derived human interleukin 1 and inhibitor(s). J. Clin. Invest. 78, 1120–1124.

Barak, V., Peritt, D., Flechner, I., Yanai, P., Halperin, T., Treves, A.J. and Dinarello, C.A. (1991). The specific IL-1 inhibitor from the human M20 cell line is distinct from the IL-1 receptor antagonist. Lymphokine Cytokine Res. 10 437–442.

Barak, V., Treves, A.J., Yanai, P., Halperin, M., Wasserman, D., Biran, S. and Braun, S. (1986). Interleukin 1 inhibitory activity secreted by a human myelomonocytic cell line (M20). Eur. J. Immunol. 16, 1449–1452.

Baumberger, C., Ulevitch, R.J. and Dayer J.-M. (1991). Modulation of endotoxic activity of lipopolysaccharide by high-density lipoprotein. Pathobiology 59, 378–383.

Bendtzen, K., Svenson, M., Jønsson, V. and Hippe, E. (1990). Autoantibodies to cytokines – friends or foes? Immunol. Today 11, 167–169.

Bendtzen, K., Hansen, M.B., Diamant, M., Heegaard, P. and Svenson, M. (1992). In "Neuroimmunology of Fever" (eds. T. Bartfai and D. Ottason) pp. 215–224. Pergamon, Oxford.

Berman, M.A., Sandborg, C.I., Calabia, B.S., Andrews, B.S. and Friou, G.J. (1986). Studies of an interleukin 1 inhibitor: characterization and clinical significance. Clin. Exp. Immunol. 64, 136–145.

Berman, M.A., Sandborg, C.I., Calabia, B.S., Andrews, B.S. and Friou, G.J. (1987). Interleukin 1 inhibitor masks high interleukin 1 production in acquired immunodeficiency syndrome (AIDS). Clin. Immunol. Immunopathol. 42, 133–140.

Beutler, B., Han, J., Kruys, V. and Giroir, B.P. (1992). In "Tumor Necrosis Factors: The Molecules and their Emerging Role in Medicine", pp 561–574. Raven Press, New York.

Bigler, C.F., Norris, D.A., Weston, W.L. and Arend, W.P. (1992). Interleukin-1 receptor antagonist production by human keratinocytes. J. Invest. Derm. 98, 38–44.

Bird, T. A., Gearing, A.J.H. and Saklatvala, J. (1988). Murine interleukin 1 receptor. J. Biol. Chem. 263, 12063–12069.

Borth, W., Scheer, B., Urbansky, A., Luger, T. and Sottrup-Jensen, L. (1990a). Binding of IL-1β to α-macroglobulins and release by thioredoxin. J. Immunol. 145, 3747–3754.

Borth, W., Urbanski, A., Prohaska, R., Susani, M. and Luger, T.A. (1990b). Binding of recombinant interleukin-1β to the third complement component and a₂-macroglobulin after activation of serum by immune complexes. Blood 75, 2388–2395.

Brown, K.M. and Rosenstreich, D.L. (1987). Mechanism of action of a human interleukin 1 inhibitor. Cell. Immunol. 105, 45–53.

Brown, K.M., Muchmore, A.V. and Rosenstreich, D.L. (1986). Uromodulin, an immunosuppressive protein derived from pregnancy urine, is an inhibitor of interleukin 1. Proc. Natl Acad. Sci. USA 83, 9119–9123.

Cannon, J.G., Tatro, J.B., Reichlin, S. and Dinarello, C.A. (1986). α melanocyte stimulating hormone inhibits immunostimulatory and inflammatory actions of interleukin 1. J. Immunol. 137, 2232–2236.

Carter, D.B., Deibel, M.R. Jr., Dunn, C.J., Tomich, C.-S.C., Laborde, A.L., Slightom, J.L., Berger, A.E., Bienkowski, M.J., Sun, F.F., McEwan, R.N., Harris, P.K.W., Yem, A.W., Waszak, G.A., Chosay, J.G., Sieu, L.C., Hardee, M.M., Zurcher-Neely, H.A., Reardon, I.M., Heinrikson, R.L., Truesdall, S.E., Shelly, J.A., Eessalu, T.E., Taylor, B.M. and Tracey D.E. Purification, cloning, expression and biological characterization of an interleukin-1 receptor antagonist protein. Nature (London) 344, 633–638.

Caruso, A., Bonfanti, C., Colombrita, D., de Francesco, M., de Rango, C., Foresti, I., Gargiulo, F., Gonzales, R., Gribaudo, G., Landolfo, S., Manca, N., Manni, M., Pirali, F., Pollara,

P., Ravizzola, G., Scura, G., Terlenghi, L., Viani, E. and Turano, A. (1990). Natural antibodies to IFN-γ in man and their increase during viral infection. J. Immunol. 144, 685–689.

Dayer, J.-M. and Fenner, H. (1992). The role of cytokines and their inhibitors in arthritis. In "Baillière's Clinical Rheumatology", vol. 6, pp 485–516. Baillière-Tindall, London.

Dinarello, C.A. (1991). Interleukin-1 and interleukin-1 antagonism. Blood 77, 1627–1652.

Dinarello, C.A. and Thompson, R.C. (1991). Blocking IL-1: interleukin 1 receptor antagonist in vivo and in vitro. Immunol. Today 12, 404–410.

Dinarello, C.A., Rosenwasser, L.J. and Wolff, S.M. (1981). Demonstration of a circulating suppressor factor of thymocyte proliferation during endotoxin fever in humans. J. Immunol. 127, 2517–2519.

Dower, S.K., Wignall, J.M., Schooley, K., McMahan, C.J., Jackson, J.L., Prickett, K.S., Lupton, S., Cosman, D. and Sims, J.E. (1989). Retention of ligand binding activity by the extracellular domain of the IL-1 receptor. J. Immunol. 142, 4314–4320.

Drips, D.J., Brandhuber, B.J., Thompson, R.C. and Eisenberg, S.P. (1991). Interleukin-1 (IL-1) receptor antagonist binds to the 80-kDa IL-1 receptor but does not initiate IL-1 signal transduction. J. Biol. Chem. 266, 10331–10336.

Eastgate, J.A., Symons, J.A. and Duff, G. W. (1990). Identification of an interleukin-1 beta binding protein in human plasma. FEBS Lett. 260, 213–216.

Eisenberg, S.P., Evans, R.J., Arend, W.P., Verderber, E., Brewer, M.T., Hannum, C.H. and Thompson, R.C. (1990). Primary structure and functional expression from complementary DNA of a human interleukin-1 receptor antagonist. Nature. (London) 343, 341–346.

Eisenberg, S.P., Brewer, M.T., Verderber, E., Heimdal, P., Brandhuber, B.J. and Thompson, R.C. (1991). Interleukin 1 receptor antagonist is a member of the interleukin 1 gene family: evolution of a cytokine control mechanism. Proc. Natl Acad. Sci. USA 88, 5232–5236.

Englemann, H., Aderka, D., Rubenstein, M., Rotman, D. and Wallach, D. (1989). A tumor necrosis factor-binding protein purified to homogeneity from human urine protects cells from tumor necrosis factor toxicity. J. Biol. Chem. 264, 11974–11980.

Estrov, Z., Kurzrock, R., Wetzler, M., Kantarjian, H., Blake, M., Harris, D., Gutterman, J.U. and Talpaz, M. (1991). Suppression of chronic myelogenous leukemia colony growth by interleukin-1 (IL-1) receptor antagonist and soluble IL-1 receptors: a novel application for inhibitors of IL-1 activity. Blood 78, 1476–1484.

Faherty, D.A., Claudy, V., Plocinski, J.M., Kaffka, K., Kilian, P., Thompson, R.C. and Benjamin, W.R. (1992). Failure of IL-1 receptor antagonist and monoclonal anti-IL-1 receptor antibody to inhibit antigen specific immune responses in vivo. J. Immunol. 148, 766–771.

Fanslow, W.C., Sims, J.E., Sassenfeld, H., Morrissey, P.J., Gillis, S., Dower, S.K. and Widmer, M.B. (1989). Regulation of alloreactivity in vivo by a soluble form of the interleukin-1 receptor. Science 248, 739–742.

Fanslow, W.C., Clifford, K.N., Park, L.S., Rubin, A.S., Voice, R.F., Beckmann, M.P. and Widmer, M.B. (1991). Regulation of alloreactivity in vivo by IL-4 and the soluble IL-4 receptor. J. Immunol. 147, 535–540.

Fernandez-Botran, R. (1991). Soluble cytokine receptors: their role in immunoregulation. FASEB J. 5, 2567–2574.

Fernandez-Botran, R. and Vitetta, E.S. (1990). A soluble high affinity, interleukin-4-binding protein is present in the biological fluids of mice. Proc. Natl Acad. Sci. USA 87, 4202–4206.

Fernandez-Botran, R. and Vitetta, E.S. (1991). Evidence that natural murine soluble interleukin 4 receptors may act as transport proteins. J. Exp. Med. 174, 673–681.

Ferrante, A., Hauptmann, B., Seckinger, P. and Dayer, J.-M. (1991). Inhibition of tumour necrosis factor alpha (TNF-alpha)-induced neutrophil respiratory burst by a TNF inhibitor. Immunology 72, 440–442.

Firestein, G.S., Berger, A.E., Tracey, D.E., Chosay, J.G., Chapman, D.L., Paine, M.M., Yu, C. and Zvaifler, N.J. (1992). IL-1 receptor antagonist protein production and gene expression in rheumatoid arthritis and osteoarthritis synovium. J. Immunol. 149, 1054–1062.

Fomsgaard, A., Svenson, M. and Bendtzen, K. (1989). Autoantibodies to tumour necrosis factor α in healthy humans and patients with inflammatory diseases and gram-negative bacterial infections. Scand. J. Immunol. 30, 219–223.

Gaffney, E.V., Stoner, C.R., Lingenfelter, S.E. and Wagner, L.A. (1989). Demonstration of IL-1α and IL-1β secretion by the monocytic leukemia cell line, THP-1. J. Immunol. Methods 122, 211–218.

Galve-de Rochemonteix, B., Nicod, L.P., Junod, A.F. and Dayer, J.-M. (1990). Characterization of a specific 20- to 25-kD interleukin-1 inhibitor from cultured human lung macrophages. Am. J. Respir. Cell Mol. Biol. 3, 355–361.

Galve-de Rochemonteix, B., Nicod, L.P., Chicheportiche, R., Lacraz, S., Baumberger, C. and Dayer, J.-M. (1993). Regulation of IL-1ra, IL-1α and IL-1β production by human alveolar macrophages with PMA, LPS and IL-4. Am. J. Respir. Cell. Mol. Biol. 8, 160–168.

Garrone, P., Djossou, O., Galizzi, J.P. and Banchereau, J. (1991). A recombinant extracellular domain of the human interleukin 4 receptor inhibits the biological effects of interleukin 4 on T and B lymphocytes. Curr. J. Immunol. 21, 1365–1369.

Gatanaga, T., Hwang, C., Kohr, W., Cappuccini, F., Lucci J.A., III, Jeffes, E.W.B., Lentz, R., Tomich, J., Yamamoto, R.S. and Granger, G.A. (1990). Purification and characterization of an inhibitor (soluble tumor necrosis factor receptor) for tumor necrosis factor and lymphotoxin obtained from the serum ultrafiltrates of human cancer patients. Proc. Natl Acad. Sci. USA 87, 8781–8784.

Girardin, E., Grau, G.E., Dayer, J.-M., Roux-Lombard, P. and Lambert, P.H. (1988). Tumor necrosis factor and interleukin-1 in the serum of children with severe infectious purpura. N. Engl. J. Med. 18, 397–400.

Girardin, E., Roux-Lombard, P., Grau, G.E., Suter, P., Gallati, H., The J5 Study Group and Dayer, J.-M. (1992). Imbalance between tumor necrosis factor α and soluble TNF receptor concentrations in severe meningococcemia. Immunology 76, 20–23.

Giri, J.G., Newton, R.C. and Horuk, R. (1990). Identification of soluble interleukin-1 binding protein in cell-free supernatants. J. Biol. Chem. 265, 17416–17419.

Goodwin, R.G., Friend, D., Ziegler, S.F., Jerzy, R., Falk, B.A., Gimpel, S., Cosman, D., Dower, S.K. March, C.J., Namen,

A.E. and Park, L.S. (1990). Cloning of the human and murine interleukin-7 receptors: demonstration of a soluble form and homology to a new receptor superfamily. Cell 60, 941–951.

Gosset, P., Lassalle, P., Tonnel, A.B., Dessaint, J.P., Wallaert, B., Prin, L., Pestel, J. and Capron, A. (1988). Production of an interleukin-1 inhibitory factor by human alveolar macrophages from normals and allergic asthmatic patients. Am. Rev. Respir. Dis. 138, 40–46.

Gottlieb, R.A., Lennarz, W.J., Knowles, R.D., Cianciolo, G.J., Dinarello, C.A., Lachman, L.B. and Kleinerman, E.S. (1989). Synthetic peptide corresponding to a conserved domain of the retroviral protein p15E blocks IL-1 mediated signal transduction. J. Immunol. 142, 4321–4328.

Granowitz, E.V., Santos, A.A., Poutsiaka, D.D., Cannon, J.G., Wilmore, D.W., Wolf, S.M. and Dinarello, C.A. (1991). Production of interleukin-1-receptor antagonist during experimental endotoxaemia. Lancet 338, 1423–1424.

Gruaz-Chatellard, D., Baumberger, C., Saurat, J.-H, and Dayer, J.-M. (1991). Interleukin 1 receptor antagonist in human epidermis and cultured keratinocytes. FEBS Lett. 294, 137–140.

Hannum, C.H., Wilcox, C.J., Arend, W.P., Joslin, F.G., Dripps, D.J., Heimdal, P.L., Armes, L.G., Sommer, A., Eisenberg, S.P. and Thompson, R.C. (1990). Interleukin-1 receptor antagonist activity of a human interleukin-1 inhibitor. Nature (London) 343, 336–340.

Hansen, M.B., Svenson, M., Diamant, M. and Bendtzen, K. (1991). Anti-interleukin-6 antibodies in normal human serum. Scand. J. Immunol. 33, 777–781.

Hansen, M.B., Svenson, M. and Bendtzen, K. (1993). Human anti-interleukin 1α antibodies. Immunol. Lett. (in press).

Haskill, S., Martin, G., Van Le, L., Morris, J., Peace, A., Bigler, C.F., Jaffe, G.J., Hammerberg, C., Sporn, S.A., Fong, S., Arend, W.P. and Ralph, P. (1991). cDNA cloning of an intracellular form of the human interleukin 1 receptor antagonist associated with epithelium. Proc. Natl. Acad. Sci. USA 88, 3681–3685.

Hession, C., Decker, J.M., Sherblom, A.P., Kumar, S., Yue, C.C., Mattaliano, R.J., Tizard, R., Kawashima, E., Schmeissner, U., Heletky, S., Chow, E.P., Burne, C.A., Shaw, A. and Muchmore, A.V. (1987). Uromodulin (Tamm-Horsfall glycoprotein): a renal ligand for lymphokines. Science 237, 1479–1484.

Honda, M., Kitamura, K., Takeshita, T., Sugamura, K. and Tokunaga, T. (1990). Identification of a soluble IL-2 receptor β-chain from human lymphoid cell line cells. J. Immunol. 145, 4131–4135.

Isler, P., Zhang, J.-H., Vey, E. and Dayer, J.-M. (1993). Cell surface proteins expressed on activated human T cells induce production of interleukin-1 beta by monocytic cells. Eur. Cytokine Netw. 4, 15–23.

Jacobs, C.A., Lynch, D.H., Roux, E.R., Miller, R., Davis, B., Widmer, M.B., Wignall, J., VandenBos, T., Park, L.S. and Beckmann, M.P. (1991). Characterization and pharmacokinetic parameters of recombinant soluble interleukin-4 receptor. Blood 77, 2396–2403.

Jacques, Y., LeMauff, B., Godard, A., Naulet, J., Concino, M., Marsh, H., Ip, S. and Soulillou, J.-P. (1990). Biochemical study of a recombinant soluble interleukin-2 receptor. Evidence for a homodimeric structure. J. Biol. Chem. 265, 20252–20258.

James, K. (1990). Interactions between cytokines and a_2-macroglobulin. Immunol. Today 11, 163–166.

Janson, R.W., Hance, K.R. and Arend, W.P. (1991). Production of IL-1 receptor antagonist by human in vitro-derived macrophages. J. Immunol. 147, 4218–4223.

Janson, R.W., King T.E. Jr., Hance, K.R. and Arend, W.P. (1993). Enhanced production of IL-1 receptor antagonist by alveolar macrophages from patients with interstitial lung disease. Am. Rev. Resp. Dis. (in press).

Ju, G., Lbriola-Tompkins, E., Campen, C.A., Benjamin, W.R., Karas, J., Plocinski, J., Biondi, D., Kaffka, K.L., Kilian, P.L., Eisenberg, S.P. and Evans, R.J. (1991). Conversion of the interleukin 1 receptor antagonist into an agonist by site-specific mutagenesis. Proc. Natl Acad. Sci. USA 88, 2658–2662.

Kabir, S. and Wigzell, H. (1989). A novel urinary sialoglycoprotein as the inhibitor of interleukin-1. Clin. Exp. Immunol. 77, 89–96.

Kawahara, D.J., Everts, M., Buckingham, B., Sandborg, C. and Berman, M. (1991). A naturally occurring 6-9-kilodalton interleukin-1 (IL-1) inhibitor prevents IL-1-mediated islet cytotoxicity but not IL-1-mediated suppression of insulin secretion. J. Immunother. 10, 182–188.

Kemp, A., Mellow, L. and Sabbadini, E. (1986). Inhibition of interleukin 1 activity by a factor in submandibular glands of rats. J. Immunol. 137, 2245–2251.

Kimball, E.S., Pickeral, S.F., Oppenheim, J.J. and Rossio, J.L. (1984). Interleukin and IL1 inhibitor activity in normal human urine. J. Immunol. 133, 256–260.

Kleinerman, E.S., Lachman, L.B., Knowles, R.D., Snyderman, R. and Cianciolo, G.J. (1987). A synthetic peptide homologous to the envelope proteins of retroviruses inhibits monocyte-mediated killing by inactivating interleukin 1. J. Immunol. 139, 2329–2337.

Koch, A.E., Kunkel, S.L., Chensue, S.W., Haines, G.K. and Strieter, R.M. (1992). Expression of interleukin-1 and interleukin-1 receptor antagonist by human rheumatoid synovial tissue macrophages. Clin. Immunol. Immunopathol. 65, 23–29.

Korn, J.H., Brown, K.M., Downie, E., Liao, Z.H. and Rosenstreich, D.L. (1987). Augmentation of IL 1-induced fibroblast PGE_2 production by a urine-derived IL 1 inhibitor. J. Immunol. 138, 3290–3294.

Lacraz, S., Nicod, L., Galve-de Rochemonteix, B., Baumberger, C., Dayer, J.-M. and Welgus, H.G. (1992). Suppression of metalloproteinase biosynthesis in human alveolar macrophages by interleukin-4. J. Clin. Invest. 90, 382–388.

LaMarre, J., Hayes, M.A., Wollenberg, G.K., Hussanini, I., Hall, S.W. and Gonias, S.L. (1991). An α2-macroglobulin receptor-dependent mechanism for the plasma clearance of transforming growth factor-β in mice. J. Clin. Invest. 87, 39–44.

Larrick. J.W. (1989). Native interleukin 1 inhibitors. Immunol. Today 10, 61–66.

Lebsack, M.E., Paul, C.C., Bloedow, D.C., Burch, F.X., Sack, M.A., Chase, W. and Catalano, M.A. (1991). Subcutaneous IL-1 receptor antagonist in patients with rheumatoid arthritis. Arth. Rheum. 34, S45.

Lennard, A., Gorman, P., Carrier, M., Griffiths, S., Scotney, H., Sheer, D., and Solari, R. (1992). Cloning and chromosome mapping of the human interleukin-1 receptor antagonist gene. Cytokine 4, 83–89.

Lesslauer, W., Tabuchi, H. and Gentz, R. (1991). Recombinant soluble tumor necrosis factor receptor proteins protect mice from lipopolysaccharide-induced lethality. Eur. J. Immunol. 21, 2883–2886.

Liao, Z., Grimshaw, R.S. and Rosenstreich, D.L. (1984). Identification of a specific interleukin 1 inhibitor in the urine of febrile patients. J. Exp. Med. 159, 126–136.

Liao, Z., Haimovitz, A., Chen, Y., Chan, J. and Rosenstreich, D.L. (1985). Characterization of a human interleukin 1 inhibitor. J. Immunol. 134, 3882–3886.

Locksley, R.M., Crowe, S., Sadick, M.D., Heinzel, F.P., Gardner, K.D. Jr., McGrath, M.S. and Mills, J. (1988). Release of interleukin 1 inhibitory activity (contra-IL-1) by human monocyte-derived macrophages infected with human immunodeficiency virus in vitro and in vivo. J. Clin. Invest. 82, 2097–2105.

Lotz, M., Tsoukas, C.D., Fong, S., Dinarello, C.A., Carson, D.A. and Vaughan, J.H. (1986a). Release of lymphokines after infection with Epstein Barr virus in vitro. II. A monocyte-dependent inhibitor of interleukin 1 downregulates the production of interleukin 2 and interferon-γ in rheumatoid arthritis. J. Immunol. 136, 3643–3648.

Lotz, M., Tsoukas, C.D., Robinson, C.A., Dinarello, C.A., Carson, D.A. and Vaughan, J.H. (1986b). Basis for defective responses of rheumatoid arthritis synovial fluid lymphocytes to anti-CD3 (T3) antibodies. J. Clin. Invest. 78, 713–721.

Mae, N., Liberato, D.J., Chizzonite, R. and Satoh, H. (1991). Identification of high-affinity anti-IL-1α autoantibodies in normal human serum as an interfering substance in a sensitive enzyme-linked immunosorbent assay for IL-1α. Lymphokine Cytokine Res. 10, 61–68.

Maliszewski, C.R., Sato, T.A., VandenBos, T., Waugh, S., Dower, S.K., Slack, J., Beckmann, M.P. and Grabstein, K.H. (1990). Cytokine receptors and B cell functions. I. Recombinant soluble receptors specifically inhibit IL-1 and IL-4-induced B cell activities in vitro. J. Immunol. 144, 3028–3033.

Malyak, M., Swaney, R.E. and Arend, W.P. (1993). Synovial fluid interleukin-1 receptor antagonist (IL-1ra) levels in rheumatoid arthritis and other arthropathies: potential contribution from synovial fluid neutrophils. Arth. Rheum. 36, 781–789.

Matsuda, T., Muchmore, A.V. and Decker, J.M. (1986). Uromodulin. An immunosuppressive 85-kilodalton glycoprotein isolated from human pregnancy urine is a high affinity ligand for recombinant interleukin 1α. J. Biol. Chem. 261, 13404–13407.

Matsuda, T., Hirano, T., Nagasuma, S. and Kishimoto, T. (1989). Identification of α2-macroglobulin as a carrier protein for IL-6. J. Immunol. 142, 148–152.

McCarthy, D.O., Domurat, F.M., Nichols, J.E. and Roberts, N.J. Jr. (1989). Interleukin-1 inhibitor production by human mononuclear leukocytes and leukocyte subpopulations exposed to respiratory syncytial virus: analysis and comparison with the response to influenza virus. J. Leuk. Biol. 46, 189–198.

McCarthy, P.L. Jr., Abhyankar, S., Neben, S., Newman, G., Sieff, C., Thompson, R.C., Burakoff, S.J. and Ferrara, J.L.M. (1991). Inhibition of interleukin-1 by an interleukin-1 receptor antagonist prevents graft-versus-host disease. Blood 78, 1915–1918.

McColl, S.R., Paquin, R., Menard, C. and Beaulieu, A.D.

(1992). Human neutrophils produce high levels of the interleukin 1 receptor antagonist in response to granulocyte/macrophage colony-stimulating factor and tumor necrosis factor α. J. Exp. Med. 176, 593–598.

McMahan, C.J., Slack, J.L., Mosley, B., Cosman, D., Lupton, S.D., Brunton, L.L., Grubin, C.E., Wignall, J.M., Jenkins, N.A., Brannan, C.I., Copeland, N.G., Huebner, K., Croce, C.M., Cannizzarro, L.A., Benjamin, D., Dower, S.K., Spriggs, M.K. and Sims, J.E. (1991). A novel IL-1 receptor, cloned from B cells by mammalian expression, is expressed in many cell types. EMBO J. 10, 2821–2832.

Mizutani, H., Black, R., and Kupper, T.S. (1991). Human keratinocytes produce but do not process pro-interleukin 1 (IL-1) beta. J. Clin. Invest. 87, 1066–1071.

Mosley, B., Beckmann, M.P., March, C.J., Idzerda, R.I., Gimpel, S.D., VandenBos, T., Friend, D., Alpert, A., Anderson, D., Jackson, J., Wignall, J.M., Smith, C., Gallis, B., Sims, J.E., Urdal, D., Widmer, M.B., Cosman, D. and Park, L.S. (1989). The murine interleukin-4 receptor: molecular cloning and characterization of secreted and membrane bound forms. Cell 59, 335–348.

Muchmore, A.V. and Decker, J.M. (1987). Evidence that recombinant IL-1α exhibits lectin-like specificity and binds to homogeneous uromodulin via N-linked oligosaccharides. J. Immunol. 138, 2541–2546.

Nicod, L.P., El Habre, F. and Dayer, J.-M. (1992). Natural and recombinant interleukin 1 receptor antagonist does not inhibit human T-cell proliferation induced by mitogens, soluble antigens or allogeneic determinants. Cytokine 4, 29–35.

Nishihara, T., Koga, T. and Hamada, S. (1988). Production of an interleukin-1 inhibitor by cell line P388D1. Murine macrophages stimulated with Haemophilus actinomycetemcomitans lipopolysaccharide. Infect. Immun. 56, 2801–2807.

Nortier, J., Vandenabeele, P. and Noel, E. (1991). Enzymatic degradation of tumor necrosis factor by activated human neutrophils. role of elastase. Life Sci. 49, 1879–1886.

Novick, D., Engelmann, H., Wallach, D. and Rubinstein, M. (1989). Soluble cytokine receptors are present in normal human urine. J. Exp. Med. 170, 1409–1414.

Ohlsson, K., Björk, P., Bergenfeldt, M., Hageman, R. and Thompson, R.C. (1990). Interleukin-1 receptor antagonist reduces mortality from endotoxin shock. Nature (London) 348, 550–552.

Olsson, I., Lantz, M., Nilsson, E., Peetre, C., Thysell, H., Grubb, A. and Adolf, G. (1989). Isolation and characterization of a tumor necrosis factor binding protein from urine. Eur. J. Haematol. 42, 270–275.

O'Neill, L.A.J., Ikebe, T., Sarsfield, S.J. and Saklatvala, J. (1992). The binding subunit of pertussis toxin inhibits IL-1 induction of IL-2 and prostaglandin production. J. Immunol. 148, 474–479.

Paganelli, K.A., Stern, A.S. and Kilian, P.L. (1987). Detergent solubilization of the interleukin 1 receptor. J. Immunol. 138, 2249–2253.

Patterson, D., Jones, C., Hart, I., Bleskan, J., Berger, R., Geyer, D., Eisenberg, P., Smith, Jr., M. F. and Arend, W.P. (1993). The human interleukin-1 receptor antagonist gene (IL-1RN) is located in the chromosome 2q14 region. Genomics, 15, 173–176.

Peterson, C.M. and Moestrup, S.K. (1990). Interactions between cytokines and α2 macroglobulin. Immunol. Today 11, 430–431.

Pierart, M.E., Najdovski, T., Appleboom, T.E. and Deschodt-Lanckman, M.M. (1988). Effect of human endopeptidase 24.11 ("enkephalinase") on IL-1-induced thymocyte proliferation activity. J. Immunol. 140, 3808–3811.

Piguet, P.F., Grau, G.E., Vesin, C., Loetscher, H., Gentz, R. and Lesslauer, W. (1992). Evolution of the collagen arthritis in mice is arrested by treatment with anti-tumor necrosis factor (TNF) antibody or a recombinant soluble TNF receptor. Immunology 77, 510–514.

Porteu, F. and Nathan C. (1990). Shedding of tumor necrosis factor receptors by activated human neutrophils. J. Exp. Med. 172, 599–607.

Porteu, F. and Nathan, C. (1992). Mobilizable intracellular pool of p55 (type I) tumor necrosis factor receptors in human neutrophils. J. Leuk. Biol. 52, 122–124.

Porteu, F., Brockhaus, M., Wallach, D., Engelmann, H. and Nathan, C.F. (1991). Human neutrophil elastase releases a ligand-binding fragment from the 75-kDa tumor necrosis factor (TNF) receptor. J. Biol. Chem. 266, 18846–18853.

Poutsiaka, D.D., Clark, B.D., Vannier, E. and Dinarello, C.A. (1991). Production of interleukin-1 receptor antagonist and interleukin-1β by peripheral blood mononuclear cells is differentially regulated. Blood 78, 1275–1281.

Quesniaux, V.F.J. (1992). Interleukins 9, 10, and 12 and kit ligand: a brief overview. Res. Immunol. 143, 385–400.

Rambaldi, A., Torcia, M., Bettoni, S., Vannier, E., Barbui, T., Shaw, A.R., Dinarello, C.A. and Cozzolino, F. (1991). Modulation of cell proliferation and cytokine production in acute myeloblastic leukemia by interleukin-1 receptor antagonist and lack of its expression by leukemic cells. Blood 78, 3248–3253.

Roberts, N.J. Jr., Prill, A.H. and Mann, T.N. (1986). Interleukin 1 and interleukin 1 inhibitor production by human macrophages exposed to influenza virus or respiratory syncytial virus. J. Exp. Med. 163, 511–519.

Robertson, B., Dostal, K. and Daynes, R.A. (1988). Neuropeptide regulation of inflammatory and immunologic responses. The capacity of α-melanocyte-stimulating hormone to inhibit tumor necrosis factor and IL-1 inducible biologic responses. J. Immunol. 140, 4300–4307.

Rodgers, B.C., Scott, D.M., Mundin, J. and Sissons, J.G.P. (1985). Monocyte-derived inhibitor of interleukin 1 induced by human cytomegalovirus J. Virol. 55, 527–532.

Rosenstreich, D.L., Tu, J.H., Kinkade, P.R., Maurer-Fogy, I., Kahn, J., Barton, R.W. and Farina, P.R. (1988). A human urine-derived interleukin-1 inhibitor. Homology with deoxyribonuclease. Int. J. Exp. Med. 168, 1767–1779.

Ross, C., Hansen, M.B., Schyberg, T. and Berg, K. (1990). Autoantibodies to crude human leucocyte interferon (IFN), native human IFN, recombinant human IFN-alpha 2b and human IFN-gamma in healthy blood donors. Clin. Exp. Immunol. 82, 57–62.

Roux-Lombard, P., Modoux, C. and Dayer, J.-M (1989). Production of interleukin-1 (IL-1) and a specific Il-1 inhibitor during human monocyte-macrophage differentiation: influence of GM-CSF. Cytokine 1, 45–51.

Roux-Lombard, P., Modoux, C., Vischer, T., Grassi, J. and Dayer, J.-M. (1992). Inhibitors of interleukin 1 activity in synovial fluids and in cultured synovial fluid mononuclear cells. J. Rheumatol. 19, 517–523.

Roux-Lombard, P., Punzi, L., Hasler, F., Bas, S., Todesco, S., Gallati, H., Guerne, P.-A. and Dayer, J.-M. (1993). Soluble tumor necrosis factor receptors in human inflammatory synovial fluids. Arth. Rheum. 36, 485–489.

Rubin, L.A. and Nelson, D.L. (1990). The soluble interleukin-2 receptor: biology, function and clinical application. Ann. Int. Med. 113, 619–627.

Rubin, L.A., Galli, F., Greene, W.C., Nelson, D.L. and Jay, G. (1990). The molecular basis for the generation of the human soluble interleukin 2 receptor. Cytokine 2, 330–336.

Salkind, A.R., McCarthy, D.O., Nichols, J.E., Domurat, F.M., Walsh, E.E. and Roberts, N.J. Jr. (1991). Interleukin-1-inhibitor activity induced by respiratory syncytial virus: abrogation of virus-specific and alternate human lymphocyte proliferative responses. J. Infect. Dis. 163, 71–77.

Sandborg, C.I., Berman, M.A., Andrews, B.S., Mirick, G.R. and Friou, G.J. (1986). Increased production of an interleukin 1 (IL-1) inhibitor with fibroblast stimulating activity by mononuclear cells from patients with scleroderma. Clin. Exp. Immunol. 66, 312–319.

Saurat, J.H., Schifferli, J., Steiger, G., Dayer, J.M. and Didierjean, L. (1991). Anti-interleukin-1α autoantibodies in humans: characterization, isotype distribution, and receptor-binding inhibition – higher frequency in Schnitzler's syndrome (urticaria and macroglobulinemia). J. Allergy Clin. Immunol. 88, 244–256.

Scala, G., Kuang, Y.D., Hall, R.E., Muchmore, A.V. and Oppenheim, J.J. (1984). Accessory cell function of human B cells. I. Production of both interleukin 1-like activity and an interleukin 1 inhibitory factor by an EBV-transformed human B cell line. J. Exp. Med. 159, 1637–1652.

Schwab, J.H., Anderle, S.K., Brown, R.R., Dalldorf, F.G. and Thompson, R.C. (1991). Pro- and anti-inflammatory roles of interleukin-1 in recurrence of bacterial cell wall-induced arthritis in rats. Infect. Immun. 59, 4436–4442.

Schwartz, T., Urbanska, A., Gschnait, F. and Luger, T.A. (1987). UV-irradiated epidermal cells produce a specific inhibitor of interleukin 1 activity. J. Immunol. 138, 1457–1463.

Seckinger, P. and Dayer, J.-M. (1992). In "Tumor Necrosis Factors. Structure Function, and Mechanisms of Action" (eds B.B. Aggarwal and J. Vilcek), pp 217–236. Marcel Dekker, New York.

Seckinger, P., Lowenthal, J.W., Williamson, K., Dayer, J.-M. and MacDonald, H.R. (1987a). A urine inhibitor of interleukin 1 activity that blocks ligand binding. J. Immunol. 139, 1546–1549.

Seckinger, P., Williamson, K., Balavoine, J.-F., Mach, B., Mazzei, G., Shaw, A. and Dayer, J.-M. (1987b). A urine inhibitor of interleukin 1 activity affects both interleukin 1α and 1β but not tumor necrosis factor α. J. Immunol. 139, 1541–1545.

Seckinger, P., Isaaz, S. and Dayer, J.-M. (1988). A human inhibitor of tumor necrosis factor α. J. Exp. Med. 167, 1511–1516.

Seckinger, P., Zhang, J.H., Hauptmann, B. and Dayer, J.-M. (1990). Characterization of tumor necrosis factor α (TNFα) inhibitor: evidence of immunological cross-reactivity with the TNF receptor. Proc. Natl. Acad. Sci. USA 87, 5188–5192.

Shirahama, M., Ishibashi, H., Tsuchiya, Y., Kurokawa, S., Hayashida, K., Okumura, Y. and Niho, Y. (1988). Kupffer cells may autoregulate interleukin 1 production by producing interleukin 1 inhibitor and prostaglandin E$_2$. Scand. J. Immunol. 28, 719–725.

Sims, J.E., March, C.J., Cosman, D., Widmer, M.B., MacDonald, H.R., McMahan, C.J., Grubin, C.E., Wignall, J.M., Jackson, J.L., Call, S.M., Friend, D., Alpert, A.R., Gillis, S., Urdal, D.L. and Dower, S.K. (1988). cDNA expression cloning of the IL-1 receptor, a member of the immunoglobulin superfamily. Science 241, 585–589.

Sims, J.E., Acres, R.B., Grubin, C.E., McMahan, C.J., Wignall, J.M., March, C.J. and Dower, S.K. (1989). Cloning the interleukin 1 receptor from human T cells. Proc. Natl. Acad. Sci. USA 86, 8946–8950.

Steinkasserer, A., Spurr, N.K., Cox, S., Jeggo, P. and Sim, R.B. (1992). The human IL-1 receptor antagonist gene (IL-1RN) maps to chromosome 2q14-q21, in the region of the IL-1α and IL-1β loci. Genomics 13, 654–657.

Suter, P. M., Suter, S., Girardin, E., Roux-Lombard, P., Grau, G.E. and Dayer, J.-M. (1992). High bronchoalveolar levels of tumor necrosis factor and its inhibitors, interleukin-1, interferon and elastase in patients with adult respiratory distress syndrome after trauma, shock or sepsis. Am. Rev. Respir. Dis. 145, 1016–1022.

Suzuki, H., Akama, T., Okane, M., Kono, I., Matsui, Y., Yamane, K. and Kashiwagi, H. (1989). Interleukin-1-inhibitory IgG in sera from some patients with rheumatoid arthritis. Arth. Rheum. 32, 1528–1538.

Suzuki, H., Kamimura, J., Ayabe, T. and Kashiwagi, H. (1990). Demonstration of neutralizing autoantibodies against IL-1α in sera from patients with rheumatoid arthritis. J. Immunol. 145, 2140–2146.

Svenson, M. and Bendtzen, K. (1988). Inhibitor of interleukin 1 in normal human urine. Different effects on mouse thymocytes and on a murine T-cell line. Scand. J. Immunol. 27, 593–599.

Svenson, M., Poulsen, L.K., Fomsgaard, A. and Bendtzen, K. (1989). IgG autoantibodies against interleukin 1α in sera of normal individuals. Scand. J. Immunol. 29, 489–492.

Svenson, M., Hansen, M.B. and Bendtzen, K. (1990). Distribution and characterization of autoantibodies to interleukin 1α in normal human sera. Scand. J. Immunol. 32, 695–701.

Svenson, M., Hansen, M.B., Kayser, L., Rasmussen, A.K., Reimert, C.M. and Bendtzen, K. (1992). Effects of human anti-IL-1α autoantibodies on receptor binding and biological activities of IL-1. Cytokine 4, 125–133.

Symons, J.A. and Duff, G.W. (1990). A soluble form of the interleukin-1 receptor produced by a human B cell line. FEBS Lett. 272, 133–136.

Symons, J.A., Eastgate, J.A. and Duff, G.W. (1990). A soluble binding protein specific for interleukin 1β is produced by activated mononuclear cells. Cytokine 2, 190–198.

Symons, J.A., Eastgate, J.A. and Duff, G.W. (1991). Purification and characterization of a novel soluble receptor for interleukin 1. J. Exp. Med. 174, 1251–1254.

Teodorescu, M., McAfee, M., Skosey, J.L., Wallman, J., Shaw, A. and Hanly, W.C. (1991). Covalent disulfide binding of human IL-1β to α₂-macroglobulin: inhibition by D-penicillamine. Mol. Immunol. 28, 323–331.

Thompson-Snipes, L.A., Dhar, V., Bond, M.W., Mosmann, T.R., Moore, K.W. and Rennick, D.M. (1991). Interleukin 10: a novel stimulating factor for mast cells and their progenitors. J. Exp. Med. 173, 507–510.

Thornberry, N.A., Bull, H.G., Calaycay, J.R., Chapman, K.T., Howard, A.D., Kostura, M.J., Miller, D.K., Molineaux, S.M., Weidner, J.R., Aunins, J., Elliston, K.O., Ayala, J.M., Casano, F.J., Chin, J., Ding, G.J.-F., Egger, L.A., Gaffney, E.P., Limjuco, G., Palyha, O.C., Raju, S.M., Rolando, A.M., Salley, J.P., Yamin, T.-T., Lee, T.D., Shively, J.E., MacCross, M., Mumford, R.A., Schmidt, J.A. and Tocci, M.J. (1992). A novel heterodimeric cysteine protease is required for interleukin-1β processing in monocytes. Nature (London) 356, 768–774.

Tiku, K., Tiku, M.L., Liu, S. and Skosey, J.L. (1986). Normal human neutrophils are a source of a specific interleukin 1 inhibitor. J. Immunol. 136, 3686–3692.

Tsudo, M., Karasuyama, H., Kitamura, F., Tanaka, T., Kubo, S., Yamamura, Y., Tamatani, T., Hatakeyama, M., Taniguchi, T. and Miyasaka, M. (1990). The IL-2 receptor β-chain (p 70). Ligand binding ability of the cDNA-encoding membrane and secreted forms. J. Immunol. 145, 599–606.

Tucci, A., James, H., Chicheportiche, R., Bonnefoy, J.Y., Dayer, J.-M. and Zubler, R.H. (1992). Effects of eleven cytokines and of IL-1 and tumor necrosis factor inhibitors in a human B cell assay. J. Immunol. 148, 2778–2784.

Van Zee, K.J., Kohno, T., Fischer, E., Rock, C.S., Moldawer, L.L., and Lowry, S.F. (1992). Tumor necrosis factor soluble receptors circulate during experimental and clinical inflammation and can protect against excessive tumor necrosis factor α *in vitro* and *in vivo*. Proc. Natl. Acad. Sci. USA 89, 4845–4849.

Vey, E., Zhang, J.-H. and Dayer, J.-M. (1992). IFN-γ and 1,25(OH)₂D₃ induce on THP-1 cells distinct patterns of cell surface antigen expression, cytokine production, and responsiveness to contact with activated T cells. J. Immunol. 149, 2040–2046.

Wakabayashi, G., Gelfand, J.A., Burke, J.F., Thompson, R.C. and Dinarello, C.A. (1991). A specific receptor antagonist for interleukin 1 prevents *Escherichia coli*-induced shock in rabbits. FASEB J. 5, 338–343.

Walsh, L.J., Seymour, G.J. and Powell, R.N. (1986). Modulation of gingival Langerhans cell T6 antigen expression *in vitro* by interleukin 1 and an interleukin 1 inhibitor. Clin. Exp. Immunol. 64, 334–341.

Walsh, L.J., Lander P.E., Seymour, G.J. and Powell, R.N. (1987). Isolation and purification of ILS, an interleukin 1 inhibitor produced by human gingival epithelial cells. Clin. Exp. Immunol. 68, 366–374.

Watrous, D.A., Andrews, B.S., Levonian, P.J. and Friou, G.J. (1990). Effects of human 17 kDa interleukin 1, 25–31 kDa thymocyte stimulating activity and the 6–9 kDa interleukin 1 inhibitor on calcium release in the newborn murine calvarial assay. J. Rheum. 17, 1142–1147.

Wong, G.H.W., Kamb, A., Elwell, J.H., Oberley, L.W. and Goeddel, D.V. (1992). In "Tumor Necrosis Factors: The Molecules and their Emerging Role in Medicine", pp 473–484. Raven Press, New York.

Wright, S.D., Ramos, R.A., Tobias, P.S., Ulevitch, R.J. and Mathison, J.C. (1990). CD14, a receptor for complexes of lipopolysaccharide (LPS) and LPS binding protein. Science 249, 1431–1433.

8. Soluble Immunopeptides in Inflammatory Arthritis

Julian A. Symons and Gordon W. Duff

1. Introduction

In RA, as in other inflammatory diseases, a wide range of soluble immunopeptides have been found to be correlated with conventional measures of disease activity. Some of these, for example the major monocyte-derived cytokines, may be involved directly in aspects of pathogenesis, while others, such as soluble forms of leucocyte "cell surface" molecules, may be related to the inflammatory process in an indirect manner being, for instance by-products of leucocyte activation. Even these may contribute to the net outcome of an inflammatory response. As an example, certain cytokine receptors in soluble form appear to bind to their cytokines and block their biological activities.

Cytokines, soluble cytokine receptors and similar molecules can usually be measured in biological fluids with relative ease using immunoassays and may therefore provide new opportunities for monitoring different aspects of disease activity *in vivo*. They might also shed light on the cellular interactions underlying the disease process.

In this chapter we describe briefly some of the better studied soluble immunopeptides that may be informative in inflammatory arthritis, particularly RA. They include some interleukins, tumour necrosis factor, cytokine receptors and soluble forms of lymphocyte CD antigens.

2. Interleukin 1

IL-1 is a peptide hormone with important activities in the regulation of immune and inflammatory reactions. Early characterization of IL-1 began with the demonstration of a protein factor in the blood of animals made febrile with bacterial endotoxin, (Atkins, 1960). This circulatory pyrogen, termed endogenous pyrogen, was later found to be similar to a factor able to augment thymocyte proliferation in response to plant lectins, termed lymphocyte-activating factor (Gery and Waksman, 1972). Other factors were also described the activities of which have since been ascribed to IL-1, including osteoclast activating factor (Dewhirst *et al.*, 1985), mononuclear cell factor, which causes prostaglandin and collagenase production from synovial fibroblasts (Mizel *et al.*, 1981), and catabolin, a factor that induces cartilage breakdown (Saklatvala, 1981). The debate on how many biological activities attributed to IL-1 are due to the action of a single molecule were largely resolved with the cloning of murine and human cDNAs coding for IL-1 and their expression as proteins. Two nucleotide sequences for murine and human IL-1 cDNAs were reported in 1984 (Lomedico *et al.*, 1984; Auron *et al.*, 1984); both encoded approximately 270-amino acid polypeptide precursors with molecular masses of 31 kDa which lacked a classical signal sequence. Both molecules

Immunopharmacology of Joints and Connective Tissue
ISBN 0–12–206345–7

were cleaved to form 17 kDa mature molecules. The two nucleotide sequences revealed a 20% homology at the peptide level and 45% homology at the nucleotide level. A second human IL-1 gene was then cloned (March *et al.*, 1985). This molecule was found to have 62% homology to the mouse IL-1 and was therefore given the name IL-1α and the other called IL-1β.

In the mid-1980s inhibitors of IL-1 action were first reported in the literature (Arend *et al.*, 1985; Balavoine *et al.*, 1986). These reports led to the cloning of a third member of the IL-1 gene family (Eisenberg *et al.*, 1990) termed IL-1Ra. The IL-1Ra has a 26% homology with IL-1β and 19% homology with IL-1α and binds to both IL-1 receptors but elicits no cellular responses.

IL-1α, IL-1β and IL-1Ra have have been characterized at the gene level, all three genes being localized on the long arm of chromosome 2 in the same chromosomal region (q13-q21). Analysis of the human IL-1α and IL-1β genes shows that the two have comparable exon length and splice site locations and it has therefore been proposed that the IL-1β gene arose by duplication (retrotransposition) of the IL-1α gene (Clark *et al.*, 1986). The 3' region of the IL-1Ra gene has a similar intron–exon organization to the agonist genes; however, the 5' region appears to be derived from a different part of the genome, possibly explaining the different biological activities (Eisenberg *et al.*, 1991).

Pro-IL-1β mRNA is rapidly induced in human PBMCs or monocytic cell lines when stimulated with endotoxin or phorbol esters. Message levels peak at 2–3 h, after which they fall to a low level. This decrease results from a specific transcriptional repression of the gene 2 h after stimulation, probably mediated by a newly synthesized protein because cycloheximide addition results in superinduction and stabilization of message levels (Fenton *et al.*, 1987). In addition to transcriptional regulation, IL-1 gene expression is also controlled at the post-transcriptional level. Stabilization of IL-1β message occurs when cells are stimulated with phorbol ester, whereas the message has a much shorter half-life when induced by endotoxin. In PBMCs, IL-1β gene transcription occurs at a greater rate than IL-1α; however, this is not true for all cell types, as in keratinocytes, IL-1α transcription predominates.

IL-1 is produced by many cell types, the most studied being the PBMC. However, a wide range of more specialized cell types such as T and B lymphocytes, smooth muscle, endothelial and various cells of the central nervous system are capable of synthesizing IL-1. Interestingly, the amount of IL-1α and IL-1β varies between different cell types. In blood monocytes stimulated with LPS, IL-1β mRNA is found to be 10–50 times more abundant than IL-1α mRNA. However, total IL-1α protein often exceeds that of IL-1β (Endres *et al.*, 1989) and this presumably reflects differential translational efficiency or protein stability. Acute T cell leukaemia cell lines have also been shown to produce IL-1; however, the IL-1

activity was only neutralizable with anti-IL-1α and IL-1β mRNA was undetectable.

IL-1α and IL-1β are both produced as 31 kDa precursors which are cleaved at specific sites to produce the mature 17 kDa molecules. Incorrect processing, leaving or deleting extra amino acids, results in reduced bioactivity. Most work has focused on the cleavage of IL-1β, as the propeptide has little receptor binding or biological activity whereas the IL-1α precursor retains receptor-binding activity (Mosley *et al.*, 1987). The pro-IL-1β molecule is processed to the 153-amino acid mature form at Asp-116–Ala-117. As mature 17 kDa IL-1β is rarely found intracellularly, it has been suggested that a cell surface or secreted enzyme is responsible for proteolytic cleavage; however, processing activity has been found in both membrane and cytosolic preparations. The presence of unprocessed 31 kDa IL-1β in culture supernatants has strengthened the notion that the enzyme responsible for cleavage is either located at the cell surface or is secreted by the cell.

Recently, the enzyme responsible for cleavage of pro-IL-1β has been purified and cloned (Cerretti *et al.*, 1992). The 45 kDa precursor ICE undergoes proteolysis at both N- and C-termini possibly by an autocatalytic route to generate an active heterodimer composed of 20 kDa and 10 kDa subunits. The ICE has the biochemical properties of a cysteine protease, but its sequence is unlike any other known cysteine protease. The importance of IL-1β cleavage in the induction of a host inflammatory response is highlighted by the finding that the pox viruses produce a 30 kDa protein encoded by the *crmA* gene which specifically inhibits the action of ICE (Ray *et al.*, 1992).

Little is known about the mechanisms involved in the secretion of IL-1 from the cell as neither IL-1 molecule has a recognizable hydrophobic signal sequence. A number of secretory pathways for IL-1 have been proposed. The presence of membrane IL-1 has resulted in the theory that a membrane-linked intermediate may play a role in the release of IL-1α; however, the existence of membrane IL-1 is controversial. Protein modification may play a role in IL-1 secretion and both phosphorylation and myristoylation may help to localize IL-1 for secretion. Evidence for a novel pathway for IL-1 secretion has been suggested (Rubartelli *et al.*, 1990) proposing that IL-1 is selectively located within intracellular vesicles which are part of the endocytic pathway. These fuse with the plasma membrane in a temperature- and calcium-dependent manner and propeptide molecules are cleaved upon release.

2.1   THE ROLE AND MEASUREMENT OF IL-1 IN RA

IL-1 has been implicated as an important mediator in a number of inflammatory diseases; however, particular attention has been directed at the role of IL-1 in inflammatory joint diseases such as RA. IL-1 is one of the most potent bone-resorbing agents known (Gowan *et al.*, 1983), and it is thought that IL-1 stimulates osteoblasts to produce a soluble factor which in turn, causes osteoclast activation. Osteoclasts then degrade the bone by generating a low-pH environment containing lysosomal proteinases over the bone matrix. As well as bone resorption, IL-1 also degrades cartilage. The actions of IL-1 have been investigated predominantly in organ culture systems, where IL-1 causes a dose-dependent release of proteoglycan which is dependent on the presence of live chondrocytes (Gowan *et al.*, 1984). IL-1 also inhibits the production of new cartilage proteoglycan via inhibition of protein synthesis. The mechanism of IL-1-induced proteoglycan breakdown is still uncertain; however, proteolytic enzymes, especially the IL-1 induced metalloproteinase stromelysin, have been implicated. In contrast with its catabolic activities described above, IL-1 augments fibroblast proliferation and collagen synthesis. IL-1 effects on cellular proliferation are influenced by prostaglandin production, and large amounts of PGE_2 produced by some fibroblasts may inhibit proliferation. The characterization of IL-1 as a factor stimulating PGE_2 produced from synovial fibroblasts was first described by Dayer and co-workers (Dayer *et al.*, 1986). The PGE_2 produced by fibroblasts may have an important role in local joint inflammation observed in RA, causing local vasodilatation and enhancing the effect of pain mediators such as bradykinin and substance P.

The availability of purified recombinant IL-1 has allowed the evaluation of IL-1 as a mediator of inflammation *in vivo*. Human IL-1 causes PMN accumulation when injected into the rabbit knee joint (Pettipher *et al.*, 1986). After a single injection of IL-1 into the joint cavity, both PMNs and monocytes accumulate, with the peak occurring 6 h after injection. Infiltration of the synovial membrane by monocytes is also seen. Single injections of IL-1 result only in acute synovitis; however, repeated injections in animals pretreated with streptococcal peptidoglycan–polysaccharide fragments leads to pannus formation in about 50% of animals (Stimpson *et al.*, 1988). The mechanism of IL-1-induced PMN accumulation appears not to involve changes in vascular permeability as, after IL-1 injection, no evidence of swelling or oedema is seen. IL-1 probably causes leucocyte infiltration by its action on the endothelium, inducing expression of adhesion proteins and by induction of chemotactic peptides of which IL-8 is a likely candidate, having been detected at high levels in certain RA joint effusions (Brennan *et al.*, 1990). Intra-articular injection of IL-1 also causes proteoglycan degradation in animals. This cartilage damage occurs independently of leucocyte infiltration, as proteoglycan degradation also occurs in leucopenic animals, and cartilage explants from these animals produce large quantities of collagenase and stromelysin.

To understand the pathogenic mechanisms of IL-1 in RA, it is important to be able to define the cellular sources of IL-1 within the joint. Resting monocytes contain no IL-1 mRNA or protein, suggesting that the gene is not constitutively expressed. However, following stimulation with endotoxin, IL-1 mRNA accumulates rapidly and IL-1 protein can be detected after 30 min (di Giovine *et al.*, 1991). Confirmation that IL-1 is produced locally within the rheumatoid joint has come from mRNA studies using Northern blotting and *in situ* hybridization combined with immunohistochemistry (Wood *et al.*, 1992a, b). These studies demonstrated that the predominant cell type producing IL-1β mRNA in the rheumatoid synovium is the CD14+ macrophage (Plate 2). Cells expressing the IL-1β gene were especially frequent in the "transitional" areas of the synovial membrane that contain macrophages, lymphocytes and plasma cells. Macrophages within the lining area also contained IL-1β mRNA.

Initial reports of IL-1 bioactivity in synovial fluid appeared in the early 1980s (Fontana *et al.*, 1982). These early demonstrations required some chromatographic fractionation before the samples yielded reliable measurements. The bioassays used were unable to distinguish between IL-1α and IL-1β and were often inhibited by biological fluids, so it was not until the development of specific immunoassays that the reliable measurement of synovial fluid IL-1 became possible (Symons *et al.*, 1989; di Giovine *et al.*, 1990). However, technical problems still occurred; these were probably due to the fact that, *in vivo*, IL-1 is carried bound to a number of soluble binding proteins. Two proteins known to bind IL-1β in the synovial fluid and plasma are α_2-macroglobulin (Borth and Luger, 1989) and the recently described natural soluble IL-1 receptor (Symons *et al.*, 1990a). Owing to the presence of these and other interfering substances, a number of extraction procedures have been developed that probably expose antibody-recognition sites. Cannon *et al.* (1988) developed a chloroform extraction procedure which results in the appearance of both bioactive and immunoreactive IL-1α and IL-1β with a molecular mass below 30 kDa. Using the Cannon extraction protocol on plasma samples collected into EDTA with protease inhibitors from patients with RA and controls, we were able to measure both IL-1β and IL-1α.

Immunoreactive levels of IL-1β were higher in patients with RA than in healthy volunteers. More importantly, the IL-1 concentrations correlated with clinical (Ritchie index, morning stiffness, pain score) and laboratory erythrocyte sedimentation rate ((ESR), haemoglobin) evidence of disease activity within the group of patients. There was a large variation in the plasma IL-1β level between individual RA patients; however, in hospital patients tested serially over a period of several weeks (Fig. 8.1), we found that IL-1β levels were related to clinical disease activity (Eastgate *et al.*, 1988). No such

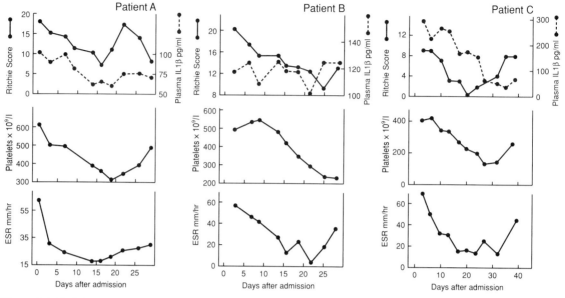

Figure 8.1 Serial measurements of plasma IL-1β, Ritchie articular index, platelets and ESR in three patients with active RA during hospital admission. (Data from Eastgate *et al.* (1988).)

correlations were found cross-sectionally in a group of RA patients tested for plasma IL-1α (Eastgate *et al.*, 1991). Indeed, between the patient and control groups there were significant correlations between the indices of inflammation and levels of IL-1α within individual patients with active disease who were tested at regular intervals over a 4–5-week period. The reason for the differences between plasma IL-1α and IL-1β are unclear; however, monocytes stimulated *in vitro* produce both IL-1α and IL-1β. The latter is rapidly released but, in contrast, IL-1α remains predominantly cell associated. Alternatively, production of IL-1α by different cell types could explain the similar blood levels in patients and control groups. A large cell population such as the skin keratinocytes secreting predominantly IL-1α (Kupper *et al.*, 1986) may lead to detectable blood levels in healthy individuals, and increased production from cells at a site of inflammation would appear as a relatively small increase over the high background.

Both forms of IL-1 have been identified in the synovial fluid (Symons *et al.*, 1989; di Giovine *et al.*, 1990) of patients with RA and other rheumatic diseases using immunoassays. However, no significant correlations with disease activity were found, probably because of the large interindividual variation in the production of IL-1. To overcome this problem, synovial fluid from patients with symmetrical and asymmetrical knee joint inflammation was obtained and local disease activity documented using the Ritchie articular index and joint circumference. In patients with symmetrical joint involvement almost identical levels of IL-1β were detected in the right and left knee joints. In contrast, in patients exhibiting asymmetrical knee joint involvement, IL-1β levels in the

inflamed joints were significantly higher than in the contralateral joints (Rooney *et al.*, 1990).

3. *Interleukin-2*

IL-2 is a genetically unrestricted peptide growth factor produced by T cells following activation with either mitogen or antigen. This activation process involves the presentation of antigen by APCs (in association with MHC products) to the T cell in the presence of IL-1. This induces the coordinate synthesis and secretion of IL-2 and expression of high- and low-affinity receptors for IL-2. Subsequent interaction of IL-2 with high-affinity IL-2 receptors produces T cell proliferation, thus expanding the small clonal population of antigen-responsive T cells. As with many other cytokines, IL-2 exhibits considerable size and charge heterogeneity. Human IL-2 is secreted as a single polypeptide (15–17 kDa) with a range of pI from 6.5 to 8.2. Initially it was thought that these differences represent multimolecular forms of IL-2, but it is now known that the heterogeneity is due to variable levels of sialic acid which does not affect the bioactivity of the molecule (Robb and Smith, 1981). A single gene for IL-2 is present in the human genome located on chromosome 4. This gene is 8 kb long with four exons and three introns. The first exon encodes the 20-amino acid hydrophobic leader sequence and the 5′ untranslated region. The three remaining exons contain the sequences for the mature peptide (Mita *et al.*, 1986). The amino acid sequence of human IL-2 predicted from the cDNA encodes a 15.4 kDa protein (Taniguchi *et al.*, 1983). Although

IL-2 is a key T cell growth factor, it is not restricted to this role. IL-2 induces other T cell lymphokines such as IFNα. This cytokine has a range of immune functions which include stimulation of NK cell activity, generation of cytotoxic T lymphocytes, macrophage activation and increased expression of MHC antigens. Studies have also shown that IL-2 causes an increase in NK cell activity beyond that attributable to induction of IFNα. IL-2 also stimulates B-cell growth indirectly by inducing other B cell growth factors such as IL-4 from T cells and also directly via IL-2 receptors on B cells. Other work also suggests that IL-2 augments the cytotoxicity of human monocytes.

IL-2 can be regarded as one of the most important humoral factors in the regulation of cellular immunity, and many human disease states are characterized by deficient production and/or responsiveness to IL-2. In chronic inflammatory conditions, a deficient production of IL-2 or defective response is seen in systemic lupus erythematosus (SLE), RA and Sjögren's syndrome (Miyasaka et al., 1984). These in vitro defects can often be reversed by the addition of exogenous IL-2 or by the removal of suppressor cells (Linker-Israeli et al., 1985).

IL-2 is difficult to measure in vivo, where it is produced and rapidly internalized. However, factors able to maintain T cell clones have been described in RA synovial fluid, and, using a sensitive immunoassay, we were able to measure significant levels of IL-2 in synovial fluid (Symons et al., 1989). Interestingly, we were able to correlate the levels of synovial fluid IL-2 with synovial levels of IL-1β ($r = +0.82$; $P < 0.001$; $n = 31$). No correlation was found between synovial fluid IL-1α and IL-2 levels and this difference may again be due to the differential translocation of the IL-1 peptides.

3.1 THE IL-2R

IL-2R is composed of three different polypeptide chains (α, β and γ) each capable of binding IL-2 with different affinities. The α chain, also known as CD25, binds IL-2 with a low affinity ($K_d = 10^{-8}$M, whereas the β chain binds IL-2 with an intermediate affinity ($K_d = 10^{-9}$M). The association of the three IL-2R chains results in the high-affinity form of the receptor ($K_d = 10^{-11}$M) with the γ chain being responsible for the internalization of the ligand (Weissman et al., 1986). The IL-2R β chain is constitutively expressed on PBMCs and its expression is only increased 2.5-fold after mitogen stimulation (Hatekeyama et al., 1989). This expression pattern is quite different from that of the α chain, the expression of which is strictly dependent on mitogenic or antigenic stimulation of the cells.

The human IL-2R α chain was cloned using the anti-Tac antibody to purify the receptor (Leonard et al., 1984). The deduced amino acid sequence shows a 251-amino acid receptor protein with a 21-amino acid N-terminal signal peptide, a 19-residue transmembrane domain and a 13-amino acid cytoplasmic domain. This region is so short that it is highly unlikely that it would possess signalling capacity. The gene for the IL-2R α chain is located on chromosome 10 at bands p14 to p15. The gene consists of eight exons and seven introns with a length of over 25 Kb. Interestingly, exon 4 can be alternatively spliced to yield an mRNA that would encode a protein lacking 72 amino acids. However, transfection of a cDNA corresponding to this message does not result in the expression of cell surface IL-2R, and the role of this gene product is unknown (Leonard et al., 1985). Although the IL-2R α chain is encoded by a single gene, multiple mRNA species are produced. Northern blotting reveals two major bands at 3500 and 1500 bases, each of which can be translated into functional IL-2R protein. As previously discussed, the IL-2R α chain is indirectly expressed after activation with antigen or mitogen. IL-2R is detectable within 4–8 h of stimulation, increasing to about 60 000/cell within 48–72 h. Transcription of the gene begins within 3 h of activation and peaks at 9 h, mRNA levels peak at 12 h and then decline (Leonard et al., 1985).

In addition to expressing α chain on their surface, activated T lymphocytes also release a soluble form of this protein (sIL-2R) (Rubin et al., 1985). The mechanism of release appears to be proteolytic cleavage at the cell surface, and the rate of release is in proportion to its cell surface expression. The released receptor is 10 kDa smaller than the 55 kDa cell surface protein because of its lack of a transmembrane domain and cytoplasmic region. The sIL-2R retains the ability to bind IL-2 and has a similar affinity for the cell surface protein (Robb and Kutny, 1987). As sIL-2R α chain is only expressed on activated MNCs and its rate of release is proportional to the cell's activation status, we postulated that levels of sIL-2R in vivo would correlate with immune activation in diseases such as RA. Further, as the sIL-2R binds to IL-2 we predicted that it could potentially affect IL-2-driven immune responses which may be important in the immunoregulation of many autoimmune diseases.

Initially we demonstrated that sera from patients with RA had higher levels of sIL-2R than patients with OA and healthy controls (Symons et al., 1988). In the RA population, paired synovial fluid samples contained even higher levels of sIL-2R, indicating that the proliferating synovial tissue is the likely source of the sIL-2R detected in the serum. Consistent with this was the high spontaneous production of sIL-2R from freshly isolated synovial fluid mononuclear cells whilst only relatively low levels were released from autologous blood MNC populations. Sequential studies of individual patients during periods of fluctuating disease activity revealed that serum levels of sIL-2R correlated with disease activity. On admission to hospital, all patients had significantly elevated serum IL-2 levels compared with age-matched healthy controls. Following therapy, a marked fall in serum sIL-2R level occurred in each patient and preceded clinical improvement by 4–8 days. Similar changes in serum sIL-2R levels were seen whether clinical remission was associated with treatment or without the use of remission-inducing drugs (Fig. 8.2).

We found that serum sIL-2R levels correlated significantly with several conventional clinical and laboratory measures of disease activity. These included the Ritchie articular index, duration of early morning stiffness, patient pain score and the physician's global assessment of disease activity. Of the laboratory measurements, only ESR and platelet count were significantly correlated with serum sIL-2R (Wood et al., 1988).

In four of 13 patients with RA, after clinical improvement, serum sIL-2R levels again began to rise (Fig. 8.3). In each of these patients a subsequent exacerbation of rheumatoid symptoms occurred. This second rise in serum sIL-2R level began 6–13 days before the observed clinical deterioration (Wood et al., 1988). These results indicate that, in individual patients, rising levels of serum sIL-2R might predict increased clinical disease activity in inflammatory arthritis. It also raises the possibility that, in some cases, clinical exacerbation may be avoided by early immunosuppressive therapy started at the time of sIL-2R increase. As previously discussed, IL-1 appears to play an important role during the immune response. IL-1 augments the maturation and proliferation of both B and T cells and their differentiation into antibody-producing B cells or into lymphokine-producing T cells. IL-1 does not act as a direct growth factor for T cells, but enhances

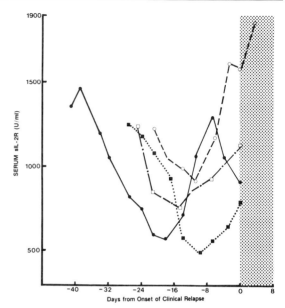

Figure 8.3 Serial sIL-2R serum levels in four RA patients whose levels initially fell preceding temporary clinical improvement and subsequently increased again preceding "clinical relapse". (Data from Wood et al. (1988).)

production of IL-2 and the IL-2 receptor. As well as finding a positive correlation between IL-2 and IL-1β in RA synovial fluid, comparison of synovial fluid sIL-2R levels with IL-1β also revealed a significant correlation ($r - +0.62$; $P < 0.007$; $n = 30$). The association of IL-2R and IL-1β is also found within the RA synovium. *In situ* localization of IL-1β and IL-2R α chain using monoclonal antibodies on RA synovia demonstrated that both are expressed in the same cellular aggregates (Duff, 1989). Further, addition of increasing concentrations of IL-1β to freshly isolated synovial fluid MNCs caused a dose-dependent potentiation of sIL-2R into the supernatant (Symons *et al.*, 1989). Taken together, the evidence would suggest that IL-1β may play a role in the potentiation of IL-2 and IL-2R production within the rheumatoid synovium and thus lead to an increase in immune-mediated inflammation.

To test the functional significance of sIL-2R in synovial fluid, we measured the inhibitory activity of synovial fluid on IL-2 driven proliferation of cytotoxic T cells and compared this with the sIL-2R level in the same fluids. There was a highly significant correlation ($r = + 0.77$; $P < 0.001$; $n = 42$) between sIL-2R concentration and the ability of synovial fluid to inhibit the proliferative response of the cytotoxic T cells to IL-2. In support of the idea that sIL-2R released into the synovial fluid mediated the inhibition of IL-2 responses we found that inhibition could be overcome by adding supraoptimal concentrations of IL-2 to the cultures and that, upon gel filtration chromatography of synovial fluid, functional

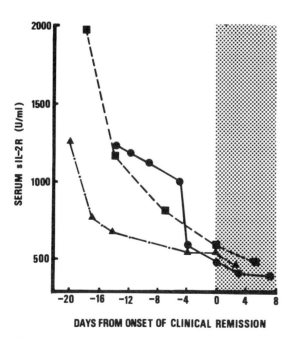

Figure 8.2 Longitudinal studies of serum sIL-2R in three patients with RA. Clinical improvement indicated by the stippled area was assessed by both standard laboratory tests and subjective and objective clinical evaluation. (Data from Symons et al. (1988).)

inhibition of the IL-2 response and immunoreactive sIL-2R were eluted as a single peak at approximately 100 kDa. As the molecular mass of the sIL-2R is approximately 45 kDa it was surprising to find IL-2R α chain immunoreactivity at 100 kDa. However, it appears that synovial fluid facilitates oligomerization or heterobinding of monomeric sIL-2R. Rodent studies (Honda et al., 1990) have shown that the β chain of IL-2R is also released. The sIL-2R β chain is a molecule of 50–55 kDa and combination of both α and β chains in solution would presumably form a high-affinity soluble IL-2 inhibitor.

4. Soluble CD4 and CD8

CD4 and CD8 are nonpolymorphic, cell surface glycoprotein members of the immunoglobulin gene superfamily expressed on distinct populations of T lymphocytes. Initially it was thought that CD8 and CD4 were markers of phenotypic function, CD4 being the helper subset and CD8 being the suppressor/cytotoxic subset. While the majority of cytotoxic T cells express CD8, many helper T cells also express CD8 (Swain, 1981). In contrast, CD4-bearing T cells can exhibit both suppressor and cytotoxic functions (Krensky et al., 1982). The widely held view now is that CD4 and CD8 are weakly associated with T cell function but strongly with MHC restriction. T cells expressing CD4 recognize antigen presented by MHC class II molecules, whereas CD8+ T cells recognize antigen in the context of class I MHC (Swain, 1983). CD4 and CD8 may therefore increase the activity of lymphocyte–APC interactions by directly binding to non-polymorphic determinants on appropriate MHC molecules. However, the role of CD4 and CD8 in T cell function is not restricted to enhancing T cell receptor contact with presented antigen. Both CD4 and CD8 are physically associated with $p56^{lck}$, a member of the Src family of cellular TPK which is expressed exclusively in lymphoid cells (Barber et al., 1989). CD4, CD8 and $p56^{lck}$ all undergo phosphorylation on serine residues when cells are activated, although regulation of the TPK may differ in the two subsets.

4.1 THE CD4 MOLECULE

The membrane-associated human CD4 protein is a single-chain 55 kDa molecule consisting of external immunoglobulin-like domains, a hydrophobic transmembrane region and a 40-residue cytoplasmic tail. The four extracellular domains are homologous to an immunoglobin V region. Upon comparison of the murine, rat and human CD4 molecules, the most impressive aspect is the evolutionary conservation of the 40-amino acid cytoplasmic tail. Of this first 32 residues, 29 are identical in human and mouse and there is only a single amino acid difference between the mouse and rat

cytoplasmic domains. The finding of strong conservation in the cytoplasmic domain of CD4 argues that this sequence is essential for the function of the molecule and is responsible for signal transduction. Other conserved sites include the two sites for N-linked glycosylation and the six extracellular cysteines that are located in pairs in three of the external domains. The human CD4 gene has been mapped to the short arm of chromosome 12 and therefore is not linked to any known immunoglobulin gene family loci (Isobe et al., 1986). This region shows high homology to the distal segment of mouse chromosome 6, and the murine CD4 gene located on this segment of chromosome 6 would be linked to the Lyt 2, Lyt 3 (CD8) and Ig–k loci.

The expression of CD4 glycoprotein is not restricted to T lymphocytes; cells of the macrophage and neutrophil lineage, as well as lymphoblastoid B cell lines can all express CD4 (Jefferies et al., 1985). Large amounts of CD4 mRNA can also be found in the brain, and as CD4 T lymphocytes are extremely rare in healthy individuals, it is likely that the source of CD4 is from bone-marrow-derived macrophages or microglia. Brain parenchymal cells may also express CD4. In the mouse, T cells express a 3.2 kb transcript whereas only a 2.4 kb mRNA is found in the brain. The brain-specific transcript is a truncated form of the T cell message which is initiated within the exon encoding the third extracellular domain of the T cell CD4. The function of this brain-specific transcript is unknown.

The mechanism of cell surface CD4 release is unknown. However, "anchor minus" cDNA clones have yet to be reported so it is likely that release occurs through proteolytic cleavage at the cell surface. Indeed, incubation of activated PBMCs, which release relatively high levels of sCD4, with the serine protease inhibitor, aprotinin, results in inhibition of CD4 release (J.A. Symons, unpublished data). As CD4 release is an activation-associated event, in vivo levels of sCD4 may allow measurement of the activation status of the subset of cells expressing this molecule.

4.2 THE CD8 MOLECULE

Unlike CD4, which is found as a monomer on human cells, the human 34 kDa CD8 molecule (or α chain) forms disulphide-linked homodimers and homomultimers on the surface of peripheral T cells (Kavathas et al., 1984). In addition, a second CD8 chain (CD8β), the human homologue of the Lyt 3 molecule is also expressed on the surface of blood T cells (Shire et al., 1988). The CD8 complex is expressed either as an α/β heterodimer or as an α homodimer. It appears that expression of CD8β is dependent on cell surface expression of CD8α chain (diSanto et al., 1988). Membrane-bound CD8α consists of an extracellular immunoglobulin-like domain which displays homology with other members of the immunoglobulin gene superfamily. This Ig-like domain is followed by a short proline, serine and threonine hinge sequence. This region also contains sites for O-linked glycosylation. After the hydrophobic transmembrane domain, both human and murine CD8 molecules have a 28-amino acid cytoplasmic tail which exhibits 55% homology.

In addition to expressing the 34 kDa α chain on their surface, activated T cells also release a soluble form of this protein (sCD8) (Fujimoto et al., 1983). The release of this molecule occurs by two distinct mechanisms. A labelled 27 kDa CD8α molecule is released from T cells following cell surface iodination and probably represents specific cleavage of the membrane-bound molecule (Fujimoto et al., 1984). Additionally, during the cloning of the CD8α gene, clones were found that had spliced out the exon encoding the transmembrane domain (Norment et al., 1989). This finding suggests that the soluble form of CD8α may arise by alternative splicing of the transmembrane domain. S$_1$ nuclease studies demonstrated that between 15 and 30% of the CD8α mRNA may be accounted for in T cell lines. The secreted CD8 protein forms homodimers composed of 27 kDa peptides; whether this protein has any immunoregulatory function remains to be determined.

Interestingly, CD8β chain transcripts have also been found lacking the sequences coding for a transmembrane domain, raising the possibility that CD8β protein may also be released and form soluble CD8α/β heterodimers.

4.3 Soluble CD4 and CD8 in RA

Extensive analysis of T cell subsets has been performed in active RA (Duke et al., 1983; Thoen et al., 1989), immunophenotyping of T cell subsets being performed in the peripheral blood, synovial fluid and synovial membrane of patients with RA. It is generally found that CD4+ lymphocytes predominate in the synovial membrane, however, the synovial fluid contains high numbers of CD8+ cells. It has been suggested that this represents selective passage of CD8+ cells from the synovium as these cells do not interact with dendritic cells to the same extent as CD4+ T lymphocytes. Some studies have described high CD4/CD8 ratios in the blood of RA patients which are associated with high levels of disease activity and subsequently return to normal after treatment. However, other studies have often found that the CD4/CD8 ratio returns to normal during active disease. Measurement of T cell subsets does not, however, provide any information on the activational status of these cell subsets. As the level of sCD4/sCD8 has been shown to be related to the activity of the particular cell types, we measured sCD4 and sCD8 during the course of active RA (Symons et al., 1990b, 1991).

Levels of both sCD4 and sCD8 were raised in the sera of patients with RA compared with age-matched healthy controls. As in the case of sIL-2R (Symons et al., 1988), synovial fluid levels of sCD4 and sCD8 were significantly

higher than the corresponding serum levels, compatible with a synovial tissue source of the soluble cell surface markers. Consistent with this was the high spontaneous production of sCD4 and sCD8 from freshly isolated synovial fluid MNCs and low spontaneous release by blood MNCs which could only produce similar levels to the synovial fluid MNCs after stimulation with mitogenic lectin. Interestingly, although sera and synovial fluid from OA patients contained lower levels of sCD4 than from RA patients, they were still higher than healthy age-matched controls. This was not a surprising result as the predominant cellular infiltrate in OA is of the macrophage type and the products of activated macrophages can be detected in the synovial fluid of OA patients (di Giovine et al., 1990). Additionally, immunophenotyping of OA synovial tissue revealed that most CD14+ tissue macrophages were also CD4+ (J.F. McCulloch et al., unpublished observations). In contrast, serum sCD8 levels in OA patients were not significantly different from age-matched controls and OA synovial fluid levels were significantly lower than the corresponding serum levels. This is probably related to the lack of T cell infiltrate in the OA synovium.

In prospective sequential studies of patients with active RA, serum levels of sCD4 were high upon admission to hospital. Following therapy, a marked fall in serum CD4 occurred in each patient which preceded clinical improvement. In a group of patients who, after initial clinical improvement, exhibited a subsequent clinical relapse,

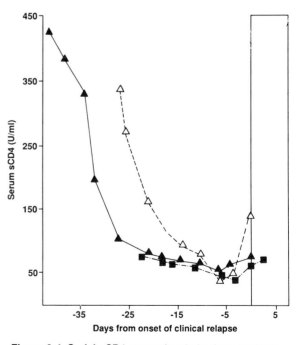

Figure 8.4 Serial sCD4 serum levels in three patients who relapsed after a period of clinical improvement. Clinical relapse is indicated by the vertical bar. (Data from Symons et al. (1991).)

serum sCD4 levels began to rise 3–5 days before the onset of clinical exacerbation (Fig. 8.4). The levels of serum CD4 followed very closely that of the sIL-2R levels, suggesting that they may be released from similar mononuclear cell types. Consistent with this idea was the finding that sIL-2R and sCD4 levels correlated with each other when measured in synovial fluid ($r = 0.79$; $P < 0.001$; $n = 22$). However, no correlation was found with sCD8. Serum sIL-2R levels, however, rose to a much greater extent than sCD4, possibly suggesting that the CD4+ MNC population is activated during the initial phase of the immune response within the joint but that IL-2R+/CD4− cells contribute more to the inflammation seen during active RA.

In contrast with sCD4, sCD8 levels, although high on admission, a rising serum CD8 was associated with the onset of clinical remission whereas falling levels were associated with the onset of clinical exacerbation (Fig. 8.5). Upon examination of synovial fluid MNC populations, it was found that either cells produced high levels of sCD8 and low levels of sIL-2R or vice versa. This, together with the differential serum levels, indicates that the size or activity of the CD8+ T cell population in the rheumatoid synovium is inversely related to the activity of the IL-2R+ MNCs. These observations may result from transient fluctuations in the activity of different populations of infiltrating MNCs. The IL-2R (α) chain appears to be expressed on the majority of activated MNCs; therefore, exacerbation of RA may result

from a general inflammatory reaction that is subsequently suppressed by the activation of a CD8+ T cell.

The function of sCD4 and sCD8 is unknown. Whether sCD4 and sCD8 retain the ability to bind to their respective MHC molecules is yet to be determined. Clearly, if the soluble molecules bind to cell surface MHC molecules, the interaction of T cell and APC may be inhibited. In the case of sCD4, a recombinantly engineered form has clinical potential in the treatment of HIV-infected patients. *In vitro* this molecule does not inhibit class II MHC–T cell interactions.

5. Tumour Necrosis Factor

In humans, TNF-α is a 17 kDa molecule which forms non-covalent biologically active trimers. The molecule was originally identified in the mid-1970s by its ability to induce cachexia in bacteria-infected animals and its cytotoxicity for certain tumour cell lines. The TNF-α gene is located on chromosome 6 in humans, just over 1000 bp from the lymphotoxin or TNF-β gene, and both genes reside within the MHC (Nedwin *et al.*, 1985). The lymphotoxin protein exhibits 30% homology to TNF; however, despite this limited sequence homology, lymphotoxin exerts almost identical biological activities. The two molecules share the same cell surface receptors, binding with comparable affinity (Aggarwal *et al.*, 1985).

TNF-α is an inducible gene product which is controlled at many levels (Sariban *et al.*, 1988). Interestingly, many of its biological effects are similar to those of IL-1. TNF has been shown to stimulate the resorption of proteoglycan in cartilage (Saklatvala, 1986) and to stimulate bone resorption *in vitro* (Bertolini *et al.*, 1986). It appears that IL-1 and TNF-α synergize in the bone resorption assay, although IL-1 is far more potent than TNF-α. TNF-α plays a major role in the activation of the immune response. TNF-α induces the expression of HLA-DR antigen and IL-2R α, and hence TNF-α-treated T cells exhibit enhanced proliferation to IL-2. Its immuno-potentiating effects have also been documented *in vivo* where TNF-α has been shown to play an important role in septic shock and GVHD. Intra-articular injection of TNF-α into animal joints has similar effects to IL-1, inducing monocyte accumulation and also synergizing with IL-1.

With relevance to RA, the presence of TNF has been demonstrated in synovial fluid by both bioassay (di Giovine *et al.*, 1988a) and immunoassay (di Giovine *et al.*, 1988b). However, no correlations with any disease parameters have been found and longitudinal studies are clearly called for. *In situ* hybridization has also been used to identify TNF-α mRNA in rheumatoid synovial tissue and expression seems to be localized to cells in the perivascular regions (Duff *et al.*, 1988). Recent data obtained using a TNF-α transgenic mouse shows that deregulated expression of TNF leads to the development

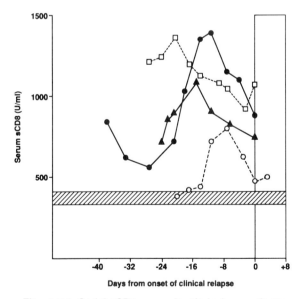

Figure 8.5 Serial sCD8 serum levels in four patients who relapsed following a period of clinical improvement. Clinical relapse is indicated by the vertical bar. Mean (± S.E.M) serum sCD8 concentration in 16 healthy age-matched controls is indicated by the cross-hatched bar. (Data from Symons et al. (1990b).)

of chronic inflammatory polyarthritis which can be suppressed with anti-TNF-α antibodies. Therefore expression of TNF-α in the RA joint may be of major pathogenic significance (Keffer *et al.*, 1991).

6.   Interleukin 6

IL-6 is a multifunctional cytokine produced by both lymphoid and non-lymphoid cells. IL-6 was previously known as β2-interferon, B cell stimulatory factor 2, 26 kDa protein, hybridoma growth factor and hepatocyte-stimulating factor. The cloning of the IL-6 cDNA (Hirano *et al.*, 1986) demonstrated that all these biological activities were mediated by the same protein.

The human IL-6 gene has been mapped to chromosome 7 at 7p21. The complete gene is approximately 5 kb in length, consisting of five exons and four introns (Yasukawa *et al.*, 1987). Comparison of the human and mouse IL-6 genomic clones reveals a high degree of homology extending approximately 350 bp upstream of the transcriptional start site, suggesting a common transcriptional regulation.

IL-6 is produced by a wide range of cell types such as T cells, B cells, monocytes, chondrocytes, fibroblasts, keratinocytes, endothelial and a variety of tumour cell lines. As with many other cytokines, IL-6 production is transcriptionally regulated and neither protein nor mRNA are expressed in resting cells. IL-6 has multiple biological activities which include growth-promoting and differentiation-inducing activities. IL-6 induces IgG, IgA and IgM production from activated B cells and it has been demonstrated that IL-6 is essential for immunoglobulin production (Muraguchi *et al.*, 1988). Furthermore, IL-6 is an autocrine growth factor for human multiple myeloma cells. IL-6 induces IL-2 receptor on T cells and hence potentiates T cell function. The effects of IL-6 are synergistic with IL-1 and TNF-α, and, as well as inducing proliferation, it induces differentiation of cytotoxic T cells. One of the most important roles for IL-6 *in vivo* is the induction of acute phase proteins from the liver. IL-6 can induce a variety of acute phase reactants such as fibrinogen, serum amyloid A, C-reactive protein and α_1-antitrypsin and also has a role in down-regulating albumin expression.

Bioactive and immunoreactive IL-6 has been demonstrated in RA synovial fluid, with lower levels being present in OA exudate fluids (Hirano *et al.*, 1988; Wood *et al.*, 1992). *In situ* hybridization studies have shown that IL-6 mRNA is present in both the lymphocyte-rich aggregates and adjacent to small blood vessels (Plate 3) and is most often associated with T cells (Wood *et al.*, 1992a, b). There are also significant correlations between serum IL-6 activity and levels of acute phase proteins and synovial fluid IL-6 levels and IgG concentration. However, unlike IL-1 and TNF, IL-6 does not induce either cartilage or bone resorption. IL-6 is produced by chondrocytes and may play a protective role in RA. In individual patients tested serially after admission to hospital, serum IL-6 was initially raised and, unexpectedly, increased with clinical improvement (Wood *et al.*, 1992a, b). The acute phase response produces a large number of protease inhibitors and potential cytokine inhibitors and these may suppress both systemic and local immune responses. Additionally, it has been reported that IL-6 can inhibit the production of both IL-1 and TNF at the transcriptional level (Schindler *et al.*, 1990). Therefore, IL-6 may provide a negative feedback signal to limit the cytokine cascade within the RA joint.

7.   Interleukin 8

Neutrophil accumulation in the joints of patients with RA is characteristic of active inflammation. Recently, a number of novel leucocyte-derived chemotactic cytokines have been described. Initially, it was thought that IL-1 and TNF had neutrophil chemotactic activity. However, using gel filtration it was possible to separate the chemotactic activity from these cytokines. Subsequently, neutrophil chemotactic factor (NCF) was purified to homogeneity and molecularly cloned (Matsushima *et al.*, 1988). After finding that NCF was produced by many different cells and had multiple targets, the molecule was renamed interleukin 8 (IL-8). The IL-8 cDNA is 1.6 kb including a 1.2 kb 3′ untranslated region. The cDNA encodes a 99-amino acid IL-8 precursor of which the first 27 amino acids are cleaved upon secretion. The estimated molecular mass of IL-8 on SDS-PAGE is 8 kDa, but it appears that IL-8 forms dimers in solution. IL-8 can be produced from many human cell types, including blood MNCs, skin fibroblasts, chondrocytes, endothelial cells and keratinocytes when stimulated with endotoxin or IL-1 and TNF. Interestingly, T cells stimulated with PHA also produce IL-8. In addition to chemotaxis, IL-8 stimulates neutrophils to release superoxide anions and lysosomal enzymes. IL-8 is also chemotactic for human basophils and stimulates the release of histamine from these cells. *In vivo* IL-8 causes local neutrophil accumulation (Furuta *et al.*, 1989) while intravenous administration of IL-8 causes neutrophilia and rapid plasma leakage. However, IL-8 does not induce fever or acute phase protein synthesis. Recently it has been reported that IL-8 biological activity (Brennan *et al.*, 1990) and immunoreactive protein (Symons *et al.*, 1992) are present in the synovial fluid of patients with RA. To date no correlations with disease activity or chemotactic activity in synovial fluid have been found. Additionally, IL-8 was undetectable in the serum from normal healthy controls or patients with RA and OA, even in those from patients with high synovial fluid levels. The absence of IL-8 from the blood, points to rapid elimination and/or receptor binding probably mediated by a receptor present on red blood cells. The finding of IL-8 in RA synovial fluid is relevant to the pathogenesis of disease, as accumulation of neutrophils producing oxygen radicals and cartilage-degrading enzymes is thought to contribute to joint damage. However, its absence from the serum makes it unlikely that measurement of IL-8 will be used in the future management of RA.

8. Conclusions

Although much information is now available on the basic biochemistry and biology of the soluble immunopeptides discussed in this chapter, there is, as yet, little known about their role in normal immune responses or the mediation of chronic inflammatory diseases such as RA. Measurement of these molecules does, however, offer the opportunity to monitor immune activation *in vivo* in a way that has not been possible before. Additionally, cytokine antagonists such as the IL-1Ra, soluble IL-1 and TNF receptors appear to have considerable therapeutic potential and the outcome of trials with these agents in RA are eagerly awaited.

9. References

Aggarwal, B.B., Eessalu, T.E. and Hass, P.E. (1985). Characterization of receptors for human tumour necrosis factor and their regulation by gamma interferon. Nature (London) 318, 665–667.

Arend, W.P., Joslin, F.G. and Massoni, R.J. (1985). Effects of immune complexes on production by human monocytes of interleukin 1 or an interleukin-1 inhibitor. J. Immunol. 134, 3868–3875.

Atkins, E. (1960). Pathogenesis of fever. Physiol. Rev. 40, 580–646.

Auron, P.E., Webb, A.C., Rosenwasser, L.J., Mucci, S.F., Rich, A., Wolff, S.M. and Dinarello, C. A. (1984). Nucleotide sequence of human monocytic interleukin-1 precursor cDNA. Proc. Natl. Acad. Sci. USA 82, 7907–7911.

Balavoine, J.-F., DeRochemonteix, B., Williamson, K., Seckinger, P., Cruchland, A. and Dayer, J.-M. (1986). Prostaglandin E₂ and collagenase production by fibroblasts and synovial cells is regulated by urine-derived human interleukin 1 inhibitor(s). J. Clin. Invest. 78, 1120–1124.

Barber, E.K., Dasgupta, J.D., Schlossman, S.F., Trevillyon, J.M. and Rudd, C.E. (1989). The CD4 and CD8 antigens are coupled to a protein-tyrosine kinase (p56[lck]) that phosphorylates the CD3 complex. Proc. Natl. Acad. Sci. USA 86, 3277–3281.

Bertolini, D.R., Nedwin, G., Bringman, T., Smith, D. and Mundy, G.R. (1986). Stimulation of bone resorption and inhibition of bone formation *in vitro* by human tumour necrosis factor. Nature (London) 319, 516–518.

Borth, W. and Luger, T.A. (1989). Identification of alpha₂ macroglobulin as a cytokine binding protein; binding of interleukin-1 beta to "F" alpha₂ macroglobulin. J. Biol. Chem. 264, 5818–5825.

Brennan, F.M., Zacharie, C.O.C., Chantry, D., Larsen, C.G., Turner, M., Maini, R.N., Matsushima, K. and Feldmann, M. (1990). Detection of interleukin-8 biological activity in synovial fluids from patients with rheumatoid arthritis and production of interleukin 8 mRNA by isolated synovial cells. Eur. J. Immunol. 20, 2141–2144.

Cannon, J.G., Van der Meer, J.W.M., Kwiatowski, D., Endres, S., Lonneman, G., Birke, J.F. and Dinarello, C.A. (1988). Interleukin 1 beta in human plasma; optimisation of blood collection, plasma extraction and radioimmunoassay methods. Lymphokine Res. 7, 457–467.

Cerretti, D.P., Kozlosky, C.J., Mosely, B., Nelson, N., Ness, K.V., Greenstreet, T.A., March, C.J., Kronheim, S.R., Druck, T., Cannizzaro, L.A., Hueber, K. and Black, R.A. (1992). Molecular cloning of the interleukin-1 beta converting enzyme. Science 256, 97–100.

Clark, B.D., Collins, K.L. Gandy, M.S., Webb, A.C. and Auron, P.E. (1986). Genomic sequence for human prointerleukin 1 beta: possible evolution from a reverse transcribed prointerleukin 1 alpha gene. Nucleic Acids Res. 14, 7897–7914.

Dayer, J.M., Rochemonteix, B, de., Burrus, B., Dermczuk, S. and Dinarello, C.A. (1986). Human recombinant interleukin-1 stimulates collagenase and prostaglandin E₂ production by human synovial cells. J. Clin. Invest. 77, 645–648.

Dewhirst, F.E., Stashenko, P.P., Mole, J.E. and Tsurumachi, T. (1985). Purification and partial sequence of human osteoclast activating factor: identity with interleukin 1 beta. J. Immunol. 135, 2562–2568.

Di Giovine, F.S., Meager, A., Leung, H. and Duff, G.W. (1988a). Immunoreactive tumour necrosis factor alpha and biological inhibitor(s) in synovial fluids from rheumatic patients. Int. J. Immunopathol. Pharmacol. 1, 17–26.

Di Giovine, F.S., Nuki, G. and Duff, G.W. (1988b). Tumour necrosis factor in synovial exudates. Ann. Rheum. Dis. 47, 768–772.

Di Giovine, F.S., Poole, S., Situnayake, R.D., Wadhwa, M. and Duff, G.W. (1990). Absence of correlations between indices of systemic inflammation and synovial fluid interleukin 1 (alpha and beta) in rheumatic diseases. Rheumatol. Int. 9, 259–264.

Di Giovine, F.S., Symons, J.A. and Duff, G.W. (1991). Kinetics of IL-1 beta mRNA and protein accumulation in human mononuclear cells. Immunol. Lett. 29, 211–218.

Di Santo, J.P., Knowles, R.W. and Flomenberg, N. (1988). The human Lyt-3 molecule requires CD8 for cell surface expression. EMBO J. 7, 3465–3470.

Duff, G.W. (1989). In "Interleukin 1 Inflammation and Disease", (ed. R. Bomford and B. Henderson), pp 243–255. Elsevier, Oxford.

Duff, G.W., Dickens, E.M., Wood, N.C., Manson, J., Symons, J., Poole, S. and di Giovine, F.S. (1988). In "Progress in Leukocyte Biology" (ed. J.J. Oppenheim, C.A. Dinarello, M. Kluger), pp 387–392. Alan Liss, New York.

Duke, O., Panayi, G.S., Janossy, G., Poulter, L.W. and Tidman, N. (1983). Analysis of T cell subsets in the peripheral blood and synovial fluid of patients with rheumatoid arthritis by means of monoclonal antibodies. Ann. Rheum. Dis. 42, 357–361.

Eastgate, J.A., Symons, J.A., Wood, N.C., Grinlinton, F.M.,

di Giovine, F.S. and Duff, G.W. (1988). Correlation of plasma interleukin 1 levels with disease activity in rheumatoid arthritis. Lancet ii, 706–709.

Eastgate, J.A., Symons, J.A., Wood, N.C., Capper, S.J. and Duff, G.W. (1991). Plasma levels of interleukin-1-alpha in rheumatoid arthritis. Br. J. Rheumatol. 30, 295–297.

Eisenberg, S.P., Evans, R.J., Arend, W.P., Verderber, E., Brewer, M.T., Hannum, C.H. and Thompson, R.C. (1990). Primary structure and functional expression from complementary DNA of a human interleukin-1 receptor antagonist. Nature (London) 343, 341–346.

Eisenberg, S.P., Brewer, M.T., Verderber, E., Heindal, P., Brandhuber, B.J. and Thompson, R.C. (1991). Interleukin-1 receptor antagonist is a member of the interleukin-1 gene family: evolution of a cytokine control mechanism. Proc. Natl Acad. Sci. USA 88, 5232–5236.

Endres S., Cannon, J.G., Ghorbani, R., Dempsey, R.A., Sisson, S.D., Lonnemann, G., Van der Meer, J.W.M., Wolff, S.M. and Dinarello, C.A. (1989). In vitro production of IL-1 beta, IL-1 alpha, TNF and IL-2 in healthy subjects: distribution, effect of cycloxygenase inhibition and evidence of independent gene regulation. Eur. J. Immunol. 19, 2327–2333.

Fenton, M.J., Clark, B.D., Collins, K.L., Webb, A.C., Rich, A. and Auron, P.E. (1987). Transcriptional regulation of the human prointerleukin 1 beta gene. J. Immunol. 138, 3972–3979.

Fontana, A., Hengartner, H., Weber, E., Fehr, K., Grob, P.J. and Cohen, G. (1982). Interleukin 1 activity in the synovial fluid of patients with rheumatoid arthritis. Rheumatol. Int. 2, 49–53.

Fujimoto, J., Levy, S. and Levy, R. (1983). Spontaneous release of the Leu-2 (T8) molecule from human T cells. J. Exp. Med. 159, 752–766.

Fujimoto, J., Stewart, S.J. and Levy, R. (1984). Immunochemical analysis of the released Leu-2 (T8) molecule. J. Exp. Med. 160, 116–124.

Furuta, R., Yamagishi, J., Kotani, H., Sakamota, F., Fukui, T., Matsui, Y., Sohmura, Y., Yamada, M., Yoshimura, T., Larsen, C.G. and Oppenheim, J.J. (1989). Production and characterisation of recombinant human neutrophil chemotactic factor. J. Biochem. (Tokyo) 106, 436–442.

Gery, I. and Waksman, B.H. (1972). Potentiation of the T lymphocyte response to mitogens. II The cellular source of potentiating mediator(s). J. Exp. Med. 136, 143–155.

Gowan, M., Wood, D.D., Ihrie, E.J., McGuire, M.K.B. and Russell, R.G.G. (1983). An interleukin 1-like factor stimulates bone resorption in vitro. Nature (London) 306, 378–380.

Gowan, M., Wood, D.D., Ihrie, E.J., Meats, J.E. and Russell, R.G.G. (1984). Stimulation by human interleukin-1 of cartilage breakdown and production of human collagenase and proteoglycanase by human chondrocytes but not by human osteoblasts in vitro. Biochim. Biophys. Acta 797, 186–193.

Hatekeyama, M., Tsudo, M., Minamoto, S., Kono, T., Doi, T., Miyata, T., Miyasaka, M. and Taniguchi, T. (1989). Interleukin 2 receptor β chain gene: generation of three receptor forms by cloned human α and β chain cDNAs. Science 244, 551–556.

Hirano, T., Yasukawa, K., Harada, H., Taga, T., Watanabe, Y., Matsuda, T., Kashiwamura, S., Nakajima, K., Koyama, K., Iwamatsu, A., Tsunasawa, S., Sakiyama, F., Matsui, H.,

Takahara, Y., Taniguchi, T. and Kishimoto, T. (1986). Complementary DNA for a novel human interleukin (BSF-2) that induces B lymphocytes to produce immunoglobulin. Nature (London) 324, 73–76.

Hirano, T., Matsuda, T., Turner, M., Miyasaka, M., Buchan, G., Tang, B., Sato, K., Shimizu, M., Maini, R., Feldmann, M. and Kishimoto, T. (1988). Excessive production of interleukin 6/B cell stimulatory factor-2 in rheumatoid arthritis. Eur. J. Immunol. 18, 797–807.

Honda, M., Kitamura, K., Takeshita, T., Sugamura, K. and Tokunaga, T. (1990). Identification of a soluble IL-2 receptor β-chain from human lymphoid cell line cells. J. Immunol. 415, 4131–4135.

Isobe, M., Huebner, K., Maddon, P.J., Littman, D.R., Axel, R. and Croce, C. (1986). The gene encoding the T cell surface protein T4 is located on human chromosome 12. Proc. Natl Acad. Sci. USA 83, 4399–4402.

Jefferies, W.A., Green, J.R. and Williams, A.F. (1985). Authentic T helper CD4 (W3/25) antigen on rat peritoneal macrophages. J. Exp. Med. 162, 117–127.

Kavathas, P., Sukhatma, V.P., Herzenberg, L.A. and Parnes, J.R. (1984). Isolation of the gene encoding for the human T lymphocyte differentiation antigen Leu-2 (T8) by gene transfer and cDNA subtraction. Proc. Natl Acad. Sci. USA 81, 7688–7692.

Keffer, J., Probert, L., Cazlaris, H., Georgopoutos, S., Kaslaris, E., Kioussis, D. and Kollias, G. (1991). Transgenic mice expressing human tumour necrosis factor: a predictive genetic model of arthritis. EMBO J. 10, 4025–4031.

Krensky, A.M., Reiss, C.S., Mier, J.W., Strominger, J.L. and Burakoff, S.J. (1982). Long term human cytolytic T cell lines allospecific for HLA-DR6 antigen are OKT4+. Proc. Natl Acad. Sci. USA 79, 2365–2369.

Kupper, T.S. and McGuire, J. (1986). Hydrocortisone reduces both constitutive and UV-elicited release of epidermal thymocyte activating factor (ETAF) by cultured keratinocytes. J. Invest. Dermatol. 87, 570–573.

Leonard, W.J., Depper, J.M., Crabtree, G.R., Rudikoff, S., Pumphrey, J., Robb, R.J., Kronke, M., Svetlik, P.B., Peffer, N.J., Waldmann, T.A. and Greene, W.C. (1984). Molecular cloning and expression of cDNAs for the human interleukin-2 receptor. Nature (London) 311, 626–635.

Leonard, W.J., Depper, J.M., Kanehisa, M., Kronke, M., Peffer, N.J., Svetlik, P.B., Sullivan, M. and Greene, W.C. (1985). Structure of the human interleukin 2 receptor gene. Science 230, 633–639.

Linker-Israeli, M., Bakke, A.C., Quismorio, F.P. and Horwitz, D.A. (1985). Correction of interleukin 2 production in patients with systemic lupus erythematosus by removal of spontaneously activated suppressor cells. J. Clin. Invest. 75, 762–768.

Lomedico, P.T., Gubler, U., Hellmann, C.P., Dukovich, M., Giri, J.G., Yu-Ching, E.P., Collier, K., Semionow, R., Chua, A.O. and Mizel, S.B. (1984). Cloning and expression of murine interleukin-1 cDNA in E. coli. Nature (London) 312, 458–461.

March, C.J., Mosley, B., Larsen, A., Ceretti, D.P., Braedt, G., Price, V., Gillis, S., Henney, C.S., Kronheim, S.R., Grabstein, K., Conlon, P.J., Hopp, T.P. and Cosman, D. (1985). Cloning, sequence and expression of two distinct human interleukin-1 complementary DNAs. Nature (London) 315, 641–647.

Matsushima, K., Morishita, K., Yoshimura, T., Lavu, S., Kobayashi, Y., Lew, W., Apella, E., Kung, H.F., Leonard, E.J. and Oppenheim, J.J. (1988). Molecular cloning of a human monocyte-derived neutrophil chemotactic factor (MDNCF) and the induction of MDNCF mRNA by interleukin-1 and tumour necrosis factor. J. Exp. Med. 167, 1883–1893.

Mita, S., Maeda, S. and Shimada, K. (1986). Characterisation of human genomic DNA sequences homologous to the interleukin 2 cDNA. Biochem. Biophys. Res. Commun. 138, 966–973.

Miyasaka, N., Nakamura, T., Russell, I.J. and Talal, N. (1984). Interleukin 2 deficiencies in rheumatoid arthritis and systemic lupus erythematosus. Clin. Immunol. Immunopathol. 31, 109–117.

Mizel, S.B., Dayer, J.M, Krane, S.M. and Mergenhagen, S.E. (1981). Stimulation of rheumatoid synovial cell collagenase and prostaglandin production by partially purified lymphocyte-activating factor/interleukin-1. Proc. Natl Acad. Sci. USA 78, 2474–2477.

Mosley, B., Dower, S.K., Gillis, S. and Cosman, D. (1987). Determination of the minimum polypeptide lengths of the functionally active sites of human interleukins 1α and 1β. Proc. Natl Acad. Sci. USA 84, 4572–4576.

Muraguchi, A., Hirano, T., Tang, B., Matsuda, T., Horii, Y., Nakajima, K. and Kishimoto, T. (1988). The essential role of B cell stimulatory factor 2 (BSF-2/IL-6) for the terminal differentiation of B cells. J. Exp. Med. 167, 332–344.

Nedwin, G.E., Naylor, S.L., Sakaguchi, A.Y., Smith, D., Jarrett-Nedwin, J., Pennica, D., Goeddel, D.V. and Gray, P.W. (1985). Human lymphotoxin and tumour necrosis factor genes: structure, homology and chromosomal localization. Nucleic Acids Res. 13, 6361–6373.

Norment, A.M., Lonberg, N., Lacy, E. and Littman, D.R. (1989). Alternatively spliced mRNA encodes a secreted form of human CD8α: characterisation of the human CD8α gene. J. Immunol. 142, 3312–3319.

Pettipher, E.R., Higgs, G.A., and Henderson, B. (1986). Interleukin 1 induces leukocyte infiltration and cartilage proteoglycan degradation in the synovial joint. Proc. Natl Acad. Sci. USA 85, 8749–8753.

Ray, C.A., Black, R.A., Kronheim, S.R., Greenstreet, T.A., Sleath, P.R., Salveson, G.S. and Pickup, D.J. (1992). Viral inhibition of inflammation: Cowpox virus encodes an inhibitor of the interleukin-1 beta converting enzyme. Cell 69, 597–604.

Robb, R.J. and Smith, K.A. (1981). Heterogeneity of human T cell growth factor(s) due to variable glycosylation. Mol. Immunol. 18, 1087–1094.

Robb, R.K. and Kutny (1987). Structure-function relationships for the IL-2-receptor system IV Analysis of the sequence and ligand binding properties of soluble Tac protein. J. Immunol. 139, 855–862.

Rooney, M., Symons, J.A. and Duff, G.W. (1990). Interleukin 1 beta in synovial fluid is related to local disease activity in rheumatoid arthritis. Rheumatol. Int. 10, 217–219.

Rubartelli, A., Cozzolino, F., Talio, M. and Sitia, R. (1990). A novel secretory pathway for interleukin 1 beta, a protein lacking a signal sequence. EMBO J. 9, 1503–1510.

Rubin, L.A., Kurman, C.C., Fritz, M.E., Biddison, W.E., Boutin, B., Yarchoan, R. and Nelson, D. L. (1985). Soluble

interleukin 2 receptors are released from activated human lymphoid cells in vitro. J. Immunol. 135, 3172–3177.

Saklatvala, J. (1981). Characterisation of catabolin, the major product of pig synovial tissue that induces resorption of cartilage proteoglycan in vitro. Biochem. J. 199, 705–714.

Saklatvala, J. (1986). Tumour necrosis factor alpha stimulates resorption and inhibits synthesis of proteoglycan in cartilage. Nature (London) 322, 547–549.

Sariban, E., Imamura, K., Luebbers, R. and Kufe, D. (1988). Transcriptional and post transcriptional regulation of tumour necrosis factor gene expression in human monocytes. J. Clin Invest. 81, 1506–1510.

Schindler, R., Mancilla, J., Endres, S., Ghorbani, R., Clark, S.C. and Dinarello, C.A. (1990). Correlations and interactions in the production of IL-6, IL-1 and tumour necrosis factor (TNF) in human blood mononuclear cells: IL-6 suppresses IL-1 and TNF. Blood 75, 40–47.

Shire, L. Gorman, S.D. and Parnes, J.R. (1988). A second chain of human CD8 is expressed on peripheral blood lymphocytes. J. Exp. Med. 168, 1993–2005.

Stimpson, S.A., Dalldorf, F.G., Otterness, I.G. and Schwab, J.M. (1988). Exacerbation of arthritis by IL-1 in rat joints previously injured by peptidoglycan-polysaccharide. J. Immunol. 140, 2964–2969.

Swain, S.L. (1981). Significance of Lyt phenotypes: Lyt 2 antibodies block activities of T cells that recognise class I major histocompatibility complex antigens regardless of their function. Proc. Natl Acad. Sci. USA 78, 7101–7105.

Swain, S.L. (1983). T cell subsets and the recognition of MHC class. Immunol. Rev. 74, 129–142.

Symons, J.A., Wood, N.C., Di Giovine, F.S. and Duff, G.W. (1988). Soluble IL-2 receptor in rheumatoid arthritis: correlation with disease activity, IL-1 and IL-2 inhibition. J. Immunol. 141, 2612–2618.

Symons, J.A., McDowell, T.L., Di Giovine, F.S., Wood, N. C., Capper, S.J. and Duff, G.W. (1989). Interleukin 1 in rheumatoid arthritis: potentiation of immune responses within the joint. Lymphokine Res. 8, 365–372.

Symons, J.A., Eastgate, J.A. and Duff, G.W. (1990a). A soluble binding protein specific for interleukin 1β is produced by activated mononuclear cells. Cytokine 2, 190–198.

Symons, J.A., Wood, N.C., Di Giovine, F.S. and Duff, G.W. (1990b). Soluble CD8 in patients with rheumatic diseases. Clin. Exp. Immunol. 80, 354–359.

Symons, J.A., McCulloch, J.F., Wood, N.C. and Duff, G.W. (1991). Soluble CD4 in patients with rheumatoid arthritis and osteoarthritis. Clin. Immunol. Immunopathol. 60, 72–82.

Symons, J.A., Wong, W.L., Palladino, M.A. and Duff, G.W. (1992). Interleukin 8 in rheumatoid and osteoarthritis. Scand. J. Rheumatol. 21, 92–94.

Taniguchi, T., Matsui, H., Fujita, T., Takaoka, C., Kashima, N., Yoshimoto, R. and Hamuro, J. (1983). Structure and expression of a cloned cDNA for human interleukin 2. Nature (London) 302, 305–310.

Thoen, J., Waalen, K., Forre, O., Kvarnes, L. and Natvig, J.B. (1989). Inflammatory synovial T cells in different activity subgroups of patients with rheumatoid arthritis and juvenile rheumatoid arthritis. Scand. J. Rheumatol. 18, 77–88.

Weissman, A.M., Harford, J.B., Svetlik, P.B., Leonard, W L., Depper, J.M., Waldmann, T.A., Greene, W.C. and

Klausner, R.D. (1986). Only high-affinity receptors for interleukin 2 mediate internalisation of ligand. Proc. Natl Acad. Sci. USA 83, 1463–1469.

Wood, N.C., Symons, J.A. and Duff, G.W. (1988). Serum interleukin-2 receptor in rheumatoid arthritis: a prognostic indicator of disease activity? J. Autoimmun. 1, 353–361.

Wood, N.C., Dickens, E., Symons, J.A. and Duff, G.W. (1992a). *In situ* hybridisation of interleukin-1 in CD14-positive cells in rheumatoid arthritis. Clin. Immunol. Immunopathol. 62, 295–300.

Wood, N.C., Symons, J.A., Dickens, E. and Duff, G.W. (1992b). *In situ* hybridization of IL-6 in rheumatoid arthritis. Clin. Exp. Immunol. 87, 183–189.

Yasukawa, K., Hirano, T., Watanabe, Y., Muratani, K., Matsuda, T., Nakai, S. and Kishimoto, T. (1987). Structure and expression of human B cell stimulatory factor 2 (BSF-2/IL-6) gene. EMBO J. 6, 2939–2945.

9. Inflammatory Reactions in Arthritis

Hans-Georg Fassbender

Immunopharmacology of Joints and Connective Tissue
ISBN 0–12–206345–7

1. Inflammation

1.1   INTRODUCTION

The integrity of the human organism may be endangered by a multitude of harmful agents. The organism therefore attempts to maintain effective barriers against such noxious substances. If these barriers fail or if the body is attacked by any other means, the degree of damage is further limited by humoral and cellular reactions, which together constitute inflammation.

Foreign material, altered "self", or damaged body cells stimulate afferent detection mechanisms. This stimulation leads, via a cascade of reactions, to the formation or activation of effectors which function to clear the tissue of such material. The tissue homeostatis is effected by cell lysis, phagocytosis, enzyme hydrolysis and free-radical-generating mechanisms. If removal or neutralization of the trigger substances occurs, inflammation ceases and a repair process takes over. The immune system may be involved in the inflammatory process. It allows for specific recognition and removal of complex substances alien to the body. It is dependent on the nature of the inducing agent and the duration of inflammation, but its relative importance is, however, only recognized in the latter part of the inflammatory process. The inflammatory process constitutes a sequence of different reaction cascades which are very closely interconnected. Inflammation has three main phases: (1) exudatio, (2) infiltration and (3) proliferation. The blood vessels play a central role in the inflammatory process as a transport system for the humoral and cellular defence mechanisms. Depending on the extent of the lesion, the organism responds via an alteration of the plasma constituents which is manifested by the "acute-phase response".

The organism tries to adapt its defence processes against specific triggers, both qualitatively and quantitatively. This behavioural efficiency ensures that the border between the physiologically necessary regulation and the pathological inflammatory process is, as far as possible, not overstepped. As long as the reaction remains within a physiological framework, a proportional balance between irritation and a defence reaction is maintained. The inflammatory process also has a tendency to self-limitation: pathogenicity overrides the inflammatory process if (1) the quality, extent and duration of the injury necessitates defence reactions that also destroy local host tissue and (2) if the defence mechanism reacts against "self" because of an error in identification (autoimmune reaction).

1.2   HUMORAL REACTIONS

At the beginning of the inflammatory process the humoral, complement and coagulation/fibrinolysis/kinin-forming systems play a particularly important role.

The human plasma coagulation system consists of 15 different clotting factors, the activation of which is mediated by limited proteolysis. The coagulation cascade can be initiated both exogenously and endogenously. Both methods of activation lead finally to the formation of thrombin from prothrombin. Activated Hageman factor simultaneously catalyses the formation of kallikrein which leads to the formation of the vasoactive kinins, bradykinin and kallidin. Thrombin cleaves fibrinogen at specific sites to release the fibrinopeptides A and B. Subsequently the fibrin molecules aggregate forming a loose meshwork. Through the effect of Factor III, intermolecular cross-links are formed which reinforce the meshwork. At the same time, fibrinolysis is activated by plasmin. The conversion of plasminogen to plasmin is catalysed by both a t-PA and a u-PA. Activation of u-PA from the inactive proform is effected by kallikrein and plasmin. t-PA is primarily located in the endothelial cells and can be released by a variety of stimuli.

The complement system is built up in a cascade-like fashion from 20 plasma components. Its most important functions are the strengthening of antigen recognition by the immune system, facilitation of phagocytosis by opsonization of particles, solubilization of immune complexes and their transport to the phagocytic system, as well as the recruitment of leukocytes by leukotactic factors. The activation of C3 by the classical or alternative pathways initiates the formation of the membrane-attack complex as an effector on the surface of cells, which leads to cell death. The activation of C3 leads simultaneously to the coating of particles and immune complexes with C3b. This opsonization prevents precipitation of the immune complexes in the tissue and enables transport to the complement receptors on the cells of the mononuclear phagocytic system. The C5a formed by cleavage of C5 produces a strong chemoattractant for macrophages and can also be generated by other proteases.

1.3 CELLULAR REACTIONS

In addition to the reactions of the humoral system, cellular reactions play an important role either via phagocytosis and/or by the secretion of mediators.

All cells, except erythrocytes, have the ability to synthesize prostaglandins, thromboxanes and leukotrienes, which are arachidonate derivates, termed eicosanoids. These substances are not stored in the cell and have only a short biological half-life (in the region of minutes). The first stage of their formation is the release of arachidonic acids by phospholipase as a result of stimulation or membrane damage. Prostaglandins and thromboxanes are produced in interim stages by the action of cyclooxygenase, and the production of leukotrienes is initiated by the action of lipoxygenase. The amount and type of product is determined by the enzyme repertoire of the cells and tissues. Prostaglandins, leukotrienes and thromboxanes influence the tone and permeability of the blood vessels and have, to some extent, a leukotactic action on other cells.

The main characteristic of granulocytes is their chemotactic and phagocytotic ability. Important chemotactic factors for these processes are (a) C5a, C5,6,7, C3bBb, (b) fibrin fragments, (c) kallikrein, (d) collagen fragments, (e) bacterial cell wall components, (f) LTB_4. Granulocytes have the capability to ingest bacteria and other foreign bodies by phagocytosis and to digest them intracellularly. Phagocytosis is facilitated by opsonins (C3b and IgG), as recognition is via specific receptors for complement (CR1) and the Fc portion of the IgG molecule on the cell surface.

Furthermore, granulocytes can be activated by different signalling substances and react in two ways. On the one hand they accelerate oxygen consumption (respiratory burst) and generate oxygen-derived free radicals, which are extremely toxic to bacteria as well as being harmful to host tissue. On the other hand, degranulation leads to release of hydrolytic enzymes which effect tissue clearance in the surrounding area.

Macrophages become activated in response to cytokines from other cells, or by contact with antigen or complement. Following an appropriate stimulus, the macrophage is able to respond, releasing a number of secretory products such as lysosomal enzymes which are able to kill bacteria and degrade altered tissue. The macrophage is also an important source of pro-inflammatory cytokines (IL-1, TNF, IFN etc). The most important function of the macrophages is phagocytosis of foreign or damaged material which is processed intracellularly and then presented to the cells of the immune system. Phagocytosis may be facilitated by opsonization or, alternatively, as with PMNs, may be accompanied by a respiratory burst resulting in release of oxygen free radicals. The respiratory burst may also occur without simultaneous phagocytosis, being triggered by soluble factors (immune complexes, C5a). Parallel to this, release of arachidonic acid-oxidation products, such as TxA_2, LTB and LTC, occurs.

Lymphocytes are components of the humoral and cellular immune system. They are responsible for the specific recognition and removal of foreign and altered "self" material. Their antigen specificity provides an extremely efficient defence mechanism. Because of the time required for recognition and processing, the immune system dominates only during the later stages of the inflammatory reaction.

In contrast with macrophages, these effector cells of the immune system are not evenly distributed in the tissue but are localized in lymphoid organs (bone-marrow, spleen, lymph nodes). Some circulate in the lymph and blood.

1.4 TISSUE REACTIONS

1.4.1 Exudation

The first event in the process of an inflammatory reaction is the detection of damage. The initial changes recognized morphologically are the reactions of the local capillary network and the postcapillary venules as a result of mediator release. The most important are histamine (from mast cells and basophils), 5-HT (from platelets), bradykinin (through activation of coagulation) and arachidonic acid metabolites (from damaged or activated cells).

The first reaction of the microcirculation is an increase in blood flow to the irritated area, which results in the observed reddening and overheating of the tissue. Plasma enters the tissue via the enlarged gaps between the endothelial cells lining the capillaries (Fig. 9.1). The inflow of water caused by alteration of the osmotic balance leads to swelling.

1.4.2 Infiltration

A new stage in the inflammatory reaction begins with cell infiltration into the irritated area. The endothelial cells lining the blood vessels play an active role in this biphasic process (Pober, 1988; Kaul et al., 1991). The first cells to infiltrate the inflamed area are the granulocytes, followed in the second stage by the mononuclear cells (monocytes, macrophages, lymphocytes and plasma cells).

The infiltration of the tissue is controlled by the binding of cell surface receptors on lymphocytes (integrins) to ligands expressed on the surface of endothelial cells (adhesion molecules). Expression of integrins by leukocytes is augmented by antigen contact or under the influence of mitogens. The pattern of adhesion molecule expression on endothelial cells is controlled by cytokines. The combined effect of the resultant infiltration is therefore determined by the type of activation. For example, IFNγ regulates the adhesion of lymphocytes and IL-1 promotes infiltration of PMNs and lymphocytes.

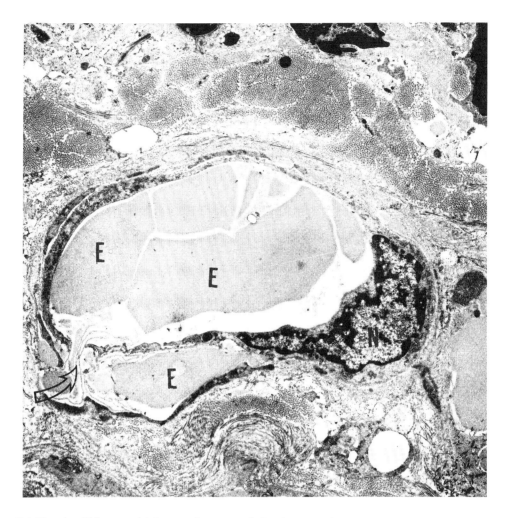

Figure 9.1 Venule within synovial tissue: plasma exudation between the extensions of two endothelial cells (arrow). N, endothelial cell nucleus; E erythrocyte.

1.4.2.1 Infiltration of PMNs

Simultaneous activation of the endothelium and slowing of blood flow through the capillaries and venules allows binding of PMNs to the vessel walls. Attracted by chemotactic factors, the PMNs then migrate into the tissue through gaps between the endothelial cells. The binding of PMNs to the endothelial cell is mediated by the integrin, CD11b/CD18 (Mac-1). This binds to ICAM-1 (inducible) and ICAM-2 on the endothelial cell surface. Further binding of PMNs is transmitted by ELAM-1 following activation of the endothelial cell by IL-1, TNF or LPS. The activation of endothelial cells leads to the synthesis of colony-stimulating factors which induce the production and release of further granulocytes from the bone marrow. Long-term stimulation results in reduced ability of the PMNs to adhere, and the infiltration phase terminates.

1.4.2.2 Infiltration of Lymphocytes

The inflammatory process acquires a new dimension by the switching-on of the cell-mediated response, morphologically represented by the accumulation of monocytes, T and B lymphocytes and plasma cells. The infiltration of the tissue by lymphocytes begins with the expression of adhesion ligands on the activated endothelial cells. The expression is initiated by IL-1, IL-4, TNF and IFNγ, appears later than with PMNs and is longer lasting. The interactions between LFA-1 and ICAM-1 and ICAM-2 as well as between VLA-4 and VCAM are well known. Further binding occurs after induction of ELAM-1. Additional control of lymphocyte circulation is effected by interaction of homing receptors on the lymphocyte with addressins, the corresponding ligands.

A turning point and critical step in the infiltration stage is the processing of antigens by MHC class II-positive cells. Macrophages and B cells contribute to this step, but other cells (endothelial cells, fibroblasts, chondrocytes) can also be stimulated by IFNγ to express MHC class II. Foreign substances are phagocytosed and processed within the cell. With the help of the class II molecule, small peptide fragments are presented to T lymphocytes for recognition by the T cell receptor. Upon antigenic stimulation, T lymphocytes respond by the secretion of mediator (including IL-2) which stimulates other lymphocytes to proliferate and become effector cells. Plasma cells develop from B lymphocytes and produce antibodies. After proliferation, another subset of B cells differentiate into resting antigen-reactive cells which serve as an immunological memory. T lymphocyte proliferation produces cytotoxic T cells which are capable of destroying the body's own cells. The secretion of MIF and MAF promotes the recruitment of further macrophages to the irritated area.

1.5   PATHOPHYSIOLOGICAL ASPECTS OF INFLAMMATION

From a pathological point of view, inflammation is a time- and self-limiting process with the aim of re-establishing the disturbed integrity. This corresponds to the term "acute inflammation". So-called "chronic inflammation," although an established term, is, however, pathologically incorrect if it is simply based on evidence of mononuclear cell infiltration into the synovial tissue.

It is important to make a distinction between genuine inflammation and the chronic immunological process because the two processes require different therapeutic treatment. This is well demonstrated by the fact that conventional antiphlogistic therapy, whilst suitable for the true inflammatory stage, is totally ineffective during the subacute chronic phase. It is a common misinterpretation to conclude that monocytic infiltration is proof of "chronic inflammation" as, for example, in the use of the term "chronic synovitis". In this process the synovial membrane manifests infiltration by cells morphologically characteristic of an immune reaction. As the experiments of Hanly et al., 1990) show, the infiltrating cells in patients with RA consist of up to 92% CD4+ lymphocytic memory cells.

Systemic immunological diseases such as RA are characterized by episodic inflammatory bursts which are triggered from time to time by the systemic immune process. Our observations show that, during the intervals between these episodes, the infiltration of tissues by lymphocytes and plasma cells is indicative of an expression of the continuing basic immunological process.

The fact that within all kinds of joint processes mononuclear infiltrates (monocytes, lymphocytes, plasma cells) are found after a short time, especially in the synovial villi, confirms that fundamentally (1) the inflammatory process never occurs without immunological participation, (2) the synovial membranes, especially the synovial villi, are particularly suited for the local immune reactions and (3) infiltration of lymphocytes and plasma cells is not specific for the disease. Consequently, the inflammatory reactions can be viewed as having two different aspects. (1) The reaction is a physiological, localized and self-limiting mechanism which is required for self-preservation of the organism. (2) Although the time-course over which this physiological reaction occurs is short, severe reactions are still capable of causing extensive structural damage.

If the control of antigenic and non-antigenic stimuli requires an increase in both qualitative (PMNs, elastase, collagen) and quantitative (macrophages, fibroblastic proliferation) activity, then biological tolerance will be broken, particularly if the immune process manifests itself in episodic bursts. As a consequence, the primarily physiological inflammatory process becomes pathological in nature, requiring the corresponding therapeutic intervention, in particular if the defensive motivation is lost, as is the case with chronic immune diseases.

In concert, the cell elements involved in the inflammatory process (PMNs, basophils, eosinophils, macrophages, lymphocytes, plasma cells), together with the complement cascade and the secondarily triggered cell proliferation (of the synovial membrane), constitute an impressive arsenal of defence mechanisms. However, they also represent weapons that not only damage localized structures but can also endanger life under certain conditions.

2.   *Osteoarthritis (Osteoarthrosis) (OA)*

2.1   DEFINITION

Osteoarthritis is the expression that dominates the Anglo–American literature and is a term reflective of clinical practice as a result of inflammatory symptoms in an arthrotic joint. The term osteoarthrosis is based on morphological–pathogenetical findings taking into account accompanying changes in adjacent bone structure, and currently is widely used in Europe.

Contrary to RA, which is a systemic disease with predilection for the joints, OA may run an asymptomatic course for many years and is exclusively characterized by the pathological changes at one or more joints. Signs of systemic inflammation are not a feature of OA. Sometimes the cartilage may be mechanically eroded down to the bone inducing pain which is not necessarily coupled with inflammation. It is only with the onset of a secondary synovitis ("inflammatory episodes") that OA becomes apparent. In 1985 a NIH (National Institutes of Health)-sponsored workshop defined the disease as follows: "osteoarthritis, the most common human joint disease, is of diverse aetiology and obscure pathogenesis and is a dynamic, but slowly progressive, non-inflammatory degenerative disease of cartilages and other tissues of joints, primarily in older individuals with intermittent, inflammatory episodes" (Mankin *et al.*, 1985). To summarize: "inflammation transforms the arthrotic into an arthritic".

2.2 PATTERNS OF OA

OA, predominantly affecting the large weight-bearing joints of the lower extremities, needs to be distinguished from the Heberden-associated OA of the finger joints of different aetiology and pathogenesis. Primary osteoarthritis without local disposition has to be separated from the secondary form. To the latter group belong osteoarthritic changes subsequent to pre-existing abnormalities as well as in the context of systemic diseases, e.g. RA.

2.3 STRUCTURE AND FUNCTION OF ARTICULAR CARTILAGE

The biophysical characteristics of adult articular cartilage, which is only a few millimetres thick, and its surrounding connective tissue enable the joint to withstand the strain of large and complex biomechanical forces over the course of decades. Implicit in this quality is the ability of the cartilage to bear loads many times that of body weight. This unique biomechanical property is due to the extreme swelling pressures generated by the hydrophilic nature of the proteoglycan molecules within the matrix which are underhydrated, and the special architecture of the collagen network.

Articular cartilage contains remarkably few cells. The only living element, the chondrocyte, comprises only 2–5% of the adult tissue volume, depending on age and topographical location within the joint (Stockwell, 1979). It is a highly and terminally differentiated mesenchymal cell recognizable as early as the 6th week in the developing embryo. The advanced differentiation is reflected in the complex ultrastructure of the cartilage cell.

The chondrocyte in the adult is differentiated from all other cells of mesenchymal origin by the following characteristics.

1. It can live in a largely anoxic (anaerobic) milieu.
2. It lives in an avascular environment and receives its nutrients and eliminates its waste products by diffusion through the extracellular matrix.
3. The adult chondrocyte seems to be a postmitotic cell and thus cannot be adequately replaced if lost.
4. It lives without direct cell-to-cell contact.

With the completion of the growing phase, the articular cartilage loses contact with the blood vessels of the bone marrow through the calcified zone. From this point on the nutritional requirements for the synthetic and other metabolic processes of hyaline cartilage are provided by diffusion through synovial fluid and have to take the following route:

- from the capillaries in the synovial membrane
- through the synovial stroma and the lining cells
- through the synovial fluid
- through the cartilage matrix
- ultimately to the chondrocyte

In comparison with the more direct blood supply of other tissues, the rather long supply line of cartilage is much more precarious and is vulnerable to interruption at any of the above stages. The removal of cellular waste products also takes place by diffusion through the cartilage matrix, the synovial fluid, the synovial stroma, finally to the lymphatic system.

The chondrocyte lives suspended in its own matrix, which affords the cell a certain protection from environmental changes in pressure. Currently it is recognized that chondrocytes in culture are able to synthesize and release the following substances:

1. predominantly collagen type II and up to 10% of minor collagens such as IX, X, XI and small amounts of type VI;
2. populations of aggregating (aggrecan) and non-aggregating (e.g. dermatan sulphate-containing) proteoglycans;
3. cartilage matrix proteins;
4. proteases;
5. protease inhibitors.

Proteins are synthesized in the RER, and the polysaccharides are added principally in the Golgi apparatus. The collagens are formed intracellularly as procollagens and polymerized extracellularly. In similar fashion, the intracellularly elaborated proteoglycan monomers attain their final aggregated structure outside the cell.

2.3.1 Cellular Heterogeneity

Adult articular cartilage can be divided, from the surface inwards, into three non-mineralized zones (I–III), which are sharply separated from a calcified zone (IV) by an interface, the tidemark.

Zone I. The tangential (superficial) layer shows the highest cell density. The most superficial chondrocytes are predominantly flattened and discoid and lie parallel to the surface. They have fewer organelles than the more deeply located chondrocytes of this layer, which show a less flattened shape. Consistent with their limited activity, the cell membrane of the upper tangential cells has only a few filopodia, in contrast with the deeper tangential chondrocytes and those found in the deeper zones.

Zone II. The typical functional active chondrocytes are found in the transitional (intermediate) layer where they exhibit characteristic ultrastructure. The round to oval cells with prominent cytoplasm are arranged singly or in small groups and are randomly distributed throughout the matrix. They have a round eccentric nucleus with a smooth membrane and frequently one nucleolus. The cell nucleus is surrounded by microfilament bundles arranged in parallel, which adjoin the nuclear membrane: this comprises a contractile structural protein. The remaining cytoplasm contains numerous free ribosomes, abundant RER and mitochondria. The Golgi apparatus is situated in a paranuclear position and consists of lamellar and vesicular structures. The chondrocytes also contain paraplasmic inclusions, mainly consisting of glycogen and lipid droplets representing stores for the predominantly anaerobic metabolic processes. The cell membrane of the active chondrocyte in the transitional zone shows a scalloped surface in the form of short finger-like processes which detach from the cell in the form of vesicles. Further away from the chondrocyte, these matrix vesicles lose their membranes.

Zone III. The chondrocytes found in the territorial matrix of the very deep layer of the radial (basal) cartilage zone are mainly ellipsoid and lie with their long axes vertical to the articular surface. They are grouped in a unit of radially arranged columns of two to six cells which is called the chondron (Aydelotte and Kuettner, 1992; Poole et al., 1988).

Zone IV. Between non-mineralized and calcified cartilage, an interface (tidemark) is recognizable even after decalcification. Without decalcification, this tidemark is characterized by a narrow band of vertical striation. In the electron micrograph, this corresponds to clusters of minerals that protrude 1–2 mm deep into the fibrillar space of zone III. After decalcification, the tidemark stains preferentially with a variety of dyes indicating the presence of a specialized extracellular matrix probably containing glycoproteins and lipids.

2.3.2 Collagens

To date, five different types of collagen have been identified in hyaline articular cartilage. Type II collagen is the predominant fibrous component, and most minor (types VI, IX, X and XI) collagens undoubtedly have important functions in determining the unique properties of the tissue (Eyre et al., 1987, 1992).

It is known from the studies of Benninghoff (1939) that collagen fibres assume an arcade-like structure at the surface of articular cartilage. However, in the deeper layers, these fibres form a tissue-specific three-dimensional framework in which constituents, such as proteoglycans or glycoproteins, are enmeshed or attached. Such interactions reinforce the stability of this network. It is thought that two of the minor collagens are involved in the fibril formation process in the cartilage matrix. Type IX collagen has been localized at intersection points between collagen fibrils. As it is covalently bound to type II collagen, it may function as a "connector" or "glue" molecule between type II fibrils (Mayne and Burgeson, 1987; Vaughan et al., 1988; Eyre et al., 1987). As a consequence, the type II collagen fibres

become less extensible. Type IX collagen is assembled from three different peptide chains and, to one of them, a single chondroitin sulphate chain is covalently bound, making it a proteoglycan as well (Mayne and Burgeson, 1987). It has been postulated that the type II collagen fibrous network becomes less rigid if these "connector" molecules are altered or diminished. As a result, the tissue is able to swell and its biomechanical properties are altered. Type IX collagen is also closely associated with the type II collagen fibrils, being localized within the fibres, and may be involved in determining their diameters (Mendler et al., 1989; van der Rest and Mayne, 1988). Type X collagen (Schmid and Linsenmayer, 1987) is synthesized only by hypertrophic chondrocytes and may play a role in the calcification process of the cartilage matrix. Small amounts of type VI collagen have been identified in articular cartilage especially in OA cartilage but not in other cartilages.

2.3.3 Proteoglycans

Most of the proteoglycans within the cartilage matrix are present as large aggregates, composed of proteoglycan monomers ("aggrecan"), hyaluronan (hyaluronate) and a link protein (Hascall, 1988; Heinegard and Oldberg, 1989). A proteoglycan monomer consists of a core protein to which large numbers of anionic glycosaminoglycan chains (predominantly chondroitin sulphate and keratan sulphate) as well as N-linked and O-linked oligosaccharides are covalently bound. Proteoglycan monomers can interact specifically and non-covalently with a small segment of a long polymer of hyaluronan via its specific binding region. Up to 200 proteoglycan monomers can interact with a single hyaluronan molecule of 1×10^6 Da and thus form aggregates of 5×10^7 to 5×10^8 Da which is more than 2 nm long as measured by electron microscopy (Rosenberg and Buckwalter, 1986; Thonar and Kuettner, 1987). A third component of the aggrecan aggregate, the link protein, binds to both the hyaluronan and the proteoglycan core protein, and stabilizes the attachment of each proteoglycan monomer (Kimura and Kuettner, 1986).

Several non-aggregating proteoglycans are also present in the cartilage matrix, including two smaller proteoglycans substituted with one or two dermatan sulphate side chains named "decorin" and "biglycan" respectively (Heinegard and Sommarin, 1987).

Owing to their high negative charge density, proteoglycans are characterized by their tremendous capacity to bind water. The hydroelastic effect of hyaline articular cartilage operates through a pump effect which results in the dissipation of energy after dynamic or passive loading. As proteoglycans are present in an underhydrated form (about 20% of its actual volume is remitted within the tissue fluid) in cartilage, they attract water, providing a swelling pressure of several atmospheres within the tissue. The collagenous network restrains the mobility of proteoglycans within the matrix and the pressure provides the stiffness and shape of the tissue. When load is applied to the cartilage, water is extruded from the loaded region. However, the movement of this water is retracted by the proteoglycans that are already in an incompletely soluble state. Through this loading and the removal of the water, the proteoglycans, and thus their highly charged side chains, are also forced closer together thereby increasing the effective charge density. Ultimately, the deformation of the tissue reaches an equilibrium when the load forces are counterbalanced by the swelling pressure of the proteoglycans. When the load is removed, the compressed proteoglycans attract water mostly from the synovial fluid and the tissue regains its original form when the equilibrium between the restricting collagen fibres and the swelling pressure of the proteoglycans is re-established. This pump system affords the removal of cellular waste products during loading and imbibing of nutrients for the chondrocytes during unloading. This process also represents a simple but ideal solution to the problem of shock absorption, enabling the articular cartilage, which is only a few millimetres thick, to protect the structure and function of the joint throughout life.

2.4 ATTEMPTED REPAIR PROCESSES

The potential of slow remodelling of the articular cartilage is retained throughout life. Characteristic features of repair processes in response to tissue damage in OA are, for example, the formation of chondrocyte clusters (cell nests, pathological chondrons) and osteophytes as well as the remodelling of the calcified cartilage zone.

2.4.1 Chondrocyte Clusters

Although the chondrocyte is regarded as a long-lived postmitotic cell which lacks reproductive function, chondrocyte clusters are observed in the vicinity of fissures in OA cartilage of the transitional and radial zones (Fig. 9.2.). The site of these cell clusters suggests that the

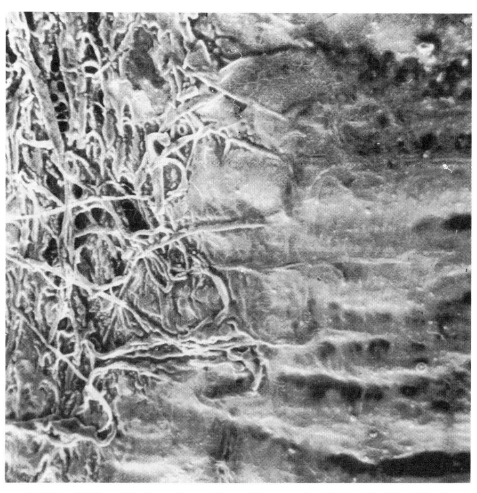

Figure 9.2 Incipient OA (knee joint): cartilage collagen fibres are denuded on the left, while they are still embedded in the proteoglycan-enriched matrix on the right-hand side of the picture. (Scanning electron micrograph.)

pathological increase in the cartilage surface in close contact with the synovial fluid may favour the proliferation of chondrocytes. However, these multicellular clusters are unable to synthesize normal matrix components. Thus, these components do not contribute to a functionally intact matrix capable of bearing load. Therefore, in spite of the quite impressive cellular hyperplasia, little repair of the cartilaginous network occurs.

2.4.2 Osteophytes

The formation of marginal new bone which follows the original lines of the joint surface can be observed as part of the bone remodelling processes characteristic of OA. The centre of the osteophyte consists of crude compact bone and an abnormal spongiosa with irregular bone trabeculae of varying thickness. The osteophyte is covered by rapidly growing newly synthesized fibrous cartilage. The structural integrity of the cartilage matrix, which is critical for the biomechanical function of the joint, may be compromised by the following external and internal factors.

The chondrocyte produces enzymes not only for matrix synthesis but also for its degradation. There is no danger to matrix integrity as long as these enzymes play their assigned role in the cycle of matrix turnover. The maintenance of structural integrity of articular cartilage depends upon a balance between matrix synthesis and degradation. These processes are regulated not only by chondrocyte-derived enzymes (such as metalloproteinases) (Murphy *et al.*, 1981; Morales and Kuettner, 1982) and enzyme inhibitors (such as TIMP) (Hembry *et al.*, 1985) but, most probably, also by growth factors, hormones and vitamins as suggested by *in vitro* and animal experiments. Experiments performed by Dingle and colleagues (1979) have shown that inflammatory mediators such as IL-1 ("catabolin") released by SM act on the chondrocytes, leading to an uncontrolled release of proteolytic enzymes. In addition, the mediators also downregulate proteoglycan synthesis, thus disrupting the fine balance between anabolism and catabolism which results in chondrocytic chondrolysis (Aydelotte *et al.*, 1986).

External proteases, singularly or in combination, can destroy extracellular matrix components. Chondrocyte-derived and external collagenases, however, specifically attack collagen types II and XI in cartilage (Gadher *et al.*, 1988). Enzymic attack on the collagen network is only likely when it is exposed through loss of the protective proteoglycan coat, and is thus secondary to extensive degradation of the proteoglycan molecule. Hyaluronidase can theoretically degrade the hyaluronan and most of the other glycosaminoglycans; however, no endogenous hyaluronidase has been found in cartilage. Proteoglycan degradation is mostly attributed to metalloproteinases, especially stromelysin, which cleaves the proteoglycan core protein. The resulting fragments diffuse out of the matrix. It is noteworthy that

stromelysin can also degrade the telopeptides of type II collagen and the associated type IX collagen, thereby loosening the collagenous network of the tissue. The decrease in proteoglycan concentration and the loosening of the fibrillar structure lead to an increase in water content and thus a decrease in biomechanical properties of the tissue.

In contrast with this primarily biochemical viewpoint, Maroudas and colleagues (1986) consider that the primary event leading to the systematic degradation of matrix components is unphysiological dynamic loading, leading to overstressing of the collagen fibre network. Rupture of the collagen network induces a release of proteoglycans and causes an increased water influx followed by failure of the hydroelastic system. A summary of the various factors that may compromise the integrity of hyaline articular cartilage includes:

1. destruction of the collagen network secondarily to mechanical overloading and physical trauma;
2. loosening of the collagen network following enzymic degradation of type IX and/or type II collagen by stromelysin;
3. excessive release of chondrocyte proteases, mostly metalloproteinases, induced by mediators such as IL-1 derived from the inflamed synovial tissue;
4. toxic damage risk to the chondrocytes by disease-modifying agents, such as dexamethasone and some NSAIDs;
5. damage to the chondrocytes due to inadequate nutrition secondarily to interruption of the supply route between synovial capillaries and chondrocytes;
6. alteration of specific non-collagenous matrix proteins, the function of which is currently incompletely understood.

Singly or in combination, these mechanisms ultimately lead to a qualitative deterioration of hyaline articular cartilage. This deterioration may be critical for loaded joints where an imbalance can arise between the quality of the matrix and the mechanical load, leading to cartilage failure.

Although the aetiology of OA is still not completely understood, it is unlikely that a single cause will be found to be responsible. More probably the different factors listed above may combine during the course of the OA disease process, with the predominance of nutritional, toxic, enzymic or physical causes in individual cases. This mosaic of factors responsible for the OA process is reflected in the clinical heterogeneity of OA and is a major impediment to the evaluation of therapy in this disease.

Biochemical and biophysical deficiencies in the matrix predominantly affect the quality of the superficial structure of the hyaline cartilage. The earliest morphological sign of this structural insufficiency is an incipient denudation of the collagen fibre network, marking the first step toward mechanical damage (Fig. 9.2). Small areas of roughness develop in the joint surface which, with increasing friction, expand in area. Subsequently, fissures develop, increasing in number and depth over the course of time. Owing to the arcade-like structure of the collagen fibres, these fissures initially run parallel to the surface and then orient vertically in the deeper layer above the tidemark. Meachim and Brooke (1984) described small horizontal fissures arising secondarily to loading between the calcified and non-calcified zones.

Complete denudation of the collagen fibres leads to a progressive phase. The joint surface becomes roughened with fissures and cartilage separation and may advance to complete abrasion of the cartilage substance. In this way, the smooth joint surface becomes fibrillated, and, during this process, flakes of cartilage which are partially free are moved by joint activity. Such fragments become strangulated and detached from their origin and float freely in the synovial fluid.

2.5 SYNOVIAL PROCESSES

During the attrition of cartilage in the degradative phase, fragments of collagen fibres, proteoglycans and calcium hydroxyapatite crystals may be found in the synovial fluid. Inflammation may then develop in the synovial membrane, and, through the action of mediators, phagocytic degradative enzymes are released.

Synovitis found secondary to OA or in trauma develops from an irritation of the lining cells which undergo mild proliferation. Thereby, club-shaped villi are formed which are initially delicate, then become solid with the development of a sparse stroma with occasional blood vessels. These dainty villi are often found in large numbers in OA and traumatic synovitis. In contrast with the "fibrinous villi" seen in systemic synovitis (e.g. in RA) (see page 180), we call these villi "proliferative villi". With the course of time, these villi increase in volume; they become distended and can be recognized by their loose transparent stroma containing relatively few blood vessels (Fig. 9.3). The secondary synovitis in OA is not only painful but also endangers, by release of IL-1, the synthesis of the matrix in the still intact articular cartilage (Dingle *et al.*, 1991). As the secondary synovitis subsides, lymphocytic infiltrates may persist in the stroma of the villi in the form of small round follicles with a central small blood vessel or sometimes with real germinal centres (Fig. 9.4). These lymphocytic foci suggest the processes of antigen presentation and antibody formation and may bear witness to the triggering of immunological mechanisms also within the context of OA.

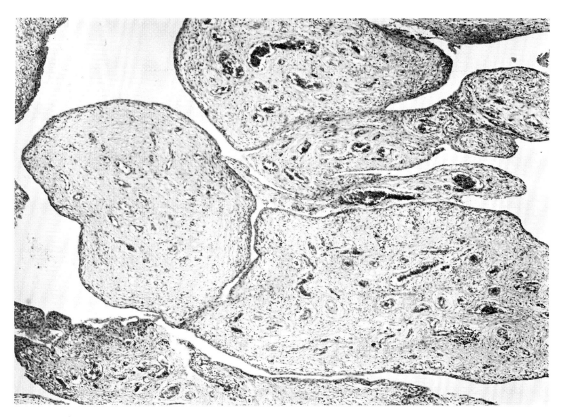

Figure 9.3 Secondary synovitis with hyperplasia in OA (knee joint): distended synovial villi with transparent stroma (vitreous "glass" villi).

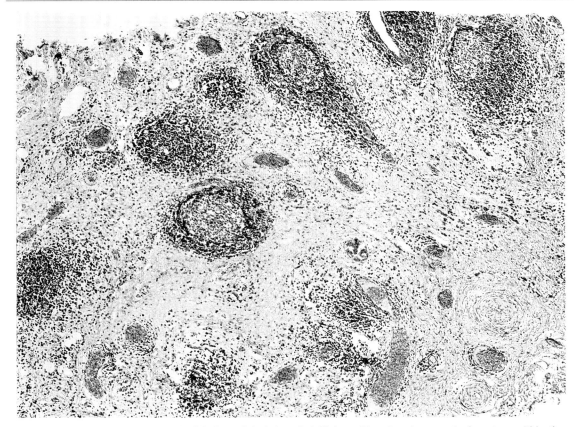

Figure 9.4 Secondary synovitis in OA (knee joint): lymph follicles with extensive germinal centres within the stroma of synovial villi.

3. RA

3.1 INTRODUCTION

Numerous studies have shown an increased association between RA and HLA-DR4. Twin studies, however, have failed to show a clear indication of strong genetic influence (Engleman *et al.*, 1983; Lawrence and Shulman, 1984). However, the importance of HLA-DR4 is not to be overlooked. Thus, the studies of Gran *et al.* (1983) and Calin *et al.* (1989) show a significant association of HLA-DR4 with seropositive RA (65% or 69% respectively) and with seronegative RA (55% or 60%) in comparison with the frequency in healthy individuals (27% or 36% respectively). Besides, HLA-DR4 seems to play a pathogenetic role in joint destruction in RA.

As, in the final analysis, immunopathological hypotheses fail to provide an adequate explanation, pathogens such as mycoplasma, clostridia and viruses have been proposed as possible triggers for RA (Alarncón, 1986). The evidence from viral antigens, viral genomes and viral products make a slow viral infection more likely than a conventional viral infection (Ziegler *et al.*, 1989).

It is estimated that the worldwide prevalence of RA in the general population lies between 0.3% and 2.0%. The incidence is thought to be 0.9%–1.5%/1000 per year (Lawrence and Shulman, 1984). However, the prevalence and incidence are higher in the urban black population in South Africa and among certain North American Indians (Yakima and Chippewa). RA affects women and men in the ratio 2–3 : 1. The peak incidence of the adult form of RA corresponds to the third and fourth decade of life, but RA can also occur in the second decade and as late as the eighth or ninth decade.

The term rheumatoid arthritis in reality hides a complex systemic disease which, although predominantly affecting the joints, may also involve other structures such as tendon sheaths, tendons, pericardium, myocardium, pleura, lungs, skin, sclerae, blood vessels and the cervical spine, and may progress under certain circumstances to a life-threatening condition.

The clinical diagnosis may be based on a number of features, which in general suffice to identify RA (Table 9.1).

3.2 STRUCTURAL CHANGES IN RA

As RA is characterized by damage and destruction of various tissues, a systematic examination of the

Table 9.1   The American Rheumatism Association 1987 revised criteria for the classification of RA

Criterion	Definition
1. Morning stiffness	Morning stiffness in and around the joints lasting at least 1 h before maximal improvement
2. Arthritis of three or more joint areas	At least three joint areas have simultaneously had soft-tissue swelling of fluid (not bony overgrowth alone) observed by a physician. The 14 possible joint areas are right or left PIP, MCP, wrist, elbow, knee, ankle and MTP joints
3. Arthritis of hand joints	At least one joint area swollen as above in a wrist, MCP or PIP
4. Symmetric arthritis	Simultaneous involvement of the same joint areas (as in 2) on both sides of the body (bilateral involvement of PIPs, MCPs or MTPs is acceptable without absolute symmetry)
5. Rheumatoid nodules	Subcutaneous nodules, over bony prominences, or extensor surfaces, or in justarticular regions, observed by a physician
6. Serum rheumatoid factor	Demonstration of abnormal amounts of serum rheumatoid factor by any method that has been positive in less than 5% of normal control subjects
7. Radiological changes	Radiological changes typical of RA on PA hand and wrist roentgenograms, which must include erosions or unequivocal bony decalcification localized to, or most marked adjacent to, the involved joints (OA changes alone do not qualify)

Abbreviations: PIPs; proximal interphalangeal joints; MCPs; metacarpophalangeal joints; MTPs, metatarsophalangeal joints; PA, posteroanterior.
Arnett *et al.* (1988).

morphological process is required. Therefore, joint tissue from patients with different rheumatic diseases should be compared by the following morphological features: (a) fibrin, (b) lymphocytes, (c) lymph follicles, (d) plasma cells, (e) PMNs, (f) siderophages, (g) villous formation, (h) lining cell proliferation, (i) giant cells, (j) stromal cell proliferation, (k) tumour-like proliferation, (l) joint destruction, (m) RA necroses and (n) fibrous stratum.

3.3   THE JOINT PROCESS

The processes occurring in the joint in RA are initiated from the synovial tissue. The normal unchanged synovial membrane has the following characteristics. (1) The surface is folded but has no villi. (2) The lining cell layer is single layered and comprises flattened lining cells. (3) The synovial stroma consists of a loose collagen fibre network sparsely populated with cells. The few fibroblasts are spindle-shaped, with small dense nuclei. Occasional macrophages may be found. (4) Blood vessels are thin-walled and sparse.

The dynamics of RA are reflected in the phasic nature of the morphological processes. The synovial processes may essentially be divided into four different phases which, during the course of the disease, merge with each other and may be repeated after every exacerbation.

3.3.1   The Exudative Stage

1. The synovial surface is smooth or contains villi resulting from the previous fibrinous phase. 2. The lining cell layer elaborates fresh deposits of fibrin. In contrast

with bacterial arthritis, the fibrin is not lamellar and only contains occasional PMNs. 3. In the area of fibrin deposition, the lining cells mainly die. The lining cell layer will then later regenerate in single to multiple layers, the cells becoming cuboid or high-cylindrical. 4. The synovial stroma demonstrates variable cell density because of hypertrophy and hyperplasia of the synovial fibroblasts. During this phase, lymphocytes and plasma cell numbers can vary from sparse to moderate, with the appearance of occasional macrophages. PMNs, if seen at all, are found singly in contact with the fibrin deposits.

The fibrinous exudate is a hallmark of clinical exacerbation of the underlying systemic process in RA. The response of the mesenchymal cell elements to the acute exudative phase is one of proliferation.

3.3.2   The Proliferative Stage

3.3.2.1   Proliferative Phase

1. The synovial surface is smooth or contains villi resulting from a previous exudative phase (see page 179). 2. The lining cell layer is dispersed with sparse membranous deposits of fibrin. Larger disorganized deposits of fibrin may, however, become detached from the surface and enter the joint cavity. 3. The lining cell layer is multigraded, and the regenerated cells are either cuboid or high-cylindrical in shape. Bud-like outgrowths of the lining cells can be seen. In the synovial tissue, frequently multinuclear synoviogenous giant cells, occasionally seen in large numbers, lie in close contact with the lining cell layer. These giant cells do not contain foreign bodies

(see page 180). 4. The synovial stroma appears to be extended. Areas are seen in which the synovial fibroblasts are hypertrophic, markedly increased in numbers and densely packed. On the margin of these proliferative zones, a few lymphocytes may be found together with occasional widely dispersed macrophages; no PMNs are evident (Fig. 9.5).

The degree of proliferation depends upon the extent and time point of the preceding fibrinous exudation. Synoviocyte proliferation may be focal or may involve large areas or all of the synovial membrane.

3.3.2.2 Tumour-like Proliferation

Proliferation of the synovial stroma cells occurring in association with the exudative phase may take on excessive proportions. At the peak of the proliferative stage, the demarcation line between the lining cell layer and the synovial stroma disappears. In extreme cases the proliferation of the synovial stroma is such that one cell lies next to another. This appearance can be very similar to that seen with malignant tumours. In agreement with the Deutsches Krebsforschungszentrum (German Cancer Research Centre) in Heidelberg and the Abteilung für Krebsforschung am Pathologischen Institut der Universität Zürich (Department of Cancer Research in

the Institute of Pathology of the University in Zurich), we have called this phenomenon TLP (Fassbender et al., 1980).

In their quiescent state, the normally unremarkable synovial stroma cells are oval to spindle-shaped. Similarly, the nucleus is elongated to oval in form, relatively small and stains darkly with haematoxylin. With increasing degrees of proliferation, the cells become progressively rounded, with an increasing nucleus/plasma ratio. The nuclear structure becomes less dense, the nuclei are round and vesicular with one or two nucleoli. At this stage, mitoses are also found. Occasional macrophages may be evident at the edges of the zone of proliferation (Fig 9.6).

In these extremely proliferating cells (TLP), we found high expression of the following oncogenes: myb in nine, myc in eight, ras in eleven, and fos in ten of 13 patients with seropositive RA. In contrast, myb, myc and ras were not detected in the synovium of patients with OA, and only two of five patients expressed fos. The fact that the nuclear oncoproteins Myb, Myc and Fos have immortalizing activity rescuing primary cells from senescence and the ability to cooperate with an activated ras gene in the transformation of primary cells indicates that these oncogenes are associated with the TLP cells found at the

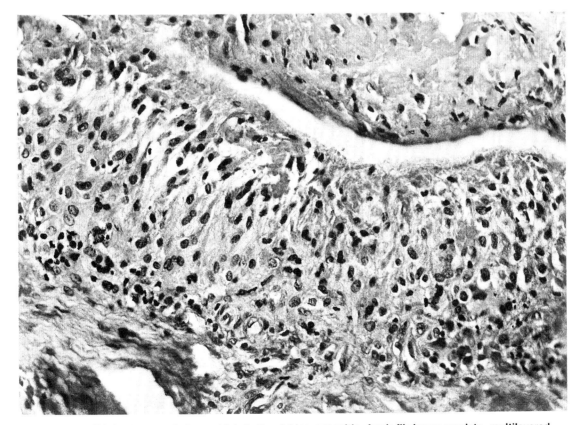

Figure 9.5 RA (metacarpophalangeal joint): flourishing synovitis, fresh fibrinous exudate, multilayered proliferation of synovial cells, solitary lymphocytes.

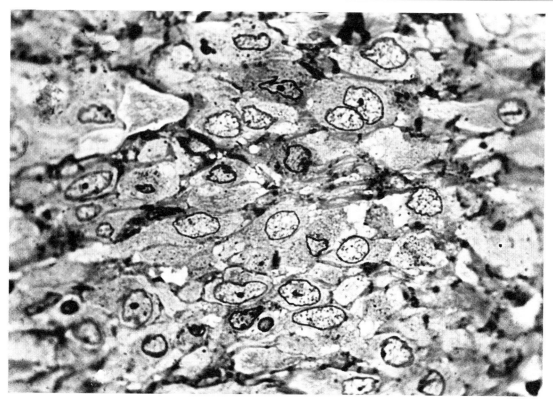

Figure 9.6 RA (proximal interphalangeal joint): compact TLP mass. The cells are oval to polyhedral and sometimes multinuclear. The nuclei are large and vesicular containing up to two nucleoli.

site of joint destruction in RA (Gay *et al.*, 1989; Trabandt *et al.*, 1991).

The endothelial cells of the arterioles and venules also participate in the proliferation process. In the region of the TLP, the lymphocytic and plasma cell infiltrates largely or completely disappear. These infiltrates, however, tend to persist in the synovial villi which rarely or to only a small extent participate in the proliferation process. In our experience, remnants of the exudative process are still evident during the TLP stage. We feel therefore that there is a causal relationship between fibrin exudation and TLP.

Our studies have shown that in seropositive RA patients, the TLP phase is correlated with a high ESR. Fibrin exudation followed by excessive synovial proliferation is thus the morphological equivalent of the acute flare up in the involved joint (Misskampf, 1984).

3.3.3 The Transition Stage

Our extensive studies on a large number of synovial specimens from patients with well-documented clinically typical RA has led us to the conclusion that the changes seen in the synovial membrane represent a dynamic process corresponding to the exacerbations and remissions characteristic of the clinical disease course. And so the TLP phase of the stroma cells is followed by a waning

of the TLP cells and the transition into a resting phase for the synovial membrane. This transition phase is characterized by the following features.

1. Old fibrin is found at the surface in the state of villous remodelling.
2. The lining cell layer becomes a single cell layer once again; the cells vary between flat and cuboid in shape.
3. The TLP cells decrease in size and number. They lose their round form and there is a reduction in the nucleus/plasma ratio. Single giant cells are only seen very occasionally.
4. Lymphocytes and plasma cells reappear together with occasional macrophages and a small number of mast cells.
5. Newly formed small-calibre blood vessels are found in the stroma, and there is a slight increase in collagen.

3.3.4 The Quiescent Stage

This phase is characterized by a lack of exudative and proliferative phenomena in addition to synovial fibrosis. 1. On the surface, villi are found with a fibrosed stroma and newly formed blood vessels. There is no fibrin deposition. 2. The lining cell layer is single graded; the cells are flattened. No giant cells are seen. 3. The synovial stroma is moderately fibrosed and contains newly formed blood vessels, predominantly venules. Only a few slender fibroblasts are evident. In contrast, large numbers of lymphocyte aggregates are found; occasionally, mainly in the synovial villi, lymph follicles with pale germinal centres are also to be seen. Perivascular plasma cells may be found occasionally. They are more diffusely spread and very rarely may be found in dense aggregates. PMNs are not found! 4. The subsided exudative–proliferative phase leaves iron-laden macrophages (siderophages) behind, which are grouped at the border of the fibrous stroma around small blood vessels. (This is in contrast with villonodular synovitis, in which siderocytes may be spread throughout the entire synovial membrane, and with haemarthros, in which the haemosiderin is stored in the lining cells.)

It is understandable from the episodic nature of RA that the remnants of the local processes summate with every exacerbation of the disease. In this way, villous formation, fibrosis and the formation and size of blood vessels increase with each flare up.

3.4 FEATURES OF THE SYNOVIAL PROCESS IN RA

3.4.1 Fibrin Organization and Granulation Tissue (In General)

Except in RA, fibrinous exudate is generally organized by the surrounding mesenchymal tissue, i.e. with the penetration of PMNs, fibroblasts and angioblasts into the fibrin. Penetration is followed by enzymic fibrin degradation by PMNs and the formation of a granulation tissue within the loosely structured fibrinous mass. Granulation tissue is characterized by a disordered network of newly formed collagen fibres and capillaries. Within this network, a rich variety of cells is found, including macrophages, fibroblasts, PMNs, mast cells and occasional lymphocytes. It is the role of the granulation tissue to enzymically digest and resorb the fibrinous exudate and to organize new tissue. As this process proceeds, the cellular content diminishes and the collagen fibre frame becomes increasingly dense. The result of organization by the granulation tissue is the collagenous scar.

In order to appreciate the unusual nature of the synovial process, it is interesting to imagine what the result would be if the events described above also occurred in the SM in RA. In this case, the fibrin deposits, which are often extensive, would be transformed into collagenous scars within the synovial tissue. This would lead to destruction of the synovial architecture and a compromise of function. On the one hand, normal synovial reactions would come to an end, as there would no longer be any reactive tissue available for exudation or proliferation, and, on the other hand, the SM would lose its nutritional role for articular cartilage. With this background, the uniqueness of the synovial reaction in RA and other non-

bacterial arthritides becomes clear. In these conditions the process is as follows.

After the exudation of plasma, fibrinogen polymerizes to fibrin on the synovial surface. The lining cells underneath die. The synovial stroma fails to react by forming granulation tissue but instead reacts by proliferating homogeneous oval synovial fibroblasts with large nuclei. These cells penetrate and migrate through the overlying fibrin and form a new lining cell layer on the fibrin surface. By avoiding the formation of scar tissue, limited deposits of fibrin are thus integrated into the genuine structure.

3.4.2 Lining Cells

The lining cells vary in form and arrangement. In a phase of quiescence, they are flat to cuboid. With irritations of various aetiology, they react by increasing volume and forming a multigraded lining cell layer. Under these circumstances, they may form structures reminiscent of high-cylindrical glandular epithelium.

Barland et al. (1964) described two types of lining cells: (1) the macrophage-like A-cell with numerous microvesicles, various inclusions, lysosomes and a dense nucleus; (2) the secretory fibroblast-like B-cell with a RER and a loosely structured nucleus. According to observations of Ghadially and Roy (1967) the percentage of B-cells in synovitis of patients with RA is increased in comparison with the normal population. This is in contrast with studies of Stofft et al. (1988), who found, in patients with RA, an increase in A-cells in comparison with the normal population. It is uncertain whether these two cell types merely represent different functional stages of the same stem cell, especially as an intermediate stage, the C-cell, can also be observed. According to the studies of Zschäbitz and Stofft (1988), it is questionable whether the A-cells originate from the bone marrow, as they are negative for peroxidase and OKM-1 and do not bind any lectins. However, there is a high probability that monocytes emigrate into the lining cell layer during acute inflammation of the synovial membrane.

3.4.3 Synovial Villi

Synovial cells also migrate through large deposits of fibrin without the formation of granulation tissue. Although a new lining cell layer forms on the fibrin surface, the central deposits of fibrin remain intact over a long period. It is only after weeks or months that the base of the fibrin deposit comes into contact with the vessels of the SM. Blood vessels, fibroblasts and macrophages grow into the deposit. The fibrin core is slowly resorbed and a new synovial stroma develops under the lining cell layer. In this manner, fibrin exudate deposits are integrated into the SM, maintaining a functional synovial structure, which may be the stage for another exudative episode. This is the typical way in which synovial villi form. As previously mentioned, these villi are not part of the original structure of the normal SM. In every case, they are the product and relics of synovial proliferative processes. They arise in RA and other types of exudative synovitis through the integration of fibrin deposits into the synovial structure and lead to a massive increase in the synovial surface area.

3.4.4 Synovial Stroma Cells

Normally, the synovial stroma is deficient in cells. The loosely structured collagen fibre frame contains only a few dispersed fibroblasts with relatively small elongated nuclei. In RA, however, excessive proliferation of the stroma cells may occur, which then in a destructive manner may encroach on adjacent structures (see pp. 177, 182).

3.4.5 Inflammatory Cells and PMNs

Essentially, lymphocytes and plasma cells are not specific for RA. They may be found to a variable extent in all types of synovitis, from RA to post-traumatic synovitis. Lymphocytes are principally found in groups, which, in patients with RA, consist of up to 92% of CD4+ memory cells (Hanly *et al.*, 1990).

According to Natvig and colleagues (1988) the distribution of inflammatory cells in RA is as shown in Table 9.2.

In contrast, plasma cells are scattered, and occasionally found in aggregates. Focal concentrations of lymphocytes, occasionally even lymph follicles with germinal centres, are preferably found in the synovial villi (Fig. 9.7). It should be emphasized that, although this follicle formation is very common in RA, it is in no way specific. In our experience, follicle formation is also quite frequently seen in synovitis accompanying OA. It should also not be considered as a characteristic feature for

continuing inflammation, but rather as the expression of the immunological reaction of the organism to antigenic material.

PMNs appear during the exudative phase and rapidly migrate through the SM, which lacks a basement membrane, penetrating into the synovial fluid where, in RA, 2000–75 000 leucocytes may be be found. More than 50% of these cells are PMNs (Schumacher, 1985). PMNs are not essentially part of the synovial process in RA. They may be found very occasionally, if at all, in the area adjacent to a fresh fibrin deposit. The concentration of PMNs in the synovial membrane in RA is indicative of bacterial superinfection (Herbert *et al.*, 1990).

3.4.6 Giant Cells

Numerous synovial-derived giant cells are often seen particularly in RA in the area of the proliferating lining cell layer mainly after fibrin exudation. These giant cells do not contain any foreign bodies. Although they are commonly seen in RA and, according to Grimley and Sokoloff (1966), more frequently in seropositive than in seronegative patients, they are, however, also seen in synovitis of other aetiology.

After operations, particularly prothesis implantation, foreign body giant cells may be seen in great numbers. Their cytoplasm contains foreign material, which may sometimes be refractile depending on its nature.

3.5 DYNAMICS OF THE SYNOVIAL PROCESS IN RA

A photomicrograph entitled ''RA synovitis'' could suggest the concept of a definitive picture characteristic or even specific for RA and thereby of a stationary process.

Table 9.2 Inflammatory cells in rheumatoid synovitis

Dendritic cells (2–4%)
    CD45+, HLA-DR, DP, DQ+
    Antigen-presenting cells
    Induce MLRs
    Make clusters with T cells
T cells (70–80%)
    Mostly CD4+ T helper cells, but also CD8+ T suppressor cells
    T cells activated *in vivo*, HLA-DR+, IL-2R+ TfR+ (20–40% positive for these activation markers)
    Spontaneously produce and consume interleukins (IL-2)
    T help augmented, T suppression decreased
B cells (10–15%)
    Activated *in vivo*, develop into plasma cells
    Spontaneously produce Ig and antibodies (e.g. rheumatoid factor)
    Immune complex formation from antibodies (e.g. IgG rheumatoid factor) with activation of complement cascade
Macrophages (5–10%)
    Activated *in vivo* with phagocytosis of IgG and IgM complexes and ADCC-type cytotoxic reactions
    Antigen processing and presentation
    Collaboration with dendritic cells (?)

Abbreviation TfR; transferrin receptor.
Natvig *et al.* (1988).

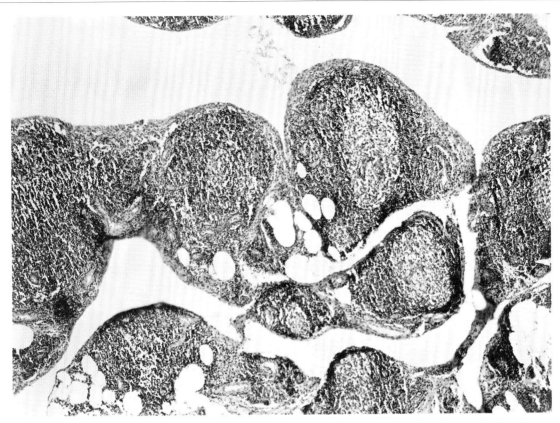

Figure 9.7 RA (knee joint): synovial villi with large lymph follicles containing extensive germinal centres.

In reality, a more or less dramatic process occurs in the synovial tissue, especially in RA but also in other arthritides, with a changing scenario which reflects the dynamics of the individual process. The photographic reproduction of lymphocyte and plasma cell infiltrates, lining cell proliferation and villi formation could be a snapshot of not only RA synovitis but also other non-bacterial joint diseases. (Only the evidence of RA necrosis, which is rarely seen in the synovial tissue, is specific for RA (see page 186).)

In the same way that one chord cannot represent a Beethoven symphony, a single histological "snapshot" cannot represent the synovial process in RA. The systemic illness moulds and directs the synovial process. In this way, the SM proves an extremely variable stage. Three components are involved: (1) fibrin exudation, (2) cellular infiltration and (3) cellular proliferation. Any of these three components may dominate the current picture.

3.6 HYPOTHESES OF JOINT DESTRUCTION IN RA

It seems plausible that joint destruction in RA arises secondarily to joint inflammation, which has been well documented clinically, immunologically, biochemically and morphologically. However, this concept is not compatible with the experience that, although pain and inflammation can be controlled with the available arsenal of steroids and non-steroidal anti-inflammatory agents, the process of joint destruction, as evident on the radiograph, is not influenced. When considering the possible pathogenetic mechanisms, it must be borne in mind that the destructive process not only involves the articular cartilage, but preferentially cortical bone, as our investigations have shown (see page 185).

At present, different hypotheses with regard to joint destruction in RA are being discussed.

3.6.1 Polymorphonuclear Neutrophils (PMNs)

The possible leading role of PMNs in joint destruction in RA is being discussed (Weissmann, 1971; Mohr and Menninger, 1979). There can be no doubt that the collagenases and elastases of the PMNs are able to degrade hyaline articular cartilage as is the case in septic arthritis. In contrast with RA in which the number of PMNs is not so high, in septic arthritis masses of PMNs are found in the synovial fluid, the enzymes of which can digest whole sequesters of the joint surface. The amount of PMN enzymes released in RA does not exceed the capacity of the inhibitors in synovial fluid (Kleesiek *et al.*, 1983).

In 1987, Jasin stated that, in RA, inflammatory cell concentrations are relatively low and hydrolytic enzymes and mediators are usually inactive because of the presence of inhibitors in excess. According to our observations, PMN occurrence is a rare finding in synovial membranes in RA, as Bywaters and Ansell pointed out as early as 1965. If, hypothetically, PMN enzymes affected articular cartilage in RA, destruction all along the joint convexity that comes into contact with synovial fluid would be expected, as is the case in purulent arthritis. Consequently the articular surface in RA would be extensively destroyed. Under no circumstances could we expect the simultaneous existence of intact cartilaginous surface and destroyed cortical bone, as we were able to show in 49% of our cases (see page 185).

3.6.2 Macrophages and Immune Complexes

In every inflammatory process, macrophages play an important role as producers of cytokines. As a direct attack of macrophages on healthy body tissue is hard to imagine, immune complexes deposited in articular cartilage have been ascribed a possible conditioning role. Cooke et al. (1975) and Menninger et al. (1983) have proved the existence of immune complexes in articular cartilage in both RA and OA. The latter study detected immune complexes in articular cartilage in six of 12 RA joints as well as in two of five OA joints, both with a similar pattern of distribution.

The question still to be answered is whether the macromolecular immune complexes can force their way into a cartilage matrix that is still intact. The avascular articular matrix is without doubt very suitable for the deposition of immune complexes; the vascularized bone, however, is not predisposed to such a process.

3.6.3 Macrophages and Cytokines

Of special interest is a possible immunologically mediated activity of macrophages for the destruction of articular cartilage. It has been presumed that macrophages are stimulated by T cells with the aid of IFNγ and other cytokines to release IL-1 and TNF-α. Thus fibroblasts and chondrocytes are stimulated to produce collagenases and other neutral proteinases (Arend and Dayer, 1990).

We have to take into consideration the fact that the release of IL-1 and TNF-α is a non-specific process that takes place in every inflammatory episode in general but in arthritides and thus also OA in particular. RA, however, has its own specific clinical and morphological profile, which is characterized with regard to quality and quantity. In particular, the primary destruction of cortical bone in RA can hardly be explained by this hypothesis. On the contrary, in accordance with Bromley and Woolley (1984), we have found single macrophages and some mast cells scattered in the region of subchondral bone destruction in RA, but only at a relatively late stage, i.e. when vascularization has taken place.

3.6.4 Chondrocytic Chondrolysis

On the basis of studies of Dingle et al. (1979), chondrocytic proteases are also considered responsible for the destruction of articular cartilage (Jasin, 1987; Arend and Dayer, 1990). There are numerous in vitro analyses of chondrocytic chondrolysis, especially with regard to the genesis of OA (Aydelotte et al., 1986). Occasionally, we were able to prove a minimal circular degradation of the territorial matrix in OA and RA, but these minor changes cannot be spatially connected to joint destruction. Furthermore, radiographic analyses by Mohr and Hummler (1986) demonstrated that the chondrocytes morphologically and functionally remain intact until they come into contact with the site of invasion by synoviogenous cell masses. From the quantitative point of view, the possible destructive role of chondrocytes should be doubted considering the fact that the cartilage cell forms only 0.1% of the total cartilage (Vignon et al., 1977). With regard to the destruction of cortical bone, the hypothetical role of chondrocytes being involved becomes irrelevant.

3.6.5 Osteoclasts

Many authors (e.g. Leisen et al., 1988; Salisbury et al., 1987) ascribe the collapse of the cortical bone in RA to osteoclasts. However, we have never found osteoclasts in the region where the destructive attack by synoviogenous cell masses takes place. In a study on 100 capitulae of metatarsal and metacarpal joints from patients with definite RA showing florid destruction of bone, no more than 12 showed single osteoclasts and they were found exclusively in the area where dead bone fragments were located and where remodelling was in progress (Fassbender, 1986b).

In agreement with Bromley and Woolley (1984), we detected single osteoclasts in the region of the breakthrough of the subchondral osseous lamella underneath a still intact articular cartilage. In this region, scattered chondroclasts in subchondral "pockets" could also be found (see page 186). However, this represents a relatively late stage already exhibiting cell deficiency and numerous blood vessels marking the beginning of pannus formation.

3.6.6 Invasion by Tumour-like Synovial Cell Masses

As long as granulation tissue or pannus at variable stages was the sole finding in the area of destruction in RA, there was understandably room for various hypotheses, all based on the premise that the destruction was secondary to inflammation.

In 1973 we described for the first time the appearance of compact groups of cells in the normally loose and relatively acellular synovial tissue in patients with RA. We could follow at the same time a stepwise change in the qualitative and quantitative behaviour of the synovial fibroblasts (synoviocytes). These cells, normally scattered and sparse, increase dramatically in number and lose their original spindle shape. They become oval and then round. This process can progress to such an extent as to give rise to a compact homogeneous mass of cells, which lie in contact with one another. At this time, a moderate number of mitoses can be demonstrated. In two studies of synovial tissue in 100 (Botzenhardt, 1975) and 265 (Misskampf, 1984) patients with clinically defined RA, we demonstrated that this proliferation of synovial cells corresponded to flare up of the disease and an increase in blood sedimentation rate. Subsequently, the synovial cells return to a fibroblastic form.

We reached a decisive stage in the explanation of joint destruction, however, when in 1978 we observed the continuous encroachment of such a compact cell mass from the synovial membrane along the "bare" area of bone on to hyaline articular cartilage. In contrast with the "pannus" known until this point, this was a synoviogenous compact homogeneous cell mass, which contained no fibres and, importantly, no blood vessels! (Fig. 9.8 and 9.9). We could clearly demonstrate and document the penetration of these cell masses into the cartilage matrix (Fassbender *et al.* 1980). These were the same large nucleated cells that we had described in the

TLP of the synovial tissue (see page 177). With invasion of the cartilage, the first step is degradation of the proteoglycans; the denuded collagen fibres remain intact, but with further progression they are also destroyed (Fig. 9.10). The cells adopt a radial formation at the invasion front as they penetrate between the fibres. The neighbouring chondrocytes remain intact until they are also caught up in the destructive process (Mohr and Hummler, 1986).

Size and nuclear structure of these densely packed cells are indicative of high metabolic activity. As may be expected, these compact cell masses have only a very short life span as they are avascular and the partial pressure of oxygen in synovial fluid is low. Because of inefficient supply of oxygen and lack of blood vessels, these cell masses lack equivalent life conditions on the joint surface and consequently the cells rapidly die. For this reason, the demonstration of this florid TLP stage in joint tissue is very difficult.

We could demonstrate the remnants of necrotic TLP cells using electron microscopy. The majority of the surviving cells show maturation to fibroblasts, although cell shape, nucleus and the presence of one to two nucleoli betray their origin as TLP cells. In between, single TLP

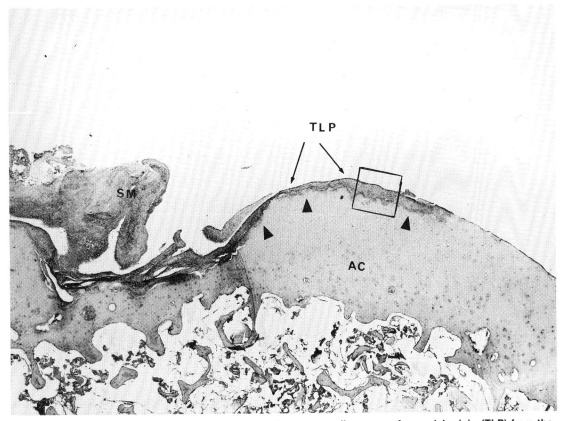

Figure 9.8 RA (metacarpophalangeal joint): attack of compact cell masses of synovial origin (TLP) from the synovial recess on to the left part of the articular surface, and invasion into the cartilaginous matrix. ▲, Site of invasion; AC, articular cartilage. SM in this instance refers to the synovial membrane. The area in the box is shown in more detail in Fig. 9.9.

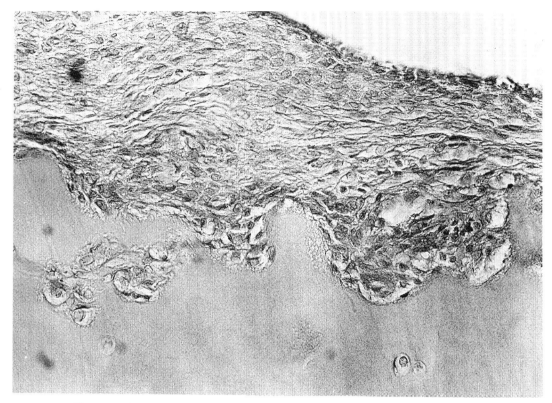

Figure 9.9 RA, detail from Fig. 9.8: compact avascular synovial cell mass (TLP).

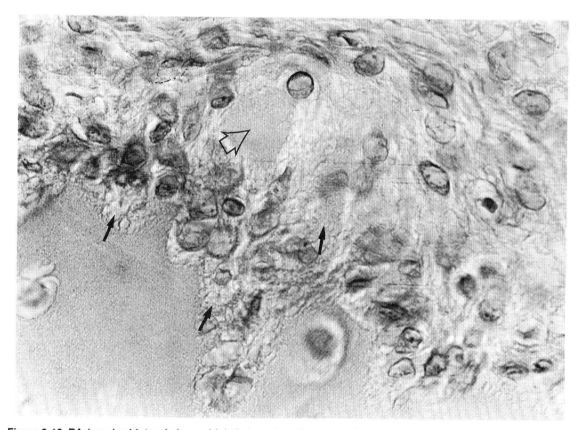

Figure 9.10 RA (proximal interphalangeal joint): invasion of macromolecular TLP cells into the articular cartilage.
→, denuded collagen fibres at the invasion front; ⇒, articular cartilage remnant.

cells are observed with their original form and structure. By light microscopy, a few penetrated blood vessels and macrophages as well as occasional single lymphocytes, PMNs and mast cells are detected at this phase. Those cells in contact with the invasion front now mainly lie along the cartilage surface, in contrast with the TLP phase. Only sporadically, cells with large nuclei (TLP) are found in the "attack position" described above, between the collagen fibres of the cartilage (Type II). The isolated macrophages that appear concurrently with the blood vessels are only engaged in a "clearance operation". We have never been able to demonstrate the penetration of macrophages into cartilaginous tissue in the region of the invasion front.

In this intermediate phase, it is possible to recognize for the first time the synthesis of collagen fibres by the fibroblast-like cells. This represents the beginnings of later pannus formation. This development is characterized by increasing deposition of collagen fibres (Type I) and a decreasing cellular content.

Pannus is a scar tissue that does not damage the articular cartilage. It seems likely that pannus acts like a shield to protect the underlying cartilage from further invasion from the synovium. The transition of destructive TLP tissue to well-recognized pannus (over cartilage and bone) may be divided into three stages: 1, tumour-like proliferation; 2, intermediate phase; 3, persistent pannus.

The term "tumour-like proliferation" raises the question as to how far these synovial cell structures compare and contrast with an MT. The differences between these two tissues are the following. (1) An MT grows slowly and its growth is coordinated with the accompanying vascularization. The MT accordingly has an adequate blood supply. In contrast, TLP tissue develops so rapidly that a vascular network has insufficient time to develop. (2) The MT has a long life span because of an adequate blood supply. In contrast, the TLP mass is fated to die quickly as, on the one hand, the highly active cell masses are avascular and, on the other hand, the multilayered densely packed cell mass in the joint space has insufficient oxygen. (3) An essential difference lies in the way in which the cell mass destructively penetrates the articular cartilage and juxta-articular bone. An invasion of tumour cells into the extracellular matrix faces a dense meshwork of collagen fibres embedded in proteoglycan gel. This sealed architecture forms a barrier which can only be breached by matrix-degrading enzymes. According to the studies of Fidler *et al.* (1978), Pauli *et al.* (1983), Woolley (1984) and Weiss and Ward (1983), membrane-associated factors of tumour cells induce synthesis and release of matrix-degrading enzymes in the surrounding mesenchymal cells. Collagenolysis occurs secondarily to a physical alteration of the matrix caused by an accumulation of glycosaminoglycans and is accompanied by an increase in water content (Knudson *et al.*, 1990). Cathepsin B plays a particular role in this

regard and is synthesized and released by stimulated host cells under the influence of tumour cells and activates collagenase (Graf *et al.*, 1981; Trabandt *et al.*, 1991). Sloane *et al.*, (1981) have demonstrated synthesis of cathepsin B in carcinoma metastases. In this manner, a pathway is cleared before the invasion of tumour cells.

In contrast, the relatively acellular cartilage matrix possesses only limited capabilities for degradation. On the other hand, the mildly proliferating synoviocytes in RA already synthesize metalloproteinases (i.e. collagenase and stromelysin) (Werb *et al.* 1986). It can therefore be assumed that the highly actively secreting TLP cells have a much higher potential for enzyme production, enabling active penetration into the articular cartilage and juxta-articular bone.

In the "bare area", between the start of the synovium and the border of articular cartilage, the TLP tissue is able to invade the cortical bone, penetrate the neighbouring marrow space and destroy the bone trabeculae. This penetration into bone corresponds to the radiological finding of the marginal erosion. The region of bone invasion next to synovium is soon surrounded by newly formed bone trabeculae; the point of penetration becomes filled by collagenous scar tissue after the TLP tissue has died away and remains recognizable.

The pannus scar protects the underlying joint cartilage from further invasion, but the destructive process may continue in the subchondral region (see page 186).

3.6.7 The Pathways of Joint Destruction in RA

According to the conventional concept of "inflammatory" destruction of the joint in RA, interest is focused on hyaline articular cartilage. However, with the experience of examining a large number of joint resection specimens (predominantly metacarpal and metatarsal heads), we gained the impression that the non-inflammatory TLP cell masses chiefly attack cortical bone in the "bare area".

Therefore we have examined the different pathways leading to joint destruction by studying 219 metatarsal and 69 metacarpal heads obtained during surgery from patients with definite RA (Fassbender *et al.*, 1992). The evaluation of these specimens revealed three pathways of aggression: A, in 15%, aggression on the articular cartilage only; B, in 49% direct invasion exclusively into the cortical bone; C, in 36% a "pincer-like" aggression, a combination of A and B in which the joint is attacked from both sides. In contrast with the hitherto conventional concepts, the findings of this study reveal a clear preference of the synovial aggression for the cortical bone rather than articular cartilage (pathway B).

The affinity of the TLP cell masses for bone tissue is of particular pathogenetic interest for the following reasons. (1) The observation that antigen and immune complexes may persist in avascular cartilage offers a theoretical basis for cartilage death (see page 182). (2) The demonstration of type II collagen fragments in the serum of RA patients raises the possibility of an immune reaction against this collagen type. Both these premises do not apply to bone. The structure of bone does not permit an accumulation of immune complexes. Moreover, bone contains fibres of type I collagen, so neither hypothesis finds support from our findings.

After destruction of the zone of contact, the TLP masses penetrate the structure of the joint in the following ways.

(1) Starting at the cartilage surface:
    (a) marginal cartilage destruction with centripetal expansion following the subchondral bone lamellae
    (b) marginal cartilage destruction with destruction of the subchondral bone lamellae and rupture into the marrow space with undermining of the joint cartilage.
(2) Starting at the cortical bone:
    (a) expansion of subchondral "pincers" (together with 1b) (Fig. 9.11)
    (b) spread into adjacent marrow space.

The TLP cell masses are only demonstrable over a few days; however, the persisting scar tissue remains as a permanent mark of synovial aggression. Although the invasive TLP masses, concomitant with their short life, are only seldom found in the marrow space, we regularly observe little subchondral "pockets" of newly formed blood vessels together with a variety of cells including fibroblasts, occasional TLP cells, macrophages and multinucleate giant cells ("chondroclasts", Bromley and Woolley, 1984) and collagen fibres during the intermediate phase. Rarely, occasional lymphocytes and PMNs are also seen. The ratio of cells to the newly formed collagen fibrils is soon altered in favour of an ever increasing dense fibre net. This smouldering subchondral process persists for a while after the TLP phase has subsided. Its destructive potential is, however, minimal.

Joint destruction secondary to aggressive TLP tissue can be explained by the demonstration of enzymes that have the potential to degrade cartilage and bone (Harris, 1976).

3.6.8 Rheumatoid Necroses (Rheumatoid Nodules)

In the field of general morphology, the rheumatoid nodule is considered to be an uncommon phenomenon. Its development is outlined in various hypotheses. One hypothesis claims a vascular occlusion to be the under-

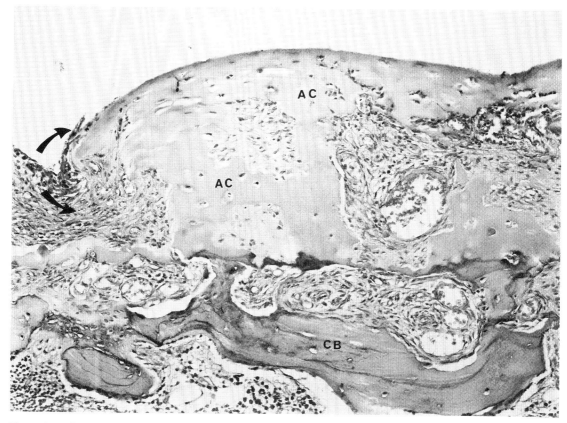

Figure 9.11 RA (metatarsophalangeal joint): undermining of the articular cartilage by marginal penetrated TLP masses (arrows). AC here denotes articular cartilage; CB, cancellous bone.

lying process. If this were the case, macrophages, fibroblasts and angioblasts would immediately infiltrate the necrotic area, as is the case in any infarction, but this has never been observed in rheumatoid nodules. The fact that the necrotic centre is surrounded by a dense palisade of fibroblasts which never penetrate the boundary line into the necrotic area (Fig. 9.12) as well as the configuration of the rheumatoid nodule do not support this hypothesis.

Another hypothesis, which claims that the development of rheumatoid necroses is caused by PMNs, is not valid, as no PMNs are found in the early developmental phases of the rheumatoid nodule. Furthermore, tissue destruction caused by PMNs would result in the formation of an abscess instead of acellular destruction of collagen fibres. The presence of immune complexes within the rheumatoid nodules does not offer an explanation for the devitalization of the connective tissue without corresponding cell involvement.

Nevertheless, humoral–immunological components must take part in the development of rheumatoid necroses, as, in principle, they are linked to the presence of IgM or IgG rheumatoid factors. (Re-evaluation of histological specimens of clinically defined rheumatoid nodules in seronegative patients showed them to be granuloma anularia.)

Another pathogenetic component is seen in minor tissue lesions predominantly found at mechanically exposed areas. Over a period of 10 years, we examined cutis and subcutis from the forefoot of 366 patients with seropositive RA, and in 71% we found rheumatoid nodules. We believe that the focal death of compact collagenous tissue of type I can only be explained by high local collagenase activity. However, as fibroblasts capable of collagenase secretion appear only after fibre dissolution, we have produced the following hypothesis: mechanically induced irritation facilitates the influx of serum containing rheumatoid factors into the tissue.

The observation that rheumatoid necroses never occur in rheumatoid factor-positive individuals who are not suffering from RA may be explained by the studies of Natvig and colleagues (1988). They found differences between the rheumatoid factors of patients with RA and those of healthy seropositive individuals. The latter virtually all show rheumatoid factor antibodies of the IgM type, whereas, in patients with RA, IgM and IgG antibodies are found. It is quite likely that only the IgG rheumatoid factors are pathogenetic, whereas the IgM

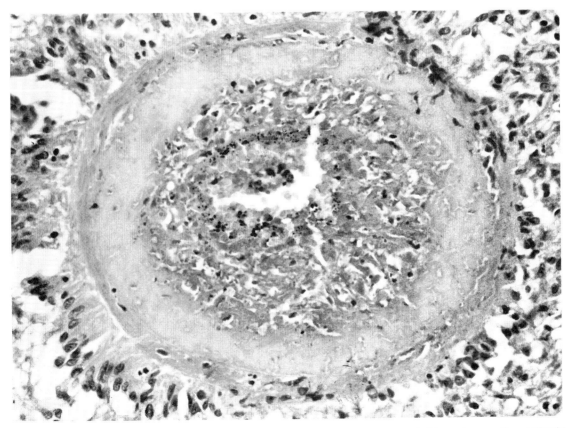

Figure 9.12 RA: total necrosis of all layers of a renal interlobular artery surrounded by a demarcating palisade consisting of connective tissue cells.

rheumatoid factors appear to escape into the blood circulation where they probably do not cause much harm.

The fact that necrotic processes are generally known only to be found in skin nodules has led to an underestimate of their importance to the patient. According to the site of involvement, nodules can simply be a cosmetic problem or they may give rise to more serious functional problems, destruction of a tendon, for example. Rarely, when the heart or blood vessels are affected, their occurrence may be life-threatening.

4.   Seronegative Spondylarthritides (SSA)

4.1   REA – A MEMBER OF THE SERONEGATIVE SPONDYLARTHRITIDES

REA is an acutely occurring painful arthritis which is primarily mono- or oligo-articular. In contrast with RA, the joints are afflicted asymmetrically, with the joints of the lower extremities, in particular the knee and ankle, being most affected. The term REA implies a causal association with a previous infection by certain micro-organisms. In general, the time period between infection and the subsequent arthritis is 1–2 months. REA generally develops in a self-limiting manner. In most cases, acute arthritis subsides after 3–5 weeks, sometimes only after a year; only rarely does it become chronic. Approximately two-thirds of patients with acute *Yersinia* arthritis have exhibited mild joint symptoms as late as 4–5 years after infection (Aho *et al.*, 1976; Kalliomäki and Leino, 1979; Marsal *et al.*, 1981).

Whereas with acute septic arthritis the causative organisms are found in the joints, it is a fundamental characteristic of REA that no organisms can be detected in the inflamed joint. This constitutes, however, a negative definition, which should be treated with caution because it may merely be limited by the present state of methodology. To date, only antigens of *Chlamydia*, *Yersinia*, *Shigella* and *Salmonella* have been identified in the synovial membrane and synovial fluid (Leirisalo *et al.*, 1982; Keat *et al.*, 1983; Taylor-Robinson *et al.*, 1988; Granfors *et al.*, 1989).

4.2   AETIOLOGY

There can be no doubt that the basis of REA is an immune mechanism, triggered by reaction of circulating antibodies to antigenic deposits in the synovial membrane. Briem *et al.* (1980) discovered circulating immune complexes in 13 of 14 patients with enteritis complicated by REA, but only in 26 of 44 patients without joint symptoms. In this context, the cross-reactions of antibodies against bacterial antigens with tissue antigens must be taken into consideration. For example, apparent cross-reactivity between antigenic components related to

HLA-B27 and materials derived from several Gram-negative bacterial strains (including *Klebsiella*, *Shigella* and *Yersinia*) has been demonstrated (Van Bohemen *et al.*, 1984). The Reiter–Fiessinger–Leroy's triad (Reiter's syndrome), arthritis, urethritis and conjunctivitis, was seen as the prototype of REA. However, among the REA it holds a special position in so far as, in most cases, arthritis is not time-limited, but becomes resident or chronic.

4.3   THE ROLE OF THE HISTOCOMPATIBILITY ANTIGEN HLA-B27

The presence of genetic traits of HLA-B27 seems to dictate whether or not REA will develop following an infection. Evidence for this has been obtained from the following observations. (1) 80–90% of patients with REA are HLA-B27-positive (Aho *et al.*, 1974; Håkanson *et al.*, 1975; Sairanen and Tiilikainen, 1975; Leirisalo *et al.*, 1982; Calin, 1984a,b). (2) *Yersinia* or similar intestinal infections do not normally lead to REA in individuals who are HLA-B27-negative. (3) Carriers of HLA-B27 genetic traits can develop reactive-type arthritides without previous microbiologically or serologically identifiable infection (Woodrow, 1985).

4.4   THE GROUP OF THE SERONEGATIVE SPONDYLARTHRITIDES (SSA)

Through the strict association with HLA-B27, REA was first assigned to the group of SSA as defined by Wright and Moll (1976). Spondylarthritides or spondarthropathies as they are called today have been characterized by Arnett (1986) as follows: (1) oligo- or poly-arthritis, (2) involvement of the skeletal axis with sacroiliitis and/or spondylitis, (3) absence of serum rheumatoid factors, (4) lack of rheumatoid nodules, (5) frequent inflammatory involvement of tendon and fascial insertions (enthesiopathy), (6) tendency to extra-articular manifestations including anterior uveitis, aortitis and skin lesions, (7) onset predominantly in young adults and children, (8) strong familial aggregation and close genetic association with HLA-B27.

By belonging to the group of HLA-B27-associated SSA, REA, which was originally characterized only by the direct relationship between infection and arthritis, now gains the extra dimension of an immunologically triggered systemic disease. The following diseases are included in the SSA group: ankylosing spondylitis, REA (including Reiter's syndrome), psoriatic arthritis, oligoarticular juvenile rheumatoid arthritis type II, Behçet's syndrome, Whipple's disease, ulcerative colitis and Crohn's disease. Rheumatic fever might well be categorized as REA because (i) it develops within a defined time period following a previous A-streptococcus infection and (ii) no reactive material is detected in the joint. However, rheumatic fever has no association with HLA-B27 and, furthermore, the focus of the disease is not in the joints but in the myocardium and endocardium. In contrast with arthritis associated with HLA-B27, the pathological mechanism of rheumatic fever has essentially been elucidated (Kaplan, 1963; Kaplan and Suchy, 1964; Fassbender, 1963).

Lyme disease should also not be categorized in the REA group even though the connection with a previous *Borrelia* infection is indisputable. The infectious agent *Borrelia burgdorferi* has indeed been identified in both synovial fluid and synovial tissue (Valesova *et al.*, 1989) but the lag time between infection and development of arthritis is extremely variable. As with rheumatic fever, no association has been found between Lyme disease and HLA-B27.

4.4.1 SSA and HLA-B27

Ankylosing spondylitis exhibits the whole spectrum of the SSA characteristics. Patients present with a wide range of joint involvement including ankylosing tendency in spine, hips, shoulders and lower extremities which may be partly asymmetrical, and have an almost

obligatory association with HLA-B27 (90%). In other diseases of the SSA group, there is frequent association with HLA-B27 but less involvement of the spinal and sacroiliac joints. For example, 80–90% of REA patients (including Reiter's syndrome) are HLA-B27-positive but only 20–30% of these exhibit uni- or bi-lateral sacroiliitis (Sairanen *et al.*, 1969; Marsal *et al.*, 1981; Leirisalo *et al.*, 1982). In contrast, the occurrence of HLA-B27 in psoriatic arthritis (20–35%) corresponds to exhibition of sacroiliitis with syndesmophyte formation (20–25%) (Schilling and Stadelmann, 1986). But interestingly, in psoriatic arthritis, approximately 60% of patients with skeletal axis involvement show association with HLA-B27 whereas those with only peripheral joint involvement show no significant association.

4.4.2 Pathology of the SSA

Although the pathological process amongst the various SSA is, in many respects, similar, it does, however, differ quantitatively. While the disease process in RA is distinguished by exudation, inflammation, synovial-induced destruction and primary necrosis, the pathological picture in SSA is determined essentially by metaplastic processes in different structures, namely the bony

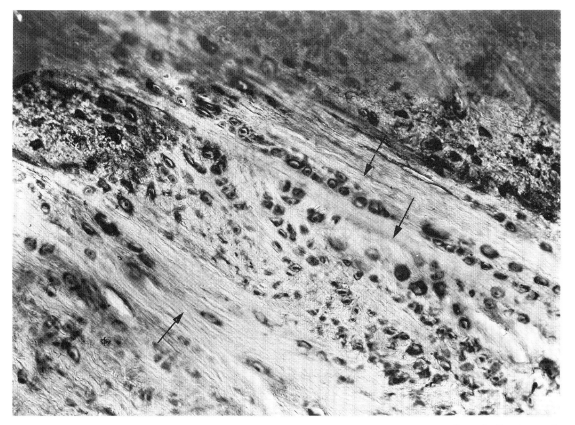

Figure 9.13 Ankylosing spondylitis: osseous transformation in the area of a hip joint. Upper half: advanced osseous transformation. Middle and lower half: chondroid transformation of the collagenous tendon tissue. Arrows, remaining collagenous tendon structure.

metaplasia marks the so-called spondylar processes (Fig. 9.13).

4.4.3   Synovial Processes

The histological picture of the synovial membrane of patients with SSA shows similarities which, in most cases, enables it to be clearly distinguished from the synovial processes occurring in RA, OA and other synovitides. The histological picture of the synovitis associated with SSA is in no way constant. Lacking the static unchanging nature of OA on the one hand and the dynamic ever-changing scene in RA on the other, it reflects to a far greater extent the course of the disease process.

In the early stages or in the area of the inflamed exacerbation, the lining cells show modest proliferation, and become cuboidal to cylindrical in shape and are multi-layered. At this stage, the remaining fibrin exudate is found on the surface of the synovial membrane. Generally, however, fibrin exudation is minimal in SSA compared with RA. Except during these short bursts of inflammation, the lining cells are flat and single-layered. The cell infiltration is variable and reflects the changing process. In active cases various combinations of lymphocytes and plasma cells infiltrate, particularly the subsynovial surface of the villi. In the course of time they retreat and, with the increasing build-up of fibrosis, they become less numerous and eventually disappear. We have never observed true lymphoid follicles. PMNs do not participate in SSA synovitis.

The overall impression of the events in the synovial membrane in SSA is of a low-grade smouldering process with only traces of short-lived exudative–proliferative inflammatory phases which leave behind fibrosis and an increased formation of villi. In no way does this process warrant the description "chronic synovitis". On the contrary, lymphocytes and plasma cells are evidence of the systemic immunological process. In patients with SSA, we have never seen high-grade proliferation of immature synovial cells such as occurs in RA ("tumour-like proliferation") (see page 177). This supports the observation that in the SSA group of diseases, no synovial-induced destruction of cartilage and bone takes place. It is noteworthy that we, in agreement with Espinoza *et al.* (1982), could demonstrate no more than minimal exudation and proliferation during the inflammatory process in synovial tissue in SSA, which now raises the question as to how the impressive bony processes came to be described, and by which these diseases are characterized.

4.4.4   Bone Processes

In contrast with RA, the cartilage on the joint surface in SSA is neither completely or even partially destroyed, nor replaced by scar pannus. The hyaline cartilage often changes to fibrocartilage. In some cases, we observed, by means of polarizing optics, a continuous transformation of radially running collagen fibres into the texture of a fibrous ankylosis. Such a picture would be inconceivable for a scar pannus resulting from inflammatory or synovial-induced cartilage destruction. The subchondral lamellar bone narrows and shows irregular zones of breakthrough and transformation. We have never found invasive pathways as seen in RA.

In contrast, the changes that we observed in spongy and cortical bone material from patients with psoriatic arthritis were surprising and documented a unique bone process which we have divided into four phases as follows (Fassbender, 1979, 1986a).

1. The first phase is marked by a focal loss of the minerals and the proteoglycan substance of the lamellar bone. The matrix, consisting of collagen fibres, is preserved in this process and characterizes the original localization of the bone lamellae. The delineation between intact bone and unmasked collagen fibre matrix is initially blurred and appears fringed. The exposed collagen fibre framework, stripped of proteoglycan, is at first fine; however, in time, the collagen fibres become coarse, in the presence of fibrocytes. The characteristic process in spongy bone is especially clearly recognizable. The network of spongiosa is broken through at several points with no consistent pattern. These breakthroughs are completely irregular and unsystematic. Although a large part of the spongiosa appears to be intact, localized areas are changed through total proteoglycan loss. The masked collagen fibres of the matrix indicate the original position of the lamellar trabeculae. Instead of the Haversian canals, one sees expanded blood vessels (Fig. 9.14). In the area of the cortical compact bone, this process does not become as evident as is the case with spongy bone. This is understandable, as the bone lamellae here lie parallel to the surface. Break-offs, as is the case in the delicate structure of the spongiosa, would therefore not be expected.

2. The loss of the proteoglycan-containing interstitial substance of the localized bone section is noted by the surrounding connective tissue, and the blurred circumscribed areas resulting from the loss of proteoglycan become settled by osteoblast chains. The osteoblasts position themselves between the remaining collagen fibre bundles and use these as a building frame for the remodelling which now begins. Depending on the age of the osteoblast chains, newly formed osteoid may be found here, smoothly covering over the raw break-off surface between the fibres at various levels.

3. The third phase is characterized by the formation of new bone in the area of the proteoglycan loss. In contrast with the specific building pattern of the original lamellar spongiosa, this newly formed bone shows a disordered connective tissue matrix. The osteocytes of these new bones are, in contrast with lamellar bones, larger and tend to be rounded. The preserved collagen fibre matrix has, to a large extent, the effect of determining the form of the remodelling of the bone. In fact, newly formed bone is considerably coarser, bulkier and really only a caricature of the genuine structure. While the

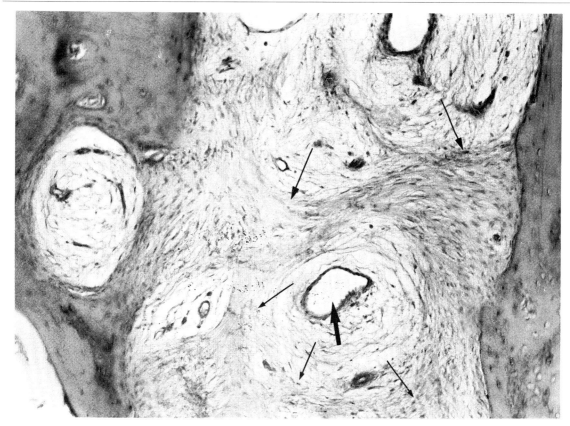

Figure 9.14 Psoriatic arthritis (distal phalanx): proteoglycan loss zone in the spongy bone. The preserved collagen fibres mark the original spongiosa structure (→). On both sides proteoglycan-containing trabeculae are still preserved.   ➡ indicates an expanded vessel as the remnant of a Haversian canal.

remodelling in the area of the spongiosa adapts itself approximately to the forms of the original network, the new bone formation in the area of the compact bone occurs parallel to the outer surface area (Fig. 9.15).

4. In all probability, the described proteoglycan loss and the new bone formation occurs very gradually, as we have had situations in which the acute collagen fibre unmasking, osteoblast activity and new bone formation were not observable and in which rather a gravel-like pagetoidal development of disordered fusion lines and a surface area of irregular appearance indicate the partially healed condition. On the cortical surface, small osteophytes may develop (Fig. 9.16). In no single case could we identify osteoclasts or lacunae as an indication of early osteoclast activity in the area of these bone processes. We considered it particularly important to establish that we could never find any traces of inflammation. The described process ensued with no participation of lymphocytes, plasma cells, PMNs or macrophages and, additionally, it is clear that enzymic degradation resulting from osteoclast activity or inflammation would never selectively release proteoglycan and leave the collagen fibre structure of the bones intact. For these reasons, we have no doubt that a unique bone process is taking place

here, in which no inflammatory or immunological reactions can be identified. These findings have now been extended to bone tissues from patients with ankylosing spondylitis, Reiter's syndrome and other REAs (Fassbender and Fassbender, 1992).

4.4.5   Pathomechanisms of SSA

We are convinced that this bone process mechanism is able to explain many of the clinical and radiological phenomena observed in the SSA diseases for the following reasons. (1) The actual synovial inflammatory process is low grade, episodic and time-limited. (2) In the areas of bone near the joints that we examined, the process was non-inflammatory and characterized by proteoglycan loss, unmasking of collagen fibrils and bone restructuring. The proteoglycan and mineral-depleted areas have the appearance of erosions or cysts in X-ray pictures.

We consider it an important observation that the bony remodelling primarily follows the form of previous structures. However, it should be remembered that these intermittently occurring breakdown and remodelling processes can lead to a negative balance in the bone structure resulting finally in osteolysis.

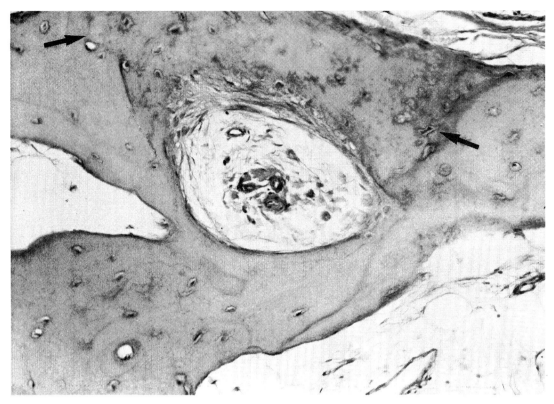

Figure 9.15 Psoriatic arthritis (distal phalanx): extensive remodelling of the spongiosa structure through insertion of newly formed reticular bone between the old spongiosa residue. The arrows mark the delineation between old lamellar and newly formed reticular bone.

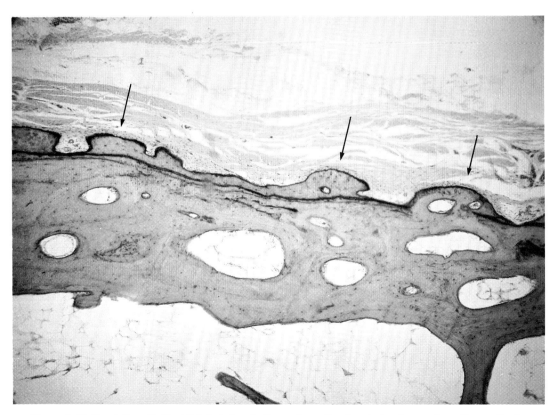

Figure 9.16 Psoriatic arthritis (distal phalanx): Several small osteophytes (arrows) on the corticalis.

4.4.6 The Role of Inflammation in the SSA

In consensus with other authors (von Swaay, 1950; Aufdermaur, 1953; Ott and Wurm, 1957) we have discarded an inflammatory cause of ossification in the axial skeleton (Fassbender, 1975) for the following reasons. Sparse clusters of lymphocytes, isolated plasma cells and newly formed blood vessels are the only findings described in the sacroiliac joints and at the connections of the annulus fibrosus of the disc cartilage with the edge of the spine. Corresponding processes are to be found in enthesiopathic rebuilding zones. Phenomena of this type are consistently found in the region of tissue destruction. These findings, in our opinion, do not warrant the description "inflammatory" and we conclude that the cause of ossification cannot be deduced with certainty, as there is no known analogous process in general pathology. Additionally, the bony ankylosing process observed in the large joints in ankylosing spondylitis is out of proportion to the low-grade episodic synovitides, and on the other hand, despite high-grade inflammation, bony ankylosis in RA is extremely rare.

4.4.7 The Role of Infection in Ankylosing Spondylitis

Despite the almost obligatory association of ankylosing spondylitis with HLA-B27, only about 20% of the carriers of this genetic trait develop the disease. This fact, together with the observation of discordance between monozygotic twins (Arnett, 1984), supports the concept that environmental factors act as "triggers". Indeed, the implication of *Yersinia*, *Shigella*, *Salmonella*, *Campylobacter* and *Chlamydia* in the initiation of REA in HLA-B27 carriers supports the idea that, in a similar way, bacteria play a significant role in the pathogenesis of ankylosing spondylitis. In this context, it is of interest to consider the two hypotheses put forward by Woodrow (1988). The "cross-tolerance" or "molecular mimicry" hypothesis infers that development of disease is a consequence of structural homology between *Klebsiella* antigens in the case of ankylosing spondylitis (and other organisms in the case of REA) and a part of the sequence of the heavy chain which determines HLA-B27 specificity (Ebringer, 1983). It is suggested that this results in the breaking of tolerance to the shared epitope, leading to disease via an autoimmune mechanism. The second hypothesis is that a plasmid-like structure, originating in *Klebsiella* and other gut organisms, gains entry to the genome of the cells of affected individuals, thereby coding for a product which becomes associated in the cell membrane with HLA-B27 molecules, thus providing a target for T cell cytotoxicity (Geczy *et al.*, 1985). It is clear that these two hypotheses offer quite different models for the pathogenesis of ankylosing spondylitis.

5. *Morphological Aspects of Therapeutic Intervention*

5.1 INTRODUCTION

When addressing the question of how morphological analysis of arthritic processes can assist therapy, one has first to consider that the arthritides, whatever their nature, derive from structural processes which can, to a large extent, be elucidated by morphology. In contrast, their causative mechanisms are elucidated by genetics, immunology and biochemistry.

The therapy of arthritis is based on two completely different concepts. On the one hand, systematic pharmacological development is aimed at well-defined or assumed pathological processes. Conversely, substances are used which were originally intended for totally different diseases, for example, gold for tuberculosis, Resochin for malaria, D-penicillamine for Wilson's disease and cytotoxic immunosuppression for tumour therapy. Clearly, the rationale for using these substances in arthritis therapy is lacking. Because of their observed influence on the progress of chronic arthritis, these substances are described with careful optimism as "disease-modifying anti-rheumatic drugs" (DMARDs).

In contrast, the targetted pharmacological development of antirheumatic drugs has demonstrated, in animal studies, defined and measurable effects on structural components of the inflammatory process, as for example effects on capillary permeability in the carageenin test and effects on fibroblast proliferation and collagen fibre formation in the cotton pellet test. The explanation and influence of the inflammatory and pain mediators are the objectives of biochemical research.

If the inflammatory process is viewed as the final stage in the hierarchical system of genetic factors, immunological disturbances and biochemical mediators, then the activation of capillaries and connective tissue, which is a result of preceding non-bacterial, exudative and proliferative events, can be determined morphologically. Thus, consideration of these aspects in the study of the structural changes in OA, RA and SSA will provide a starting point for therapeutic intervention.

5.2 OSTEOARTHRITIS (OA)

5.2.1 Articular Cartilage Lesion

The basic process of OA is recognized by a progressive deterioration of the cartilage matrix, increased erosion of the joint surface and loss of ground substance due to cartilage wearing. Decades of attempts to influence this process by local or systemic administration of various glycosaminoglycan preparations have produced only contentious results. This may be due to the fact that these therapies were carried out under scientifically unsound conditions (as, for example, "the formation of new matrix by administration of deficient substrate"). Alternatively, the inconsistencies may result from the vast variation in the arthrotic processes inherent in OA, making collection of comparable and reliable patient data difficult. The question therefore remains open as to whether the enthusiastic reports from orthopaedic surgeons of the success of these therapies will, in the future, attain scientifically plausible and clinically impartial ratification.

5.2.2 Secondary Synovitis

OA synovitis, which is caused by cartilage breakdown products, is an acute non-purulent sporadically painful inflammation (see page 169). The process is characterized by slight exudation as shown by the moderate deposits of fibrin. Antiphlogistic substances with antiexudative potency would therefore be expected to be effective on the synovial capillaries.

The proliferative stage is entirely restricted to the lining cell layer. The synovial stroma cells do not proliferate in OA. This complies with the "extrinsic" character of the accompanying synovitis, where the external irritation (i.e. from the joint areas), affects the synovial tissue. The increase in villous hyperplasia which occurs in OA is probably only of limited importance in the nutrition of the undamaged hyaline cartilage, because the fibrotic reactions do not occur in the villous stroma – as opposed to the situation in RA or SSA – so that the transport route from the synovial capillaries to the joint space is not occluded.

The fight against secondary synovitis involves not only the relief of pain, but also prevention of the production of IL-1 and other cytokines which are themselves responsible for the release of proteases from chondrocytes (Dingle *et al.*, 1979, 1991). Antiphlogistic drugs serve here to protect the remaining cartilage. Damaging effects of these drugs on the chondrocytes have been assessed by electron microscopy, with the finding that the modern NSAIDs have no adverse effects. In contrast, however, dexamethasone and, to a lesser extent, phenylbutazone are known to damage the nuclei and organelles of these cells (Annefeld and Fassbender, 1983). Clearly, any hypothetical chondrocyte damage must be weighed against the risk of injury to the cartilage threatened by secondary synovitis when using the NSAIDs available today.

5.2.3 Secondary Immunological Phenomena

The fact that, in OA, lymphocytes accumulate and lymphoid follicles with germinal centres (see page 174) can persist for months or years in the synovial membrane indicates that immunological processes are occurring. The question as to what extent these immune phenomena endanger the remaining cartilage is not yet answered, and at present there is no indication for the use of drugs other than the NSAIDs.

5.3 RA

The basis of RA is a complex of various pathomechanisms comprising entirely different processes which, only when combined, present the complete picture of the disease.

5.3.1 Inflammatory Process

The true inflammatory process manifests itself on the synovial membrane and the serous membranes. It is sporadic and activated episodically by the overriding immune process. The morphological aspect of synovitis and serositis, namely fibrin exudation and lining cell proliferation, is uncharacteristic and does not differ qualitatively from the inflammatory processes of OA and SSA. It is, however, more intense and more episodic. Fibrin exudation and lining cell proliferation can be effectively treated with conventional NSAID therapy.

As already mentioned, homotypic and heterotypic cell interactions are dependent on the presence of adhesion molecules at the surface of cells. Because key steps in the inflammatory cascade require adhesion of, for example, lymphocytes to endothelial cells, blocking of this interaction by use of monoclonal antibodies is another strategy to control inflammation-associated events. In common concepts of the pathogenesis of RA, T lymphocytes play an important role by recognition of antigens and secretion of cytokines. An adhesive receptor–ligand pair involved in the binding of T cells to antigen-presenting cells or endothelial cells is LFA-1 and ICAM-1. Thus, antibodies (1A29, mouse IgG1) against ICAM-1 have been shown to exert a strong suppressive effect on adjuvant arthritis in rats. Using this antibody treatment, not only the production of arthritogenic lymphocytes in donors but also the progression of arthritis in recipients can be influenced (Iigo *et al.*, 1991). Theoretically, the intercellular adhesion molecules offer promising starting points for therapeutic interventions.

5.3.2 Destructive Process

The overwhelming importance attributed to joint destruction in RA is not a consequence of synovial inflammation. The damage to joint structures results from homogeneous aggregations of immature synovial cells which invade the cartilage and adjacent bone, degrading the proteoglycans and collagen by enzymic action (TLP see page 177). This immature neoplastic cell fusion has no inflammatory components and therefore cannot be treated antiphlogistically. This explains why joint destruction is not prevented by conventional therapy. Our observations show that TLP–cell fusion is extremely short-lived and then changes into scar pannus, thereby losing its aggressive nature, a process that is repeated in episodic bursts. Cytotoxic drugs may well be effective against this process but only during the florid stage of proliferation. However, because this stage cannot be anticipated or recognized clinically, as it is not connected with the inflammatory exacerbation, cytotoxic therapy remains a problem of targeting. The question as to whether substances such as gold, D-penicillamine and other DMARDs can influence this oncological process remains unresolved. Because their mechanisms of action are unknown, the answer must be left to medical empiricism.

5.3.3 Necrotizing Process

A specific characteristic of RA is the primary necrotizing process. We have established by systematic morphological analysis that these tissue necroses proceed with no previous inflammatory involvement. Because of this, RA necroses, which can have remarkable clinical significance depending on their location, are not receptive to antiphlogistic therapy. It is interesting to note, however, that these specific necroses appear only in RA patients positive for rheumatoid factor. The obligatory association of rheumatoid factor with the immune complexes present in the necroses indicates an immunological basis for these phenomena. Hypothetically one may deduce plausible grounds for immunosuppressive therapy.

5.4 SERONEGATIVE SPONDYLARTHRITIDES (SSA)

5.4.1 Synovitis

Whereas in OA the joint process is primarily local and restricted, in RA and SSA it is the last step of a hierarchical series of stages. Mediators released probably because of an immunological error can themselves trigger a synovitis with morphological alterations.

The inflammatory process in the synovial tissue in SSA is short lived and low grade. In the early stages, slight fibrin exudation occurs together with a distinct proliferation and hypertrophy of the lining cells. The reactivity of the lining cells declines as the fibrosis of the synovial stroma increases. Although described as "intrinsic" arthritis as opposed to that seen in OA, these inflammatory exacerbations may, nevertheless, respond to conventional non-steroidal therapy. Incidentally, these short-lived synovitides never attack the cartilage or bone and therefore represent no danger to the joint itself.

5.4.2 Metaplastic Bone Processes

During our analyses of true pathognomic phenomena such as cartilage destruction and bony metaplasia (which characterizes ankylosing spondylitis and psoriatic arthritis), we have never found any evidence of inflammatory involvement. Conventional antiphlogistic therapy would therefore be unsuitable for these phenomena, but may, however, be effective in treating the accompanying osteoblast proliferation. Theoretically, efficacy of the cytotoxic drugs, e.g. methotrexate, would also be anticipated.

The often long-lasting dense infiltration of the synovial stroma by lymphocytes and plasma cells indicates continuation of an immune process possibly justifying immunosuppressive therapy.

Consequently, we find that morphological analysis of the SSA reveals three foci for therapeutic intervention: (1) the episodic uncharacteristic synovitides requiring only NSAIDs, (2) the osteoblast activity associated with bony metaplasia which potentially should respond to antiproliferative and possibly cytotoxic drugs, and (3) the systemic immune processes which may theoretically be treated with immunosuppressants, as in RA.

6. *References*

Aho, K., Ahvonen, P., Lassus, A., Sievers, K. and Tiilikainen, A. (1974). HL-A27 in reactive arthritis and Reiter's disease. Arth. Rheum. 17, 521–526.

Aho, K., Ahvonen, P., Lassus, A. Sievers, K. and Tiilikainen, A. (1976). In "Infection and Immunology in the Rheumatic Diseases" (ed D.C. Dumonde), pp 341–344. Blackwell, Oxford.

Alarcón, G.S. (1986). "Rheumatology and Immunology", 2nd edn (ed A.S. Cohen and J.C. Bennett), pp 196–214. Grune & Stratton, Orlando, Florida.

Annefeld, M. and Fassbender, H.G. (1983). Ultrastrukturelle Untersuchungen zur Wirksamkeit antiarthrotischer Substanzen. Z. Rheumatol. 42, 199–202.

Arend, W.P. and Dayer, J.-M. (1990). Cytokines and cytokine inhibitors or antagonists in rheumatoid arthritis. Arth. Rheum. 33, 305–315.

Arnett, F.C. (1984). In "Spondylarthropathies" (ed A. Calin), pp 297–321. Grune & Stratton, Orlando, Florida.

Arnett, F.C. (1986). In "Rheumatology and Immunology", 2nd edn (eds. A.S. Cohen and J.C. Bennett), pp 221–228. Grune & Stratton, Orlando, Florida.

Arnett, F.C., Edworthy, S.M., Block, D.A., McShane, D.J., Fries, J.F., Cooper, N.S., Healey, L.A., Kaplan, S.R., Liang, M.H., Luthra, H.S., Medsger, T.A., Mitchell, D.M., Neustadt, D.H., Pinals, R.S., Schaller, J.G., Sharp, J.T., Wilder, R.L. and Hunder, G.G. (1988). The American Rheumatism Association 1987 revised criteria for the classification of rheumatoid arthritis. Arth. Rheum. 31, 315–324.

Aufdermaur, M. (1953). Spondylitis ankylopoetica. Pathologische Anatomie. Documenta Geigy, H 2, Basel.

Aydelotte, M.B., Schleyerbach, R., Zeck, B.J. and Kuettner, K.E. (1986). In "Articular Cartilage Biochemistry" (ed K.E. Kuettner, R. Schleyerbach and V.C. Hascall), pp 235–256. Raven Press, New York.

Aydelotte, M.B. and Kuettner, K.E. (1993). In "Cartilage Degradation: Basic and Clinical Aspects" pp. 37–65. (ed J.F. Woessner jr. and D.S. Howell). Marcel Dekker, New York, Basel and Hong Kong.

Barland, P., Novikoff, A.B. and Hamerman, D. (1964). Fine structure and cytochemistry of the rheumatoid synovial membrane with the special reference to lysosomes. Am. J. Pathol. 44, 853–859.

Benninghoff, A. (1939). In "Lehrbuch der Anatomie des Menschen" 1. Bd. J.F. Lehmanns, München and Berlin.

van Bohemen, C.G., Rumet, F.C. and Zanen, H.C. (1984). Identification of HLA-B27 M1 and -M2 cross-reactive antigens in *Klebsiella*, *Shigella*, and *Yersinia*. Immunology 52, 607–616.

Botzenhardt, C. (1975). Fibroblastäre Proliferation und lymphozytäre Infiltration des Stratum synoviale bei chronischer Polyarthritis in Beziehung zur klinischen Aktivität der Erkrankung. Inauguraldissertation, Johannes-Gutenberg-Universität, Mainz.

Briem, H., Norberg, R., Jonsson, M., et al. (1980). Circulating immune complexes in patients with intestinal infections. J. Infect. 2, 215–220.

Bromley, M. and Woolley, D.E. (1984). Histopathology of the rheumatoid lesion – identification of cell types at sites of cartilage erosion. Arth. Rheum. 27, 857–863.

Bywaters, E.G.L. and Ansell, B.M. (1965). Monoarticular arthritis in children. Ann. Rheum. Dis. 24, 116–121.

Calin, A. (1984a). In "Spondylarthropathies" (ed A. Calin), pp 119–149. Grune & Stratton, Orlando, Florida.

Calin, A. (1984b). In "Spondylarthropathies" (ed A. Calin), pp 1–8. Grune & Stratton, Orlando, Florida.

Calin, A., Elswood, J. and Klouda, P.T. (1989). Destructive arthritis, rheumatoid factor, and HLA-DR4. Susceptibility versus severity, a case-control study. Arth. Rheum. 32, 1221–1225.

Cooke, T.D., Richter, S., Hurd, E. and Jasin, H.E. (1975). Localization of antigen antibody complexes in intraarticular collagenous tissues. Ann. NY Acad. Sci. 256, 10–24.

Dingle, J.T., Saklatvala, J., Hembry, R., Tyler, J., Fell, H.B. and Jubb, R. (1979). A cartilage catabolic factor from synovium. Biochem. J. 184, 177–180.

Dingle, J.T., Horner, A. and Shield, M. (1991). The sensitivity of synthesis of human cartilage matrix to inhibition by IL-1 suggests a mechanism for the development of osteoarthritis. Cell Biochem. Funct. 9, 99–102.

Ebringer, A. (1983). The cross tolerance hypothesis, HLA-B27 and ankylosing spondylitis. Br. J. Rheum. 22, Suppl. 2, 53–66.

Engleman, E.P., Bombardier, C. and Hochberg, M.C. (1983). Conference on epidemiology of rheumatic diseases. Specific needs of the developing countries. J. Rheumatol. 10, 1–107.

Espinoza, L.R., Vasey, F.B., Espinoza, C.G., Bocanegra, T.S. and Germain, B.F. (1982). Vascular changes in psoriatic synovium. Arth. Rheum. 25, 677–683.

Eyre, D.R., Wu, J.-J. and Apone, S. (1987). A growing family of collagens in articular cartilage: identification of 5 genetically distinct types. J. Rheumatol. 14, 25–27.

Eyre, D.R., Wu, J.-J. and Woods, P. (1992). In "Articular Cartilage and Osteoarthritis" (ed K.E. Kuettner, R. Schleyerbach, J.G. Peyron and V.C. Hascall), pp 119–131. Raven Press, New York.

Fassbender, H.G. (1963). Nosologische Typen des rheumatischen Granuloms und ihre biologische Bedeutung. Frankf. Zschr. Pathol. 72, 586–604.

Fassbender, H.G. (1975). Pathologie rheumatischer Erkrankungen. Springer, Berlin, Heidelberg and New York.

Fassbender, H.G. (1979). Extra-articular processes in osteoarthropathia psoriatica. Arch. Orthop. Traumat. Surg. 95, 37–46.

Fassbender, H.G. (1986a). In "Arthritis und Spondylitis psoriatica" (ed F. Schilling), pp 31–44. Steinkopff, Darmstadt.

Fassbender, H.G. (1986b). In "Cartilage Biochemistry" (ed K.E. Kuettner, R. Schleyerbach and V.C. Hascall), pp 371–389. Raven Press, New York.

Fassbender, H.G. and Fassbender, R. (1992). Synovial characteristics of seronegative spondarthritides. Clin. Invest. (in press).

Fassbender, H.G., Simmling-Annefeld, M. and Stofft, E. (1980). Transformation der Synovialzellen bei Rheumatoider Arthritis. Verh. Dtsch. Ges. Path. 64, 193–212.

Fassbender, H.G., Hebert, T.D. and Seibel, M. (1992). Pathways of joint destruction in MTP- and MCP joints in rheumatoid arthritis. Scand. J. Rheumatol. 21, 10–16.

Fidler, I.J., Gersten, D.M. and Hart, I.R. (1978). The biology of cancer invasion and metastasis. Adv. Cancer Res. 28, 149–250.

Gadher, S.J., Eyre, D.R., Duance, V.C., Wotton, S.F., Heck, L.W., Schmid, T.M. and Woolley, D.E. (1988). Susceptibility of cartilage collagens type II, IX, X, and XI to human synovial collagenase and neutrophil elastase. Eur. J. Biochem. 175, 1–7.

Gay, S., Huang, G-q., Ziegler, B., Fassbender, H.G. and Gay, R.E. (1989). Expression of myb, myc, ras and fos oncogenes in synovial cells of patients with rheumatoid arthritis (RA) or osteoarthritis (OA). Arth. Rheum. 32, (S), No. 4, 59.

Geczy, A.F., Prendergast, J.K., Sullivan, J.S., Upfold, L.I., Edmonds, J.P. and Bashir, H.V. (1985). In "Advances in Inflammation Research, Vol. 9 The Spondylarthropathies" (ed M. Ziff and S.B. Cohen), pp 129–137. Raven Press, New York.

Ghadially, F.N. and Roy, S. (1967). Ultrastructure of synovial membrane in rheumatoid arthritis. Ann. Rheum. Dis. 26, 426–443.

Graf, M., Baici, A. and Sträuli, P. (1981). Histochemical localization of cathepsin B at the invasion front of the rabbit V2 carcinoma. Lab. Invest. 45, 587–596.

Gran, J.T., Husby, G. and Thorsby, E. (1983). The association between rheumatoid arthritis and HLA antigen DR4. Ann. Rheum. Dis. 42, 292–296.

Granfors, K., Jalkanen, S., von Essen, R., Lahesmaa-Rantala, R., Isomäki, O., Pekkola-Heino, K., Merilahti-Palo, R., Saario, R., Isomäki, H. and Toivanen, A. (1989). Yersinia antigens in synovial fluid cells from patients with reactive arthritis. N. Engl. J. Med. 320, 216–221.

Grimley, P.M. and Sokoloff, L. (1966). Synovial giant cells in rheumatoid arthritis. Am. J. Pathol. 49, 931–943.

Håkansson, U., Löw, B., Eitrem, R., and Winblad, S. (1975). HLA-27 and reactive arthritis in an outbreak of salmonellosis. Tissue Antigens 6, 366–367.

Hanly, J.G., Piedger, D., Parkhill, W., Roberts, M. and Gross, M. (1990). Phenotypic characteristics of dissociated mononuclear cells from rheumatoid synovial membrane. J. Rheumatol. 17, 1274–1279.

Harris, E.D. jr. (1976). Recent insights into the pathogenesis of the proliferative lesion in rheumatoid arthritis. Arth. Rheum. 19, 68–72.

Hascall, V.C. (1988). Proteoglycans: The chondroitin sulfate/keratan sulfate proteoglycan of cartilage. ISI Atlas of Science: Biochemistry 12, 189–198.

Hebert, T.D., Siebert, G. and Fassbender, H.G. (1990). Bakterielle Superinfektion (BSI) bei chronischen Gelenkerkrankungen. Z. Rheumatol. 49, Suppl. 1, V–28.

Heinegard, D. and Sommarin, Y. (1987). In "Methods of Enzymology, Structural and Contractile Proteins, Part D. Extracellular Matrix, Vol. 144" (ed L.W. Cunningham), pp 305–319. Academic Press, Orlando, Florida.

Heinegard, D. and Oldberg, A. (1989). Structure and biology of cartilage and bone matrix noncollagenous macromolecules. FASEB J. 3, 2042–2051.

Hembry, R.-M., Murphy, G. and Reynolds, J.J. (1985). Immunolocalization of tissue inhibitor of metalloproteinases (TIMP) in human cells: Characterization and use of a specific antiserum. J. Cell Sci. 73, 105–119.

Iigo, Y., Takashi, T., Tamatani, T., Miyasaka, M., Higashida, T., Yagida, H., Okumura, K. and Tsukada, W. (1991). ICAM-1-dependent pathway is critically involved in the pathogenesis of adjuvant arthritis in rats. J. Immunol. 147, 4167–4171.

Jasin, H.E. (1987). Intra-articular antigen–antibody reactions. Rheum. Dis. Clin. North Am. 13 (2), 179–189.

Kalliomäki, J.L. and Leino, R. (1979). Follow-up studies of joint complications in Yersiniosis. Acta Med. Scand. 205, 512–525.

Kaplan, M.H. (1963). Immunologic relation of streptococcal and tissue antigens. I. Properties of an antigen in certain strains of group A streptococci exhibiting an immunologic cross reaction with human heart tissue. J. Immunol. 90, 595–606.

Kaplan, M.H. and Suchy, M.L. (1964). Immunologic relation of streptococcal and tissue antigens. II. Cross reactions of antisera to mammalian heart tissue with a cell wall constituent of certain strains of group A streptococci. J. Exp. Med. 119, 643–650.

Kaul, A., Blake, D.R. and Pearson, J.D. (1991). Vascular endothelium, cytokines, and the pathogenesis of inflammatory synovitis. Ann. Rheum. Dis. 50, 828–832.

Keat, A.C., Thomas, B.J. and Taylor-Robinson, D. (1983). Chlamydial infection in the etiology of arthritis. Br. Med. Bull. 39, 168–174.

Kimura, J.H. and Kuettner, K.E. (1986). In "Articular Cartilage Biochemistry" (ed K.E. Kuettner, R. Schleyerbach and V.C. Hascall), pp 257–272. Raven Press, New York.

Kleesiek, H., Neumann, S. and Greiling, H. (1983). In "Theoretische und klinische Befunde der Knorpelforschung, 3. Symposion für Bindegewebsforschung" (ed N. Dettmer et al., pp 134–141. Eular, Basel.

Knudson, W., Subbaiah, S. and Pauli, B. (1990). Proteoglycan synthesis by normal and neoplastic human transitional epithelial cells. J. Cell. Biochem. 43, 255–279.

Lawrence, R.C. and Shulman, L.E. (1984). Proceedings of the Fourth International Conference, National Institutes of Health. Gower Medical Publishing, New York.

Leirisalo, M., Skylv, G., Kousa, M., Voipio-Pulki, L.M., Suoronta, H., Nissila, M., Hvidman, L., Nielsen, E.D., Sveijgard, A., Tiilikainen, A. and Laitinen, O. (1982). Follow-up study on patients with Reiter's disease and reactive arthritis with special reference to HLA-B27. Arth. Rheum. 25, 249–256.

Leisen, J.C., Duncan, H., Riddle, J.M. and Pitchford, W.C. (1988). The erosive front: a topographic study of the junction between the pannus and the subchondral plate in the macerated rheumatoid metacarpal head. J. Rheumatol. 15, 17–22.

Mankin, H.J., Brandt, T.K. and Shulman, L.E. (1985). Workshop on etiopathogenesis of osteoarthritis: Proceedings and recommendations. 13, 1126–1160.

Maroudas, A., Katz, E.P., Wachtel, E.J., Mizrahi, J. and Soudry, M. (1986). In "Articular Cartilage Biochemistry" (ed K.E. Kuettner, R. Schleyerbach and V.C. Hascall), pp 311–327. Raven Press, New York.

Marsal, L., Windblad, S. and Wollheim, F.A. (1981). Yersinia enterocolitica arthritis in southern Sweden: a four year follow-up study. Br. Med. J. 283, 101–103.

Mayne, R. and Burgeson, R. (1987). "Structure and Function of Collagen Types". Academic Press, Orlando, Florida.

Meachim, G. and Brooke, G. (1984). In "Osteoarthritis: Diagnosis and Management" (ed R.W. Moskowitz, D.S. Howell, V.M. Goldberg and H.J. Mankin), pp 29–42. W.B. Saunders, Philadelphia.

Mendler, M., Eich-Bender, S.G., Vaughan, L., Winterhalter, K.H. and Bruckner, P. (1989). Cartilage contains mixed fibrils of collagen types II, IX, and XI. J. Cell Biol. 108, 191–197.

Menninger, H., Lambusch, M., Mohr, W. and Wessinghage, D. (1983). Immunkomplexe: Mediatoren für die Bildung von entzündlichem Granulationsgewebe? Z. Rheumatol. 42, 7–15.

Misskampf, H.J. (1984). Zusammenhang zwischen Synovialstromazellproliferation bei CP- und Arthrose- Patienten und klinischen Daten unter besonderer Berücksichtigung der Rheumafaktoren. Inauguraldissertation, Johannes-Gutenberg-Universität, Mainz.

Mohr, W. and Menninger, H. (1979). Neutrophile Granulozyten bei der entzündlich-rheumatischen Knorpeldestruktion. Bull. Schweiz. Akad. Med. Wiss. 35, 443–451.

Mohr, W. and Hummler, N. (1986). Zerstört das Pannusgewebe bei der chronischen Polyarthritis einen Knorpel mit vitalen Granulozyten? Akt. Rheumatol. 11, 162–168.

Morales, T.I. and Kuettner, K.E. (1982). The properties of the neutral proteinase released by primary chondrocyte cultures and its action on proteoglycan aggregate. Biochem. Biophys. Acta 705, 92–101.

Murphy, G., McGuire, M.B., Russell, R.G.G. and Reynolds, J.J. (1981). Characterization of collagenase, other metalloproteinases and an inhibitor (TIMP) produced by human synovium and cartilage in culture. Clin. Sci. 61, 711–716.

Natvig, J.B., Førre, Ø., Randen, I., Steinitz, M., Thompson, K. and Waalen, K. (1988). B lymphocytes, B cell clones and rheumatoid factor antibodies in rheumatoid inflammation. Scand. J. Rheumatol. 76 (S), 217–227.

Ott, V.R. and Wurm, H. (1957). "Spondylitis ankylopoetica". Steinkopff, Darmstadt.

Pauli, B.U., Schwartz, D.E., Thonar, E.J.-M. and Kuettner, K.E. (1983). Tumor invasion and host extracellular matrix. Cancer Metast. Rev. 2, 129–152.

Pober, J.S. (1988). Cytokine-mediated activation of vascular endothelium. Am. J. Pathol. 133, 426–433.

Poole, C.A., Ayad, S. and Schofield, J.R. (1988). Chondrons from articular cartilage: (1) Imunolocalization of type VI collagen in the pericellular capsule of isolated canine chondrons. J. Cell Sci. 90, 635–643.

van der Rest, M. and Mayne, R. (1988). Type IX collagen proteoglycan from cartilage is covalently cross-linked to type II collagen. J. Biol. Chem. 263, 1615–1618.

Rosenberg, L.C. and Buckwalter, J.A. (1986). In "Articular Cartilage Biochemistry" (ed K.E. Kuettner, R. Schleyerbach and V.C. Hascall), pp 39–58. Raven Press, New York.

Sairanen, E. and Tiilikainen, A. (1975). HL-A27 in Reiter's disease following Shigellosis. Scand. J. Rheumatol. 8 (S) 30–11.

Sairanen, E., Paronen, I. and Mäkönen, H. (1969). Reiter's syndrome: A follow-up study. Acta Med. Scand. 185, 57–63.

Salisbury, A.K., Duke, O. and Paulter, L.W. (1987). Macrophage-like cells of the pannus area in rheumatoid arthritis joints. Scand J. Rheumatol. 16, 263–272.

Schilling, F. and Stadelmann, M.-L. (1986). In "Arthritis und Spondylitis Psoriatica" (ed F. Schilling), pp 1–21. Steinkopff, Darmstadt.

Schmid, T.M. and Linsenmayer, T.F. (1987). In "Structure and Function of Collagen types" (ed R. Mayne and R.E. Burgeson), pp 223–259. Academic Press, Orlando, Florida.

Schumacher, H.R. (1985). In "Textbook of Rheumatology" Vol. 2, 2nd edn (ed W. Kelley, E. Harris Jr., S. Ruddy and C.B. Sledge), pp 561–568. W.B. Saunders, Philadelphia, London, Toronto, Mexico City, Rio de Janeiro, Sydney and Tokyo.

Sloane, B.F., Dunn, J.R. and Honn, K.V. (1981). Lysosomal cathepsin B with metastatic potential. Science 212, 1151–1153.

Stockwell, R.A. (1979). In "Biological Structure and Function", Vol. 7 (ed R.J. Harrison and R.M.H. McMinn), pp 67–69. Cambridge University Press, Cambridge.

Stofft, E., Zschäbitz, A., Pöttgen, K., Kunt, T. and Nissen, A. (1988). Zur Morphologie und Morphometrie der Synovialiszellen bei Arthrose und rheumatoider Arthritis. Z. Rheumatol. 47, 271.

van Swaay, H. (1950). Spondylitis ankylopoetica. Een pathogenetische studie. Diss. med., Leiden.

Taylor-Robinson, D., Thomas, B.J., Dixey, J., Osborn, M.F., Furr, P.M. and Keast, A.C. (1988). Evidence that *Chlamydia trachomatosis* causes seronegative arthritis in women. Ann. Rheum. Dis. 47, 295–299.

Thoar, E.J-M.A. and Kuettner, K.E. (1987). In "The Biology of Extracellular Matrix: Proteoglycans" (ed T.N. Wight and R.P. Mecham), pp 211–246. Academic Press, New York.

Trabandt, A., Aicher, W.K., Gay, R.E., Sukhatme, V.P., Nilson-Hamilton, R.T., Fassbender, H.G. and Gay, S. (1990). Expression of the collagenolytic and ras-induced cysteine protease cathepsin L and proliferation-associated oncogenes in synovial cells of MRL/l-mice and patients with rheumatoid arthritis. Matrix 10, 349–361.

Trabandt, A., Gay, R.E., Fassbender, H.G. and Gay, S. (1991). Cathepsin B in synovial cells at the site of joint destruction in rheumatoid arthritis. Arth. Rheum. 34, 1444–1451.

Vaughan, L., Mendler, M., Huter, S., Bruckner, P., Winterhalter, K.H., Irwin, M. and Mayne, R. (1988). D-periodic distribution of collagen type IX along cartilage fibrils. J. Cell Biol. 106, 991–997.

Valesova, M., Trnavsky, K., Hulinska, D., Alusik, S., Janousek, J. and Jirons, J. (1989). Detection of *Borrelia* in the tissue from a patient with Lyme borreliosis by electron microscopy. J. Rheumatol. 16, 1502–1505.

Vignon, E., Arlot, M. and Vignon, G. (1977). Étude de la cellularité du cartilage articulaire fissuré. Comparaison des lésions liées et de l'âge des lésions arthosiques de la tête femorale humaine. Pathol. Biol. 25, 29–32.

Weiss, L. and Ward, P.M. (1983). Cell detachment and metastasis. Cancer Metast. Rev. 2, 111–127.

Weissmann, G. (1971). In "Rheumatoid Arthritis" (ed W. Müller, H.-G. Harweth and K. Fehr), pp 141–154. Academic Press, London and New York.

Werb, Z., Hembry, R.M., Murphy, G. and Aggeler, J. (1986). Commitment to expression of the metalloendopeptidases collagenase and stromelysin: Relationship of inducing events to changes in cytoskeletal architecture. J. Cell Biol. 102, 697–702.

Woodrow, J.C. (1985). In "Clinics in Rheumatic Diseases, Vol 11, No. 1: Seronegative Spondylarthropathies" (ed G.S. Panayi), pp 1–24. W.B. Saunders, London, Philadelphia and Toronto.

Woodrow, J.C. (1988). In "Baillière's Clinical Rheumatology Vol. 2/No. 3: Genetics of Rheumatic Diseases" (ed D.M. Greenan), pp 603–622. Baillière-Tindall, London, Philadelphia, Sydney, Tokyo and Toronto.

Woolley, D.E. (1984). In "Invasion. Experimental and Clinical Implications" (eds M.M. Mareel and K.C. Calman), pp 228–251. Oxford University Press, Oxford, New York and Tokyo.

Wright, V. and Moll, J.M.H. (1976). "Seronegative Polyarthritis". North-Holland Publishing Company, Amsterdam, New York and Oxford.

Ziegler, B., Gay, R.E., Huang, G.-q., Fassbender, H.G. and Gay, S. (1989). Immunohistochemical localisation of HTLV-I p19- and p24-related antigenes in synovial joints of patients with rheumatoid arthritis. Am. J. Pathol. 135, 1–5.

Zschäbitz, A. and Stofft, E. (1988). The lectin binding pattern of normal and pathologically altered synovial tissue. Histol. Histopathol. 3, 419–424.

10. Connective Tissue Destruction in Rheumatoid Arthritis: Therapeutic Potential of Selective Metalloproteinase Inhibitors

Brian Henderson and Simon Blake

1. Introduction

Rheumatoid arthritis is a bewilderingly complex disease in which chronic inflammation in the synovial lining is associated with the destruction of the extracellular matrices of articular cartilage and subchondral bone. This tissue destruction takes a number of forms (Fig. 10.1). The articular cartilage in rheumatoid joints is normally thinner than in unaffected joints. This is recognized in radiographs as a decrease in the joint space. Centripetal erosion of the articular cartilage is also a common sight at operation. This localized damage is associated with the growth of synovial pannus, a granulation tissue which grows over and, apparently, into the articular cartilage replacing the cartilage matrix. Localized changes in bone are also a common feature of rheumatoid arthritis. The most commonly recognized change in the bone of the rheumatoid joint is juxta-articular erosion. These erosions occur in the bone immediately adjacent to the inflamed synovium and mainly affect the cortical bone. In

Immunopharmacology of Joints and Connective Tissue
ISBN 0-12-206345-7

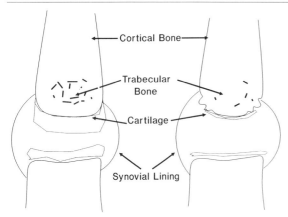

Figure 10.1 Schematic diagram showing the major sites of tissue destruction in the rheumatoid joint. The left hand drawing is of a normal joint showing the cartilage, trabecular and cortical bone in relation to the synovial lining. The right hand drawing represents an arthritic joint and shows the thinning of articular cartilage, centripetal erosion of cartilage and bone and the localized osteoporosis found in both cortical and trabecular bone.

addition to this localized bone loss there is also a diffuse osteoporosis, involving both cortical and trabecular bone.

Other intra-articular structures such as menisci may also show signs of degradation. In contrast, the inflamed synovial lining rarely shows signs of damage. Indeed one of the major features of this tissue is the fibrotic growth of the synovial lining. The pathological changes occurring in arthritic joints have been reviewed by Henderson and Edwards (1987).

A large number of drugs are used clinically for the treatment of rheumatoid arthritis. NSAIDs are widely used to relieve pain and suppress inflammation by their inhibitory action on the enzyme cyclooxygenase. Glucocorticoids, once widely used, are now used sparingly because of the appearance of side effects and the uncertainty about their efficacy (Byron and Kirwan, 1986). A variety of so-called slow-acting agents, e.g. gold, penicillamine and chloroquine, are in common use. Their mechanism of action is still the subject of debate. While showing efficacy in a proportion of patients, they can also produce severe side effects. Immunosuppressants are increasingly used in treating rheumatoid arthritis. Azathioprine has been used for many years and newer agents such as methotrexate and cyclosporine have been tested. While all of these agents may reduce pain and swelling in affected joints, it is clear that they have little, if any, effect on the process of joint destruction (Ianuzzi et al., 1983). Indeed, there is growing evidence that NSAIDs can exacerbate the destruction of articular cartilage in patients with osteoarthritis (Rashad et al., 1989). Indomethacin administration has also been found to accelerate the loss of cartilage proteoglycan in rabbits with antigen-induced

arthritis, a model closely resembling rheumatoid arthritis (Pettipher et al., 1989).

There is a pressing need to develop drugs that can inhibit joint destruction in rheumatoid arthritis. The dogma that rheumatoid arthritis is an autoimmune disease has resulted in attention being focused on the development of agents that inhibit the activity of T lymphocytes. However, the primacy of the role of the T lymphocyte in the pathogenesis of rheumatoid arthritis has recently become the subject of active debate (Firestein and Zvaifler, 1990). An alternative strategy would be to inhibit the final process(es) that leads to destruction of the extracellular matrices of the joint. The gross pathology and histopathology of the rheumatoid joint are consistent with the hypothesis that progressive enzymic destruction of the macromolecular components of cartilage and bone is occurring. Therefore, at least in theory, the simplest way of inhibiting this tissue breakdown would be to inhibit the lytic enzymes responsible. The nature of the enzymes responsible for joint destruction and the therapeutic potential of inhibiting such enzymes is the subject of this chapter.

2.   Eukaryotic Proteinases

Our current understanding of the enzymology of proteinases owes a great deal to groups such as those at the Strangeways Research Laboratory in Cambridge, whose *raison d'être* was (and still is) to decipher the mechanisms responsible for joint damage in arthritis. Many hundreds of proteinases have now been discovered and, on the basis of their catalytic mechanisms and evolutionary origin, have been classified into four major groups. This classification is based on the chemical groups present in the enzyme's active site responsible for the catalytic activity. At present, proteinases are divided into four catalytic families: serine, cysteine, aspartic and metalloproteinases. There are also some proteinases for which the catalytic mechanism is at present unknown (Table 10.1; Barrett and Rawlings, 1991).

3.   Proteinases Involved in Joint Destruction in Rheumatoid Arthritis

The specialized biomechanical properties of articular cartilage are due to the structure and interactions of the collagens and proteoglycans of which cartilage is composed. The collagens form the fibrous structural framework which in combination with proteoglycan and its associated water gives cartilage its resilience to compressive loading. The biomechanical properties of cartilage are dependent upon the maintenance of this collagen network and the retention within it of high concentrations of proteoglycan. Loss of either of these components can compromise the structure and function of cartilage. The

Table 10.1 Proteinase classification

	Aspartic	Cysteine	Serine	Metallo-	Unknown
Examples	Pepsin, cathepsins D and E, HIV endopeptidase, renin	Papain, cathepsins B,H,L,S, calpains	Trypsin, chymotrypsin, elastases, cathepsin G, plasmin, plasminogen activators	Thermolysin, collagenase, stromelysins, gelatinases, EC 24.11, EC 24.15, ACE	Eukaryotic leader peptidase Bacterial leader peptidase I
pH range of activity	3–6	3–7	6–10	6–9	
Inhibitors	Pepstatin	Leupeptin, thiol-blocking agents	Dip-F, PMS-F	EDTA, 1,10-phenan-throline, TIMP-1 and -2 phosphor-amidon	
Major plasma inhibitors		α_2M	α_1PI α_2M	α_2M	

Abbreviations: Dip-F, di-isopropyl fluorophosphate; PMS-F, phenylmethanesulphonyl fluoride; α_2M, α_2-macroglobulin; α_1PI, α_1-proteinase inhibitor; TIMP, tissue inhibitor of metalloproteinases; ACE, acetyl cholinesterase.

major connective tissue macromolecule in bone is type I collagen which becomes calcified. The localized loss of bone in rheumatoid arthritis is presumably related to the loss of this collagen. The study of the enzymic mechanisms responsible for joint destruction has concentrated largely on articular cartilage.

All the major classes of proteinases have, at one time or another, been implicated in the process of rheumatoid joint destruction (as reviewed by Henderson and Edwards, 1987). Our current understanding of the enzymology of joint breakdown can be traced back to pioneering work at the Strangeways Laboratory in the early 1950s in which it was shown that high concentrations of vitamin A would cause resorption of the matrix of cultured embryonic chicken or mouse long bones (Fell and Mellanby, 1952). In a separate study Lewis Thomas demonstrated that intravenous injection of papain into young rabbits caused their ears to lose their natural stiffness and droop like those of a spaniel. Sections of papain-treated rabbit ears revealed that the cartilage had lost its normal basophilia (Thomas, 1956; McCluskey and Thomas, 1958). The similarity between the effects induced by papain or by hypervitaminosis A on cartilage suggested that the mechanism of action of vitamin A on cartilage was due to the activation of proteases similar to papain (Fell and Thomas, 1960).

Further *in vitro* studies of limb bone cartilage suggested that matrix degradation was due to the action of the lysosomal enzyme cathepsin D, an aspartic proteinase which had only recently been described (reviewed by Dingle, 1962). Examination of synovial lining from rheumatoid patients revealed that it contained elevated levels of various lysosomal lytic enzymes (Luscombe, 1963). Using a specific antiserum to cathepsin D, it was demonstrated that explants of rheumatoid synovial lining released this enzyme and that it was located extracellularly at the pannus/cartilage junction in tissue sections. Injection of this anti-cathepsin D antibody into the joints of live rabbits with chronic experimental arthritis also demonstrated the release of the enzyme *in vivo* (Poole *et al.*, 1976).

By the early 1970s, the evidence supporting the hypothesis that lysosomal proteinases, and in particular cathepsin D, were responsible for joint destruction appeared strong. This was in spite of the fact that cathepsin D had no activity at neutral pH and did not cleave native collagen. However, the finding that a selective inhibitor of cathepsin D did not inhibit cartilage matrix breakdown in culture finally disproved this hypothesis (Hembry *et al.*, 1982). This latter study showed the value of selective inhibitors in testing hypotheses concerning the role of different classes of proteinases in joint destruction in rheumatoid arthritis.

3.1 INVOLVEMENT OF COLLAGENASE AND OTHER METALLOPROTEINASES IN JOINT DESTRUCTION

The collagens, in particular the fibrous collagens, constitute approximately 50% of the protein of adult vertebrates. Type I collagen is the predominant fibre-forming collagen in bone and type II collagen is the major form of collagen in hyaline articular cartilage (Van der Rest and Garrone, 1991). These fibre-forming or interstitial collagens are composed of triple-helical polypeptide chains with each chain comprising just over

1000 amino acids. There are three amino acids per turn of the helix and every third amino acid is glycine. The amino acid sequence of the individual collagen α chains is therefore Gly-X-Y and there is an abundance of proline and hydroxyproline. The structure of the collagen triple helix renders it resistant to the action of most proteases.

It was only in 1962 that the first vertebrate collagenase was described in the cultures of tadpole tail fins (Gross and Lapiere, 1962). These workers defined the criteria of identity for a true collagenase as "a proteinase that acts in a specific manner on native (i.e. undenatured) collagen at neutral pH" (Gross and Lapiere, 1962). Thirty years on, we now know that collagenase is simply one of a growing family of related metalloproteinases (also termed MMPs or the matrixins). The structure and function of these enzymes will be defined in a later section.

The discovery of a vertebrate collagenase that had the capacity to degrade native collagen at physiological temperature and pH opened a new chapter in the study of the mechanism of rheumatoid joint destruction. Before detailing the evidence for the role of these enzymes in rheumatoid joint pathology, it is worthwhile reminding the reader of the criteria used by pharmacologists to define the pathogenetic role of a particular mediator (Dale's criteria). Firstly, it must be found at the site of the disease or there must be evidence of its activity in lesional sites (with the MMPs this would be specific cleavage products). Secondly, the injection of the mediator must reproduce symptoms of the disease. Injection of human collagenase into rabbit knee joints does produce an arthritis (reviewed by Steffen, 1980). A more satisfactory test would be to produce transgenic animals in which overproduction of MMPs in joint tissues could be induced. Thirdly, antagonists or inhibitors of the mediator (MMP inhibitors) must be able to inhibit the disease or pathological state.

There is ample evidence for the presence of collagenase and other metalloproteinases in the rheumatoid joint. Evanson and co-workers were the first to demonstrate that explants of rheumatoid synovial lining released collagenase into the culture medium (Evanson et al., 1967). Since this report, many other groups have shown that inflamed synovial lining (from a number of arthritic lesions) produces collagenase and other metalloproteinases (e.g. Martel-Pelletier et al., 1988; reviewed by Henderson and Edwards, 1987; Murphy et al., 1991a). In contrast, normal synovial lining tends to produce little metalloproteinase activity (McGuire et al., 1981). The cells within the synovial lining producing these metalloproteinases appear to be activated fibroblasts (including synovial lining type B cells) and mesenchymal cells. This has been shown using both immunocytochemical (Okada et al., 1989; Murphy et al., 1991a) and in situ (Case et al., 1989a; Firestein et al., 1991; Gravallese et al., 1991; McCachren, 1991) labelling. This confirms the findings from the study of disaggregated rheumatoid synovial lining which identified the

collagenase-producing cells as activated fibroblast-like cells (Dayer et al., 1976, 1979; reviewed by Henderson and Edwards, 1987).

In animal models of rheumatoid arthritis, the inflamed synovial lining also expresses large amounts of collagenase and other MMPs (Cambray et al., 1981; Murphy et al., 1989; Case et al., 1989b; Hasty et al., 1990). In rabbits with antigen-induced arthritis, a model widely held to most closely resemble the joint pathology of rheumatoid arthritis, it is possible to immunolocalize collagenase, stromelysin and gelatinase in the inflamed synovial lining within 1 day of induction of disease. Non-inflamed synovial lining contains little, if any, enzyme (B. Henderson, G. Murphy, R.M. Hembry and J.J. Reynolds, unpublished data).

It is therefore abundantly clear that the synovial lining of the rheumatoid diarthrodial joint synthesizes large amounts of MMPs. However, the relevance of this synthesis to the pathogenesis of joint destruction is not immediately clear. Measurement of MMPs in synovial fluid is difficult because of the presence of inhibitors and other constituents which affect the assay. Cawston and co-workers, taking care to remove such inhibitors, found active collagenase in only 12–25% of rheumatoid synovial fluids examined. Moreover, latent enzyme was found only in 50–65% of such fluids (Cawston et al., 1984). More recently, immunoassays have been developed which can detect proforms and active forms of the MMPs (Walakovits et al., 1992). Using such assays, large amounts of collagenase and stromelysin have been detected in rheumatoid synovial fluids. Again the enzymes detected were the inactive proforms and were therefore unable to cause damage to the extracellular matrices of cartilage or bone. As the source of these enzymes is believed to be the inflamed synovium, it is unlikely that the synovial MMPs contribute significantly to the destruction of cartilage and bone. The role that these synovial MMPs play in the pathology of rheumatoid arthritis is therefore, at present, obscure.

The demonstration that damaged (i.e. minced) synovial lining released a factor (termed catabolin; now presumed to be the cytokine, IL-1) that stimulated the release of proteoglycans from cartilage explants (Fell and Jubb, 1977) gave rise to the current paradigm of joint damage in rheumatoid arthritis. Cartilage, and possibly also bone, are believed to be responding to cytokines produced by cells in the inflamed synovial lining. These cytokines stimulate the chondrocytes to synthesize MMPs which then degrade the cartilage matrix. The ability of cytokines such as IL-1 and TNF-α to cause proteoglycan release from cartilage explants or to stimulate isolated chondrocytes to synthesize MMPs has been well documented (reviewed by Henderson et al., 1987; Henderson and Lewthwaite, 1991). Intra-articular injection of IL-1 into the rabbit knee joint induces an acute synovitis and loss of proteoglycan from articular cartilage (Pettipher et al., 1986; Henderson and Pettipher, 1988). This loss of proteoglycan appears to be a direct effect of IL-1 on chondrocytes, as it is unaffected when leucocyte entry into joints is blocked (Pettipher *et al.*, 1988). Rheumatoid cartilage has been assayed for MMP activity and been shown to contain increased levels of activity (Martel-Pelletier *et al.*, 1988). Similarly elevated levels of MMPs have also been extracted from human osteoarthritic cartilage (Pelletier *et al.*, 1987).

Using an antiserum that reacts with unwound type II collagen α chains, Poole and co-workers have reported that, when bovine nasal cartilage was cultured in the presence of IL-1, it showed an increase in pericellular and intercellular staining for this epitope. This same antibody was found to stain sections of rheumatoid and osteoarthritic cartilage but showed little reactivity with normal cartilage. Rheumatoid cartilage stained intensely in a narrow rim at the surface and intense staining was also seen around chondrocytes in the mid and deep zones of cartilage. This is the first demonstration of collagen degradation in rheumatoid arthritis at sites distant from the synovium and joint fluid (Dodge and Poole, 1989; Dodge *et al.*, 1991). Of course, the enzymes responsible for the collagenolysis cannot be identified by this technique. Damage at the cartilage surface was speculated to be caused by neutrophil elastase or cathepsin G.

The role of MMPs in bone resorption is still the subject of debate. The best evidence for the role of such enzymes in the resorption of bone in culture has come from the use of selective inhibitors (reviewed in detail by Sakamoto and Sakamoto (1988) and discussed in Section 5.4).

3.2 EVIDENCE AGAINST THE ROLE OF KNOWN MMPs IN JOINT DESTRUCTION

There is strong evidence supporting the hypothesis that destruction of the extracellular matrices of articular cartilage and subchondral bone in chronic arthritis is due to local stimulation of MMP synthesis. However, there are certain experimental findings that do not support this hypothesis. The IL-1-driven breakdown of articular cartilage in culture cannot be inhibited by TIMP-1 (see Section 4.3 for definition) (Saklatvala, 1989), and very high concentrations of potent MMP inhibitors are needed to inhibit this process (Caputo *et al.*, 1987: reviewed in more detail in Section 5.5.2). If this *in vitro* cartilage breakdown was due to the action of MMPs, then much lower concentrations of such inhibitors would be thought to be needed. Substantial amounts of proteoglycan are lost from the articular cartilages of rabbits with polycation-induced arthritis (Page-Thomas, 1977) or antigen-induced arthritis (Dumonde and Glynn, 1962). In polycation-induced arthritis, both the synovial lining and the articular cartilage from the inflamed joints have the capacity to synthesize and secrete MMPs (Cambray *et al.*, 1981; Murphy *et al.*, 1981; Henderson *et al.*,

1990a). In contrast, in the antigen-induced model, the inflamed synovial lining has elevated levels of MMPs but the articular cartilage fails to synthesize or secrete MMPs. This has been shown by both the failure to measure the synthesis of MMP activity by arthritic cartilage (Henderson *et al.*, 1990a) and negative immunolocalization results of the MMPs in sections of articular cartilage (B. Henderson, G. Murphy, R.M. Hembry and J.J. Reynolds, unpublished studies). This study shows that it is possible to lose a substantial amount of proteoglycan from articular cartilage without the involvement of MMPs. The loss of cartilage proteoglycan in this model is not due to the activity of infiltrating leucocytes in the joint cavity. Thus, proteoglycan loss is restricted to the mid-zone of the cartilage (Beesley *et al.*, 1992), and inhibition of leucocyte entry into inflamed joints does not inhibit cartilage damage (Pettipher *et al.*, 1988).

Recent studies of the aggrecan (aggregating cartilage proteoglycan)-cleavage products produced by IL-1-stimulated cartilage suggest that breakdown of the aggrecan is not catalysed by stromelysin or related MMPs. The MMPs including stromelysin and the 72 and 95 kDa gelatinases cleave between the G1 and G2 domains in proteoglycan at Asp^{341} and Phe^{342}. In IL-1-stimulated bovine cartilage, however, the major cleavage site is between Glu^{373} and Ala^{374} (Sandy *et al.*, 1991; Flannery *et al.*, 1991; Fosang *et al.*, 1991, 1992). This suggests that some enzyme other than the known MMPs (which has been termed aggrecanase) is responsible for the loss of cartilage proteoglycan (Fig. 10.2). Of course it is likely that this aggrecanase is also a metalloproteinase.

Increased breakdown of the extracellular matrices of the joint tissues may not be the only mechanism at work to cause joint damage. There is growing evidence that cytokines can inhibit the synthesis of connective tissue macromolecules in tissues such as articular cartilage (Tyler and Saklatvala, 1985; see review by Henderson and Lewthwaite, 1991). This inhibition of synthetic capacity may synergize with the increased rate of breakdown to produce tissue pathology.

The only way to definitively test the hypothesis that joint damage in rheumatoid arthritis is due to the degradative activity of MMPs is to develop selective inhibitors of these enzymes and to test them in relevant models of arthritis and then eventually in man. The rest of this chapter is devoted to the nature of the MMPs and the development and use of such inhibitors.

4. *The Matrix Metalloproteinases*

It is now 30 years since the initial discovery of the first MMP, collagenase (Gross and Lapiere, 1962). Early studies of this family of enzymes was hampered by the small amounts of enzyme produced by cells and tissues. Our current understanding of this growing family of enzymes owes much to the techniques of molecular

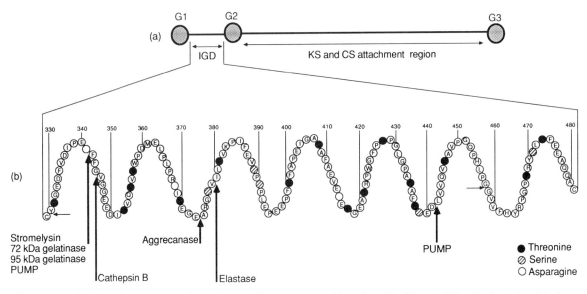

Figure 10.2 (a) Domain structure of porcine cartilage aggrecan (domains G1, G2 and G3) with the interglobular domain (IGD) between G1 and G2. Cleavage of aggrecan occurs in this interglobular domain. (b) Sequence of the IGD with the cleavage points for the MMPs, cathepsin B, elastase and the putative proteinase, aggrecanase. This diagram is reproduced by permission of Drs A. Fosang and T. Hardingham.

biology. Gene cloning has enabled the diversity of the MMPs to be recognized, and the ability to express large amounts of these enzymes has allowed structural studies to be made. A number of reviews on various aspects of the MMPs have been published in recent years (Birkedal-Hansen, 1988; Alexander and Werb, 1989; Emonard and Grimaud, 1990; Docherty and Murphy, 1990; Matrisian, 1990; Henderson *et al.*, 1990b; Murphy *et al.*, 1991a; Woessner, 1991).

At the present time there are seven well-characterized MMPs (Table 10.2). Additional enzymes have been recognized in cDNA libraries, although the putative enzymes may not have been isolated (e.g. Basset *et al.* (1990) have described an enzyme termed stromelysin

3 or MMP11 expressed in uterus, placenta and embryonic limb bud). The cDNA and protein sequences of these enzymes all show homology to that of interstitial collagenase.

The characterized enzymes are secreted as zymogens which can be activated by proteinases (e.g. plasmin), organomercurials or chaotropic agents. Activation is accompanied or followed by the loss of a 10 kDa N-terminal domain. The catalytic mechanism depends upon the zinc ion present in the catalytic centre, and this family of enzymes can cleave all of the extracellular components of the connective tissue matrix with the possible exception of elastin.

Table 10.2 Matrix metalloproteinase (MMP) family

Enzyme	Molecular mass (kDa) (SDS-PAGE)		Major substrates
	Latent	Active	
Collagenase (MMP1)	55	45	Collagen types I, II, III, VII, X
Neutrophil collagenase (MMP8)	75	58	Collagen types I, II, III
Stromelysin (MMP3)	57	48	Proteoglycan, fibronectin, laminin, collagens III, IV, V, IX, link protein, gelatin
Stromelysin-2 (MMP10)	57	48	Proteoglycan, fibronectin, gelatins
PUMP-1 (MMP7)	28	20	Proteoglycan, fibronectin, gelatins, all activate procollagenase
72 kDa gelatinase (MMP2)	72	66	Collagens IV, V, VII, X, gelatin, fibronectin
92 kDa gelatinase (MMP9)	95	88	Collagens IV, V, gelatin

4.1   STRUCTURE AND ACTIVATION OF THE MMPs

The MMPs have a surprisingly complex structure. For example the largest known MMP – 92 kDa gelatinase (MMP9) – has seven domains (Fig. 10.3). Beginning with the signal peptide there is, in turn: (i) a propeptide domain which is lost during activation; (ii) an active-site domain which is separated from the zinc-binding domain by a fibronectin-like domain; (iii) a type V collagen-like domain and finally a C-terminal haemopexin-like domain. The fibronectin, collagen and haemopexin domains are not required for proteolytic activity and are absent from MMP7 (PUMP-1), the smallest and simplest of the MMP family (Woessner and Taplin, 1988; Quantin *et al.*, 1989). The haemopexin domain is believed to be involved in determining substrate specificity, as its removal from collagenase leaves this protein able to cleave various proteins but unable to cleave collagen (Clark and Cawston, 1989). The function of the fibronectin-like and collagen-like domains may be to facilitate binding of the enzymes to their macromolecular substrates.

The mechanism responsible for the activation of the MMPs has puzzled investigators for many years. A diverse collection of agents such as aminophenylmercuric acetate, chaotropic agents, hypochlorous acid and proteinases such as plasmin and trypsin have been used for years to activate these enzymes. One likely possibility was the involvement of a sulphydryl group(s) in a relatively inaccessible position within the enzymes. All the MMPs possess a perfectly conserved 8–10-amino acid sequence, including one of the three conserved cysteines found in these enzymes, in the catalytic domain. It is likely that these conserved residues play a part in directing the specificity of the enzyme reaction (Sanchez-Lopez *et al.*, 1988). Van Wart and co-workers have proposed a model to account for this cysteine group in activation. The conserved cysteine in the catalytic domain is coordinated to the zinc atom in the catalytic centre, thus excluding water which must be the fourth substituent in the active site to allow full enzymic activity (see Section 5.2). Conversion of this cysteine to a non-bonding form, either chemically or by use of chaotropic agents to change the peptide conformation breaking the cysteine–zinc coordination, results in autocatalytic cleavage of the N-terminal propeptide and activation (Springman *et al.*, 1990). Proteases such as plasmin are believed to cleave off sufficient of the propeptide to "loosen" the binding of the cysteine to the zinc thus allowing autolytic cleavage and permanent activation of the MMP. Although proteases can activate collagenase, further cleavage of collagenase by stromelysin (MMP3) results in a marked increase in catalytic activity (reviewed by Woessner, 1991). It is proposed that stromelysin plays a key role in the *in vivo* activation of collagenase.

4.2   SUBSTRATE SPECIFICITY OF THE MMPs

Collagenase, or as it should more correctly be called interstitial collagenase, cleaves the three interstitial (fibre-forming) collagens – type I, II and III. These are distinguished from the other collagens in which there are non-helical domains (see review by Van der Rest and Garrone, 1991). This enzyme will also cleave α_2-macroglobulin with a k_{cat}/K_m 1–2 log orders greater than that for cleavage of the interstitial collagens (Enghild *et al.*, 1989). The gelatinases will cleave gelatin, fibronectin and collagens containing non-triple-helical domains such as type IV, V, VII and X. The 72 kDa gelatinase also has some weak elastolytic activity. The stromelysins have a wide substrate specificity being able to cleave proteoglycan, link protein, fibronectin, laminin, gelatin and types II, IV, V and IX collagen. In addition, these enzymes can cleave procollagenase (Table 10.2).

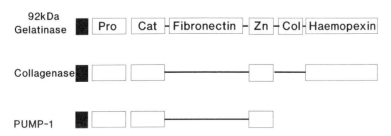

Figure 10.3 The domain structure of the MMPs. The boxes represent regions of amino acid similarity between the various enzymes. Collagenase and stromelysin have the same domain structure and the 72 kDa gelatinase is similar to the 92 kDa gelatinase but lacks the type V collagen domain. The shaded box is the signal peptide domain. The Pro domains are cleaved when the enzymes are converted to their active forms. The catalytic Cat domain contains a conserved region with three histidine residues which is believed to be the zinc-binding region and is denoted Zn. All enzymes with the exception of PUMP-1 contain the haemopexin domain. The gelatinases contain a fibronectin domain which has similarities to the collagen-binding domain of fibronectin. The 92 kDa gelatinase also contains a domain with sequence similarities to the α_2 chain of type V collagen (denoted Col).

4.3   Natural Inhibitors of the MMPs

The release of a potent inhibitor of collagenase by cultured fetal rabbit bone was reported by Sellers et al. (1977). The inhibitor was of molecular mass 30 kDa (by gel filtration), was heat sensitive and was inactivated by the action of trypsin or chymotrypsin. Further work showed that this inhibitor blocked the activity of rabbit bone metalloproteinases that degraded proteoglycan and gelatin (Sellers et al., 1979). This inhibitor was subsequently named TIMP (Cawston et al., 1981). On cloning, TIMP was shown to consist of 184 amino acids with a molecular mass of around 21 kDa. Glycosylation accounts for the greater molecular mass of the native inhibitor (28 kDa) (Docherty et al., 1985). There are 12 highly conserved cysteine residues which form six disulphide bonds organizing the molecule into a two-domain structure (Williamson et al., 1990). The MMP-inhibitory activity resides in the N-terminal domain, as shown by full retention of activity in a truncated version of the molecule in which the C-terminal domain was omitted (Murphy et al., 1991b). TIMP purified from rabbit bone forms a 1:1 complex with MMPs. The binding is reversible but the affinity of binding is high with a minimum K_i of approximately 10^{-10} M (Cawston, 1986).

A second inhibitor has been isolated from cultured human melanoma cells as a 21 kDa protein bound to the proform of 72 kDa gelatinase (Stetler-Stevenson et al., 1989). This molecule, called TIMP-2, has been cloned, and, although the primary sequence identity is only 40%, the cysteine residues that form the six disulphide bonds in TIMP (i.e. TIMP-1) are completely conserved (Boone et al., 1990). TIMP-1 has been shown to be a more potent inhibitor of collagenase, stromelysin and 72 kDa gelatinase than TIMP-2 (Ward et al., 1991). However, TIMP-2 has been reported to bind to rabbit interstitial 52 kDa procollagenase and inhibit the conversion to the 42 kDa active enzyme initiated by organomercurials. It also partially inhibited procollagenase activation induced by plasmin (De Clerck et al., 1991a). A high molecular mass TIMP-like inhibitor (large inhibitor of metalloproteinases (LIMP)) has been purified from culture supernatants of WI-38 fibroblasts. This molecule, although antigenically distinct from TIMP, formed inhibitory complexes with collagenase, stromelysin and 72 kDa gelatinase (Cawston et al., 1990). As far as is known, these inhibitors do not inhibit other metalloproteinases. How many more natural inhibitors of the MMPs await discovery remains to be determined. Information obtained from study of the interaction of natural inhibitors with the MMPs should be useful in the design of synthetic inhibitors.

5.   Development of Low Molecular Mass MMP Inhibitors as Therapeutic Agents

Enzyme inhibitors are widely used as drugs. The most successful drug of all time, aspirin, acts by irreversibly inhibiting the enzyme cyclooxygenase. However, the development of such inhibitors as drugs is no trivial task. Schnebli (1985) has postulated five criteria to be met by a proteinase inhibitor in order to have therapeutic potential (Table 10.3). The inhibitor must be specific. In the context of MMP inhibition, the requirement may be for inhibitors that block all members of this enzyme family or, alternatively, for compounds specifically blocking only one enzyme. The efficiency/potency means that not only should the inhibitor be extremely potent (have a low K_i) but that it should also have a high association rate constant and a low dissociation constant. That is, the inhibitor must interact rapidly with the enzyme to form an inhibitor complex and the complex should be stable for optimal effect. These requirements for pharmacological rather than biochemical inhibition are discussed in detail by Bieth (1980). The need for low toxicity is obvious. Whether or not this can be achieved with the MMPs will be discussed in Section 6. As has been described, there are a number of natural inhibitors of the MMPs. These molecules could have therapeutic potential but one problem with them is their potential immunogenicity. If patients were to mount an immune response to say TIMP, then this would preclude the further use of the molecule.

The final criterion, bioavailability, is also the one most difficult to achieve. Active compounds must not only inhibit the enzyme of interest, they must (i) be absorbed into the blood, (ii) reach the site in the organism where the enzyme is active, (iii) achieve a therapeutic concentration and (iv) maintain this concentration for a reasonable period. No matter how therapeutically useful a compound is, if it has to be taken frequently, then patient compliance diminishes.

Table 10.3   Criteria for development of therapeutic proteinase inhibitors

(1) Specificity (must only inhibit selected proteinase(s))
(2) Efficiency/potency (must be highly potent)
(3) Low toxicity
(4) Non-antigenic (problem with proteinaceous inhibitors)
(5) Bioavailabilty (must gain access to sites of proteinase activity)

5.1 CURRENT METALLOPROTEINASE INHIBITOR DRUGS

In spite of the difficulties in developing proteinase inhibitors as therapeutic agents, there is an increasing number of drugs on the market that inhibit metalloproteinases. Inhibitors of the metalloproteinase, ACE, are used in the treatment of hypertension. ACE is a zinc-containing carboxypeptidase which converts angiotensin I to the highly active vasoconstrictive peptide angiotensin II. Inhibition of ACE blocks the generation of angiotensin II. Captopril, a thiol-containing compound, was the first ACE inhibitor to be marketed. The development of this compound has been reviewed (Ondetti and Cushman, 1982; Petrillo and Ondetti, 1982). A number of distinct compounds are now on the market (Wingard et al., 1991). Inhibitors of the plasma membrane ectoenzyme neutral metalloendopeptidase (also called neutral endopeptidase (NEP), membrane metalloendopeptidase, enkephalinase or EC 3.4.24.11) have been developed and are in clinical trial as analgesics, anti-diarrhoeal agents and for various cardiovascular complaints (Chipkin, 1986; Erdos and Skidgel, 1989; Schwartz et al., 1990). More recently, inhibitors of a second membrane metalloendopeptidase, EC 3.4.24.15, have been shown to significantly lower blood pressure in the spontaneously hypertensive rat (Genden and Molineaux, 1991). These examples show that it is possible to develop clinically useful metalloproteinase inhibitors.

5.2 DEVELOPMENT OF LOW MOLECULAR MASS MMP INHIBITORS: GENERAL BACKGROUND

A number of pharmaceutical companies including Roche, SmithKline Beecham, Merck Sharp & Dohme, Searle (Monsanto) and Squibb and biopharmaceutical companies such as Celltech, British Biotechnology, Synergen and Chiron have programmes to develop synthetic or natural inhibitors of the MMPs as therapeutic agents. The major strategy taken by the pharmaceutical companies has been to develop low molecular mass competitive inhibitors.

The development of selective inhibitors of mammalian metalloproteinases owes much to Matthews and co-workers, who have extensively studied the catalytic mechanism of the bacterial enzyme thermolysin (EC 3.4.24.4). This is a thermostable calcium-binding zinc endopeptidase of molecular mass 35 kDa produced by the thermophilic bacterium *Bacillus thermoproteolyticus*. The three-dimensional structure of the enzyme has been determined to a nominal resolution of 1.6 Å and the binding of various inhibitors to thermolysin has also been determined crystallographically with similar resolution (reviewed by Matthews, 1988). Modelling of the active

sites of ACE, NEP and the MMPs has been based on data obtained from thermolysin. There is increasing doubt as to the value of such modelling because the homology between thermolysin and the MMPs is low. However, in the absence of detailed structural information on the MMPs, the proposed mechanism of peptide bond cleavage has been of value in designing inhibitors. A schematic diagram showing the key features of the proposed mechanism of action of thermolysin is shown in Fig. 10.4 with a detailed description of the mechanism. In simple terms, in the free enzyme, the zinc ion is coordinated to the side chains of His^{142}, His^{146} and Glu^{166} with a water molecule serving as the fourth ligand. The carbonyl oxygen of the incoming peptide substrate coordinates to the zinc ion in the catalytic centre. The water molecule is displaced toward Glu^{143} but is not totally excluded from coordination with the zinc ion. There is then a nucleophilic attack by the water molecule on the carbonyl carbon of the substrate. The attacking water is thought to be activated by interactions with both Glu^{143} and the zinc ion. In the presumed transition state, the carbonyl carbon of the substrate is tetrahedral and the zinc ion is coordinated to five ligands rather than to four in the free enzyme. The importance of the zinc ion in this catalytic mechanism is obvious.

Phosphoramidon, a naturally occurring potent inhibitor of thermolysin (and other metalloproteinases such as NEP), is thought to be a transition state analogue. Information derived from crystallographic studies of thermolysin and of thermolysin–phosphoramidon complexes has led to the synthesis of extremely potent inhibitors of thermolysin such as carbobenzoxy-L-Phe^P-L-Leu-L-Ala (ZF^{P}LA) which has a K_i of 70 pM (Holden et al., 1987). Moreover, such studies have related the structure of the inhibitors to the kinetics of their binding, and slow- and fast-binding inhibitors have been synthesized (Holden et al., 1987; Bartlett and Marlowe, 1987). This information may be of use in designing MMP inhibitors which bind rapidly to the enzyme active site, a requirement for pharmacological activity discussed in the previous section.

From the X-ray structures of the various classes of proteinases, it has been found that the catalytic site lies in a cleft on the surface of the enzyme molecule. The substrate polypeptide chain lies along the active-site cleft, and on either side of the catalytic site are so-called specificity subsites adapted to binding particular amino acid side chains, or the polypeptide backbone. This is the part of the enzyme that will be responsible for substrate recognition and in which there will be differences between different metalloproteinases. Such differences in substrate binding allow the design of selective metalloproteinase inhibitors. A system for referring to these subsites was developed by Berger and Schechter (1970) and is now in common usage (Fig. 10.5).

In designing ACE inhibitors, it was found that some simple dipeptide analogues such as Val-Trp were reasonably potent competitive inhibitors (e.g. the K_i for

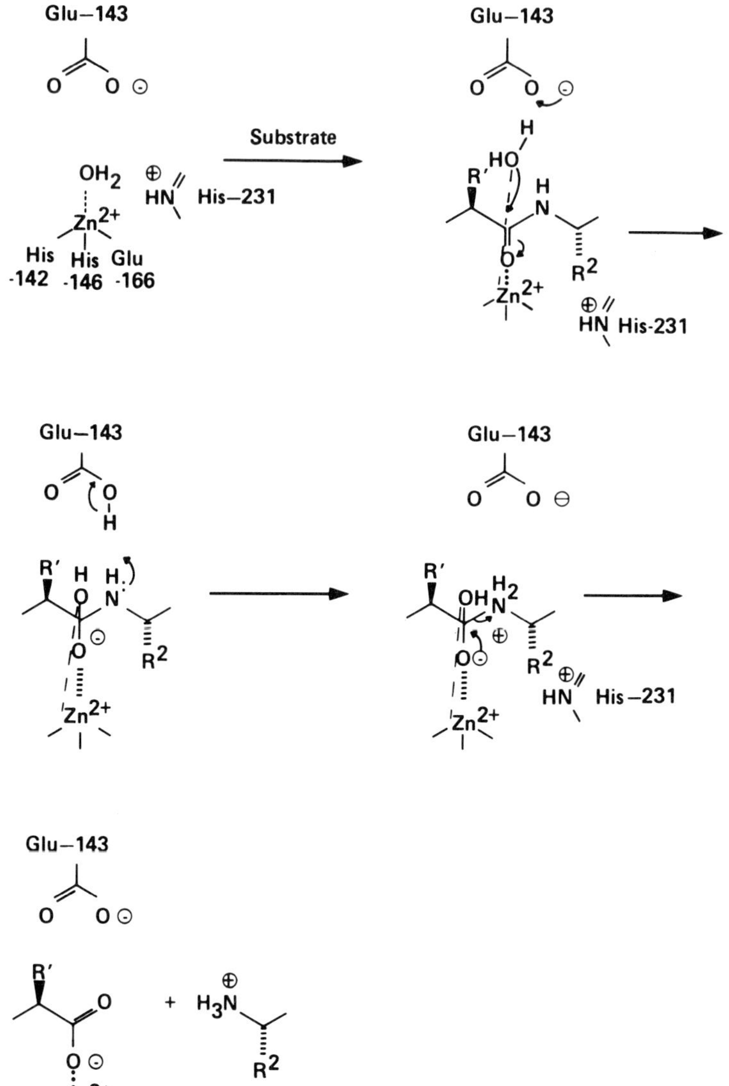

Figure 10.4 Schematic diagram representing the proposed mechanism of action of the bacterial enzyme thermolysin. The drawing on the top left shows the active site in the free enzyme with the zinc ion coordinated to the side chains of His[142], His[146] and Glu[166] with a water molecule serving as the fourth ligand. An incoming peptide is presumed to displace the zinc-bound water molecule toward Glu[143], forming a pentacoordinate complex (top right). The carbonyl group of the scissile bond is further polarized by coordination of its oxygen to the zinc, rendering the carbonyl carbon more susceptible to nucleophilic attack. The displaced water molecule, activated by the carboxylate of Glu[143], attacks the carbonyl group of the scissile bond to give a tetrahedral intermediate (left middle). The oxyanion is stabilized by coordination to the zinc and by hydrogen-bonding to the side chains of Tyr[157] and His[231]. The proton abstracted from the water molecule by Glu[143] is then presumed to be transferred to the nitrogen of the scissile bond (right middle). Collapse of the tetrahedral intermediate then gives a primary amine and a carboxylic acid and thus a zinc-bound carboxylate and primary ammonium species after proton transfer (bottom). After release of the protonated amine, a water molecule becomes the fifth zinc ligand, and expulsion of the product carboxylic acid and movement of the water molecule to its native position completes the cycle. (Reproduced from Henderson et al. (1991) with permission.)

SPECIFICITY SUBSITES OF PROTEINASES : TERMINOLOGY

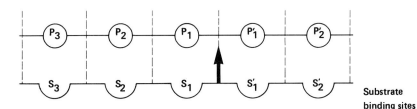

Figure 10.5 Terminology used to identify the specificity subsites of proteinases and the complementary features of the substrate. In this scheme, for the active site of an endopeptidase the substrate-binding sites are considered to be located on either side of the catalytic group in the enzyme active site. The subsites are numbered S_1, S_2 etc., away from the catalytic site towards the N-terminus of the substrate and $S'_1 S'_2$ etc., towards the C-terminus. The subsites are normally thought of as binding the side chains of the amino acid residues of the substrate. The amino acid residues in the substrate are correspondingly numbered P_1, P_2 etc. (N-terminal) and P'_1, P'_2 etc. (C-terminal). (After Berger and Schechter, 1970.)

Val-Trp is 0.3 μM). However, as would be expected, given the importance of zinc in the active site, dipeptide analogues containing strong zinc-binding ligands are much more potent inhibitors. Zinc-binding ligands used in the synthesis of ACE and also MMP inhibitors include thiols, hydroxamic acids, carboxylate and phosphonic acid. The interaction of the thiol ligand in captopril and the carboxylate ligand in the more potent enalapril with the zinc in the binding site of ACE is shown in Fig. 10.6. Further details of the chemistry and enzymology of

metalloproteinase inhibitors (although written too early to consider the MMP inhibitors in detail) is given in the excellent review by Powers and Wade Harper (1986).

5.3 DEVELOPMENT OF SYNTHETIC MMP INHIBITORS

To date the main strategy used in the development of inhibitors of the MMPs has been to incorporate a

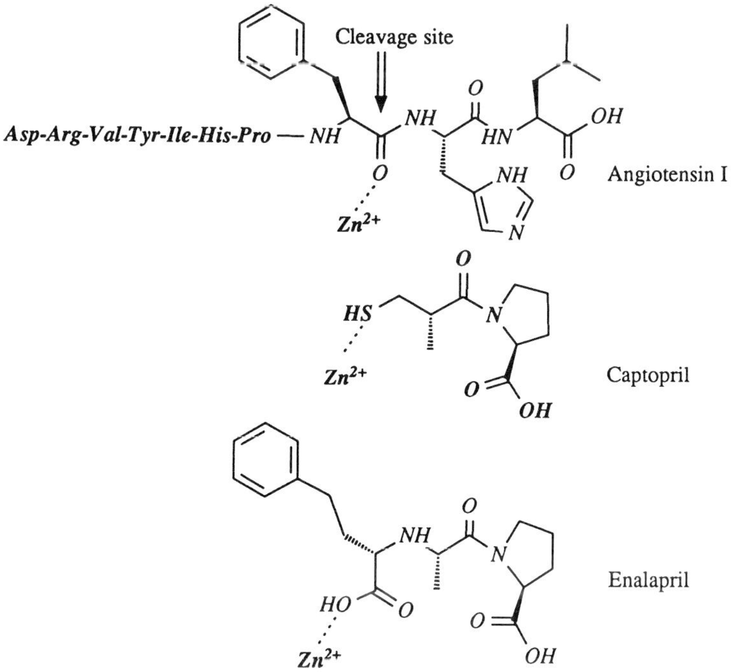

Figure 10.6 Inhibitors of ACE, captopril and enalapril, showing their relationship to the natural substrate angiotensin I. Note the similarity of these inhibitors to the dipeptide cleavage product and the binding of the zinc ligand in these molecules to the zinc ion in the enzyme's active site. (Reproduced from Henderson et al. (1991) with permission.)

zinc-binding group into a peptide framework which is modelled on the sequence of the substrate-cleavage site. Most attention has focused on the cleavage sites in the interstitial collagens (Fig. 10.7). However, the increasing knowledge of the MMP cleavage site in aggrecan (Fig. 10.2) could also be used in design studies. Most groups developing synthetic MMP inhibitors have screened their compounds using crude or semi-purified enzymes acting on macromolecular substrates (collagen for collagenase, casein or crude proteoglycan for stromelysin). The design of inhibitors depends on the accuracy and precision of the assay and on the derivation of kinetic information. In the widely used collagen fibril assay for collagenase (Cawston and Barrett, 1979), it is not easy to manipulate the concentration of collagen and so it cannot be used for deriving kinetic data (e.g. K_i values). The use of synthetic substrates or of the soluble collagenase assay developed by Van Wart's group (Mallya *et al.*, 1986) is needed in order to gain information about the kinetics of the inhibitors being designed.

Gray and colleagues were the first to rationally design collagenase inhibitors using metal-binding peptide analogues of the C-terminal sequence of the collagenase-cleavage site. The most active compound was 2-mercapto-4-methylpentanoyl-Ala-Gly-Gln-D-Arg-NH$_2$. Compare this structure with the collagen-cleavage site shown in Fig. 10.7. This compound had an IC$_{50}$(the concentration of inhibitor required to inhibit the enzyme activity by 50%) of 10 μM.

Since this early attempt to develop collagenase inhibitors, the major advances (as far as can be gathered from the literature) have been made by groups at Searle (now Monsanto and British Biotechnology), Stuart Pharmaceuticals (a subsidiary of ICI apparently no longer involved in this work) and Roche, England. Extensive investigations have been made of the subsite requirements of the collagenase active site using peptides based on the collagen-cleavage site and containing a variety of zinc-binding ligands. The zinc-binding ligand has been incorporated on to either side of the collagen-cleavage site or into the centre of the peptide as is shown in Fig. 10.8. This is the same approach that was used in the development of ACE inhibitors (Petrillo and Ondetti, 1982). These groups can be attached to the N-terminal or C-terminal residues or placed in the middle of the substrate sequence to produce what are termed left hand side (LHS), right hand side (RHS) or combination inhibitors respectively (Fig. 10.8). The design of such inhibitors has

Collagen		P$_4$		P$_3$		P$_2$		P$_1$	Cleavage site	P$'_1$		P$'_2$		P$'_3$
Bovine α_1	(I)	Gly	—	Pro	—	Gln	—	Gly		Ile	—	Ala	—	Gly
Bovine α_2	(I)	Gly	—	Pro	—	Gln	—	Gly		Leu	—	Leu	—	Gly
Bovine α_1	(II)			Unknown			—	Gly		Ile	—	Ala	—	Gly
Human α_1	(I)	Gly	—	Pro	—	Gln	—	Gly		Ile	—	Ala	—	Gly
Human α_1	(II)			Unknown			—	Gly		Ile	—	Ala	—	Gly
Human α_1	(III)	Gly	—	Pro	—	Leu	—	Gly		Ile	—	Ala	—	Gly

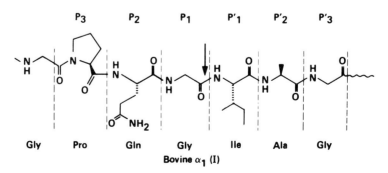

Figure 10.7 The cleavage site in mammalian interstitial collagens catalysed by collagenase (MMP1). The lower diagram shows the amino acid sequence around the cleavage site in the bovine α_1 (I) chain. As described in Fig. 10.5, the individual amino acid residues are numbered P$_1$, P$_2$ etc. away from the catalytic site towards the N-terminus and P$'_1$, P$'_2$ etc. toward the C-terminus.

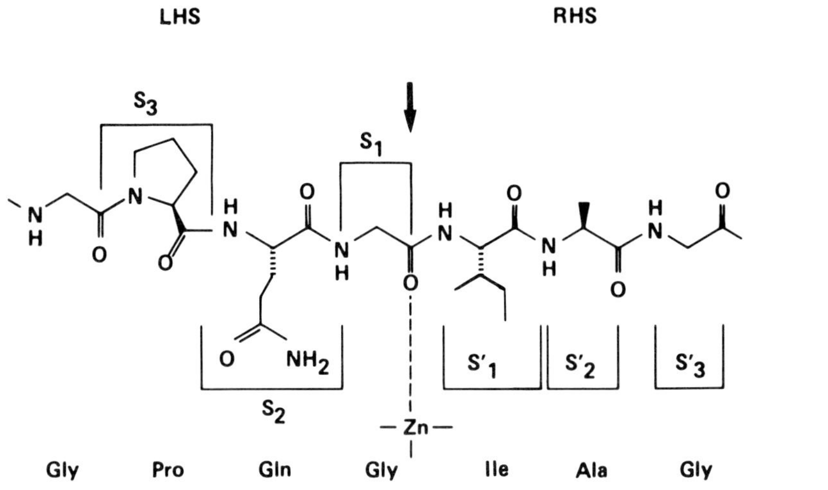

LHS Inhibitors (N–terminal) $P_3 - P_2 - P_1$ – Zinc binding group

RHS Inhibitors (C–terminal) Zinc binding group $P'_1 - P'_2 - P'_3$

LHS + RHS $P_3 - P_2 - P_1$ – Zinc binding group – $P'_1 - P'_2 - P'_3$

Figure 10.8 Three types of metalloproteinase peptide analogue inhibitors. The linear sequence of substrate amino acids at the active site in collagenase with the substrate-binding sites enumerated is shown in the upper diagram. The lower diagram shows that zinc-binding ligands can be attached to peptides derived from the P_3–P_1 side of the substrate to produce left hand side (LHS) inhibitors (also termed N-terminal inhibitors) or to the P'_3–P'_1 side to produce right hand side (RHS) or C-terminal inhibitors. In addition the zinc ligand can be attached to the centre of the peptide amino acid sequence. (Reproduced from Henderson and Davies (1991) with permission.)

been reviewed by Johnson *et al.* (1987) (see also Henderson and Davies, 1991).

A number of groups have investigated the LHS inhibitors. Compounds containing thiols (DiPasquale *et al.*, 1986) or hydroxamic acids (Johnson *et al.*, 1987) as zinc-binding ligands have been synthesized. Such compounds are weak inhibitors with I_{50} values in the micromolar range.

Thiol-containing peptides were the first RHS inhibitors described (Donald *et al.*, 1986). However, it was soon shown that hydroxamic acid-containing inhibitors were significantly more active and did not suffer from oxidative inactivation (Dickens *et al.*, 1986; Johnson *et al.*, 1987; Darlak *et al.*, 1990). A comparison of the activities of peptide inhibitors containing carboxyalkyl, thiol or hydroxamate zinc-binding groups is shown in Table 10.4 (see Shaw *et al.*, 1988). These compounds were synthesized by Stuart Pharmaceuticals and have been tested for activity against neutral proteoglycan- and collagen-degrading enzymes released from IL-1-stimulated rabbit articular chondrocytes. The hydroxamic acid-containing compounds show a log order difference in their ability to inhibit collagenase and the proteoglycan-degrading activity (presumably stromelysin and gelatinase).

In addition to investigating the role of the zinc ligand in determining potency, the effect of modifying the C-terminal P'_1 to P'_4 peptide side chains has also been investigated (Fig. 10.9). In collagen, the P'_1 is Leu/Ile. Altering the stereochemistry, removing the side chain or replacing the P'_1 isobutyl side chain by methyl or benzyl groups resulted in inactive compounds. At P'_2, a number of replacements for the natural residue, alanine, can be made to produce more activity. At P'_3 the natural amino acid, glycine, could be replaced by alanine to give increased activity. Most other replacements led to loss of activity. Finally, changes in the P'_4 position had little influence on activity. Further improvement in activity was observed when the amide bond between P'_3 and P'_4 was replaced by a carboxylic acid or an ester. When all these optimizations in structure had been made, the final inhibitor shown in Fig. 10.9 was obtained (Johnson *et al.*, 1987). A comparison of the activities of the most active hydroxamic acid-containing inhibitors from Searle, Roche and Stuart pharmaceuticals is shown in Fig. 10.10.

Table 10.4 Comparison of the activity of metalloproteinase inhibitors synthesized by Stuart Pharmaceuticals

		$IC_{50}(M)$	
Class	Compound	collagenase	stromelysin
Carboxyalkyl			
	HOOCCH (i-Bu)LeuLeuLeuOH	$>10^{-4}$	5.3×10^{-6}
	HOOCCH (i-Bu)LeuLeuPheNH$_2$	$>10^{-4}$	5.2×10^{-6}
	HOOCCH (i-Bu)LeuPheNH$_2$	$>10^{-5}$	1.9×10^{-6}
Thiol	Ac Phe NHCH(i-Bu)CH$_2$SH	10^{-6}–10^{-5}	10^{-6}–10^{-5}
	Ac Ser NHCH(i-Bu)CH$_2$SH	10^{-6}–10^{-5}	10^{-6}–10^{-5}
	Ac Trp NHCH(i-Bu)CH$_2$SH	1.6×10^{-6}	10^{-6}–10^{-5}
Hydroxamate			
	HONHCOCH$_2$CH(n-pentyl)COLeuPheNH$_2$	4.8×10^{-6}	1×10^{-7}
	HONHCOCH$_2$CH(n-pentyl)COLeuAlaNH$_2$	$>10^{-6}$	1.2×10^{-7}
	HONHCOCH$_2$CH(i-Bu)COLeuPheNH$_2$	4.1×10^{-7}	4.2×10^{-8}
	HONHCOCH$_2$CH(n-pentyl)COValAlaNH$_2$	4.5×10^{-7}	3.4×10^{-8}

From DiPasquale *et al.* (1986).

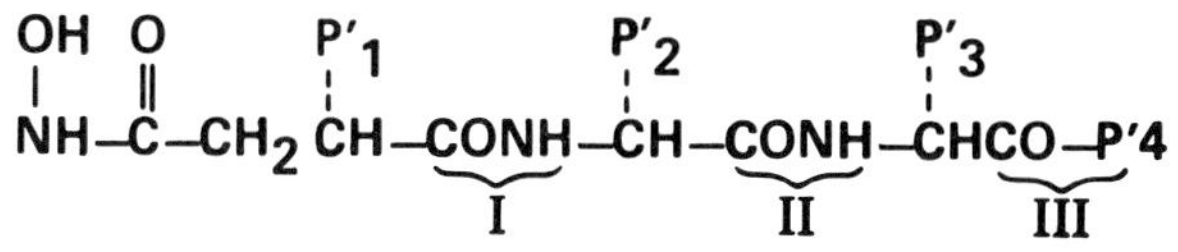

P'_1 Limited to Leu/Ile

P'_2 Leu, Tyr(OMe), Lys (Boc), Val but not Pro can replace Ala to give more active compounds

P'_3 Replacement of glycine normally leads to inactive compounds. However, replacement by L–alanine improved activity.

P'_4 Little effect of a variety of replacements.

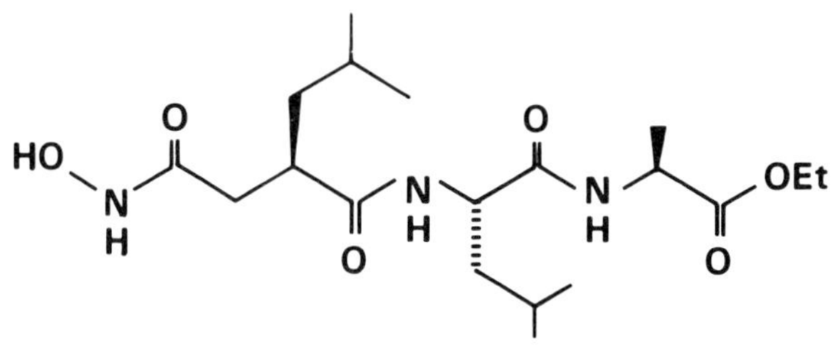

$$IC_{50} = 8.5 \times 10^{-9} M$$
$$Ki = 5.0 \times 10^{-9} M$$

Figure 10.9 The effect on inhibitor potency of modifying the side chains in the RHS inhibitors synthesized by Roche. The effect of the various side chain replacements is described, and the final compound, which has incorporated these favourable modifications, has an IC_{50} value of 8.5 nM against collagenase. (Reproduced from Henderson and Davies (1991) with permission.)

Hydroxamic Acid Based Collagenase Inhibitors

Company	Structure	Activity (nM) IC$_{50}$

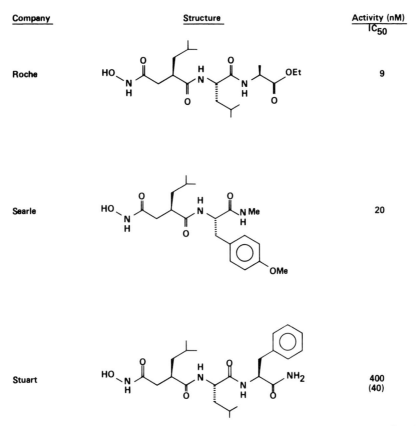

Roche		9
Searle		20
Stuart		400 (40)

Figure 10.10 Hydroxamic acid-based peptide analogue inhibitors synthesized by Roche, Searle and Stuart Pharmaceuticals. The compounds are the most active of the respective series. The Stuart compound is 10-fold more active against rabbit chondrocyte proteoglycanase (stromelysin and gelatinase) than against rabbit collagenase. (Reproduced from Henderson and Davies (1991) with permission.)

The RHS compounds described are believed to be competitive inhibitors of the MMPs. However, there is little information available on the enzyme kinetics of such inhibitors. A recent study by Gray and co-workers of potent thiol-based compounds reported that their mode of inhibition, as defined by use of Dixon plots, could not be clearly defined (Darlak *et al.*, 1990). A similar problem was also reported in studies of neutrophil collagenase and was explained as being due to interactions of the inhibitor with the collagen (Mookhtiar *et al.*, 1987). The binding of inhibitors to the extracellular matrix in cartilage or bone may be a problem in the therapeutic use of these inhibitors.

The Roche Group (Welwyn Garden City, UK) have made further modifications to their inhibitors to increase *in vivo* stability. Building in a lactam ring into the right hand side of the hydroxamic acid shown in Fig. 10.11 had minimal effect on activity but should increase stability in the body. In addition to increasing the stability of the molecule, the Roche group have also developed compounds that are transition state analogues. The

acceleration of the rates of specific reactions by enzymes is attributed to the stabilization of the transition state at the catalytic centre. As a consequence, inhibitors that partially mimic this transition state bind more tightly than the equivalent substrate. Very potent transition state analogue inhibitors of proteases such as thermolysin (Matthews, 1988), renin (Blundell *et al.*, 1987) and elastase (Trainor, 1987) have been developed in recent years. The Roche compound is a phosphinic acid transition state analogue containing the lactam ring which had been optimized in earlier studies (top structure in Fig. 10.11). It is claimed that the structure confers almost total metabolic stability to this inhibitor (Brown, 1991).

5.4 FUTURE DEVELOPMENTS IN INHIBITOR DESIGN

As far as we can tell from the literature, the majority of synthetic MMP inhibitors synthesized to date are peptide

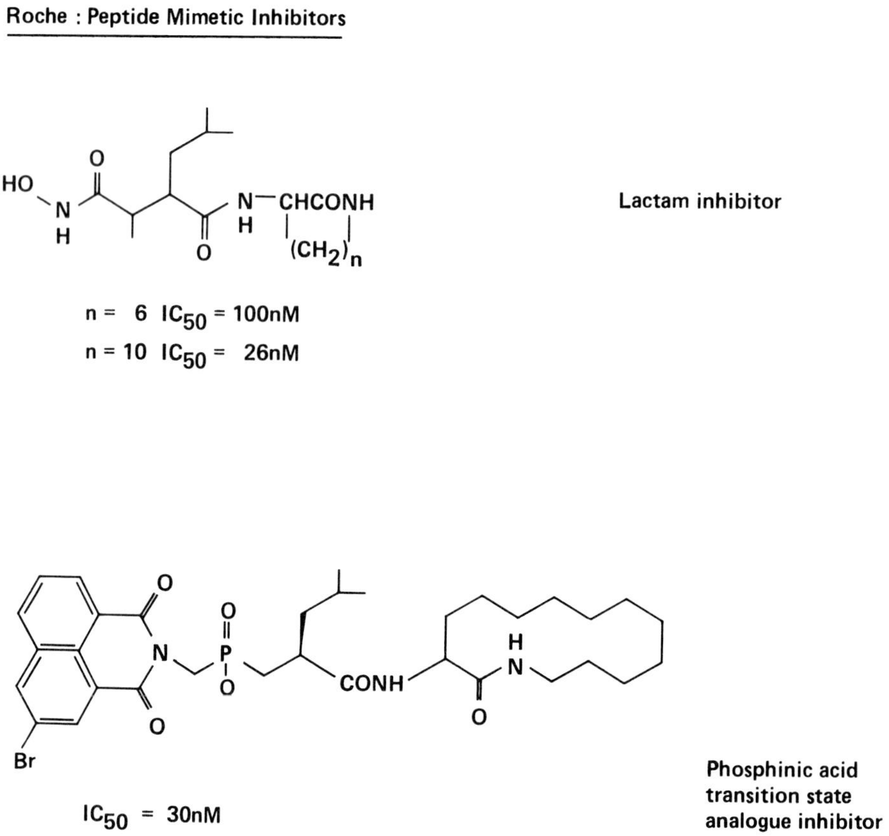

Roche : Peptide Mimetic Inhibitors

Lactam inhibitor

n =   6 IC_{50} = 100nM
n = 10 IC_{50} =   26nM

IC_{50} = 30nM

Phosphinic acid
transition state
analogue inhibitor

Figure 10.11 Development, by Roche Pharmaceuticals of peptide mimetic inhibitors containing a lactam ring (top structure) and a phosphinic acid transition state analogue inhibitor (bottom structure). These compounds have been developed to increase *in vivo* stability. (See Johnson *et al.* (1987) and Nixon *et al.* (1991).)

analogues of the collagen-cleavage site containing zinc ligands. While these compounds are potent inhibitors, they are unlikely to be particularly useful therapeutic agents. The reason for this is simple. Small peptides have very limited bioavailability because of problems of entering the blood from the gut and their rapid inactivation by tissue proteinases. Proteolytic inactivation can be minimized by replacement of the peptide bond with an isostere which is less susceptible to proteolytic cleavage. The classic peptide backbone modification is substituting D- for L-amino acids. A range of additional backbone modifications improving stability to protease attack have been developed (reviewed by Veber and Freidinger, 1985; Fauchere, 1986). Few reports of the synthesis and use of peptide isostere MMP inhibitors have yet appeared. An inhibitor containing the protease-"stable" ketomethylene bond has been described (Wallace *et al.*, 1986). Roche have developed their transition state inhibitor which is claimed to be stable *in vivo* (Brown, 1991). Therefore the next stage in the development of MMP inhibitors as drugs is to explore the synthesis of non-peptide analogues for inhibitory activity both in *in vitro* and *in vivo* systems.

To reiterate, up until the present time the emphasis of the development of MMP inhibitors has been to inhibit the active enzyme. Compounds that have been developed are potent inhibitors of the isolated MMPs but, as will be described in the next section, they are generally poor inhibitors of connective tissue breakdown both *in vitro* and *in vivo*. These experimental results could be explained if: (i) enzymes other than the known MMPs (and with different enzymic mechanisms) were responsible for the tissue damage; or (ii) if the concentration of connective tissue substrate at the site of enzymic breakdown is so very much greater than that of the competitive MMP inhibitor that it cannot demonstrate activity at sensible concentrations. It is obvious that the concentration of proteoglycan and collagen in articular cartilage is much higher than is ever used in test-tube assays of MMP inhibitor activity. If this latter explanation is valid, then it may require the development of very much more potent compounds and/or compounds with different mechanisms of inhibition.

An additional approach that could be taken to the design of inhibitors of the MMPs is to target the activation of these enzymes. If the process of activation of the proenzymes could be inhibited, then this would attain the same goal as inhibition of the active enzyme. This approach would not suffer from the problems just indicated with regard to the enzyme substrate ratios in connective tissue. The amounts of proenzyme produced by activated cells is low and so competitive inhibitors would be effective. The recent report that TIMP-2 inhibits the activation of procollagenase (DeClerk et al., 1991a) suggests that this is a viable approach. Knowledge of the three-dimensional structure of TIMP-2–procollagenase complexes would be invaluable in the design of such "proenzyme inhibitors". Unfortunately, to date, only porcine interstitial collagenase has been crystallized and only a low-resolution X-ray crystal structure has been obtained (Lloyd et al., 1989).

5.5 BIOLOGICAL ACTIVITY OF MMP INHIBITORS

The ultimate test of the hypothesis that a particular disease state is due to the actions of a specific enzyme or group of enzymes is to inhibit the enzyme(s). If this proves beneficial, then the hypothesis is supported and a new and effective therapy is on the horizon. This is the current situation with the MMPs. There are a number of diseases in which the pathology is believed to depend on the actions of specific MMPs or of all of the MMPs acting in concert. In the arthritic diseases, it is believed that stromelysin and the gelatinases are responsible for the breakdown of aggrecan (although this is now questionable – see Section 3.2) and that collagenase breaks down the collagen network. In tumour metastasis, it is thought that the 72 and 92 kDa gelatinases are important in the passage of cells across the basement membranes of blood vessels (Testa and Quigley, 1991). Corneal damage due to trauma is believed to be the result of the stimulation of synthesis of interstitial collagenase by corneal epithelial cells (Berman, 1980). There is now a growing body of studies in which inhibitors of the MMPs have been tested both in vitro and in vivo to determine if they can block tissue pathology. The discussion will first concentrate on studies with TIMP and then will focus on low molecular mass inhibitors.

5.5.1 TIMP

The ability of natural or recombinant human TIMP (rhTIMP, mainly TIMP-1) to inhibit the breakdown of collagen matrices by mesenchymal cells or inhibit tumour cell migration through human amnion or reconstituted basement membranes (Matrigel) has been established. Thus rhTIMP has been shown to inhibit the degradation of radioactively labelled collagen films by vitamin-D-stimulated osteoblasts (Thomas et al., 1987) and by IL-1-stimulated chondrocytes or epithelial cells (Gavrilovic et al., 1987). These cells are presumed to release MMPs when stimulated. TIMP has also been reported to inhibit

the breakdown of porcine synovial tissue stimulated by colchicine (Reynolds et al., 1988). However, TIMP was apparently unable to block the release of proteoglycan from bovine nasal cartilage stimulated by IL-1 (Saklatvala, 1989).

Cultured neonatal murine calvaria or fetal rat long bones are routinely used to investigate the mechanisms of bone turnover. Sakamoto et al. (1984) found that a TIMP-like inhibitor isolated from bone or an anti-collagenase antibody inhibited parathyroid hormone-stimulated bone resorption.

TIMP-1 inhibits the invasion of human amnion by M5076 sarcoma cells (Thorgeirsson et al., 1982) or B16 cells (Mignatti et al., 1986; Schultz et al., 1988). In more recent years it has been shown that TIMP-2 can also inhibit tumour cell invasion. Invasion of a reconstituted basement membrane by HT-1080 tumour cells was inhibited by approximately 85% by TIMP-2 (Albini et al., 1991). This inhibition was related to the inhibition of the 72 kDa gelatinase. DeClerk and co-workers demonstrated the inhibitory activity of rhTIMP-2 on the invasion of cultured smooth muscle cell monolayers by HT-1080 cells and by a ras-transformed rat fibroblast line, 4R. This latter cell line secretes mainly the 92 kDa gelatinase (DeClerk et al., 1991b). These studies show that TIMP can inhibit tumour cell migration by blockade of either of the known gelatinases.

Angiogenesis is a key event in normal remodelling, wound healing and various diseases. Tumour growth depends on neovascularization, and in rheumatoid arthritis the pannus is a granulation tissue. Selective inhibition of angiogenesis could therefore be of therapeutic importance. The finding that TIMP can inhibit experimental angiogenesis in the chick yolk sac membrane is therefore of interest (Takigawa et al., 1990).

TIMP has also shown some inhibitory activity in in vivo studies. The assumption is that the effects seen are due to inhibition of MMPs. However, TIMP may have other actions which give rise to the observed effects. Lark et al. (1990) have demonstrated that injection of rhTIMP into the rat pleural cavity before the injection of stromelysin inhibited the ability of the enzyme to degrade injected aggrecan monomer. Significant inhibition occurred at TIMP/stromelysin molar ratios of 2:1 and 1:1 with less inhibition at molar ratios of 0.5:1 and 0.25:1. The serine proteinase inhibitor α_1-proteinase inhibitor did not inhibit stromelysin activity in the pleural cavity (Lark et al., 1990).

TIMP-1 has been reported to inhibit experimental metastasis in nude mice. In this model, animals are injected with a fixed number of a known metastatic tumour cell line, and the numbers of metastatic colonies in the lungs estimated. Schultz et al. (1988) found that treatment of mice with 1.14 mg of rhTIMP every 12 h for 5 days inhibited lung colonization by mouse B16 tumour cells by 50%. In a separate study using a ras-transfected rat embryo cell line (4R), rhTIMP-1

(0.96 mg) was given every 6 h over the first day after tumour cell injection and then every 12 h until the last administration at 84 h. Animals were killed after 2 weeks and the tumour nodules on the lungs counted. TIMP treatment was found to have inhibited colonization by 83% (Alvarez *et al.*, 1990).

These results appear impressive and suggest that TIMP-1 or -2 could have therapeutic potential in inhibiting cancer metastasis. The potential at present is unclear but a few simple calculations suggest one major problem. In order to inhibit (but not completely block) lung colonization in mice, repeated injections of around 1 mg of rhTIMP were needed. Taking an average weight for a mouse as 25 g and scaling up the doses for a standard 70 kg "man", then each dose of TIMP would be in the region of 3 g. This would have to be administered daily for many years. With a regime of four doses per day, then a patient would require 12 g per day × 365 = 4.4 kg per year. The cost of this therapy would therefore be very expensive assuming that such enormous quantities of recombinant protein could be manufactured. One other problem which could arise with the injection of such large amounts of protein is the stimulation of an untoward immune response to the TIMP.

The report that rhTIMP also inhibits collagen-induced arthritis in mice (Carmichael *et al.*, 1989) also raises the point made above as very large amounts of TIMP were administered. The other major argument against the use of TIMP in treating diseases such as rheumatoid arthritis is the need to inject the protein. This would not be such a problem in a life-threatening condition like cancer. The most likely conditions benefitting from the inhibitory activity of the TIMPs are corneal ulceration and periodontal disease. In both lesions, the TIMP can be applied locally obviating problems with systemic half-life and bioavailability.

5.5.2   Low Molecular Mass Compounds

The first description of the *in vitro* activity of a low molecular mass collagenase inhibitor was the report from Vaes's group that a Searle carboxyalkyl inhibitor (CI-1:   *N*-[3-*N*-(benzyloxycarbonyl)amino-1-(*R*)-carboxypropyl]-L-leucyl-*O*-methyl-L-tyrosine *N*-methylamide) could inhibit calvarial bone resorption induced by parathyroid hormone. The compound was a carboxyalkyl peptide analogue with an IC_{50} value of approximately 1–5 μM. Complete suppression of bone resorption was seen with 25–50 μM inhibitor and significant inhibition was obtained with as little as 10 μM (Delaisse *et al.*, 1985). This should be contrasted with the results in cartilage described below. The synthesis and release of collagenase from osteoblasts is believed to be an essential step in allowing osteoclasts to degrade the mineralized matrix of bone (reviewed by Sakamoto and Sakamoto, 1988).

A number of pharmaceutical companies have designed MMP inhibitors for the treatment of osteo- and

rheumatoid arthritis. The team at Stuart Pharmaceuticals designed some very potent hydroxamic acid inhibitors (DiPasquale *et al.*, 1986). Compounds such as U24631 (HONCOCC(*n*-phenyl)COValAlaNH$_2$) had IC_{50} values against rabbit chondrocyte proteoglycanase (presumably stromelysin and gelatinase) of 30 nM. When this same compound was tested for its ability to inhibit proteoglycan loss from retinoid-stimulated rabbit articular cartilage, it showed only minimal activity at 0.1 mM. In contrast, compound U24278 (HONCOCC(*n*-pentyl)COLeuPheNH$_2$) which was 10-fold less active than U24631 in the proteoglycanase assay almost completely inhibited proteoglycan loss from rabbit cartilage at 0.1 mM (Caputo *et al.*, 1987). Similar results have been reported by Roche with their potent hydroxamic peptide analogue compound Ro31-4724 and their transition state analogue inhibitor Ro31-7467 (Fig. 10.11). The former compound has a potency value of 10–25 nM when tested with MMPs capable of cleaving collagen, gelatin or casein. The transition state analogue inhibitor has a similar potency against collagenase but is 10-fold less active with gelatin- or casein-degrading MMPs. High concentrations of both inhibitors (0.1 mM) were required to inhibit proteoglycan loss from IL-1-stimulated bovine nasal cartilage (Nixon *et al.*, 1991).

To investigate in more detail the pathophysiological stimuli promoting joint destruction, cartilage removed from rabbits with induced "osteoarthritis" (produced by removing part of the meniscus of the knee joint) has been tested to ascertain the effect of synthetic collagenase inhibitors. In cartilage removed from operated joints, there was an increased release of proteoglycan. Potent hydroxamic acid inhibitors (active at nanomolar concentrations with purified enzyme) blocked this release of proteoglycan but the concentration reported to do this was 0.1 mM, suggesting that there was little effect at lower concentrations.

These findings with cartilage proteoglycan loss induced by IL-1, retinoids or *in vivo* pathomechanisms may have a number of explanations as discussed in the previous section: (i) the inhibitors may be unable to enter the articular cartilage because of the high concentration of connective tissue macromolecules; (ii) the compounds may bind to the cartilage matrix and be unable to interact with the MMPs; (iii) the enzyme(s) responsible for cartilage proteoglycan loss may not be those against which the inhibitors have been designed. The putative enzyme termed aggrecanase which is responsible for the cleavage of proteoglycan in IL-1-stimulated cartilage *in vitro* may not be inhibited by the MMP inhibitors designed to date. Finally, the very high ratio of substrate/inhibitor in articular cartilage may require high concentrations of inhibitor to achieve efficacy. The ability to inhibit bone resorption in culture with micromolar concentrations of a relatively inactive MMP inhibitor partly supports the last point.

The Searle hydroxamic acid inhibitor SC44463 (Fig. 10.10) has been tested for its ability to inhibit tumour cell invasion through Matrigel-reconstituted basement membrane. This process is believed to be due to the release of gelatinases and is inhibited by TIMPs. This compound would inhibit the invasion of the Matrigel by HT-1080 cells but only at relatively high concentrations. It also blocked the colonization of the lungs of experimental mice by B16 and M2 tumour cells. Significant inhibition was seen when 1 mg of inhibitor was given along with the tumour cells and 2.5 mg given 2 h later (Fig. 10.12). The inhibitor had to be given along with the tumour cells. If given 2 h later, it was ineffective (Reich et al., 1988). Again, this compound which is extremely active against purified MMPs needs to be administered at very high concentrations in order to show efficacy. To achieve almost complete inhibition of colonization, 6 mg of the drug had to be administered over a 2–3 h period. Scaling up this dosage for a 70 kg man would mean, with the same experimental protocol, the administration of 17 g of drug. MMP inhibitors have also been tested for their ability to inhibit the penetration of cultured sympathetic neurones into collagen gels. This is an in vitro model of the normal process of neurite outgrowth in the peripheral nervous system. The Searle carboxyalkyl inhibitor reported to inhibit calvarial bone

resorption, CI-1, was inactive even at 10 mM. In contrast, thiol inhibitors such as $HSCH_2$-(R,S)-$CH[CH_2CH(CH_3)_2]$-CO-Phe-NH_2 (Gray et al., 1986) inhibited neuronal migration by 50% at concentrations of 150–200 nM (a concentration close to the K_i of these inhibitors of 50–100 nM) (Pittman and Williams, 1988).

MMP inhibitors have also been used to ascertain the importance of collagenase in ovulation. The mature oocyte must penetrate a number of collagenous layers in order to escape from the Graafian follicle. The Searle hydroxamic acid peptide analogue inhibitor, SC44463 (Fig. 10.12), which has an IC_{50} against purified MMPs of approximately 20 nM (Searle data) and against rat ovarian collagenase of 3 nM (Butler et al., 1991), was tested for its ability to inhibit ovulation in perfused rat ovaries. Significant inhibition of ovulation was seen with 2.5 nM inhibitor and a concentration of 25 nM resulted in 55% inhibition. Perfusion medium was tested for the presence of this inhibitor to gain some information on its stability. After 20 h of perfusion, the medium still contained $89.8 \pm 9.1\%$ (mean $\pm$ S.E.M.; $n = 5$) of the inhibitor (Butler et al., 1991). It is unclear why these potent hydroxamic acid-containing inhibitors are so efficacious in the ovary but show such limited activity in cultured articular cartilage or in inhibiting tumour cell invasion, but the problems discussed above, including

Inhibition of Experimental Metastases by a Collagenase Inhibitor

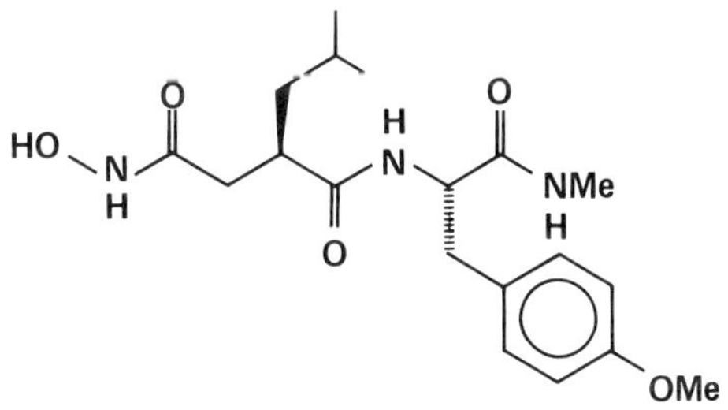

SC 44463

Mouse Group	Treatment	Lung Lesions, no/mouse mean ± SEM
1	No inhibitor	133 ± 20
2	1 mg at 0h + 2.5 mg at 2h	15 ± 4*
3	1 mg at 0h + 5 mg at 2h	5 ± 2*
4	5 mg at 2h	81 ± 20

B16–F10 cells used
*p<0.01

Figure 10.12 Inhibition of experimental metastasis in mice dosed with the Searle hydroxamic acid analogue inhibitor (SC44463). B16-F10 tumour cells were injected into mice and the animals killed 2 weeks later, and the number of tumour colonies in the lung enumerated. To determine the effect of inhibiting MMPs on tumour cell colonization, one group of animals was given 2.5 mg of inhibitor along with the cells and a second dose given 2 h later. Another group was given twice this dose. This treatment has significantly inhibited the colonization of the lung by tumour cells. (Reproduced from Reich et al. (1988) with permission.)

penetration of inhibitor, substrate concentration and enzyme specificity, may be involved.

The efficacy of MMP inhibitors in arthritis models must have been tested by a number of the leading companies but almost no results have been released. British Biotechnology have reported that a number of their compounds inhibited adjuvant arthritis in the rat. Significant improvement in joint swelling which was paralleled by substantial bone- and cartilage-sparing effects was found with administration of reasonable doses of inhibitor (Crimmin, 1991). Of course, adjuvant arthritis is a very poor model of rheumatoid arthritis, more resembling leprosy than arthritis (Gardner, 1972). Indeed this lesion, including cartilage and bone destruction, can be inhibited by non-steroidal drugs (Billingham, 1983). As has been discussed, these same drugs have no effect on tissue destruction in rheumatoid arthritis. Given the uncertainty of the pathological mechanisms in this adjuvant model it is important to relate the inhibition of cartilage and bone damage to inhibition of the MMPs.

Simple metal-binding agents such as cysteine and EDTA have been reported to have some efficacy in treating both experimental corneal ulceration and ulceration in man (reviewed by Berman, 1980). Two recent studies have utilized potent peptide-based synthetic MMP inhibitors and have shown some efficacy in the alkali-burned corneal ulceration model (Burns et al., 1990; Schultz et al., 1990). Inhibitor-treated animals showed little corneal ulceration, and few inflammatory cells were evident (Burns et al., 1990).

6. Potential Side Effects

The pharmaceutical industry is a cautious beast knowing that, if it commits itself to one therapeutic possibility, it may end up spending tens of millions of pounds just to produce a drug that has interesting, but commercially disastrous, side effects. The possibility that inhibitors of the MMPs may generate side effects will have been actively discussed within the corridors of pharmaceutical companies. However, it is too early to predict the possible side effects. Unfortunately, we know very little about the role of this growing family of enzymes in normal homeostasis. It is assumed that the MMPs are responsible for the normal remodelling of the connective tissue matrices of the various tissues and organs of the body. Inhibition of these enzymes by a general MMP inhibitor could block this remodelling and produce tissue pathology. In certain tissues such as the lung (Laurent, 1982), periodontal ligament and gingiva (Sodek, 1990), there is a rapid turnover of collagen. Inhibition of MMP activity could lead to fibrotic changes in these tissues. Bone contains an organic matrix consisting of 90% collagen and is constantly undergoing remodelling. The inhibition of this remodelling could lead to pathological changes. Wound healing must involve the activity of the

MMPs and would certainly be affected by inhibitors of these enzymes. The ability of TIMP to inhibit neovascularization, a key process in wound healing (Takigawa et al., 1990), gives some cause for concern.

Woessner et al. (1989) have proposed that ovulation requires the action of a specific collagenase to remove a collagen meshwork lying over the follicle. Evidence supporting this hypothesis includes the increased collagenase activity in gonadotrophin-treated rat ovaries and the ability to inhibit ovulation using extremely low concentrations of the Searle hydroxamic peptide inhibitor SC44463 (Woessner et al., 1989; Butler et al., 1991). Collagenase has long been recognized as a major enzyme in the involution of the postpartum uterus (Woessner, 1980). MMPs are presumably also involved in the periodic neovascularization which occurs in the endometrium during the menstrual cycle. If MMP inhibitors blocked any of these physiological activities, then they could not be prescribed for the premenopausal woman.

The above discussion has highlighted a few of the possible side effects to be expected from the use of MMP inhibitors. We still do not know if such side effects would actually occur. A similar panel of untoward reactions have probably been drawn up for most of the drugs in current use. Even if side effects are seen with MMP inhibitors, it is possible to minimize them. For example, if a particular pathological state is due to the action of only one MMP, then specific inhibitors of this enzyme could be developed. A number of companies have reported the development of inhibitors that have some limited (e.g. one log order) selectivity (discussed above). This would allow the functioning of the other members of the family and curtail toxicity. Another possibility is to target the inhibitor to the pathological tissue thereby preventing systemic problems. If these tactics fail, it may still be possible to use MMP inhibitors for conditions such as periodontal disease, corneal ulceration and skin lesions where the inhibitor can be applied topically.

7. Conclusions

During the past two decades, evidence has accumulated to support the hypothesis that collagenase and related enzymes are intimately involved in the pathology of a range of common diseases such as arthritis, cancer and periodontal disease. During this time it has become apparent that collagenase is simply one of a large, and growing, family of zinc-dependent enzymes. The inhibition of these enzymes could therefore produce therapeutic benefit or even a cure for these diseases. A number of natural inhibitors of the MMPs have also been discovered.

During the past decade a number of pharmaceutical companies and research laboratories have developed potent inhibitors of the MMPs. These inhibitors have been tested in a variety of in vitro systems involving connective tissue breakdown. The results to date have been disappointing and it is not clear why these potent compounds are so inefficacious, particularly in inhibiting breakdown of articular cartilage. Natural and low molecular mass inhibitors have been tested in animals and again have shown some effects but only at high concentrations. These problems can probably be overcome by developing more potent compounds and ensuring that the peptide bonds are replaced by non-peptidic isosteres. Once it can be shown that such modified compounds inhibit pathological tissue breakdown, the major problem will be with side effects when the compounds are given chronically. Again such problems could, in theory, be overcome by designing compounds capable of inhibiting one or a limited number of the MMPs, thus leaving some MMP activity for normal homeostatic purposes or by targetting inhibitors to the lesional tissues.

If, at the worst, the inhibitors of the MMPs prove to be too toxic for chronic use, they will at least have allowed us to test hypotheses about the role of the MMPs in the normal organism and in various disease states.

8. Acknowledgements

We would like to thank the Nuffield Trust (Oliver Bird Foundation) for support. Thanks also go to Sajeda Meghji for help with diagrams and to Val Cardinali for her typing skills. We also wish to express our thanks to Sean Nair for his constructive criticism of the review.

9. References

Alexander, C.M. and Werb, Z. (1989). Proteinases and extracellular matrix remodelling. Curr. Opin. Cell Biol. 1, 974–982.

Albini, A., Melchiori, A., Santi, L., Liotta, L.A., Brown, P.D. and Stetler-Stevenson, W.G. (1991). Tumour cell invasion inhibited by TIMP-2. J. Natl Cancer Inst. 83, 775–779.

Alvarez, O.A., Carmichael, D.F. and DeClerck, Y.A. (1990). Inhibition of collagenolytic activity and metastasis by a recombinant human tissue inhibitor of metalloproteinases. J. Natl Cancer Inst. 82, 589–595.

Barrett, A.J. and Rawlings, N.D. (1991). Types and families of endopeptidases. Biochem. Soc. Trans. 19, 707–715.

Bartlett, P.A. and Marlowe, C.K. (1987). Possible role for water dissociation in the slow binding of phosphorus-containing transition-state analogue inhibitors of thermolysin. Biochemistry 26, 8553–8561.

Basset, P., Bellocq, J.P., Wolf, C., Stoll, I., Hutin, P., Limacher, J.M., Podhajcer, O.L., Chenard, M.P., Rio, M.C. and Chambon, P. (1990). A novel metalloproteinase gene specifically expressed in stromal cells of breast carcinoma. Nature (London) 348, 699–704.

Beesley, J.E., Jessup, E., Pettipher, E.R. and Henderson, B. (1992). Microbiochemical analysis of changes in proteoglycan and collagen in joint tissues during the development of antigen-induced arthritis in the rabbit. Matrix 12, 189–196.

Berger, A. and Schechter, I. (1970). Mapping the active site of papain with the aid of peptide substrates and inhibitors. Philos. Trans. R. Soc. London Ser. B 257, 249–264.

Berman, M.B. (1980). In "Collagenase in Normal and Pathological Connective Tissues" (ed D.E. Wooley and J.M. Evanson), pp 141–174. Wiley, London.

Bieth, J.G. (1980). Pathophysiological interpretation of kinetic constants of protease inhibitors. Bull. Eur. Physiopathol. Respir. 16, (Suppl) 183–195.

Billingham, M.E.J. (1983) Models of arthritis and the search for anti-arthritic drugs. Pharmacol. Ther. 21, 389–428.

Birkedal-Hansen, H. (1988). From tadpole collagenase to a family of matrix metalloproteinases. J. Oral Pathol. 17, 445–451.

Blundell, T.L., Cooper, J., Foundling, S.J., Jones D.M., Atrash, B. and Szelke, M. (1987). On the rational design of renin inhibitors: X-ray studies of aspartic proteinases complexed with transition-state analogues. Biochemistry 26, 5585–5590.

Boone, T.C., Johnson, M.J., DeClerck, Y.A. and Langley, K.E. (1990). cDNA cloning and expression of a metalloproteinase inhibitor related to tissue inhibitor of metalloproteinases. Proc. Natl Acad. Sci. USA 87, 2800–2804.

Brown, P.A. (1991). In "Unmet Therapeutic and Diagnostic Needs in Osteoporosis, Osteoarthritis and Rheumatic Diseases". Corporate Dynamics SA. Heathrow Penta Hotel, April 1991.

Burns, F.R., Gray, R.D. and Paterson, C.A. (1990). Inhibition of alkali-induced corneal ulceration and perforation by a thiol peptide. Invest. Ophthalmol. Vis. Sci. 31, 107–114.

Butler, T.A., Zhu, C., Mueller, R.A., Fuller, G.C., Lemaire, W.J. and Woessner, J.F. (1991). Inhibition of ovulation in the perfused rat ovary by the synthetic collagenase inhibitor SC 44463. Biol. Reprod. 44, 1183–1188.

Byron, M.A. and Kirwan, J.R. (1986). Corticosteroids in rheumatoid arthritis: is a trial of their "disease modifying" potential feasible? Ann. Rheum. Dis. 46, 171–173.

Cambray, G.J., Murphy, G., Page-Thomas, D.P. and Reynolds, J.J. (1981). The production in culture of metalloproteinases and an inhibitor by joint tissues from normal rabbits and from rabbits with a model arthritis. I. Synovium. Rheumatol. Int. 1, 11–16.

Caputo, C.B., Sygowski, L.A., Wolanin, D.J., Patton, S.P., Caccese, R.G., Shaw, A., Roberts, R.A. and DiPasquale, G. (1987). Effect of synthetic metalloproteinase inhibitors on cartilage autolysis in vitro. J. Pharmacol. Exp. Ther. 240, 460–465.

Carmichael, D.F., Stricklin, G.P. and Stuart, J.M. (1989). Systemic administration of TIMP in the treatment of collagen-induced arthritis in mice. Agents Actions 27, 378–379.

Case, J.P., Lafyatis, R., Remmess, E.F., Kumkumian, G.K. and Wilder, R.L. (1989a). Transin/stromelysin expression in rheumatoid synovium. A transformation-associated metalloproteinase secreted by phenotypically invasive synoviocytes. Am. J. Pathol. 135, 1055–1064.

Case, J.P., Sano, H., Lafyatis, R., Remmess, E.F., Kumkumian, G.K. and Wilder, R.L. (1989b). Transin/stromelysin expression in the synovium of rats with experimental erosive arthritis. J. Clin. Invest. 84, 1731–1740.

Cawston, T.E. (1986). In "Proteinase Inhibitors" (ed A. Barrett and G. Salvesen), pp 589–610. Elsevier, Amsterdam.

Cawston, T.E. and Barrett, A.J. (1979). A rapid and reproducible assay for collagenase using [1-^{14}C]acetylated collagen. Anal Biochem. 99, 340–345.

Cawston, T.E., Galloway, A., Mercer, E., Murphy, G. and Reynolds, J.J. (1981). Purification of rabbit bone inhibitor of collagenase. Biochem. J. 195, 159–165.

Cawston, T.E., Mercer, E., deSilva, M. and Hazleman, B.L. (1984). Metalloproteinases and collagenase inhibitors in rheumatoid synovial fluid. Arth. Rheum. 27, 285–290.

Cawston, T.E., Curry, V.A., Clark, I.M. and Hazleman, B.L. (1990). Identification of a new metalloproteinase inhibitor that forms tight-binding complexes with collagenase. Biochem. J. 269, 183–187.

Chipkin, R.E. (1986). Inhibitors of enkephalinase: the next generation of analgesics. Drugs of the Future 11, 593–606.

Clark, I.M. and Cawston, T.E. (1989). Fragments of human fibroblast collagenase. Purification and characterization. Biochem. J. 263, 201–206.

Crimmin, M.J. (1991). In "Unmet Therapeutic and Diagnostic Needs in Osteoporosis, Osteoarthritis and Rheumatic Diseases" Corporate Dynamics SA, Heathrow Penta Hotel, April 1991.

Darlak, K., Miller, R.B., Stack, M.S., Spatola, A.F. and Gray, R.D. (1990). Thiol-based inhibitors of mammalian collagenase. J. Biol. Chem. 265, 5199–5205.

Dayer, J.-M., Krane, S.M., Russell, R.G.G. and Robinson, D.R. (1976). Production of collagenase and prostaglandins by isolated adherent rheumatoid synovial cells. Proc. Natl Acad. Sci. USA 73, 945–949.

Dayer, J.-M., Breard, J., Chess, L. and Krane, S.M. (1979). Participation of monocyte–macrophages and lymphocytes in the production of a factor that stimulates collagenase and prostaglandin release by rheumatoid synovial cells. J. Clin. Invest. 64, 1386–1392.

DeClerck, Y.A., Yean, T.D., Lu, H.S., Ting, J. and Langley, K.E. (1991a). Inhibition of autoproteolytic activation of interstitial procollagenase by recombinant metalloproteinase inhibitor. MI/TIMP-2. J. Biol. Chem. 266, 3893–3899.

DeClerck, Y.A., Yean, T.D., Chan, D., Shimada, H. and Langley, K.E. (1991b). Inhibition of tumor invasion of smooth muscle cell layers by recombinant human metalloproteinase inhibitor. Cancer Res. 51, 2151–2157.

Delaisse, J.M., Eeckhout, Y., Sear, C., Galloway, A., McCullagh, K. and Vaes, G. (1985). A new synthetic inhibitor of mammalian tissue collagenase inhibits bone resorption in culture. Biochem. Biophys. Res. Commun. 133, 483–490.

Dickens, J.P., Donald, D.K., Kneen, G. and McKay, W.R. (1986). US Patent 4599361, 1986.

Dingle, J.T. (1962). Lysosomal enzymes and the degradation of cartilage matrix. Proc. R. Soc. Med. 55, 109–111.

DiPasquale, G., Caccese, R., Pasternack, R., Conaty, J., Hubbs, S. and Perry, K. (1986). Proteoglycan- and collagen-degrading enzymes from human interleukin-1-stimulated chondrocytes from several species. Proteoglycanase and collagenase inhibitors as potentially new disease-modifying antiarthritic agents. Proc. Soc. Exp. Biol. Med. 183, 262–267.

Docherty, A.J.P. and Murphy, G. (1990). The tissue metalloproteinase family and the inhibitor TIMP: a study using cDNAs and recombinant proteins. Ann. Rheum. Dis. 49, 469–479.

Docherty, A.J.P., Lyons, A., Smith, B.J., Wright, E.M., Stephens, P.E., Harris, J.J.R., Murphy, G. and Reynolds, J.J. (1985). Sequence of human tissue inhibitor of metalloproteinases and its identity to erythroid potentiating activity. Nature (London) 318, 66–69.

Dodge, G.R. and Poole, A.R. (1989). Immunohistochemical detection and immunochemical analysis of type II collagen degradation in human normal, rheumatoid and osteoarthritic articular cartilages and in explants of bovine articular cartilage cultured with interleukin-1. J. Clin. Invest. 83, 647–661.

Dodge, G.R., Pidoux, I. and Poole, A.R. (1991). The degradation of type II collagen in rheumatoid arthritis: an immunoelectron microscope study. Matrix 11, 330–338.

Donald, D.K., Hann, M.M., Saunders, J. and Wadsworth, A.J. (1986) US Patent 4595700, 1986.

Dumonde, D.C. and Glynn, L.E. (1962). The production of arthritis in rabbits by an immunological reaction to fibrin. Br. J. Exp. Pathol. 43, 373–383.

Emonard, H. and Grimaud, J.-A. (1990). Matrix metalloproteinases: A review. Cell Mol. Biol. 36, 131–153.

Enghild, J.J., Salvesen, G., Brew, K. and Nagase, H. (1989). Interaction of human rheumatoid synovial collagenase (matrix metalloproteinase I) and stromelysin (matrix metalloproteinase 3) with human α_2-macroglobulin and chicken ovostatin. J. Biol. Chem. 264, 8779–8785.

Erdos, E.G. and Skidgel, R.A. (1989). Neutral endopeptidase 24.11 (enkephalinase) and related regulators of peptide hormones. FASEB J. 3, 145–151.

Evanson, J.M., Jeffrey, J.J. and Krane, S.M. (1967). Human collagenase: identification and characterization of an enzyme from rheumatoid synovium in culture. Science 158, 499–502.

Fauchere, J.-L. (1986). Elements for the rational design of peptide drugs. Adv. Drug Res. 15, 29–69.

Fell, H.B. and Mellanby, E. (1952). The effect of hypervitaminosis A on embryonic limb bones cultivated in vitro. J. Physiol. 116, 320–349.

Fell, H.B. and Thomas, L. (1960). Comparison of the effects of papain and vitamin A on cartilage II. The effects on organ cultures of embryonic skeletal tissue. J. Exp. Med. 111, 719–743.

Fell, H.B. and Jubb, R.W. (1977). The effect of synovial tissue on the breakdown of articular cartilage in organ culture. Arth. Rheum. 20, 1359–1371.

Firestein, G.S. and Zvaifler, N.J. (1990). How important are T cells in chronic rheumatoid synovitis. Arth. Rheum. 33, 768–773.

Firestein, G.S., Paine, M.M. and Littman, B.H. (1991). Gene expression (collagenase, TIMP, complement, and HLA-DR) in rheumatoid arthritis and osteoarthritis synovium: quantitative analysis and effect of intraarticular corticosteroids. Arth. Rheum. 34, 1094–1105.

Flannery, C., Boynton, R., Gordy, J., Neame, P. and Sandy, J.D. (1991). Specific cleavage sites in aggrecan catabolism. Abstract 12-3. International Meeting on the Biology and Pathology of the Extracellular Matrix. Lorne, Australia, Dec. 1991.

Fosang, A.J., Neame, P.J., Hardingham, T.E., Murphy, G. and Hamilton, J.A. (1991). Cleavage of cartilage proteoglycan between G1 and G2 domains by stromelysin. J. Biol. Chem. 266, 15579–15582.

Fosang, A.J., Neame, P.J., Last, K., Hardingham, T.E., Murphy, G. and Hamilton, J.A. (1992). The interglobular domain of cartilage aggrecan is cleaved by PUMP, gelatinase and cathepsin B. J. Biol. Chem. 267, 19470–19474.

Gardner, D.L. (1972). "The Pathology of Rheumatoid Arthritis". Edward Arnold, London.

Gavrilovic, J., Hembry, R.M., Reynolds, J.J. and Murphy, G. (1987). Tissue inhibitor of metalloproteinases (TIMP) regulates extracellular type I collagen degradation by chondrocytes and endothelial cells. J. Cell Sci. 87, 357–362.

Genden, E.M. and Molineaux, C.J. (1991). Inhibition of endopeptidase 24.15 decreases blood pressure in normotensive rats. Hypertension 18, 360–365.

Gravallese, E.M., Darling, J.M., Ladd, A.L., Katz, J.N. and Glimcher, L.H. (1991). In situ hybridization studies of stromelysin and collagenase messenger RNA expression in rheumatoid synovium. Arth. Rheum. 34, 1076–1084.

Gray, R.D., Miller, R.B. and Spatola, A.F. (1986). Inhibition of mammalian collagenases by thiol-containing peptides. J. Cell Biochem. 32, 71–77.

Gross, J. and Lapiere, C.M. (1962). Collagenolytic activity in amphibian tissues: a tissue culture assay. Proc. Natl Acad. Sci. USA 48, 1014–1022.

Hasty, K.A., Reife, R.A., Kang, A.H. and Stuart, J.M. (1990). The role of stromelysin in the cartilage destruction that accompanies inflammatory arthritis. Arth. Rheum. 33, 388–397.

Hembry, R.M., Knight, C.G., Dingle, J.T. and Barrett, A.J. (1982). Evidence that extracellular cathepsin D is not responsible for the resorption of cartilage matrix in culture. Biochim. Biophys. Acta 714, 307–312.

Henderson, B. and Edwards, J.C.W. (1987). "The Synovial Lining: In Health and Disease". Chapman & Hall, London.

Henderson, B. and Pettipher, E.R. (1988). Comparison of the in vivo inflammatory activities after intra-articular injection of natural and recombinant IL-1α and IL-1β in the rabbit. Biochem. Pharmacol. 37, 4171–4176.

Henderson, B. and Davies, D.E. (1991). In "Osteoarthritis: Current Research and Prospects for Pharmacological Intervention" (ed R.G.G. Russell and P. Dieppe), pp 203–215. IBC Technical Services, London.

Henderson, B. and Lewthwaite, J. (1991). Cytokines and cartilage loss in rheumatoid arthritis and osteoarthritis. Curr. Med. Lit. 10, 3–10.

Henderson, B., Pettipher, E.R. and Higgs, G.A. (1987). Mediators of rheumatoid arthritis. Br. Med. Bull. 43, 415–428.

Henderson, B., Docherty, A.J.P. and Beeley, N.R.A. (1990a). Design of inhibitors of articular cartilage destruction. Drugs of the Future 15, 495–508.

Henderson, B., Pettipher, E.R. and Murphy, G. (1990b). Metalloproteinases and cartilage proteoglycan depletion in chronic arthritis: Comparison of antigen-induced and polycation-induced arthritis. Arth. Rheum. 33, 241–246.

Holden, H.M., Tronrud, D.E., Monzingo, A.F., Weaver, L.H. and Matthews B.W. (1987). Slow- and fast-binding inhibitors of thermolysin display different modes of binding. Crystallographic analysis of extended phosphonamidate transition-state analogues. Biochemistry 26, 8542–8553.

Ianuzzi, L., Dawson, N., Zein, N. and Kushner, I. (1983). Does drug therapy slow radiographic deterioration in rheumatoid arthritis. N. Engl. J. Med. 301, 1023–1028.

Johnson, W.H., Roberts, N.A. and Borkakoti, N. (1987). Collagenase inhibitors: their design and potential therapeutic use. J. Enzyme Inhibition 2, 1–22.

Lark, M.W., Saphos, C.A., Walakovits, L.A. and Moore, V.L. (1990). In vivo activity of human recombinant tissue inhibitor of metalloproteinases (TIMP). Biochem. Pharmacol. 39, 2041–2049.

Laurent, G.J. (1982). Rates of collagen synthesis in lung, skin and muscle obtained in vivo by a simplified method using [^{3}H]proline. Biochem. J. 206, 535–544.

Lloyd, L.F., Skarzynski, T., Wonacott, A.J., Cawston, T.E., Clark, I.M., Mannix, C.J. and Harper, G.P. (1989). Crystallization and preliminary x-ray analysis of porcine synovial collagenase. J. Mol. Biol. 210, 237–238.

Luscombe, M. (1963). Acid phosphatase and catheptic activity in rheumatoid synovial tissue. Nature (London) 197, 1010.

Mallya, S.K., Mookhtiar, K.A. and Van Wart, H.E. (1986). Accurate, quantitative assays for the hydrolysis of soluble type I, II and III ^{3}H acetylated collagens by bacterial and tissue collagenases. Anal. Biochem. 158, 334–345.

Martel-Pelletier, J., Cloutier, J.-M. and Pelletier, J.-P. (1988). In vivo effects of anti-rheumatic drugs on neutral collagenolytic proteases in human rheumatoid arthritis cartilage and synovium. J. Rheumatol. 15, 1198–1204.

Matrisian, L.M. (1990). Metalloproteinases and their inhibitors in matrix remodelling. Trends Genet. 6, 121–125.

Matthews, B.W. (1988). Structural basis of the action of thermolysin and related zinc peptidases. Acc. Chem. Res. 21, 333–340.

McCachren, S.S. (1991). Expression of metalloproteinases and metalloprotease inhibitor in human arthritic synovium. Arth. Rheum. 34, 1085–1093.

McCluskey, R.T. and Thomas, L. (1958). The removal of cartilage matrix, in vivo, by papain. Identification of crystalline papain protease as the cause of the phenomenon. J. Exp. Med. 108, 371–384.

McGuire, M.B., Murphy, G., Reynolds, J.J. and Russell, R.G.G. (1981). Production of collagenase and inhibitor (TIMP) by normal, rheumatoid and osteoarthritic synovium in vitro: effect of hydrocortisone. Clin. Sci. 61, 703–710.

Mignatti, P., Robbins, E. and Rifkin, D.B. (1986). Tumour invasion through the human amniotic membrane: requirement for a proteinase cascade. Cell 47, 487–498.

Mookhtiar, K.A., Marlowe, C.K., Bartlett, P.A. and Van Wart, H. (1987). Phosphonamidate inhibitors of human neutrophil collagenase. Biochemistry 26, 1962–1965.

Murphy, G., Cambray, G.J., Virani N., Page-Thomas, D.P. and Reynolds, J.J. (1981). The production in culture of metalloproteinases and an inhibitor by joint tissues from normal rabbits and from rabbits with a model arthritis. II. Articular cartilage. Rheumatol. Int. 1, 17–20.

Murphy, G., Hembry, R.M., McGarrity, A.M., Reynolds, J.J. and Henderson, B. (1989). Gelatinase (type IV collagenase) immunolocalization in cells and tissues: use of an antiserum to rabbit bone gelatinase that identifies high and low M_r forms. J. Cell Sci. 92, 487–495.

Murphy, G., Docherty, A.J.P., Hembry, R.M. and Reynolds, J.J. (1991a). Metalloproteinases and tissue damage. Br. J. Rheumatol. 30 (Suppl. 1), 25–31.

Murphy, G., Houbrechts, A., Cockett, M.I., Williamson, R.A., O'Shea, M. and Docherty, A.J.P. (1991b). The N-terminal domain of tissue inhibitor of metalloproteinases retains metalloproteinase inhibitory activity. Biochemistry 30, 8097–8101.

Nixon, J.S., Bottomley, K.M.K., Broadhurst, M.J., Brown, P.A., Johnson, W.H., Lawton, G., Marley, J., Sedgwick, A.D. and Wilkinson, S.E. (1991). Potent collagenase inhibitors prevent interleukin-1-induced cartilage degradation *in vitro*. Int. J. Tissue Reac. 13, 237–243.

Okada, Y., Takeuchi, N., Tomita, K., Nakanishi, I. and Nagase, H. (1989). Immunolocalization of matrix metalloproteinase-3 (stromelysin) in rheumatoid synovioblasts (B cells) correlation with rheumatoid arthritis. Ann. Rheum. Dis. 48, 645–653.

Ondetti, M.A. and Cushman, D.W. (1982). Enzymes of the renin–angiotensin system and their inhibitors. Annu. Rev. Biochem. 51, 283–308.

Page-Thomas, D.P. (1977). In "Aspects of Synovial Biodegradation in Experimental Models of Chronic Inflammatory Diseases" (ed L.E. Glynn and H.D. Schlumberger), pp 353–365. Springer-Verlag, Berlin.

Pelletier, J.P., Martel-Pelletier, J., Cloutier, J.M. and Woessner, J.F. (1987). Proteoglycan-degrading acid metalloprotease activity in human osteoarthritic cartilage and the effect of intra-articular steroid injections. Arth. Rheum. 30, 541–548.

Petrillo, E.W. and Ondetti, M.A. (1982). Angiotensin-converting enzyme inhibitors: medicinal chemistry and biological actions. Med. Res. Rev. 2, 1–41.

Pettipher, E.R., Higgs, G.A. and Henderson, B. (1986). Interleukin-1 induces leukocyte infiltration and cartilage proteoglycan degradation in the synovial joint. Proc. Natl Acad. Sci. USA 83, 8749–8753.

Pettipher, E.R., Henderson, B., Moncada, S. and Higgs, G.A. (1988). Leukocyte infiltration and cartilage proteoglycan loss in immune arthritis in the rabbit. Br. J. Pharmacol 95, 169–176.

Pettipher, E.R., Henderson, B., Edwards, J.C.W. and Higgs, G.A. (1989). Effect of indomethacin on swelling, lymphocyte influx and cartilage proteoglycan depletion in experimental arthritis. Ann. Rheum. Dis. 48, 623–627.

Pittman, R.N. and Williams, A.G. (1988). Neurite penetration into collagen gels requires Ca^{2+}-dependent metalloproteinase activity. Dev. Neurosci. 11, 41–51.

Poole, A.R., Hembry, R.M., Dingle, J.T., Pinder, I., Ring, E.F.J. and Cosh, J. (1976). Secretion and localization of cathepsin D in synovial tissues removed from rheumatoid and traumatized joints. Arth. Rheum. 19, 1295–1307.

Powers, J.C. and Wade Harper, J. (1986). In "Proteinase Inhibitors" (ed A. Barrett and G. Salvesen), pp 219–298. Elsevier, Amsterdam.

Quantin, G., Murphy, G. and Breathnach, R. (1989). Pump-1 cDNA codes for a protein with characteristics similar to those of classical collagenase family members. Biochemistry 28, 5327–5334.

Rashad, S., Revell, P., Hemingway, A., Low, F., Rainsford, K. and Walker, F. (1989). Effect of non-steroidal anti-inflammatory drugs on the course of osteoarthritis. Lancet 2, 519–522.

Reich, R., Thompson, E.W., Iwamoto, Y., Martin, G.R., Deason, J.R., Fuller, G.C. and Miskin, R. (1988). Effects of inhibitors of plasminogen activator, serine proteinases, and collagenase IV on the invasion of basement membranes by metastatic cells. Cancer Res. 48, 3307–3312.

Reynolds, J.J., Lawrence, C.E. and Gavrilovic, J. (1988). In "The Control of Tissue Damage" (ed. A. Glauert), pp 281–296. Elsevier, Amsterdam.

Sakamoto, S. and Sakamoto, M. (1988). Degradative processes of connective tissue proteins with special emphasis on collagenolysis and bone resorption. Mol. Asp. Med. 10, 299–428.

Sakamoto, S., Sakamoto, M. and Horton, J.E. (1984). In "Endocrine Control of Bone and Calcium Metabolism" (ed D.V. Cohn, T. Fujita, J.T. Potts and R.V. Talmage), pp 140–143. Elsevier, Amsterdam.

Saklatvala, J. (1989). In "Interleukin-1 Inflammation and Disease" (ed R. Bomford and B. Henderson), pp 143–162. Elsevier, Amsterdam.

Sanchez-Lopez, R., Nicholson, R., Gesnel, M-C., Matrisian, L.M. and Breathnach, R. (1988). Structure–function relationships in the collagenase family member transin. J. Biol. Chem. 263, 11892–11899.

Sandy, J.D., Neame, P.J., Boynton, R.E. and Flannery, C.R. (1991). Catabolism of aggrecan in cartilage explants: identification of a major cleavage site within the interglobular domain. J. Biol. Chem. 266, 8683–8685.

Schnebli, H.P. (1985). In "Handbook of Inflammation" (ed I.L. Bonta, M.A. Bray and M.J. Parnham), Vol. 5, pp. 321–333. Elsevier, Amsterdam.

Schultz, G., Strelow, S., Stern, G., Galardy, R. and Grobelny, D. (1990). Inhibition of corneal ulceration in alkali burned rabbit corneas by a synthetic collagenase inhibitor. Invest. Ophthalmol. Vis. Sci. 31 (Suppl.), 559.

Schultz, R.M., Silberman, S. and Persky, B. (1988). Inhibition by human recombinant tissue inhibitor of metalloproteinases of human amnion invasion and lung colonization by murine B16-F10 melanoma cells *in vivo*. Cancer Res. 48, 5539–5545.

Schwartz, J.C., Gros, C., Lecomte, J.M. and Bralet, J. (1990). Enkephalinase (EC 3.4 24.11) inhibitors: protection of endogenous ANF against inactivation and potential therapeutic applications. Life Sci. 47, 1279–1297.

Sellers, A., Cartwright, E., Murphy, G. and Reynolds, J.J. (1977). Evidence that latent collagenases are enzyme–inhibitor complexes. Biochem. J. 163, 303–307.

Sellers, A., Murphy, G., Meikle, M.C. and Reynolds, J.J. (1979). Rabbit bone collagenase inhibitor blocks the activity of other neutral metalloendoproteinases. Biochem. Biophys. Res. Commun. 87, 581–587.

Shaw, A., Roberts, R.A. and Wolanin, D.J. (1988). In "Advances in Inflammation Research" Vol. 12, pp 67–79. Raven Press, New York.

Sodek, J. (1990). In "The Biology of Tooth Movement" (ed L.A. Norton and C. Burstone), pp 157–181. CRC Press, Boca Raton, Florida.

Springman, E.B., Angleton, E.L., Birkedal-Hansen, H. and Van Wart, H.E. (1990). Multiple modes of activation of latent human fibroblast collagenase: evidence for the role of a Cys^{73} active-site zinc complex in latency and a "cysteine switch" mechanism for activation. Proc. Natl Acad. Sci. USA 87, 364–368.

Steffen, C. (1980). In "Studies in Joint Disease" (ed A. Maroudas and E.J. Holborow), pp 201–226. Pitman Medical, Bath.

Stetler-Stevenson, W.G., Krutzsch, H.C. and Liotta, L.A. (1989). Tissue inhibitor of metalloproteinase (TIMP-2). A new member of the metalloproteinase inhibitor family. J. Biol. Chem. 264, 17374–17378.

Takigawa, M., Nishida, Y., Suzuki, F., Kishi, J., Yamashita, K. and Hayakiana, T. (1990). Induction of angiogenesis in chick yolk sac membrane by polyamides and its inhibition by TIMP and TIMP-2. Biochem. Biophys. Res. Commun. 171, 1264–1271.

Testa, J.E. and Quigley, J.P. (1991). Reversal of misfortune. TIMP-2 inhibits tumor cell invasion. J. Natl Cancer Inst. 83, 740–742.

Thomas, L. (1956). Reversible collapse of rabbit ears after intravenous papain, and prevention of recovery by cortisol. J. Exp. Med. 156, 245–259.

Thomas, B.M., Atkinson, S.J., Reynolds, J.J. and Meikle, M.C. (1987). Degradation of type I collagen films by mouse osteoblasts stimulated by 1,25 dihydroxyvitamin D3 and inhibited by human recombinant TIMP. Biochem. Biophys. Res. Commun. 148, 596–602.

Thorgeirsson, V.P., Liotta, L.A., Kalebic, T., Marglies I., Thomas, K. and Russo, R.G. (1982). Effect of natural protease inhibitors and a chemoattractant on tumor cell invasion in vitro. J. Natl Cancer Inst. 69, 1049–1054.

Trainor, D.A. (1987). Synthetic inhibitors of human neutrophil elastase. Trends Pharmacol. Sci. 8, 303–307.

Tyler, J. and Saklatvala, J. (1985). Pig interleukin-1 (catabolin) induces resorption of cartilage proteoglycan and prevents synthesis of proteoglycan and collagen. Br. J. Rheumatol. 24 (Suppl. 1), 150–155.

Van der Rest, M. and Garrone, R. (1991). Collagen family of proteins. FASEB J. 5, 2814–2823.

Veber, D.F. and Freidinger, R.M. (1985). The design of metabolically stable peptide analogs. Trends Neurol. Sci. 8, 392–396.

Walakovits, L., Moore V.L., Bhardwaj, N., Gallick, G.S. and Lark, M.W. (1992). Detection of stromelysin and collagenase in synovial fluid from patients with rheumatoid arthritis and post-traumatic knee injury. Arth. Rheum. 35, 35–42.

Wallace, D.A., Bates, S.R.E., Walker, B., Kay, G., White J., Guthrie, D.J.S., Blumson, N.L. and Elmore, D.T. (1986). Competitive inhibition of human skin collagenase by N-benzyloxycarbonyl-L-prolyl-L-alanyl-3-amino-2-oxopropyl-L-leucyl-L-alanylglycine ethyl ester. Biochem. J. 239, 797–799.

Ward, R.V., Hembry, R.M., Reynolds, J.J. and Murphy, G.G. (1991). The purification of tissue inhibitor of metalloproteinases-2 and tissue inhibitor of metalloproteinases-1. Biochem. J. 278, 179–187.

Williamson, R.A., Marston, F.A.O., Angal, S., Koklitis, P., Panico, M., Morris, H.R., Carne, A.F., Smith, B.J., Harris, T.J.R. and Freedman, R.B. (1990). Disulphide bond assignment in human tissue inhibitor of metalloproteinases (TIMP). Biochem. J. 268, 267–274.

Wingard, L.B., Brody, T.M., Larner, J.L. and Schwartz, A. (1991). "Human Pharmacology". London, Wolfe Publishing.

Woessner, J.F. (1980). In "Collagenase in Normal and Pathological Connective Tissues" (ed D.E. Woolley and J.M. Evanson), pp 223–239. Wiley, London.

Woessner, J.F. (1991). Matrix metalloproteinases and their inhibitors in connective tissue remodelling. FASEB J. 5, 2145–2154.

Woessner, J.F. and Taplin, C.J. (1988). Purification and properties of a small latent matrix metalloproteinase of the rat uterus. J. Biol. Chem. 263, 16918–16925.

Woessner, J.F., Morioka, N., Zhu, C., Makaida, T., Butler, T. and LeMaire, W.J. (1989). Connective tissue breakdown in ovulation. Steroids, 54, 491–499.

11. Lysosomal Cysteine Endopeptidases in the Degradation of Cartilage and Bone

David J. Buttle

1. Introduction

The extracellular matrix is maintained by the cells found within it. These cells are responsible for striking the delicate balance between the synthesis and catabolism of matrix components. Thus, even in what appears to be a static condition, matrix components are being turned over in a highly controlled way. The resorption of connective tissue is also a part of many normal physiological changes, such as growth, development and wound healing. Usually in these processes, the existing matrix has to be removed in a highly regulated manner in order to allow for new matrix to be laid down, to produce the "programmed" structural changes. An example would be the replacement of cartilage by bone during normal osteogenesis.

Many pathological processes are also associated with extracellular matrix degradation, but in these cases the destruction of connective tissue can be regarded as inappropriate and lacking the strict control characteristic of

Copyright © 1994 Academic Press Limited
All rights of reproduction in any form reserved.

normal physiological changes. Thus, the balance between synthesis and catabolism is shifted in favour of tissue destruction, as is seen in the arthritides. The tilting of the balance is usually, but not always, associated with an inflammatory reaction, which contributes to the imbalance by providing a source of inflammatory mediators, enzymes and free radicals. The destruction of the extracellular matrix could, in principle, be directly caused by the action of any of a variety of enzyme types, or non-enzymically by the action of the free radicals. Although not the principal subject matter of this chapter, the possible involvement of free radicals in bone and cartilage degradation deserves some mention.

Macrophages and neutrophils can generate superoxide free radicals by means of an "oxidative burst" involving the action of a membrane-bound NADPH oxidase. The superoxide anion may then be converted, via a series of reactions, to the hydroxyl radical and other highly reactive species that can fragment proteins (Wolff et al., 1986) including, in vitro, collagen (Monboisse et al., 1983) and proteoglycan (Dean et al., 1984). The action on proteoglycan seems to involve selective fragmentation of the protein core (Dean et al., 1985) and link proteins (Roberts et al., 1989). As well as the direct effect of cleaving matrix components, the damage done to proteins by radicals, both in terms of fragmentation and modification, makes the proteins more susceptible to enzymic hydrolysis (Wolff and Dean, 1986) and can also lead to the activation of latent endopeptidases such as neutrophil collagenase (EC 3.4.24.34) (Weiss et al., 1985). There are no clear indications as to the relative importance of oxidant damage at sites of inflammation and in the pathology of the joint, but the available evidence has been reviewed (Kleinveld et al., 1989).

Mammalian tissues are well endowed with enzymes capable of metabolizing extracellular matrix protein components. These enzymes, the peptide bond hydrolases or peptidases, can be split into two separate groups, the exopeptidases and the endopeptidases (or proteinases) (Barrett and McDonald, 1986). The exopeptidases attack proteins at the ends, removing one, two or three amino acids at a time from either a free N- or C-terminus. Endopeptidases can cleave internal peptide bonds, and are therefore much more efficient at fragmenting large proteins. For this reason, endopeptidases are likely to provide the initial (rate-determining) cleavages of matrix components, producing a greater number of free termini which may then be attacked by exopeptidases.

The endopeptidases are classified in terms of their catalytic mechanism, and conveniently described according to the chemical structure providing the catalytically essential nucleophile. There are four types of endopeptidase so far recognized: the serine-type (EC 3.4.21), cysteine-type (EC 3.4.22), aspartic-type (EC 3.4.23) and metalloendopeptidases (EC 3.4.24) (IUBMB Nomenclature Committee, 1992). The possibility that other as yet unrecognized endopeptidase types exist cannot be discounted (Barrett and Rawlings, 1991). Members of all four recognized types of endopeptidase are synthesized by the resident cells of cartilage and bone, and also by inflammatory cells, and many of these enzymes have been shown to be capable of cleaving the major protein components of cartilage and bone (proteoglycan and collagen type I in bone and collagen types II, IX, X and XI in cartilage) in vitro (for reviews see Barrett and Saklatvala, 1985; Murphy and Reynolds, 1992). There are therefore a large number of candidate enzymes that could be involved in normal and pathological breakdown of bone and cartilage, and the definition of which ones are important in particular disease processes is a subject of considerable current interest. Once a particular enzyme is implicated, the job of synthesizing and testing potential therapeutic agents directed specifically against that enzyme can begin.

The cysteine-type endopeptidases are well represented in mammalian cells. The calcium-dependent cysteine endopeptidases, the calpains (EC 3.4.22.17), are mainly cytosolic in location. All the other well-characterized mammalian cysteine endopeptidases are found principally in the lysosomes of most cell types, and their primary function is without doubt the intracellular digestion of proteins and peptides in the lysosomes (Barrett et al., 1988). However, there is now a sizeable body of evidence suggesting that the lysosomal cysteine endopeptidases may also be involved in the breakdown of the protein components of the extracellular matrix. The present chapter is intended as a brief review of this subject.

2. The Lysosomal Cysteine Endopeptidases: Properties Related to a Potential Role in Extracellular Matrix Breakdown

There are four distinct lysosomal cysteine endopeptidases about which there is a considerable amount of structural and enzymological information. These enzymes, cathepsins B (EC 3.4.22.1), H (EC 3.4.22.16), L (EC 3.4.22.15) and S (EC 3.4.22.27) are all members of the papain (EC 3.4.22.2) family, that is to say, they share an evolutionary ancestor with the plant enzyme (Fig. 11.1). Less information is available on two other potentially related enzymes, cathepsins N and T (Kirschke and Barrett, 1987). These two will not be further discussed here, although it has been reported that cathepsin N has activity against type I collagen and gelatin (Maciewicz and Etherington, 1988).

Like other lysosomal hydrolases, cathepsins B, H, L and S have acidic pH optima and are active in a reducing environment. They tend to be irreversibly denatured at pH values above about 7, although the rate at which

```
            1           2          3          4          5
                             *
        123456ABCD78901A234567890123456789012345678901234AB567890


papain    IPEYVD----WRQKG-AVTPVKNQGSCGSCWAFSAVVTIEGIIKIRTGN--LNEYSE

bovine B  LPESFDAREQWPN-CPTIKEIRDQGSCGSCWAFGAVEAISDRICIHSNGRVNVEVSA

human H   YPPSVD----WRKKGNFVSPVKNQGACGSCWTFSTTGALESAIAIATGK--MLSLAE

human L   APRSVD----WREKG-YVTPVKNQGQCGSCWAFSATGALPGQMFRKTGR--LISLSE

bovine S  LPDSMD----WREKG-CVTEVKYQGACGSCWAFSAVGALEAQVKLKTGK--LVSLSA
```

Figure 11.1 Amino acid sequence alignment around the active-site cysteine of papain and the mammalian lysosomal cysteine endopeptidases. The amino acids (single letter code) are numbered according to the sequence of papain. The active-site cysteine is marked by *. The sequence for papain is taken from Cohen et al. (1986), those for human cathepsins H and L from Ritonja et al. (1988) and those for bovine cathepsins B and S from Meloun et al. (1988) and Ritonja et al. (1991) respectively. Residues identical with those of papain are shown in white-on-black.

this occurs varies with the enzyme and the species from which it was obtained (see below). If a reducing environment is not provided, activity is reversibly lost as a result of oxidation of the thiolate anion of the active-site cysteine, often to a mixed disulphide. The enzymology and mechanism of cysteine endopeptidases in general have been comprehensively reviewed (Brocklehurst et al., 1987).

Lysosomal enzymes are synthesized on membrane-bound polysomes in the rough endoplasmic reticulum, where co-translational removal of the prepeptide is achieved by the leader peptidase. Various post-translational modifications occur, including glycosylation of some asparagine residues followed by the phosphorylation of mannose in the Golgi. This provides a ligand for binding to the mannose-6-phosphate receptors which transport the newly synthesized enzymes to a pre-lysosomal acidic compartment rather than allowing them to follow the secretory pathway. The receptors release their ligands upon reaching an acidic compartment, and are recycled. Various proteolytic cleavages occur which result in the removal of the propeptide and formation of the mature lysosomal forms of the enzyme (Kornfeld, 1986).

All the evidence to date suggests that the lysosomal cysteine endopeptidases follow this general pathway. The removal of the propeptide is thought to be accompanied by enzyme activation (but see below). Thus, like secreted endopeptidases, lysosomal endopeptidases are synthesized as inactive precursors, presumably to prevent inappropriate proteolysis during biosynthesis. Although the bulk of newly synthesized enzyme is directed to the lysosome, in some cell types, such as fibroblasts, there is a fraction that escapes capture by the trafficking mechanism and is secreted as the proenzyme (Hanewinkel et al., 1987; Erickson, 1989).

2.1   CATHEPSIN B

Cathepsin B is the most abundant of the lysosomal cysteine endopeptidases. Its concentration in lysosomes of human liver has been estimated to be about 1.5 mM (40 mg/ml) (Dean and Barrett, 1976).

In substrate specificity, cathepsin B differs from the other lysosomal endopeptidases in its efficient cleavage of synthetic substrates with arginine in the P_2 position (in the terminology of Berger and Schechter, 1970) (Barrett and Kirschke, 1981). Cathepsin B is also unique in having peptidyl dipeptidase activity (cleaving dipeptides from the C-terminus of peptides) (Aronson and Barrett, 1978; Bond and Barrett, 1980) as well as endopeptidase activity. The X-ray crystallographic structure of human liver cathepsin B has recently been solved, and there are now plausible structural explanations for these characteristics of its catalytic behaviour (Musil et al., 1991). However, cathepsin B has a very broad specificity against protein substrates that is still difficult to predict. Of the 29 peptide bonds in the oxidized B chain of insulin, ten were cleaved by cathepsin B, with eight different amino acids in P_1 and seven in P_2 (McKay et al., 1983). It is likely that some of these cleavages were the result of the enzyme's peptidyl dipeptidase activity rather than its action as an endopeptidase.

Cathepsin B cleaves proteoglycan (Morrison et al., 1973; Roughley and Barrett, 1977; Roughley, 1977; Nguyen et al., 1990) at pH 5.0 to 5.5, and link protein in vitro at pH 5.5 (Nguyen et al., 1990). It is also capable of attacking collagen types I (Burleigh et al., 1974), II, IX and XI (Maciewicz et al., 1991). Of the reactions of cathepsin B with collagen, that with type I has been most thoroughly characterized. The enzyme initially attacks the non-helical region of the collagen molecule, thus removing the cross-link. The helical portion of the molecule then becomes susceptible and is degraded to small peptides. The pH optimum for the degradation of soluble collagen is 4.5–5.0, and below 4.0 for insoluble collagen.

Cathepsin B purified from human liver is rapidly denatured above pH 7.4 (Barrett, 1973). Bovine spleen cathepsin B is slightly more stable, losing about half of its activity after 10 min at 37°C and pH 7.6 (Willenbrock and Brocklehurst, 1985).

The biosynthesis of cathepsin B has been investigated. The conversion of the preproprotein (Chan *et al.*, 1986) of $M_r = 36\,000$ to the mature $27\,000$-M_r single- and two-chain forms found in lysosomes is a multistep process. Proteolytic events, glycosylation and phosphorylation result in a number of intermediate species which can be identified in the cell by pulse–chase experiments. About 5% of the newly synthesised protein is secreted by fibroblasts in culture as the proenzyme (Hanewinkel *et al.*, 1987).

There is now evidence to suggest that some secreted precursor forms of cathepsin B are active, or activated after they leave the cell without removal of the entire propeptide. A form of the enzyme secreted by mammary glands in organ culture is active against low-M_r substrates, but is incapable of cleaving protein substrates as judged by its lack of inhibition by α_2-macroglobulin (Recklies *et al.*, 1982; Mort and Recklies, 1986), which implies an inability to cleave the "bait" region of the inhibitor (Salvesen and Barrett, 1980). A precursor form of cathepsin B found in purulent sputum is also active against low-M_r substrates (Buttle *et al.*, 1988). This form ($M_r = 37\,000$) has been shown to be produced from the inactive precursor ($M_r = 40\,000$) by the action of neutrophil elastase, and can then digest proteoglycan at pH 5.0 and bind to α_2-macroglobulin (Buttle *et al.*, 1991).

A property shared by all precursor forms of cathepsin B is stability at alkaline pH. This capacity is presumably bestowed on the molecule by the presence of all or part of the propeptide, but the structural basis for the stability of the precursor and the instability of the mature molecule is not understood.

2.2 CATHEPSIN H

The main action of cathepsin H may be as an aminopeptidase, and it is usually assayed with substrates containing an unblocked amino acid, generally arginine (Barrett and Kirschke, 1981). The ability of the enzyme to act as an endopeptidase seems to vary according to the species.

The human enzyme appears to have only weak endopeptidase activity, with no action on collagen (Kirschke *et al.*, 1980), but it is capable of releasing proteoglycan from killed bovine nasal septum cartilage. An enzyme concentration of 62 nM released 9% of proteoglycan in the cartilage in 60 min at pH 5.0, an amount not dissimilar to that released by human

cathepsins B (10%) and L (10.5%) (D.J. Buttle, unpublished). The enzyme from rabbit lung ("BANA hydrolase") is reported to be efficient at degrading acid-soluble skin collagen at pH 3.5. As is the case with cathepsin B, the non-helical regions were preferentially attacked (Singh *et al.*, 1978).

The mature lysosomal form of cathepsin H may be more tolerant of slightly alkaline media than is cathepsin B. Human cathepsin H retained 20% of its activity after exposure to a pH of 7.5 for 60 min at 22°C (Schwartz and Barrett, 1980), and the enzyme from bovine spleen lost only 50% after 30 min at 37°C and pH 7.6 (Willenbrock and Brocklehurst, 1985).

Cathepsin H is synthesized as a preproprotein (Ishidoh *et al.*, 1987) and processed in the normal way (Nishimura and Kato, 1987). An octapeptide derived from the propeptide remains attached via a disulphide bridge to the mature form of the human enzyme, but it is not known if this has any functional significance (Ritonja *et al.*, 1988). Very little is known about the properties of any secreted forms of cathepsin H.

2.3 CATHEPSIN L

Cathepsin L has powerful proteolytic activity and can be readily assayed with azocasein, even in the presence of 3 M urea to distinguish its activity from that of cathepsin B (Barrett and Kirschke, 1981). However, relatively few bonds in the oxidized B chain of insulin were cleaved by cathepsin L, compared with cathepsin B, and there was a clear preference for the hydrolysis of bonds preceded by hydrophobic residues in positions P_2 and P_3 (Kärgel *et al.*, 1980).

The cartilage proteoglycan core protein and link proteins are hydrolysed more extensively *in vitro* by cathepsin L than by cathepsin B (Nguyen *et al.*, 1990), although the relevance of the result of a limit digest *in vitro* compared with what might be happening *in vivo* is questionable. Elastin, which is refractory to degradation by many endopeptidases, is nevertheless efficiently hydrolysed by cathepsin L, with a pH optimum of 5 (Mason *et al.*, 1986). Cathepsin L also solubilizes insoluble type I collagen several times more efficiently than does cathepsin B. Although the pH optimum for this activity is 3.5, significant activity is still observed at pH 6.0. The action on collagen is qualitatively similar to that of cathepsin B, with the main effect being cleavage of the non-helical terminal regions resulting in removal of the cross-links (Kirschke *et al.*, 1982). A similar mode of attack on the collagens from cartilage has been reported, and again cathepsin L was more active than cathepsin B (Maciewicz *et al.*, 1990).

The lysosomal form of cathepsin L is unstable even below pH 7. There is some species variation, with the enzyme from man and cattle detectably losing activity at pH 5.5 and 30°C after 1 h, whereas the sheep and rabbit enzymes are stable up to pH values of 6.0 and 6.5

respectively (Mason, 1986). However, even at pH 7.0 and 37°C, the human enzyme retains 15% of the original activity after 15 min (Mason et al., 1985).

Cathepsin L is synthesized as a preproprotein, processed and delivered to the lysosome (Portnoy et al., 1986). A proportion of the proenzyme may be secreted. The amount being secreted can increase dramatically as a result of viral transformation of fibroblasts. Message levels can increase 20-fold (Stearns et al., 1990) and procathepsin L becomes the most abundant secreted protein (Mason et al., 1987). There is some debate as to whether the change in trafficking of procathepsin L upon viral transformation is due to a reduction in the number of mannose-6-phosphate receptors (Achkar et al., 1990), an alteration in protein structure resulting in impairment of receptor binding (Lazzarino and Gabel, 1990) or to the increased translation coupled with a low degree of phosphorylation of the ligand (Dong and Sahagian, 1990). There is also evidence that trafficking of procathepsin L from prelysosomes to mature lysosomes is mediated by a membrane-bound lysosomal proenzyme receptor (McIntyre and Erickson, 1991). Transformation could also affect this system. The proenzyme secreted by fibroblasts in cell culture is catalytically inactive, but becomes active if the culture medium is incubated at pH 3.0 (Mason et al., 1989) or if the proenzyme is purified. The activation can occur without any apparent change in M_r (Mason et al., 1987), although the loss of a small part of the propeptide cannot be ruled out. As with cathepsin B, proteolytically active precursor forms of cathepsin L may sometimes be found extracellularly, such as in medium conditioned by mammary gland organ cultures (Recklies and Mort, 1985).

As is the case with precursor forms of cathepsin B, the presence of all or part of the propeptide confers stability on the protein at mildly alkaline pH. The active precursor retained 90% of its activity after a 1 h incubation at pH 8.0 and 37°C (Mason et al., 1987).

2.4 CATHEPSIN S

Cathepsin S was recently shown to be distinct from cathepsin L (Kirschke et al., 1986). So far, it has only been detected in lymphoid tissue, kidney and lung (Kirschke et al., 1989), but the likelihood is that further work on this relatively newly discovered enzyme will provide evidence for a wider distribution. The specificity of cathepsin S is similar to but not identical with that of cathepsin L. Hydrolysis of the oxidized B chain of insulin demonstrated a strong preference for hydrophobic residues in P_2 and P_3, but favouring aliphatic residues as opposed to the bulky aromatic side chains preferred by cathepsin L. The use of aliphatic versus hydrophobic residues in small synthetic substrates allows the activities of these enzymes to be distinguished (Brömme et al., 1989). Cathepsin S matches cathepsin L in its efficient cleavage of most protein substrates. Against insoluble

type I collagen, however, it was only about one-third as active at pH 3.5 and 30°C (Kirschke et al., 1989). This still makes it at least as efficient as cathepsin B. The action of cathepsin S on cartilage collagens and proteoglycan has not been investigated.

Cathepsin S differs from the other lysosomal cysteine endopeptidases in being much more stable at mildly alkaline pH. Only 10% of the enzyme activity is lost following preincubation for 1 h at pH 7.5 and 40°C. Thus cathepsin S is the only lysosomal cysteine endopeptidase with proteolytic activity that can be readily detected by conventional methods above pH 7.0 (Kirschke et al., 1989).

Studies on the biosynthesis of cathepsin S have not yet been reported. However, partial cDNA clones for the enzyme (Qian et al., 1990; Wiederanders et al., 1991) and antisera against it (Kirschke et al., 1989) have now been obtained so that information on the biosynthesis and processing of this enzyme should be forthcoming. No information is yet available about secreted forms of cathepsin S.

2.5 ENDOGENOUS INHIBITORS OF THE LYSOSOMAL CYSTEINE ENDOPEPTIDASES

The endogenous inhibitors of the lysosomal cysteine endopeptidases are α_2-macroglobulin and the members of the cystatin superfamily.

α_2-Macroglobulin provides protection against inappropriate proteolysis in the bloodstream by irreversibly binding and trapping most endopeptidases, including cathepsins B, H and L (Mason, 1989). The inhibitor is too large to escape into tissues except in cases of extreme vascular permeability.

The cystatin superfamily consists of a large number of evolutionarily related tight-binding reversible inhibitors of the lysosomal cysteine endopeptidases. They are divided into three distinct families (for reviews see Barrett et al., 1986; Barrett, 1987; Turk and Bode, 1991). The family 3 cystatins are the kininogens and are principally proteins of the bloodstream (M_r 50 000–120 000), where they are involved in the control of vasodilatation and in blood clotting as well as acting as inhibitors of cysteine endopeptidases. The family 1 cystatins (stefins) are largely intracellular (cytosolic) inhibitors of M_r 11 000. One of the members of this family, cystatin A, is found in neutrophils (Davies and Barrett, 1984) and may be released from these cells in appreciable amounts at sites of inflammation (Buttle et al., 1990). The family 2 cystatins are small (M_r 13 000) proteins found extracellularly in body fluids such as saliva and seminal fluid. One of these, cystatin C, is the tightest binding of the mammalian cystatins to cathepsins B, H, L (Barrett et al., 1986) and S (Brömme et al., 1991). Its interaction with cathepsin B is the weakest, K_i being about 0.15 nM. The N-terminal portion of the inhibitor is efficiently removed by the action of neutrophil elastase and this results in a further weakening of the interaction with cathepsin B by three orders of magnitude (Abrahamson *et al.*, 1991). Thus, even in the presence of cystatins, extracellular inhibition of cathepsin B at sites of inflammation may well be far from complete, as is the case in purulent human sputum (Buttle *et al.*, 1990, 1991).

Inhibitory activity against cathepsin B has been detected in bovine nasal septum and human articular cartilages, and in both tissues the properties of the inhibitors are consistent with them being family 1 or family 2 cystatins (Roughley *et al.*, 1978; Killackey *et al.*, 1983). The origin, concentration, location and binding constants for these inhibitors are not known so that their importance in providing protection against proteolysis by the cysteine endopeptidases cannot be assessed.

3.   Cysteine Endopeptidases and Bone Resorption

Bone is a complex tissue, and its turnover is under extremely precise and complex physiological control. Agents involved in controlling bone turnover include parathyroid hormone, 1,25-dihydroxyvitamin D, prostaglandins, platelet-derived growth factor, EGF, TGFs, insulin-like growth factor-I, fibroblast growth factor, colony-stimulating factors, INFγ, calcitonin, IL-1, TNF-α and bone morphogenetic proteins (one of which, BMP-1, is a member of a family of metalloendopeptidases and expresses endopeptidase activity: Rawlings and Barrett, 1990; Dumermuth *et al.*, 1991). Various cellular interactions between the three main cell types of bone, osteoblasts, osteocytes and osteoclasts, are also thought to add yet another level of control (for reviews see Goldring and Goldring (1990) and Vaes (1988)). Perhaps the main target of the intricate controlling mechanism is the rate and site of bone resorption, and the cell type largely responsible for the resorption is the osteoclast. Over the past ten years or so, evidence has accumulated that the endopeptidases responsible for the degradation of the organic component of bone are largely of the cysteine type.

3.1   MODELS OF BONE RESORPTION

Bone resorption has generally been measured as the release of ^{45}Ca from prelabelled explants of neonatal mouse calvariae or fetal rat long bones. All the cell types responsible for bone turnover are therefore present, and these young tissues usually respond well to experimental manipulation. For the study of osteoclastic bone resorption, young animals can be kept on a calcium-free diet, which increases the rate of bone resorption and the

number of osteoclasts. For some studies on osteoclasts, it has been necessary to isolate these cells and manipulate them in cell culture.

3.2   MECHANISM OF OSTEOCLASTIC BONE RESORPTION: THE EXTRACELLULAR PHAGOLYSOSOME

The existence in bone of large multinucleated cells with some unusual anatomical features has been recognized for a very long time, and these cells were suspected of being the agents of bone resorption, and therefore called osteoclasts, as early as 1873 (Vaes, 1988). The most outstanding features of osteoclasts are the ruffled border and surrounding clear zone. The frequency of osteoclasts with a clear zone and ruffled border is altered by reagents that affect the rate of bone resorption, such as parathyroid hormone. The ruffled border and clear zone were therefore recognized to be parts of the resorbing system of the cell (Holtrop *et al.*, 1974). The ruffled border is a system of finger-like cellular projections that extend from the base of the cell to the bone surface. These are surrounded by the clear zone, where the plasma membrane of the cell lies directly on the surface of the bone, effectively sealing the area under the cell, including the ruffled border, from the surrounding extracellular environment. The biochemical makeup and cytoskeletal organization of the clear zone are unique and reflect its adhesive function (Marchisio *et al.*, 1984). Osteoclasts can fluctuate between resorptive activity and periods of quiescence, depending on the stimuli. Ruffled borders are seen only during periods of activity, and the cell may change shape at times of quiescence, in effect "storing" the membrane required to make the ruffled borders as extensive cell processes (Miller, 1977).

During periods of resorptive activity, the area under the osteoclast into which the ruffled border projects (the lacuna) is actively acidified by the osteoclast. The membrane of the ruffled border contains membrane proteins normally associated with lysosomal membranes, including the lysosomal proton pump, and lysosomal enzymes are transported into the bone-resorbing lacuna (Baron *et al.*, 1985). The presence of lysosomal membrane proteins and lysosomal hydrolases could both be explained by fusion of lysosomal membranes with the ruffled border. Microelectrode studies have demonstrated the ability of osteoclasts to rapidly acidify this extracellular compartment, at a rate of 1 pH unit/min, to a limit of pH 3.0 (Silver *et al.*, 1988). Thus, the resorptive lacunae can be considered as extracellular phagolysosomes.

The removal of the mineral phase of bone is required in order to expose the organic collagenous component. The low pH beneath the osteoclast may itself be sufficient to dissolve the mineral (Eeckhout, 1990). The question then arises of how the collagenous component is removed.

3.3 DIRECT EVIDENCE FOR THE INVOLVEMENT OF THE CYSTEINE ENDOPEPTIDASES IN BONE RESORPTION: THE USE OF TYPE-SPECIFIC ENDOPEPTIDASE INHIBITORS

Type-specific inhibitors of endopeptidases can prove invaluable in the assignation of the pathophysiological role of an enzyme or group of enzymes. If such studies provide evidence for the involvement of an endopeptidase in some important physiological or pathological process, the use of inhibitory compounds as therapeutic agents then becomes a possibility.

There are two main types of inhibition, reversible and irreversible. Reversible inhibition is characterized by the reappearance of enzyme activity after removal of all or some of the inhibitor, for example by dilution, or after the addition of another reagent, such as a substrate, which competes with the inhibitor for the active site of the enzyme. Thus, reversible inhibition is dependent primarily on the concentration of the inhibitor, and the inhibition is defined by the equilibrium constant (K_i) which is the inhibitor concentration giving 50% inhibition.

Irreversible inhibition is normally achieved by reagents reacting covalently with, and thereby inactivating, the enzyme. The extent of inhibition is dependent on time, as well as concentration, and is defined in terms of a rate constant (k) characterizing the reaction. Irreversible inhibitors can therefore also be called enzyme inactivators. (For a fuller and more exact description of the characterization of enzyme inhibition, see Knight (1986)).

In biological systems the use of fast-acting inactivators has the advantage that the enzyme is inactivated within a few minutes and does not regain activity as the concentration of inactivator falls as a result of excretion or breakdown. A fast-acting inactivator could be defined as one having a second-order rate constant (k_2) of $1000 \, \text{M}^{-1}\text{s}^{-1}$. Such an inactivator, if present at a concentration of $10 \, \mu\text{M}$, would inactivate 99% of the enzyme in about 8 min. New activity would then appear, only after the inactivator had been removed from the system, by the synthesis of new enzyme molecules or the activation of molecules that had been present as inactive zymogens while the inactivator had been present.

Both reversible inhibitors and irreversible inactivators are available for use with the serine- and cysteine-type endopeptidases, whereas only reversible inhibitors are available for the aspartic and metalloendopeptidases. This is because of differences in the catalytic mechanism. The serine- and cysteine-type endopeptidases utilize a reactive nucleophile that is a part of the enzyme molecule to form a covalent tetrahedral intermediate. In contrast, the metallo- and aspartic endopeptidases employ an activated water molecule as the nucleophile, and do not proceed via covalent intermediates (Rich, 1990).

For reversible inhibitors to be effective in biological systems, they must usually be very tight-binding, with subnanomolar K_i values, so that the inhibitor concentration can be maintained well above K_i.

A potential disadvantage of inactivators is that they contain a reactive group that may react with proteins other than the target enzyme. Therefore they may be toxic or have unwanted effects on the biological system.

Apart from toxicity, the other major complicating factor associated with the use of inhibitors is bioavailability. Many inhibitors are proteins and are potentially unstable and prone to proteolytic inactivation in biological systems. The only way in which most proteins can enter a cell is by endocytosis, followed by transport to the lysosomes and breakdown. Hydrophilic compounds, even those of moderate size, do not readily cross the plasma membrane, and so these also must normally rely upon uptake via endocytic vacuoles. Chemical conversion caused by the acidity of the lysosome (Diener *et al.*, 1986) or proteolysis in the lysosome (Kopecek and Duncan, 1987) have both been seen as potential ways of converting prodrugs to drugs after the prodrug has reached the lysosome. But usually, targetting inhibitors to intracellular compartments requires the use of small hydrophobic reagents that can traverse membranes.

Getting inhibitors to extracellular locations may also present problems. For instance, the high concentration of negative charges in cartilage could hinder the passage of positively charged compounds, or the entry of negatively charged reagents, while the solubility of hydrophobic compounds or proteins in aqueous media may be limiting. Notwithstanding all these potential problems and limitations of the method, the use of specific inhibitors provides one of very few approaches that can demonstrate a causal link between an enzyme involved in the rate-limiting step of a process and the occurrence of the process itself. In this respect it is perhaps analogous to the use of deletion mutants for exploring metabolic pathways in lower organisms.

The cysteine endopeptidases have been suspected of involvement in bone resorption for over a decade. The first report of the effects of endopeptidase inhibitors on the breakdown of bone (Delaissé *et al.*, 1980) described a series of inhibitors and inactivators that were effective at inhibiting hydroxyproline release from fetal mouse calvariae. Some of these reagents, such as leupeptin, antipain and tosyl-lysylchloromethane, inhibit or inactivate serine and cysteine endopeptidases. However, the cysteine endopeptidase-specific fast inactivator, benzyloxycarbonyl-Phe-Ala-CHN$_2$, was effective, giving 50% inhibition of hydroxyproline release at a reagent concentration of $2.6 \, \mu\text{M}$, and its effect was reversible.

The peptidyl diazomethane (above) is hydrophobic and could be expected to enter cells and the lacunae. However, the highly hydrophilic epoxidyl peptide inactivator of cysteine endopeptidases, E64 (Fig. 11.2c), was also found to be effective at reversibly inhibiting hydroxyproline release from mouse embryo calvariae, although a slightly higher concentration (5–25 μM) was required for inhibition. When leupeptin (4 mg) or E64 (2 mg) was administered to rats by intraperitoneal injection, a 50% reduction in urinary hydroxyproline was detected by 3 h, the levels returning to normal by 24 h. Pepstatin, the inhibitor of aspartic endopeptidases such as lysosomal cathepsin D, was without effect (Delaissé *et al.*, 1984).

The response of osteoclasts to the cysteine endopeptidase inactivators, benzyloxycarbonyl-Phe-Ala-CHN$_2$ and E64, was looked at more directly in a simplified system consisting of an enriched population of osteoclasts cultured on acellular dentine. Thus any effect of the inactivators on complex interactions that may be occurring in bone explants was precluded. Both inactivators, the peptidyl diazomethane at a concentration of 12.5 μM and E64 at 40 μM, reduced the number, depth and volume of resorption pits by about 75%, without affecting the appearance or mobility of the cells. There was some microscopic evidence for the formation of demineralized patches in the presence of the inactivators, but these areas were not so extensively excavated, suggesting an inhibitory effect on collagen removal rather than demineralization (Delaissé *et al.*, 1987). The latter observation was supported by the studies of Everts *et al.* (1988), in which demineralization proceeded but collagen degradation was retarded by 50 μM E64 on mouse embryo metacarpal bones in culture. Evidence therefore exists for a direct effect of the lysosomal cysteine endopeptidases on collagen breakdown by osteoclasts.

Morphometric studies of the effect of the cysteine endopeptidase inactivator Z-Phe-Ala-CH$_2$F (Fig. 11.2e) (1 μM) on osteoclasts in juvenile rabbit calvariae demonstrated a reduction in the incidence of osteoclasts exhibiting a ruffled border from 62% to 12%, perhaps indicating a non-specific or toxic effect of the reagent. Osteoclasts in cultures containing the inactivator showed an increased incidence of collagen-containing vacuoles, pointing to an inhibition of degradation of internalized collagen as well as degradation in the extracellular phagolysosome (Van Noorden and Everts, 1991).

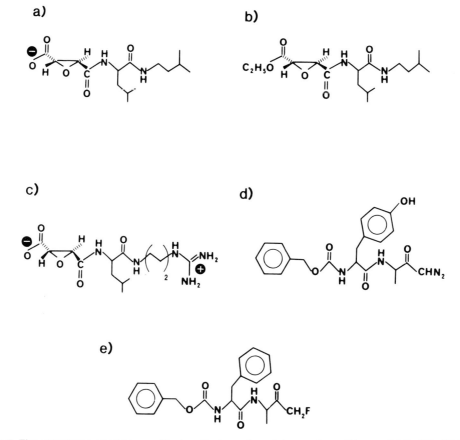

Figure 11.2 The structures of some specific inactivators of cysteine endopeptidases. (a) Ep475; (b) Ep453; (c) E64; (d) Z-Tyr-Ala-CHN$_2$; (e) Z-Phe-Ala-CH$_2$F.

The peptidyl diazomethane benzyloxycarbonyl-Phe-Phe-CHN$_2$ shows some selectivity in that it inactivates cathepsin L extremely rapidly but is only a reversible inhibitor of cathepsin B (Kirschke and Shaw, 1981). This reagent has recently been found to be effective at inhibiting the resorption of bone by isolated osteoclasts at a concentration of 1 μM, thereby implicating cathepsin L rather than cathepsin B in this process (Rifkin et al., 1991).

3.4   FURTHER EVIDENCE CONSISTENT WITH THE INVOLVEMENT OF THE CYSTEINE ENDOPEPTIDASES

Activity due to a cathepsin B-like enzyme was identified in the culture medium of mouse embryo calvariae cultured at slightly acidic, but not at slightly alkaline, pH, presumably because of lability of the enzyme above pH 7. The amount of activity was increased by parathyroid hormone, and was therefore closely correlated with hydroxyproline release and calcium loss from the explants (Delaissé et al., 1984). Cathepsin L-like activity has recently been demonstrated in isolated chicken osteoclasts (Rifkin et al., 1991). Earlier, the presence of three distinct cysteine endopeptidase activities had been demonstrated in embryonic mouse calvariae (Delaissé et al., 1986), and an attempt to isolate and characterize these has recently been made. One was found to be due to cathepsin B. The remaining two activities appeared to be those of cathepsin L-related enzymes. One appeared to be an active precursor form of cathepsin L. Its M_r and stability at pH 7.2 were consistent with this. The third activity was that of an enzyme with the catalytic characteristics of cathepsin L, but an apparent M_r of 70 000 on gel chromatography and stability up to pH 9. This enzyme reacted with an antibody to cathepsin L, but had $M_r = 25 000$ on Western blots. It may therefore be a complex between the mature lysosomal form of cathepsin L and another molecule that confers stability at alkaline pH. This high-M_r form of cathepsin L was also detected in muscle, but not in liver, spleen or kidney. It is not certain that osteoclasts were the source of these enzymes, all of which were capable of depolymerizing acid-soluble skin collagen (Delaissé et al., 1991).

There is evidence to suggest that intracellular collagen degradation by cells other than osteoclasts is mediated to some extent by the cysteine endopeptidases. Both leupeptin and E64 caused a dose-dependent increase in the numbers of lysosomal structures containing cross-banded collagen fibrils in periosteal fibroblasts in explant cultures of mouse embryo metacarpal bone rudiments. At a concentration of 100 μM, E64 produced a thirtyfold increase in the total volume made up by these organelles. The vacuoles were thought to be phagolysosomes, as their accumulation was inhibited by cytochalasin B (Everts et al., 1985).

Although most of the evidence suggests that osteoclasts can resorb bone by a mechanism that is independent of the action of interstitial collagenase (EC 3.4.24.7) (Blair et al., 1986), a role for the action of the metalloendopeptidase in the resorption of mineralized bone has not been entirely ruled out. There have been two studies of the effect of a reversible collagenase inhibitor on bone resorption. This compound, a carboxyalkyl peptide, has an IC$_{50}$ (equivalent to K_i) of about 1 μM with mammalian collagenase. In embryonic mouse calvariae the compound was reported to reversibly inhibit hydroxyproline loss by 91% and calcium release by 50% at a concentration of 50 μM (Delaissé et al., 1985). However, when added at comparable concentration to isolated osteoclasts cultured on acellular dentine, it was without effect (Delaissé et al., 1987). One possible explanation of these results is that the action of collagenase (possibly synthesized by osteoblasts: Heath et al., 1984) is required to degrade the osteoid layer of embryonic bone in order to provide a layer of mineralized bone on which the osteoclasts can act. The role of collagenase in the turnover of adult bone, which contains little or no osteoid, is still obscure. Procollagenase is present in, and can be extracted from, mineralized bone (Eeckhout et al., 1986), and it has been shown that the actions of collagenase and lysosomal extracts on insoluble bone collagen are additive at mildly acidic pH, and that the elevated calcium concentrations likely to be encountered under activated osteoclasts stimulate this additive effect (Eeckhout, 1990). Taken together with the observation that cathepsin B can activate procollagenase (Eeckhout and Vaes, 1977), these results suggest that procollagenase sequestered in mineralized bone could participate in the degradation of the organic constituent of bone occurring in osteoclast lacunae.

4.   Cysteine Endopeptidases and Cartilage Degradation

The idea that lysosomal endopeptidases may be implicated in cartilage breakdown is not new. Much of the work suggesting that the involvement of the lysosomal enzymes was at least a possibility was carried out some time ago using model organ culture systems of cartilage breakdown.

4.1   MODELS OF CARTILAGE BREAKDOWN: EFFECTS OF RETINOIDS

The first tissue culture model of cartilage breakdown was reported by Fell and Mellanby (1952). They studied the effects of high concentrations of retinoids on embryonic and fetal cartilaginous limb-bone rudiments. The vitamin caused loss of metachromasia followed by shrinkage of the tissue, without killing the cells. Suggestions that the effect may be the direct result of a chondrolytic enzyme (Fell *et al.*, 1956) were strengthened by the results of animal experiments in which reversibly oxidized papain was injected intravenously into rabbits. Loss of proteoglycan was evident after 4 h, and almost complete by 18 h (Thomas, 1956). These experiments were important, in that they demonstrated that cartilage had sufficient reducing capacity to activate a cysteine endopeptidase. In fact, when activated enzyme was injected, it had no effect on the cartilaginous tissues (McCluskey and Thomas, 1958) presumably because it was being irreversibly inactivated in the blood by α_2-macroglobulin. These results led Fell and Thomas (1960) to examine the effects of crude papain on embryonic cartilaginous tissue in organ culture, where it was clearly shown that 1 h of incubation with papain resulted in complete loss of metachromatic staining, without any obvious change in the cells.

The metabolic effects of high doses of retinoids on cartilage cultures were studied in more detail. As well as increasing the rate of loss of sulphate from cartilage, the vitamin also had the effect of reducing its rate of incorporation, demonstrating the suppression of proteoglycan synthesis as well as stimulation of its loss (Fell *et al.*, 1956). It was also found that hypervitaminosis A caused a switch in respiration by chondrocytes, from aerobic to anaerobic, resulting in the excretion by the cells of increased amounts of lactic acid (Dingle *et al.*, 1961). The discoveries that the chondrocytes contain a lysosomal enzyme that is capable of the autolytic removal of the cartilage proteoglycan at pH values from 3 to 5 (Lucy *et al.*, 1961), and that the enzyme is released from isolated lysosomes by the action of retinoids (Dingle, 1961), were made at about the same time. The presence of the same activity in the culture medium of cartilaginous rudiments grown in the presence of vitamin A added further weight to the argument that the release of a lysosomal enzyme could account for the breakdown of cartilage proteoglycan in this system (Fell and Dingle, 1963).

The effect of retinoids on collagen breakdown was much less severe than their stimulation of proteoglycan release. However, hydroxyproline release from limb-bone rudiments was found to be stimulated by the vitamin (Dingle *et al.*, 1966).

Efforts to more accurately define the properties of the enzyme(s) responsible for cartilage breakdown began. Ali (1964) and Ali *et al.* (1967) reported that the rate of autolytic breakdown of killed cartilage at pH 5.0 was increased by the addition of cysteine, and reduced in the presence of iodoacetamide and mercuric chloride. The authors suggested that cathepsin B might be partly responsible for the autolysis. Other findings implicated the aspartic-type endopeptidase, cathepsin D, in the autolytic process. The inhibitor of the aspartic-type endopeptidases, pepstatin, was capable of totally inhibiting the release of proteoglycan. Some pepstatin-resistant activity remained, however, if dithiothreitol and EDTA were also included in the incubation medium (Dingle *et al.*, 1972). The available evidence therefore suggested that the chondrocytes contained sufficient quantities of two lysosomal endopeptidases, cathepsins B and D, to effect the rapid breakdown of the surrounding cartilage proteoglycan. For these enzymes to be responsible for the chondrolytic effect induced by retinol, they must be able to confront the extracellular matrix in an environment of moderately low pH. The increased presence of cathepsin D around chondroblasts and chondrocytes of rabbit ear cartilage following stimulation with retinol was elegantly demonstrated (Poole *et al.*, 1974).

4.2   The Hypothesis of a Pericellular Site of Action

Consideration of all the evidence implicating a role for lysosomal endopeptidases in chondrocyte-mediated cartilage degradation led to the formulation of a hypothesis by Dingle (1975), suggesting that the site of proteoglycan degradation was in the pericellular zone immediately around the chondrocyte. In order for the enzymes to be located outside the cell, either in the culture medium or localized within the extracellular matrix, they may well have had to pass through an area immediately adjacent to the cell in which an acidic environment is maintained by the metabolic activities of the chondrocyte. The increased excretion of lactate by retinol-stimulated cells would favour a lowering of pH immediately around the cell, and, if the contents of lysosomes were being discharged, this too would very probably lead to a lowering of local pH. The pericellular space would therefore be a likely site of action for endopeptidases acting at mildly acidic pH. The argument was strengthened by the lack of any plausible alternative degradative agent: enzymes acting at neutral pH, such as the matrix metalloendopeptidases, were noticeably absent from cartilage cultures.

The pericellular hypothesis lacked direct experimental support, however. If a particular group of endopeptidases were responsible, then it should be possible to inhibit their action by adding type-specific inhibitors to the culture system. Attempts at this approach gave only negative results. Hembry *et al.* (1982) failed to inhibit the resorption of retinol-stimulated cartilage with the specific inhibitor of aspartic-type endopeptidases, pepstatin, even though the inhibitor was clearly capable of penetrating the tissue. Inhibitors of other types of endopeptidase were also tried, such as E64 (Fig. 11.2c) for the inhibition of the cysteine-type enzymes, tosyl-lysylchloromethane for the trypsin-like serine and cysteine endopeptidases, chymostatin for chymotrypsin-like serine and cysteine endopeptidases, and the metal chelators EDTA and 1,10-phenanthroline. The latter two were shown to inhibit via a non-specific toxic effect, and the other reagents were ineffective. The authors concluded that the enzyme(s) responsible may be acting in an environment from which the inhibitors were excluded, such as an intracellular location or a pericellular zone.

4.3 MODELS OF CARTILAGE BREAKDOWN: EFFECTS OF IL-1 AND TNF-α

The realization that the inflammatory cytokines IL-1 and TNF-α have a similar, but more dramatic, effect on cartilage to that of the retinoids, causing rapid release of proteoglycan by a chondrocyte-mediated mechanism (Saklatvala et al., 1983, 1984; Saklatvala, 1986) added pathophysiological relevance to the earlier work with the retinoids. This became even more significant once it had been demonstrated that IL-1 also stimulated proteoglycan release when injected into the joints of whole animals (Pettipher et al., 1986). The effects of the cytokines also parallelled those of vitamin A in that the synthesis of proteoglycan by cartilage explants was suppressed (Tyler, 1985; Saklatvala, 1986) and glycolysis by cells in culture was increased (Bird et al., 1987; Taylor et al., 1988). The main effect on cartilage collagen metabolism appears to be a suppression of synthesis (Tyler and Benton, 1988). A stimulatory effect on collagen degradation can only be observed at 12 days of culture, and requires relatively high doses of IL-1 (Tyler, 1988).

It is well known that isolated chondrocytes respond to IL-1 and TNF-α, in a manner similar to the response of fibroblasts and synovial cells in culture, by synthesizing increased amounts of inactive precursors of the matrix metalloendopeptidases, such as interstitial collagenase and stromelysin (EC 3.4.24.17) (Stephenson et al., 1987; Schnyder et al., 1987; Bunning and Russell, 1989). This is one response that is not generated by the action of retinoic acid, which in fact inhibits collagenase gene expression at a concentration of 5 μM (Lafyatis et al., 1990). Even so, it has become quite generally accepted that the matrix metalloendopeptidases are largely responsible for cartilage matrix turnover (Brinckerhoff, 1991) possibly after activation by plasmin generated by plasminogen activator, also synthesized in response to IL-1 by cultured chondrocytes (Bunning et al., 1987). However, direct evidence, by means of the establishment of a causal link between this (or any other) type of endopeptidase and the degradative response to the cytokines, has been hard to come by.

4.4 THE USE OF TYPE-SPECIFIC ENDOPEPTIDASE INHIBITORS IN CARTILAGE CULTURES

The first reported attempt at the use of type-specific inhibitors in cytokine-stimulated cartilage cultures was with a series of inhibitors of the matrix metalloendopeptidases. One of these, the metal chelator phenanthroline, had already been shown to act via a toxic effect (Hembry et al., 1982). The other two were both hydroxamic acid peptides with estimated IC$_{50}$ (that is, K_i) values of 0.1 μM for proteoglycan-degrading metalloendopeptidases (DiPasquale et al., 1986). At a concentration of 100 μM, these reagents virtually completely inhibited both IL-1- and retinol-stimulated proteoglycan release from cultured rabbit articular cartilage (Caputo et al., 1987).

More recently Nixon et al. (1991) reported the inhibition of IL-1-induced proteoglycan and collagen depletion of bovine nasal septum cartilage by a hydroxamic acid peptide and a phosphinic acid peptide. The hydroxamate inhibited collagenase, gelatinase and "caseinase" (probably stromelysin) with IC$_{50}$ values of 10–26 nM, and inhibited both proteoglycan and collagen loss in the culture model at concentrations of 100 μM and 1 μM respectively. The phosphinic acid exhibited specificity for collagenase, the IC$_{50}$ of about 20 nM being an order of magnitude lower than for the inhibition of the other two metalloendopeptidase activities. This reagent did not inhibit proteoglycan release from the cultures, even at 100 μM concentration, but inhibited collagen breakdown at 1 μM.

Of course, inhibitory effects can be obtained in a nonspecific way by compounds that are toxic to the cells, so that it is very important to attempt to exclude this possibility by making control experiments. The only such control experiment reported by Caputo et al. (1987) was a study of the effect of the inhibitors on the suppression of proteoglycan synthesis by retinol and IL-1. From the data given it would seem that the suppressive effect was slightly increased by the inhibitors, even 3 days after their removal. Nixon et al. (1991) reported that their reagents did not affect cell viability as measured by lactate dehydrogenase release and glucose utilization, without providing data. It would seem that the evidence available for the involvement of the matrix metalloendopeptidases in IL-1-induced cartilage collagen breakdown is currently stronger than for their involvement in proteoglycan release.

Saklatvala and Sarsfield (1988) used bovine nasal septum cartilage explants to study the effect of a number of inhibitors of all four catalytic types of endopeptidase on IL-1-stimulated proteoglycan release, with only negative results. This was somewhat surprising, in that two of the reagents they studied, the cysteine endopeptidase inhibitors leupeptin and E64, are effective at inhibiting osteoclastic bone resorption (Section 3.3). The explants also failed to secrete detectable amounts of proteoglycan-degrading activity into the culture medium of IL-1-stimulated explants. However, striking inhibition was achieved by cytochalasins B and D, suggesting that cell membrane movement and perhaps endocytosis are involved in the degradative response.

More recently it has been found that lipophilic, but not

hydrophilic, inactivators of cysteine endopeptidases inhibit IL-1-stimulated proteoglycan release from bovine nasal septum cartilage. The epoxidyl peptide Ep475 (Fig. 11.2a) is a very fast-acting hydrophilic inactivator of most cysteine endopeptidases. This, and the related rapid hydrophilic inactivator E64, were without effect on the cartilage cultures, even at a concentration of 2 mM (Saklatvala and Sarsfield, 1988). A hydrophobic pro-inactivator, the ethyl ester of Ep475, called variously Ep453, EST, E64d and loxistatin, (Fig. 11.2b) inactivates papain only very slowly *in vitro* (Tamai *et al.*, 1987). However, it is more effective at inactivating cysteine endopeptidases in cells than is Ep475, because it has the ability to pass through membranes (Wilcox and Mason, 1992) and is then converted to the active form by the action of unidentified esterases (Tamai *et al.*, 1986). Ep453 was found to inhibit the IL-1-stimulated release of proteoglycan from bovine nasal septum cartilage in a dose-dependent manner, with statistically significant inhibition occurring at an inactivator concentration of 10 μM (Fig. 11.3). Even at a concentration of 100 μM, Ep453 had no detectable effect on protein synthesis or glycolysis, and its inhibition of proteoglycan degradation was reversible. These results were taken as evidence that cysteine endopeptidases mediate the rate-limiting step in proteoglycan release in the system, but that effective inhibitors must pass through membranes (Buttle *et al.*, 1992). Supporting evidence for this hypothesis comes from the finding that a hydrophobic cysteine endopeptidase inactivator with completely different structure from that of Ep453 has a very similar inhibitory effect. This

compound, Z-Tyr-Ala-CHN2 (Fig. 11.2e), shows dose-dependent inhibition of proteoglycan release, with statistically significant inhibition being obtained at a concentration of 1 μM (Fig. 11.3) (Buttle and Saklatvala, 1992). The radioiodinated form of this inactivator has been shown to specifically label cathepsins B and L in intact fibroblasts (Mason *et al.*, 1989), and to label these enzymes in intact purified lysosomes within 10 min (Wilcox and Mason, 1989). In the cartilage culture system, the inhibitory effect of this inactivator on proteoglycan release was reversible, and no reduction in protein synthetic rate in its presence was observed. The reagent did inhibit rates of glycolysis, but this effect required higher inactivator concentrations than were needed to inhibit proteoglycan release. Thus it was concluded that the inhibition of proteoglycan release was not due to a general toxic effect.

The question of whether Ep453 and Z-Tyr-Ala-CHN2 act via an effect on IL-1 signal transduction was addressed. Neither inactivator interfered with an early IL-1-dependent phosphorylation event (EGF receptor trans-modulation) or with the IL-1-mediated increased production of IL-6 or PGE2 in fibroblasts (Buttle and Saklatvala, 1992).

Second-order rate constants for the inactivation of the individual cysteine endopeptidases by the peptidyl diazomethane have been determined. Cathepsins L, B and S are rapidly inactivated, but the reagent has no measurable effect on the activities of cathepsin H, or the cytosolic calcium-dependent cysteine endopeptidase, m-calpain (EC 3.4.22.17) (Table 11.1), thus precluding

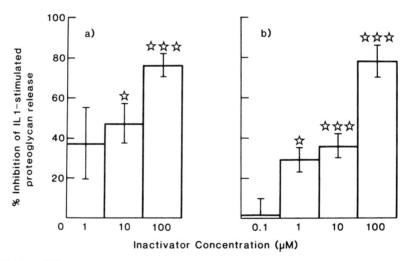

Figure 11.3 Inhibition of IL-1-stimulated proteoglycan release from bovine nasal septum cartilage by lipophilic inactivators of cysteine endopeptidases. The experiments were carried out on cartilage explants in serum-free culture medium containing 0.3 nM recombinant human IL-1α. Control levels of proteoglycan release (in the absence of IL-1) were subtracted, and the percentage inhibition due to the presence of the inactivator was calculated (± S.E.M.). (a) Ep453; (b) Z-Tyr-Ala-CHN2. The effect of the presence of inactivator was compared with the IL-1-stimulated response in the absence of inactivator by unpaired Student's t-test: $^*P < 0.05$; $^{***}P < 0.0005$.

Table 11.1 Second-order rate constants for the inactivation of cysteine endopeptidases by Z-Tyr-Ala-CHN$_2$

Cathepsin B	Cathepsin L	Cathepsin S	Cathepsin H	m-calpain
1800	120 000	1700	< 10	< 10

Second-order rate constants (k_2) were derived from k_{obs}/[I], and corrected for the presence of substrate in the assay mixture. The measurements were made at 30°C and pH 5.5 for cathepsins B and L, pH 6.0 for cathepsin H, pH 6.5 for cathepsin S and pH 7.5 for m-calpain. The enzymes were purified from bovine tissues (Buttle and Saklatvala, 1992).

an involvement of the latter two enzymes in the IL-1-stimulated degradative response. It is concluded that one or more of the lysosomal enzymes cathepsins B, L or S are responsible for the rate-limiting step in IL-1-stimulated cartilage proteoglycan degradation in bovine nasal septum cartilage explants (Buttle and Saklatvala, 1992).

Given that the evidence for the involvement of the lysosomal cysteine endopeptidases, at least in the bovine nasal septum cartilage model system, appears quite strong, various questions remain concerning the mechanism and site of action of the enzymes in chondrocyte-mediated proteoglycan breakdown. The fact that only lipophilic inactivators are effective would, at first glance, suggest that the site of action is intracellular, or at least membrane-limited in some way. But the involvement of a peri-cellular location is not necessarily ruled out. It may be necessary to inactivate the enzymes before their release, because the cleavage of proteoglycan is so fast, and both the enzyme concentration (which may be locally very high; see Section 2.1) and concentration of the substrate (up to 80 mg/ml proteoglycan concentration in cartilage) may render an extracellular inhibitor ineffective. It seems likely that an extracellular site of action would require that it be acidified to some extent, although, as pointed out in Sections 2.1–2.4, the lysosomal cysteine endopep-tidases may be transiently active even slightly above pH 7. The fact that the rate of lactic acid excretion by chon-drocytes is increased in response to IL-1 would favour the generation of a low pericellular pH, as would the extru-sion of the contents of lysosomes. Evidence now exists to suggest that metabolically active cells can rapidly generate an acidic pericellular microenvironment in the cellular contact zone where diffusion is limited (Silver et al., 1988). The cartilage matrix may limit diffusion suffi-ciently to allow an acidic environment to form around chondrocytes, or the cells might create invaginations which are then acidified. If the enzymes are indeed active outside the cells, then the question arises as to whether lysosomal or precursor forms of the enzymes are involved. Release of enzymes via the secretory pathway would lead to the involvement of precursor forms; fusion of lysosomal and plasma membranes would lead to the involvement of the mature lysosomal forms.

It is not known whether the lysosomal enzymes are acting directly on proteoglycan or through an earlier rate-determining step. For instance, cathepsin B is capable of activating prostromelysin (Murphy et al., 1992) and prourokinase-type plasminogen activator (Kobayashi et al., 1991). Cathepsin B could therefore initiate a proteo-lytic cascade resulting in the involvement of the metal-loendopeptidase stromelysin, and the serine-type endopeptidase plasmin, in proteoglycan degradation.

4.5 FINDINGS CONSISTENT WITH THE INVOLVEMENT OF THE CYSTEINE ENDOPEPTIDASES

Various other lines of research have tentatively indicated that the lysosomal cysteine endopeptidases may be involved in proteoglycan degradation, via either a chondrocyte- or synovial cell-mediated mechanism.

If the lysosomal cysteine endopeptidases are indeed involved in cartilage proteoglycan breakdown, it is of course necessary that they be present in the tissue at the time of joint damage, although the demonstration of their presence does not in itself show their involvement. Cathepsin B has been localized in joint tissues by a number of different laboratories. Mort et al. (1984) found extracellular cathepsin B at the periphery of explants of human rheumatoid synovium by the antibody-capture technique, using an antibody that only recognized denatured cathepsin B. The authors hypothe-sized that the reaction with antibody was limited to the tissue edges because the pH within the explant was suffi-ciently acidic to maintain the enzyme in its native confor-mation. Cathepsin B activity has been localized in chondrocytes of articular cartilage by histochemical methods (Van Noorden and Vogels, 1986; Van Noorden et al., 1987). No extracellular activity was detected. Van Noorden et al. (1988) investigated the involvement of the cysteine endopeptidases in an animal model of arthritis. Of cathepsins H, L and B, only activity of the latter enzyme was increased, as determined histochemically, in cells and in the extracellular matrix, by the onset of the experimental arthritis. The animals were treated with the fast-acting hydrophobic inactivator of the cysteine endopeptidases, Z-Phe-Ala-CH$_2$F (Fig. 11.2e). At a dose of 0.5 mg/kg administered i.v. or orally, the number of inflammatory cells was judged to be decreased, and at 5 mg/kg i.v. and 50 mg/kg administered orally, cartilage damage was assessed to be reduced. The authors suggested that cathepsin B, or an enzyme with cathepsin B-like activity, may be involved in the destruction of the cartilage matrix. Another study (Gabrijelcic et al., 1990) investigated the levels of cathepsin B and cathepsin H, as measured by ELISA, in sera and synovial fluids of rheumatoid arthritis patients. Levels of both enzymes were increased compared with samples from osteoarthritis or gout sufferers. The only study to report an effect of IL-1 on cysteine endopeptidase production by chondrocytes (Baici and Lang, 1990) used cells growing in monolayers. Intracellular activity trebled as a result of treatment with IL-1, without any significant increase in extracellular activity. Trabandt et al. (1991) localized cathepsin B primarily to synovial lining cells close to sites of tissue erosion in human rheumatoid arthritis, and demonstrated increased cathepsin B mRNA levels in synovial cells from rheumatoid arthritis patients. Increased cathepsin B mRNA levels have also been detected in mouse mandibular condyles undergoing osteogenesis (Friemert et al., 1991). The authors suggested that the enzyme could be involved in the breakdown of the cartilage matrix before the synthesis of bone.

Maciewicz et al. (1990) reported that rabbit hip synoviocytes, when cultured in a type I collagen gel, secreted the inactive precursor form of cathepsin L. Activation of the precursor was achieved by incubation at pH 3.25, or by incubation at pH 4.5 in the presence of a lysosomal extract or of purified lysosomal cathepsin L. Cathepsin L was detected by ELISA by Trabandt et al. (1990) in synovial cells of rheumatoid arthritis patients, near sites of joint destruction. Hybridization studies revealed greater levels of cathepsin L gene transcription by cultured synovial cells from rheumatoid arthritis patients than control fibroblasts, spleen cells, leukaemic cells or peripheral blood lymphocytes.

A distinct line of approach has been to identify the cleavage positions produced in vivo in cartilage proteins, and to try to match these to cleavages produced in vitro by purified endopeptidases. So far, the metalloendopeptidase stromelysin, the serine endopeptidase from neutrophils, cathepsin G, and cathepsin B have been shown to produce the same cleavage sites of the link protein LP3 in vitro as are found in vivo (Nguyen et al., 1991). A similar approach has been taken with regard to proteoglycan breakdown. The major site of cleavage of bovine articular cartilage proteoglycan produced in culture was located, and found to be the same with or without stimulation with IL-1, and to occur between the G1 and G2 globular domains (Sandy et al., 1991). This suggests that IL-1 increases the rate of normal proteoglycan turnover, rather than initiating a completely new process. Ilic et al. (1992) extended the study, finding the same cleavage site and two others after exposure of the cultures to retinoic acid. A surprising result was that all three cuts occurred at glutamyl bonds, which is a very unusual point of attack by known mammalian endopeptidases.

The isolated G1-G2 fragment from pig laryngeal cartilage has been used as a substrate to explore the cleavage sites produced by purified endopeptidases in vitro. So far, those produced by stromelysin (Fosang et al., 1991), the metalloendopeptidases PUMP (EC 3.4.24.23), neutrophil gelatinase (EC 3.4.24.35), tissue gelatinase (EC 3.4.24.24) and cathepsin B (Fosang et al., 1992) have been located, and none of them coincides with the bond cleaved during culture of bovine cartilage. On the face of it, this is good evidence against the involvement of any of these endopeptidases in pathological proteoglycan breakdown. But the results should perhaps be interpreted cautiously. Apart from the potential problem of species differences, the cleavage of a protein fragment may occur at a different place from that of the native molecule. In this particular instance the effects on conformation or accessibility of the interglobular region by other parts of the proteoglycan molecule, link proteins, hyaluronate or collagen, are not known. The complete proteoglycan molecule is far less susceptible to cleavage as a component of intact cartilage than when in solution, and the sites of cleavage may also change. In the case of cathepsin B, this enzyme is reported to be able to further process the products of its own endopeptidase activity by its peptidyl dipeptidase and carboxypeptidase activities in vitro (Koga et al., 1991). These points, together with an acknowledgement of our lack of understanding of the factors governing the specificity of cleavage of native proteins by these endopeptidases, may mean that we have to wait until the experiments are carried out with intact cartilage rather than a protein fragment before this approach unambiguously identifies the endopeptidase(s) involved.

5. Conclusions

There is strong evidence for the involvement of the cysteine endopeptidases in collagen breakdown in bone, and recent experiments now suggest that the same group of lysosomal enzymes may also be involved in proteoglycan breakdown in cartilage. More work on the involvement of the cysteine endopeptidases in proteoglycan release from articular cartilage in culture and from the joints of whole animals is now needed, to determine whether the findings obtained with the septum cartilage model are applicable to human disease processes.

One major difference between the bone and cartilage systems is the ability of hydrophilic inactivators to inhibit collagen breakdown in bone resorption, but not proteoglycan release from cartilage. Further work is required to investigate the reasons for this difference, and to delineate which particular enzyme(s) is involved in each system. The design and use of inactivators that are more-or-less specific for one particular cysteine endopeptidase should help to answer the question of which enzyme(s) is involved, and may then lead on to investigations into the use of cysteine endopeptidase inactivators as drugs. Although the prospect of the successful use as a drug of an inactivator of a lysosomal endopeptidase seems slim, owing to the undoubtedly essential role of these enzymes in normal cellular processes, there is a possibility that this new therapeutic approach will become a reality.

6. *References*

Abrahamson, M., Mason, R.W., Hansson, H., Buttle, D.J., Grubb, A. and Ohlsson, K. (1991). Human cystatin C. Role of the N-terminal segment in the inhibition of human cysteine proteinases and in its inactivation by leukocyte elastase. Biochem. J. 273, 621–626.

Achkar, C., Gong, Q., Frankfater, A. and Bajkowski, A.S. (1990). Differences in targeting and secretion of cathepsins B and L by BALB/3T3 fibroblasts and Moloney murine sarcoma virus-transformed BALB/3T3 fibroblasts. J. Biol. Chem. 265, 13650–13654.

Ali, S.Y. (1964). The degradation of cartilage matrix by an intracellular protease. Biochem. J. 93, 611–618.

Ali, S.Y., Evans, L., Stainthorpe, E. and Lack, C.H. (1967). Characterization of cathepsins in cartilage. Biochem. J. 105, 549–557.

Aronson, N.N. and Barrett, A.J. (1978). The specificity of cathepsin B. Hydrolysis of glucagon at the C-terminus by a peptidyl dipeptidase mechanism. Biochem. J. 171, 759–765.

Baici, A. and Lang, A. (1990). Effect of interleukin 1β on the production of cathepsin B by rabbit articular chondrocytes. FEBS Lett. 277, 93–96.

Baron, R., Neff, L., Louvard, D. and Courtoy, P.J. (1985). Cell mediated extracellular acidification and bone resorption: evidence for a low pH in resorbing lacunae and localization of a 100-kD lysosomal membrane protein at the osteoclast ruffled border. J. Cell Biol. 101, 2210–2222.

Barrett, A.J. (1973). Human cathepsin B1. Purification and some properties of the enzyme. Biochem. J. 131, 809–822.

Barrett, A.J. (1987). The cystatins: a new class of peptidase inhibitors. Trends Biochem. Sci. 12, 193–196.

Barrett, A.J. and Kirschke, H. (1981). Cathepsin B, cathepsin H, and cathepsin L. Methods Enzymol. 80, 535–561.

Barrett, A.J. and Saklatvala, J. (1985). In "Textbook of Rheumatology", 2nd edn (ed W.N. Kelley, E.D. Harris, S. Ruddy and C.B. Sledge), pp 182–196. W.B. Saunders Co., Philadelphia.

Barrett, A.J. and McDonald, J.K. (1986). Nomenclature: protease, proteinase and peptidase. Biochem. J. 237, 935.

Barrett, A.J. and Rawlings, N.D. (1991). Types and families of endopeptidases. Biochem. Soc. Trans. 19, 707–715.

Barrett, A.J., Rawlings, N.D., Davies, M.E., Machleidt, W., Salvesen, G. and Turk, V. (1986). In "Proteinase Inhibitors" (ed A.J. Barrett and G. Salvesen), pp 515–569. Elsevier Science Publishers BV, Amsterdam.

Barrett, A.J., Buttle, D.J. and Mason, R.W. (1988). Lysosomal cysteine proteinases. ISI Atlas of Science: Biochemistry 1, 256–260.

Berger, A. and Schechter, I. (1970). Mapping the active site of papain with the aid of peptide substrates and inhibitors. Philos. Trans. R. Soc. London (Biol.) 257, 249–264.

Bird, T.A., Gearing, A.J.H. and Saklatvala, J. (1987). Murine interleukin-1 receptor: differences in binding properties between fibroblastic and thymoma cells and evidence for a two-chain receptor model. FEBS Lett. 225, 21–26.

Blair, H.C., Kahn, A.J., Crouch, E.C., Jeffrey, J.J. and Teitelbaum, S.L. (1986). Isolated osteoclasts resorb the organic and inorganic components of bone. J. Cell Biol. 102, 1164–1172.

Bond, J.S. and Barrett, A.J. (1980). Degradation of fructose-1,6-bisphosphate aldolase by cathepsin B. A further example of peptidyldipeptidase activity of this proteinase. Biochem. J. 189, 17–25.

Brinckerhoff, C.E. (1991). Joint destruction in arthritis: metalloproteinases in the spotlight. Arth. Rheum. 34, 1073–1075.

Brocklehurst, K., Willenbrock, F. and Salih, E. (1987). In "Hydrolytic Enzymes" (ed A. Neuberger and K. Brocklehurst), pp 39–158. Elsevier Science Publishers B.V., Amsterdam.

Brömme, D., Steinert, A., Friebe, S., Fittkau, S., Wiederanders, B. and Kirschke, H. (1989). The specificity of bovine spleen cathepsin S. A comparison with rat liver cathepsins L and B. Biochem. J. 264, 475–481.

Brömme, D., Rinne, R. and Kirschke, H. (1991). Tight-binding inhibition of cathepsin S by cystatins. Biomed. Biochim. Acta 50, 631–635.

Bunning, R.A.D. and Russell, R.G.G. (1989). The effect of tumor necrosis factor α and gamma-interferon on the resorption of human articular cartilage and on the production of prostaglandin E and of caseinase activity by human articular chondrocytes. Arth. Rheum. 32, 780–784.

Bunning, R.A.D., Crawford, A., Richardson, H.J., Opdenakker, G., Van Damme, J. and Russell, R.G.G. (1987). Interleukin 1 preferentially stimulates the production of tissue type plasminogen activator by human articular chondrocytes. Biochim. Biophys Acta 924, 473 482.

Burleigh, M.C., Barrett, A.J. and Lazarus, G.S. (1974). Cathepsin B1. A lysosomal enzyme that degrades native collagen. Biochem. J. 137, 387–398.

Buttle, D.J. and Saklatvala, J. (1992). Lysosomal cysteine endopeptidases mediate interleukin 1-stimulated cartilage proteoglycan degradation. Biochem. J. 287, 657–661.

Buttle, D.J., Bonner, B.C., Burnett, D. and Barrett, A.J. (1988). A catalytically active high-M_r form of human cathepsin B from sputum. Biochem. J. 254, 693–699.

Buttle, D.J., Burnett, D. and Abrahamson, M. (1990). Levels of neutrophil elastase and cathepsin B, and cystatins in human sputum: relationship to inflammation. Scand. J. Clin. Lab. Invest. 50, 509–516.

Buttle, D.J., Abrahamson, M., Burnett, D., Mort, J.S., Barrett, A.J., Dando, P.M. and Hill, S.L. (1991). Human sputum cathepsin B degrades proteoglycan, is inhibited by α_2-macroglobulin and is modulated by neutrophil elastase cleavage of cathepsin B precursor and cystatin C. Biochem. J. 276, 325–331.

Buttle, D.J., Saklatvala, J., Tamai, M. and Barrett, A.J. (1992). Inhibition of interleukin 1-stimulated cartilage proteoglycan degradation by a lipophilic inactivator of cysteine endopeptidases. Biochem. J. 281, 175–177.

Caputo, C.B., Sygowski, L.A., Wolanin, D.J., Patton, S.P., Caccese, R.G., Shaw, A., Roberts, R.A. and DiPasquale, G. (1987). Effect of synthetic metalloprotease inhibitors on cartilage autolysis *in vitro*. J. Pharmacol. Exp. Ther. 240, 460–465.

Chan, S.J., San Segundo, B., McCormick, M.B. and Steiner, D.F. (1986). Nucleotide and predicted amino acid sequences of cloned human and mouse preprocathepsin B cDNAs. Proc. Natl Acad. Sci. USA 83, 7721–7725.

Cohen, L.W., Coghlan, V.M. and Dihel, L.C. (1986). Cloning and sequencing of papain-encoding cDNA. Gene 48, 219–227.

Davies, M.E. and Barrett, A.J. (1984). Immunolocalization of human cystatins in neutrophils and lymphocytes. Histochemistry 80, 373–377.

Dean, R.T. and Barrett, A.J. (1976). In "Essays in Biochemistry, vol. 12" (ed P.N. Campbell and W.N. Aldridge), pp 1–40. Academic Press, New York.

Dean, R.T., Roberts, C.R. and Forni, L.G. (1984). Oxygen-centred free radicals can efficiently degrade the polypeptide of proteoglycans in whole cartilage. Biosci. Rep. 4, 1017–1026.

Dean, R.T., Roberts, C.R. and Jessup, W. (1985). In "Progress in Clinical and Biological Research. Vol. 180. Intracellular Protein Catabolism" (ed E. Khairallah, J.S. Bond and J.W.C. Bird), pp 341–350. Alan R. Liss, New York.

Delaissé, J.-M., Eeckhout, Y. and Vaes, G. (1980). Inhibition of bone resorption in culture by inhibitors of thiol proteinases. Biochem. J. 192, 365–368.

Delaissé, J.-M., Eeckhout, Y. and Vaes, G. (1984). *In vivo* and *in vitro* evidence for the involvement of cysteine proteinases in bone resorption. Biochem. Biophys. Res. Commun. 125, 441–447.

Delaissé, J.-M., Eeckhout, Y., Sear, C., Galloway, A., McCullagh, K. and Vaes, G. (1985). A new synthetic inhibitor of mammalian tissue collagenase inhibits bone resorption in culture. Biochem. Biophys. Res. Commun. 133, 483–490.

Delaissé, J.-M., Ledent, P., Eeckhout, Y. and Vaes, G. (1986). In "Cysteine Proteinases and their Inhibitors", pp 259–268. Walter de Gruyter & Co., Berlin.

Delaissé, J.-M., Boyde, A., Maconnachie, E., Ali, N.N., Sear, C.H.J., Eeckhout, Y., Vaes, G. and Jones, S.J. (1987). The effects of inhibitors of cysteine proteinases and collagenase on the resorptive activity of isolated osteoclasts. Bone 8, 305–313.

Delaissé, J.-M., Ledent, P. and Vaes, G. (1991). Collagenolytic cysteine proteinases of bone tissue. Cathepsin B, (pro)cathepsin L and a cathepsin L-like 70 kDa proteinase. Biochem. J. 279, 167–174.

Diener, E., Diner, U.E., Sinha, A., Xie, S. and Vergidis, R. (1986). Specific immunosuppression by immunotoxins containing daunomycin. Science 231, 148–150.

Dingle, J.T. (1961). Studies on the mode of action of excess vitamin A. 3. Release of a bound protease by the action of vitamin A. Biochem. J. 79, 509–512.

Dingle, J.T. (1975). The secretion of enzymes into the pericellular environment. Philos. Trans. R. Soc. London Ser. B 271, 315–324.

Dingle, J.T., Lucy, J.A. and Fell, H.B. (1961). Studies on the mode of action of excess vitamin A. 1. Effect of excess of vitamin A on the metabolism and composition of embryonic chick-limb cartilage grown in organ culture. Biochem J. 79, 497–500.

Dingle, J.T., Fell, H.B. and Lucy, J.A. (1966). Synthesis of connective-tissue components. The effect of retinol and hydrocortisone on cultured limb-bone rudiments. Biochem. J. 98, 173–181.

Dingle, J.T., Barrett, A.J. and Poole, A.R. (1972). Inhibition by pepstatin of human cartilage degradation. Biochem. J. 127, 443–444.

DiPasquale, G., Caccese, R., Pasternak, R., Conaty, J., Hubbs, S. and Perry, K. (1986). Proteoglycan- and collagen-degrading enzymes from human interleukin 1-stimulated chondrocytes from several species: proteoglycanase and collagenase inhibitors as potentially new disease-modifying antiarthritic agents. Proc. Soc. Exp. Biol. Med. 183, 262–267.

Dong, J. and Sahagian, G.G. (1990). Basis for low affinity binding of a lysosomal cysteine protease to the cation-independent mannose 6-phosphate receptor. J. Biol. Chem. 265, 4210–4217.

Dumermuth, E., Sterchi, E.E., Jiang, W., Wolz, R.L., Bond, J.S., Flannery, A.V. and Beynon, R.J. (1991). The astacin family of metalloendopeptidases. J. Biol. Chem. 266, 21381–21385.

Eeckhout, Y. (1990). Possible role and mechanism of action of dissolved calcium in the degradation of bone collagen by lysosomal cathepsins and collagenase. Biochem. J. 272, 529–532.

Eeckhout, Y. and Vaes, G. (1977). Further studies on the activation of procollagenase, the latent precursor of bone collagenase. Biochem. J. 166, 21–31.

Eeckhout, Y., Delaissé, J.-M. and Vaes, G. (1986). Direct extraction and assay of bone tissue collagenase and its relation to parathyroid-hormone-induced bone resorption. Biochem. J. 239, 793–796.

Erickson, A.H. (1989). Biosynthesis of lysosomal endopeptidases. J. Cell. Biochem. 40, 31–41.

Everts, V., Beertsen, W. and Tigchelaar-Gutter, W. (1985). The digestion of phagocytosed collagen is inhibited by the proteinase inhibitors leupeptin and E-64. Collagen Rel. Res. 5, 315–336.

Everts, V., Beertsen, W. and Schröder, R. (1988). Effects of the proteinase inhibitors leupeptin and E-64 on osteoclastic bone resorption. Calcif. Tissue Int. 43, 172–178.

Fell, H.B. and Mellanby, E. (1952). The effect of hypervitaminosis A on embryonic limb-bones cultivated *in vitro*. J. Physiol. 116, 320–349.

Fell, H.B. and Thomas, L. (1960). Comparison of the effects of papain and vitamin A on cartilage. II. The effects on organ cultures of embryonic skeletal tissue. J. Exp. Med. 111, 719–744.

Fell, H.B. and Dingle, J.T. (1963). Studies on the mode of action of excess of vitamin A. 6. Lysosomal protease and the degradation of cartilage matrix. Biochem. J. 87, 403–408.

Fell, H.B., Mellanby, E. and Pelc, S.R. (1956). Influence of excess vitamin A on the sulphate metabolism of bone rudiments grown *in vitro*. J. Physiol. 134, 179–188.

Fosang, A.J., Neame, P.J., Hardingham, T.E., Murphy, G. and Hamilton, J.A. (1991). Cleavage of cartilage proteoglycan between G1 and G2 domains by stromelysins. J. Biol. Chem. 266, 15579–15582.

Fosang, A.J., Neame, P.J., Last, K., Hardingham, T.E., Murphy, G. and Hamilton, J.A. (1992). The interglobular domain of cartilage aggrecan is cleaved by PUMP, gelatinases and cathepsin B. J. Biol. Chem. 267, 19740–19774.

Friemert, C., Closs, E.I., Silbermann, M., Erfle, V. and Strauss, P.G. (1991). Isolation of a cathepsin B-encoding cDNA from murine osteogenic cells. Gene 103, 259–261.

Gabrijelcic, D., Annan-Prah, A., Rodic, B., Rozman, B., Cotic, V. and Turk, V. (1990). Determination of cathepsins B and H in sera and synovial fluids of patients with different joint diseases. J. Clin. Chem. Clin. Biochem. 28, 149–153.

Goldring, M.B. and Goldring, S.R. (1990). Skeletal tissue response to cytokines. Clin. Orthop. Rel. Res. 258, 245–278.

Hanewinkel, H., Glössl, J. and Kresse, H. (1987). Biosynthesis of cathepsin B in cultured normal and I-cell fibroblasts. J. Biol. Chem. 262, 12351–12355.

Heath, J.K., Atkinson, S.J., Meikle, M.C. and Reynolds, J.J. (1984). Mouse osteoblasts synthesize collagenase in response to bone resorbing agents. Biochim. Biophys. Acta 802, 151–154.

Hembry, R.M., Knight, C.G., Dingle, J.T. and Barrett, A.J. (1982). Evidence that extracellular cathepsin D is not responsible for the resorption of cartilage matrix in culture. Biochim. Biophys. Acta 714, 307–312.

Holtrop, M.E., Raisz, L.G. and Simmons, H.A. (1974). The effects of parathyroid hormone, colchicine and calcitonin on the ultrastructure and the activity of osteoclasts in organ culture. J. Cell Biol. 60, 346–355.

Ilic, M.Z., Handley, C.J., Robinson, H.C. and Mok, M.T. (1992). Mechanism of catabolism of aggrecan by articular cartilage. Arch. Biochem. Biophys. 294, 115–122.

Ishidoh, K., Imajoh, S., Emori, Y., Ohno, S., Kawasaki, H., Minami, Y., Kominami, E., Katunuma, M. and Suzuki, K. (1987). Molecular cloning and sequencing of cDNA for rat cathepsin H. FEBS Lett. 226, 33–37.

IUBMB Nomenclature Committee. Enzyme Nomenclature 1992, Academic Press, New York.

Kärgel, H.-J., Dettmer, R., Etzold, G., Kirschke, H., Bohley, P. and Langner, J. (1980). Action of cathepsin L on the oxidized B-chain of bovine insulin. FEBS Lett. 114, 257–260.

Killackey, J.J., Roughley, P.J. and Mort, J.S. (1983). Proteinase inhibitors of human articular cartilage. Collagen Rel. Res. 3, 419–430.

Kirschke, H. and Shaw, E. (1981). Rapid inactivation of cathepsin L by Z-Phe-PheCHN$_2$ and Z-Phe-Ala-CHN$_2$. Biochem. Biophys. Res. Commun. 101, 454–458.

Kirschke, H. and Barrett, A.J. (1987). In "Lysosomes: Their Role in Protein Breakdown" (ed H. Glaumann and F.J. Ballard), pp 193–238. Academic Press, New York.

Kirschke, H., Langner, J., Riemann, S., Wiederanders, B., Ansorge, S. and Bohley, P. (1980). In "Protein Degradation in Health and Disease. Ciba Foundation Symposium 75" (ed D. Evered and J. Whelan), Excerpta Medica/Elsevier North Holland, Amsterdam, pp 15–35.

Kirschke, H., Kembhavi, A.A., Bohley, P. and Barrett, A.J. (1982). Action of rat liver cathepsin L on collagen and other substrates. Biochem. J. 201, 367–372.

Kirschke, H., Schmidt, I. and Wiederanders, B. (1986). Cathepsin S. The cysteine proteinase from bovine lymphoid tissue is distinct from cathepsin L. Biochem. J. 240, 455–459.

Kirschke, H., Wiederanders, B., Brömme, D. and Rinne, A. (1989). Cathepsin S from bovine spleen. Purification, distribution, intracellular localization and action on proteins. Biochem. J. 264, 467–473.

Kleinveld, H.A., Swaak, A.J.G., Hack, C.E. and Koster, J.F. (1989). Interactions between oxygen free radicals and proteins. Implications for rheumatoid arthritis. An overview. Scand. J. Rheumatol. 18, 341–352.

Knight, C.G. (1986). In "Proteinase Inhibitors" (ed A.J. Barrett and G. Salvesen), pp 23–51. Elsevier Science Publishers BV, Amsterdam.

Kobayashi, H., Schmitt, M., Goretzki, L., Chucholowski, N., Calvete, J., Kramer, M., Günzler, W.A., Jänicke, F. and Graeff, H. (1991). Cathepsin B efficiently activates the soluble and the tumor cell receptor-bound form of the proenzyme urokinase-type plasminogen activator (pro-uPA). J. Biol. Chem. 266, 5147–5152.

Koga, H., Yamada, H., Nishimura, Y., Kato, K. and Imoto, T. (1991). Multiple proteolytic action of rat liver cathepsin B: specificities and pH-dependences of the endo- and exopeptidase activities. J. Biochem. (Tokyo) 110, 179–188.

Kopecek, J. and Duncan, R. (1987). Targetable polymeric prodrugs. J. Controlled Rel. 6, 315–327.

Kornfeld, S. (1986). Trafficking of lysosomal enzymes in normal and disease states. J. Clin. Invest. 77, 1–6.

Lafyatis, R., Kim, S.-J., Angel, P., Roberts, A.B., Sporn, M.B., Karin, M. and Wilder, R.L. (1990). Interleukin 1 stimulates and all-trans-retinoic acid inhibits collagenase gene expression through its 5′ activator protein-1-binding site. Mol. Endocrinol. 4, 973–980.

Lazzarino, D. and Gabel, C.A. (1990). Protein determinants impair recognition of procathepsin L phosphorylated oligosaccharides by the cation-independent mannose 6-phosphate receptor. J. Biol. Chem. 265, 11864–11871.

Lucy, J.A., Dingle, J.T. and Fell, H.B. (1961). Studies on the mode of action of excess vitamin A. 2. A possible role of intracellular proteases in the degradation of cartilage matrix. Biochem. J. 79, 500–508.

Maciewicz, R.A. and Etherington, D.J. (1988). A comparison of four cathepsins (B, L, N and S) with collagenolytic activity from rabbit spleen. Biochem. J. 256, 433–440.

Maciewicz, R.A., Wardale, R.-J., Wotton, S.F., Duance, V.C. and Etherington, D.J. (1990). Mode of activation of the precursor to cathepsin L: implication for matrix degradation in arthritis. Biol. Chem. Hoppe-Seyler 371, 223–228.

Maciewicz, R.A., Wotton, S.F., Etherington, D.J. and Duance, V.C. (1991). Susceptibility of the cartilage collagens types II, IX and XI to degradation by the cysteine proteinases, cathepsins B and L. FEBS Lett. 269, 189–193.

Marchisio, P.C., Cirillo, D., Naldini, L., Primavera, M.V., Teti, A. and Zambonin-Zallone, A. (1984). Cell–substratum interaction of cultured avian osteoclasts is mediated by specific adhesion structures. J. Cell Biol. 99, 1696–1705.

Mason, R,W. (1986). Species variants of cathepsin L and their immunological identification. Biochem. J. 240, 285–288.

Mason, R.W. (1989). Interaction of lysosomal cysteine proteinases with α_2-macroglobulin: conclusive evidence for the endopeptidase activities of cathepsins B and H. Arch. Biochem. Biophys. 273, 367–374.

Mason, R.W., Green, G.D.J. and Barrett, A.J. (1985). Human liver cathepsin L. Biochem. J. 226, 233–241.

Mason, R.W., Johnson, D.A., Barrett, A.J. and Chapman, H.A. (1986). Elastinolytic activity of cathepsin L. Biochem. J. 233, 925–927.

Mason, R.W., Gal, S. and Gottesman, M.M. (1987). The identification of the major excreted protein (MEP) from a transformed mouse fibroblast cell line as a catalytically active precursor form of cathepsin L. Biochem. J. 248, 449–454.

Mason, R.W., Wilcox, D., Wikstrom, P. and Shaw, E.N. (1989). The identification of active forms of cysteine proteinases in Kirsten-virus-transformed mouse fibroblasts by use of a specific radiolabelled inhibitor. Biochem. J. 257, 125–129.

McCluskey, R.T. and Thomas, L. (1958). The removal of cartilage matrix, *in vivo*, by papain. Identification of crystalline papain protease as the cause of the phenomenon. J. Exp. Med. 108, 371–384.

McIntyre, G.F. and Erickson, A.H. (1991). Procathepsins L and D are membrane-bound in acidic microsomal vesicles. J. Biol. Chem. 266, 15438–15445.

McKay, M.J., Offermann, M.K., Barrett, A.J. and Bond, J.S. (1983). Action of human liver cathepsin B on the oxidized insulin B chain. Biochem. J. 213, 467–471.

Meloun, B., Baudys, M., Pohl, J., Pavlik, M. and Kostka, V. (1988). Amino acid sequence of bovine spleen cathepsin B. J. Biol. Chem. 263, 9087–9093.

Miller, S.C. (1977). Osteoclast cell-surface changes during the egg-laying cycle in Japanese quail. J. Cell Biol. 75, 104–118.

Monboisse, J.C., Braquet, P., Randoux, A. and Borel, J.P. (1983). Non-enzymatic degradation of acid-soluble calf skin collagen by superoxide ion. Biochem. Pharmacol. 32, 53–58.

Morrison, R.I.G., Barrett, A.J., Dingle, J.T. and Prior, D. (1973). Cathepsins B1 and D. Action on human cartilage proteoglycans. Biochim. Biophys. Acta 302, 411–419.

Mort, J.S. and Recklies, A.D. (1986). Interrelationship of active and latent secreted human cathepsin B precursors. Biochem. J. 233, 57–63.

Mort, J.S., Recklies, A.D. and Poole, A.R. (1984). Extracellular presence of the lysosomal proteinase cathepsin B in rheumatoid synovium and its activity at neutral pH. Arth. Rheum. 27, 509–515.

Murphy, G. and Reynolds, J.J. (1993). In "Connective Tissue and Its Disorders: Molecular, Genetic and Medical Aspects" pp 287–316 (ed P. Royce and B. Steinmann). Wiley R. Liss, New York.

Murphy, G., Ward, R., Gavrilovic, J. and Atkinson, S. (1992). Physiological mechanisms for metalloproteinase activation. Matrix (Supplement 1), 224–230.

Musil, D., Zucic, D., Turk, D., Engh, R.A., Mayr, I., Huber, R., Popovic, T., Turk, V., Towatari, T., Katunuma, N. and Bode, W. (1991). The refined 2.15 Å X-ray crystal structure of human liver cathepsin B: the structural basis for its specificity. EMBO J. 10, 2321–2330.

Nguyen, Q., Mort, J.S. and Roughley, P.J. (1990). Cartilage proteoglycan aggregate is degraded more extensively by cathepsin L than by cathepsin B. Biochem. J. 266, 569–573.

Nguyen, Q., Liu, J., Roughley, P.J. and Mort, J.S. (1991). Link protein as a monitor *in situ* of endogenous proteolysis in adult human articular cartilage. Biochem. J. 278, 143–147.

Nishimura, Y. and Kato, K. (1987). Intracellular transport and processing of lysosomal cathepsin H. Biochem. Biophys. Res. Commun. 148, 329–343.

Nixon, J.S., Bottomley, K.M.K., Broadhurst, M.J., Brown, P.A., Johnson, W.H., Lawton, G., Marley, J., Sedgwick, A.D. and Wilkinson, S.E. (1991). Potent collagenase inhibitors prevent interleukin-1-induced cartilage degradation *in vitro*. Int. J. Tissue React. 13, 237–243.

Pettipher, E.R., Higgs, G.A. and Henderson, B. (1986). Interleukin 1 induces leukocyte infiltration and cartilage degradation in the synovial joint. Proc. Natl Acad. Sci. USA 83, 8749–8753.

Poole, A.R., Hembry, R.M. and Dingle, J.T. (1974). Cathepsin

D in cartilage: the immunohistochemical demonstration of extracellular enzyme in normal and pathological conditions. J. Cell Sci. 14, 139–161.

Portnoy, D.A., Erickson, A.H., Kochan, J., Ravetch, J.V. and Unkeless, J.C. (1986). Cloning and characterization of a mouse cysteine proteinase. J. Biol. Chem. 261, 14697–14703.

Qian, F., Frankfater, A., Miller, R.V., Chan, S.J. and Steiner, D.F. (1990). Molecular cloning of rat precursor cathepsin H and the expression of five lysosomal cathepsins in normal tissues and in a rat carcinosarcoma. Int. J. Biochem. 22, 1457–1464.

Rawlings, N.D. and Barrett, A.J. (1990). Bone morphogenetic protein 1 is homologous in part with calcium-dependent serine proteinase. Biochem. J. 266, 622–624.

Recklies, A.D. and Mort, J.S. (1985). Rat mammary gland in culture secretes a stable high molecular weight form of cathepsin L. Biochem. Biophys. Res. Commun. 131, 402–407.

Recklies, A.D., Poole, A.R. and Mort, J.S. (1982). A cysteine proteinase secreted from human breast tumours is immunologically related to cathepsin B. Biochem. J. 207, 633–636.

Rich, D.H. (1990). In "Comprehensive Medicinal Chemistry, Volume 2" (ed P.G. Sammes), pp 391–441. Pergamon, Oxford.

Rifkin, B.R., Vernillo, A.T., Kleckner, A.P., Auszmann, J.M., Rosenberg, L.R. and Zimmerman, M. (1991). Cathepsin B and L activities in isolated osteoclasts. Biochem. Biophys. Res. Commun. 179, 63–69.

Ritonja, A., Popovic, T., Kotnik, M., Machleidt, W. and Turk, V. (1988). Amino acid sequences of the human kidney cathepsins H and L. FEBS Lett. 228, 341–345.

Ritonja, A., Colic, A., Dolenc, I., Ogrinc, T., Podobnik, M. and Turk, V. (1991). The complete amino acid sequence of bovine cathepsin S and a partial sequence of bovine cathepsin L. FEBS Lett. 283, 329–331.

Roberts, C.R., Roughley, P.J. and Mort, J.S. (1989). Degradation of human proteoglycan aggregate induced by hydrogen peroxide. Biochem. J. 258, 805–811.

Roughley, P.J. (1977). The degradation of cartilage proteoglycans by tissue proteinases. Proteoglycan heterogeneity and the pathway of proteolytic degradation. Biochem. J. 167, 639–646.

Roughley, P.J. and Barrett, A.J. (1977). The degradation of cartilage proteoglycans by tissue proteinases. Proteoglycan structure and its susceptibility to proteolysis. Biochem. J. 167, 629–637.

Roughley, P.J., Murphy, G. and Barrett, A.J. (1978). Proteinase inhibitors of bovine nasal cartilage. Biochem. J. 169, 721–724.

Saklatvala, J. (1986). Tumour necrosis factor α stimulates resorption and inhibits synthesis of proteoglycan in cartilage. Nature (London) 322, 547–549.

Saklatvala, J. and Sarsfield, S.J. (1988). In "The Control of Tissue Damage" (ed A.M. Glauert), pp 97–108. Elsevier Science Publishers BV, Amsterdam.

Saklatvala, J., Sarsfield, S.J. and Pilsworth, L.M.C. (1983). Characterization of proteins from human synovium and mononuclear leucocytes that induce resorption of cartilage proteoglycan *in vitro*. Biochem. J. 209, 337–344.

Saklatvala, J., Pilsworth, L.M.C., Sarsfield, S.J., Gavrilovic, J. and Heath, J.K. (1984). Pig catabolin is a form of interleukin 1. Biochem. J. 224, 461–466.

Salvesen, G.S. and Barrett, A.J. (1980). Covalent binding of proteinases in their reaction with α_2-macroglobulin. Biochem. J. 187, 695–701.

Sandy, J.D., Neame, P.J., Boynton, R.E. and Flannery, C.R. (1991). Catabolism of aggrecan in cartilage explants. Identification of a major cleavage site within the interglobular domain. J. Biol. Chem. 266, 8683–8685.

Schnyder, J., Payne, T. and Dinarello, C.A. (1987). Human monocyte or recombinant interleukin 1's are specific for the secretion of a metalloproteinase from chondrocytes. J. Immunol. 138, 496–503.

Schwartz, W.N. and Barrett, A.J. (1980). Human cathepsin H. Biochem. J. 191, 487–497.

Silver, I.A., Murrills, R.J. and Etherington, D.J. (1988). Microelectrode studies on the acid microenvironment beneath adherent macrophages and osteoclasts. Exp. Cell Res. 175, 266–276.

Singh, H., Kuo, T. and Kalnitsky, G. (1978). In "Protein Turnover and Lysosome Function" (ed H.L. Segal and D.J. Doyle), pp 315–331. Academic Press, New York.

Stearns, N.A., Dong, J., Pan, J.-X., Brenner, D.A. and Sahagian, G.G. (1990). Comparison of cathepsin L synthesized by normal and transformed cells at the gene, message, protein and oligosaccharide levels. Arch. Biochem. Biophys. 283, 447–457.

Stephenson, M.L., Goldring, M.B., Birkhead, J.R., Krane, S.M., Rahmsdorf, H.J. and Angel, P. (1987). Stimulation of procollagenase synthesis parallels increases in cellular procollagenase mRNA in human articular chondrocytes exposed to recombinant interleukln 1β or phorbol ester. Biochem. Biophys. Res. Commun. 144, 583–590.

Tamai, M., Matsumoto, K., Omura, S., Koyama, I., Ozawa, Y. and Hanada, K. (1986). In vitro and in vivo inhibition of cysteine proteinases by EST, a new analog of E-64. J. Pharmacobio-Dyn. 9, 672–677.

Tamai, M., Yokoo, C., Murata, M., Oguma, K., Sota, K., Sato, E. and Kanaoka, Y. (1987). Efficient synthetic method for ethyl (+)-(2S, 3S)-3-[(S)-3-methyl-1-(3-methylbutyl-carbamoyl)]-2-oxiranecarboxylate (EST), a new inhibitor of cysteine proteinases. Chem. Pharm. Bull. 35, 1098–1104.

Taylor, D.J., Whitehead, R.J., Evanson, J.M., Westmacott, D., Feldmann, M., Bertfield, H., Morris, M.A. and Woolley, D.E. (1988). Effect of recombinant cytokines on glycolysis and fructose 2,6-bisphosphate in rheumatoid synovial cells in vitro. Biochem. J. 250, 111–115.

Thomas, L. (1956). Reversible collapse of rabbit ears after intravenous papain, and prevention of recovery by cortisone. J. Exp. Med. 104, 245–251.

Trabandt, A., Aicher, W.K., Gay, R.E., Sukhatme, V.P., Nilson-Hamilton, M., Hamilton, R.T., McGhee, J.R., Fassbender, H.G. and Gay, S. (1990). Expression of the collagenolytic and ras-induced cysteine proteinase cathepsin L and proliferation-associated oncogenes in synovial cells of MRL/1 mice and patients with rheumatoid arthritis. Matrix 10, 349–361.

Trabandt, A., Gay, R.E., Fassbender, H.-G. and Gay, S. (1991). Cathepsin B in synovial cells at the site of joint destruction in rheumatoid arthritis. Arth. Rheum. 34, 1444–1451.

Turk, V. and Bode, W. (1991). The cystatins: protein inhibitors of cysteine proteinases. FEBS Lett. 285, 213–219.

Tyler, J.A. (1985). Articular cartilage cultured with catabolin (pig interleukin 1) synthesizes a decreased number of normal proteoglycan molecules. Biochem. J. 227, 869–878.

Tyler, J.A. (1988). In "The Control of Tissue Damage" (ed A.M. Glauert), pp 197–219. Elsevier Science Publishers BV, Amsterdam.

Tyler, J.A. and Benton, H.P. (1988). Synthesis of type II collagen is decreased in cartilage cultured with interleukin 1 while the rate of intracellular degradation remains unchanged. Collagen Rel. Res. 8, 393–405.

Vaes, G. (1988). Cellular biology and biochemical mechanism of bone resorption. Clin. Orthop. Rel Res. 231, 239–271.

Van Noorden, C.J.F. and Vogels, I.M.C. (1986). Enzyme histochemical reactions in unfixed and undecalcified cryostat sections of mouse knee joints with special reference to arthritic lesions. Histochemistry 86, 127–133.

Van Noorden, C.J.F. and Everts, V. (1991). Selective inhibition of cysteine proteinases by Z-Phe-AlaCH$_2$F suppresses digestion of collagen by fibroblasts and osteoclasts. Biochem. Biophys. Res. Commun. 178, 178–184.

Van Noorden, C.J.F., Vogels, I.M.C., Everts, V. and Beertsen, W. (1987). Localization of cathepsin B activity in fibroblasts and chondrocytes by continuous monitoring of the formation of a final fluorescent reaction product using 5-nitrosalicylaldehyde. Histochem. J. 19, 483–487.

Van Noorden, C.J.F, Smith, R.E. and Rasnick, D. (1988). Cysteine proteinase activity in arthritic rat knee joints and the effects of a selective systemic inhibitor, Z-Phe-Ala-CH$_2$F. J. Rheumatol. 15, 1525–1535.

Weiss, S.J., Peppin, G., Ortiz, X., Ragsdale, C. and Test, S.T. (1985). Oxidative autoactivation of latent collagenase by human neutrophils. Science 227, 747–749.

Wiederanders, B., Brömme, D., Kirschke, H., Kalkkinen, N., Rinne, A., Paquette, T. and Toothman, P. (1991). Primary structure of bovine cathepsin S. Comparison to cathepsins L, H, B and papain. FEBS Lett. 286, 189–192.

Wilcox, D. and Mason, R.W. (1989). Labelling of cysteine proteinases in purified lysosomes. Biochem Soc. Trans. 17, 1080–1081.

Wilcox, D. and Mason, R.W. (1992). Inhibition of cysteine proteinases in lysosomes and whole cells. Biochem. J. 285, 495–502.

Willenbrock, F. and Brocklehurst, K. (1985). Preparation of cathepsins B and H by covalent chromatography and characterization of their catalytic sites by reaction with a thiol-specific two-protonic-state reactivity probe. Biochem. J. 227, 511–519.

Wolff, S.P. and Dean, R.T. (1986). Fragmentation of proteins by free radicals and its effect on their susceptibility to enzymic hydrolysis. Biochem J. 234, 399–403.

Wolff, S.P., Garner, A. and Dean, R.T. (1986). Free radicals, lipids and protein degradation. Trends Biochem. Sci. 11, 27–31.

Glossary

Note: This glossary is up to date for the current volume only and will be supplemented with each subsequent volume.

A Absorbance
Å Angstrom
AA Arachidonic acid
AAb Autoantibody
Ab Antibody
Ab1 Idiotype antibody
Ab2 Anti-idiotype antibody
Ab2α Anti-idiotype antibody which binds outside the antigen binding region
Ab2β Anti-idiotype antibody which binds to the antigen binding region
Ab3 Anti-anti-idiotype antibody
Ψa Apical membrane potential
Abcc Antibody dependent cytotoxic activity
ABA-L-GAT Arsanilicacid conjugated with the synthetic polypeptide L-GAT
AC Adenylate cyclase
ACAT Acyl-co-enzyme-A acyltransferase
ACAID Anterior chamber associated immune deviation
ACE Angiotensin-converting enzyme
ACh Acetylcholine
α₁-ACT α₁-antichymotrypsin
ACTH Adrenocorticotrophin hormone
ADCC Antibody-dependent cell-mediated cytotoxicity
Ado Adenosine
ADP Adenosine diphosphate
AES Anti-eosinophil serum
Ag Antigen
AGE Advanced glycosylation end-product
AGEPC 1-*O*-Alkyl-2-acetyl-*sn*-glyceryl-3-phosphocholine
AI Angiotensin I
AII Angiotensin II
AID Autoimmune disease
AIDS Acquired immune deficiency syndrome
A/J A Jackson inbred mouse strain
cAMP Cyclic adenosine monophosphate (adenosine 3′,5′-phosphate)
AM Alveolar macrophage
AML Acute myelogenous leukaemia

AMP Adenosine monophosphate
ANAb Anti-nuclear antibodies
ANCA Anti-neutrophil cytoplasmic auto antibodies
cANCA Cytoplasmic ANCA
pANCA Perinuclear ANCA
AND Anaphylactic degranulation
ANF Atrial natriuretic factor
ANP Atrial natriuretic peptide
Anti-I-A Antibody against class II molecule encoded by I-A locus
Anti-I-E Anttibody against class II MHC molecule encoded by I-E locus
anti-Ig Antibody against an immunoglobulin
anti-RTE Anti-tubular epithelium
APA B-azaprostanoic acid
APAS Antiplatelet antiserum
APC Antigen-presenting cell
APD Action potential duration
ApO-B Apolipoprotein B
APUD Amine precursor uptake and decarboxylation
ARDS Acute respiratory distress syndrome
AS Ankylosing spondylitis
4-ASA 4-aminosalicylic acid
5-ASA 5-aminosalicylic acid
ASA Acetylsalicylic acid (aspirin)
ATHERO-ELAM A monocyte adhesion molecule
ATL Adult T cell leukaemia
ATP Adenosine 3′5′ triphosphate
AUC Area under curve
AVP Arginine vasopressin

B₁receptor Bradykinin receptor subtype
B₂receptor Bradykinin receptor subtype
B₂ (CD18) A leukocyte integrin
β₂M β₂-microglobulin
BAF Basophil-activating factor
BAL Bronchoalveolar lavage
BALF Bronchoalveolar lavage fluid
BALT Bronchus-associated lymphoid tissue
B cell Bone marrow-derived lymphocyte
BCF Basophil chemotactic factor

BCG Bacillus Calmette–Guérin
bFGF Basic fibroblast growth factor
BG Birbeck granules
BHR Bronchial hyperresponsiveness
BI-CFC Blast colony-forming cells
b.i.d. *Bis in die* (twice a day)
Bk Bradykinin
BM Bone marrow
BMCMC Bone marrow cultured mast cell
BMMC Bone marrow mast cell
BOC-FMLP Butoxycarbonyl-FMLP
bp Base pair
BPB Para-bromophenacyl bromide
BPI Bacterial permeability-increasing protein
BSA Bovine serum albumin
β-TG β-thromboglobulin

CatG Cathepsin G
C1 The first component of complement
C1 inhibitor A serine protease inhibitor which inactivates C1r/C1s
C1q Complement fragment 1q (anaphylatoxin)
C1qR Receptor for C1w; facilitates attachment of immune complexes to mononuclear leucocytes and endothelium
C2 The second component of complement
C3 The third component of complement
C3a Complement fragment 3a (anaphylatoxin)
C3a₇₂₋₇₇ A synthetic carboxyterminal peptide C3a analogue
C3aR Receptor for anaphylatoxins, C3a, C4a, C5a
C3b Complement fragment 3b (anaphylatoxin)
C3bi Inactivated form of C3b fragment of complement
C4 The fourth component of complement
C4b Complement fragment 4b (anaphylatoxin)

C4BP C4 binding protein; plasma protein which acts as co-factor to factor I inactivate C3 convertase

C5 The fifth component of complement

C5a Complement fragment 5a (anaphylatoxin)

C5aR Receptor for anaphylatoxins C3a, C4a and C5a

C5b Complement fragment 5b (anaphylatoxin)

C6 The sixth component of complement

C7 The seventh component of complement

C8 The eighth component of complement

C9 The ninth component of complement

$C_\varepsilon 2$ Heavy chain of immunoglobulin E: domain 2

$C_\varepsilon 3$ Heavy chain of immunoglobulin E: domain 3

$C_\varepsilon 4$ Heavy chain of immunoglobulin E: domain 4

Ca Calcium

CAH Chronic active hepatitis

CALT Conjunctival associated lymphoid tissue

cAMP Cyclic adenosine monophosphate (adenosine 3′,5′-phosphate)

CAM Cell adhesion molecule

CBH Cutaneous basophil hypersensitivity

CBP Cromolyn-binding protein

CCK Cholecystokinin

CCR Creatinine clearance rate

CD Cluster of differentiation (a system of nomenclature for surface molecules on cells of the immune system); cluster determinant

CD1 Also known as MHC class I-like surface glycoprotein

CD1a Isoform a also known as non-classical MHC class I-like surface antigen

CD1c Isoform c also known as non-classical MHC class I-like surface antigen

CD2 Defines T cells involved in antigen non-specific cell activation

CD3 Also known as T cell receptor-associated surface glycoprotein on T cells

CD4 Defines MHC class II-restricted T cell subsets

CD5 Also known as Lyt1 in mouse

CD7 Cluster of differentiation 7.

CD8 Defines MHC class I-restricted T cell subset

CD11a Known to be α chain of LFA-1 (leucocyte function antigen-1) present on several types of leucocyte and which mediates adhesion

CD11b Known to be α chain of CR3 (complement receptor type 3) present on several types of leucocyte and which mediates adhesion

CD11c Known to be complement receptor 4 α chain.

CD18 Known to be the common β chain of the CD11 family of molecules

CD20 Known to be pan B cell

CD31 Known to be platelets, monocytes, macrophages, granulocytes and B-cells

CD34⁻ Known to be a stem cell marker

CD33⁺ Known to be a monocyte and stem cell marker

CD45 Known to be a pan leucocyte marker

CD45RO Known to be the isoform of leukosialin present on memory T cells

CD49 Cluster of differentiation 49

CD59 Known to be a low molecular weight HRf present to many haemotopoetic and non-haemotopoetic cells

CD62 Known to be present on activated platelets and endothelia cells

CDC Complement-dependent cytotoxicity

cDNA Complementary DNA

CDP Choline diphosphate

CDR Complementary-determining region

CD$_{xx}$ Common determinant xx

CEA Carcinoembryonic antigen

CETAF Corneal epithelial T cell activating factor

CF Cystic fibrosis

Cf Cationized ferritin

CFA Complete Freund's adjuvant

CFC Colony-forming cell

CFU Colony-forming unit

CFU-Eo/B Eosinophil/basophil colony-forming cell

CFU-GM Granulocyte-macrophage colony-forming cell

CFU-S Colony-forming unit, spleen

CGD Chronic granulomatous disease

cGMP Cyclic guanosine monophosphate (guanosine 3′,5′-phosphate)

CGRP Calcitonin gene-related peptide

CHO Chinese hamster ovary

CI Chemical ionization

CIBD Chronic inflammatory bowel disease

CK Creatine phosphokinase

CKMB The myocardial-specific isoenzyme of creatine phosphokinase

Cl Chloride

CL Chemiluminescent

CL18/6 Anti-ICAM-1 monoclonal antibody

CLC Charcot–Leyden crystal

CMC Critical micellar concentration

CMI Cell mediated immunity

CML Chronic myeloid leukaemia

CMV Cytomegalovirus

CNS Central nervous system

CO Cyclooxygenase

CoA Coenzyme A

CoA-IT Coenzyme A-independent Transacylase

Con A Concanavalin A

COPD Chronic obstructive pulmonary disease

COS Fibroblast-like kidney cell line established from simian cells

CoVF Cobra venom

CP Creatine phosphate

CPJ Cartilage/pannus junction

Cr Chromium

CR Complement receptor

CR1 Complement receptor type 1

CR2 Complement receptor type 2

CR3 Complement receptor type 3

CR3-α Complement receptor type 3-α

CRF Corticotrophin-releasing factor

CRH Corticotrophin-releasing hormone

CRI Cross-reactive idiotype

CRP C-reactive protein

CSA Cyclosporin A

CSF Colony-stimulating factor

CSS Churg–Strauss syndrome

CTAP-III Connective tissue-activating peptide

CTD Connective tissue diseases

C terminus Carboxy terminus of peptide

CTlp Cytotoxic T lymphocyte precursors

CTL Cytotoxic T lymphocyte

CTMC Connective tissue mast cell

ct.min⁻¹ Counts per minute

Da Dalton (the unit of relative molecular mass)

DAF Decay accelerating factor

DAG Diacylglycerol

DAO Diamine oxidase

D-Arg D-Arginine

DArg–[Hyp³,DPhe⁷]–BK Bradykinin B₂ receptor antagonist. Peptide derivative of bradykinin

DArg–[Hyp³,Thi⁵,DTic⁷,Tic⁸]–BK Bradykinin B₂ receptor antagonist. Peptide derivative of bradykinin

DC Dendritic cell

DCF Oxidized DCFH

DCFH 2′,7′-dichlorofluorescin

DEC Diethylcarbamazine

desArg⁹–BK Carboxypeptidase N product of bradykinin

desArg¹⁰KD Carboxypeptidase N product of kallidin

DFMO α-Difluoromethyl ornithine

DFP Diisopropyl fluorophosphate

DGLA Dihomo-γ-linolenic acid
DH Delayed hypersensitivity
DHR Delayed hypersensitivity reaction
DIC Disseminated intravascular coagulation
DL-CFU Dendritic cell/Langerhans cell colony forming
DLE *Discoid lupus erythematosus*
DMARD Disease-modifying anti-rheumatic drug
DMF *N,N*-Dimethylformamide
DMSO Dimethyl sulfoxide
DNA Deoxyribonucleic acid
D-NAME D-Nitroarginine methyl ester
DNase Deoxyribonuclease
DNCB Dinitrochlorobenzene
DNP Dinitrophenol
Dpt4 *Dermatophagoides pteronyssinus* allergen 4
DGW2 HLA phenotype
DR3 HLA phenotype
DR7 HLA phenotype
DREG-2 Murine IgG₁ monoclonal antibody against L-selectin
ds Double-stranded
DSCG Disodium cromoglycate
DST Donor-specific transfusion
DTH Delayed-type hypersensitivity
DTPA Diethylenetriamine pentaacetate
DTT Dithiothreitol
d*v*/d*t* Rate of change of voltage within time

ε Molar absorption coefficient
EA Egg albumin
EAE Experimental autoimmune encephalomyelitis
EAF Eosinophil-activating factor
EAR Early phase asthmatic reaction
EAT Experimental autoimmune thyroiditis
EBV Epstein–Barr virus
EC Electron capture
ECD Electron capture detector
ECE Endothelin converting enzyme
E-CEF Eosinophil cytotoxicity enhancing factor
ECF-A Eosinophil chemotactic factor of anaphylaxis
ECG Electrocardiogram
ECGF Endothelial cell growth factor
ECGS Endothelial cell growth supplement
E. coli *Escherichia coli*
ECP Eosinophil cationic protein
ED₃₅ Effective dose producing 35% maximum response
ED₅₀ Effective dose producing 50% maximum response
EDF Eosinophil differentiation factor
EDN Eosinophil-derived neurotoxin

EDRF Endothelium-derived relaxant factor
EDTA Ethylenediamine tetraacetic acid (etidronic acid)
EE Eosinophilic eosinophils
EEG Electroencephalogram
EET Epoxyeicosatrienoic acid
EFA Essential fatty acid
EFS Electrical field stimulation
EG1 Monoclonal antibody specific for the cleaved form of eosinophil cationic peptide
EGF Epidermal growth factor
EGTA Ethylene glycol-bis(β-aminoethyl ether)*N,N,N'N'*-tetraacetic acid
EI Electron impact
eIF-2 Subunit of protein synthesis initiation factor
ELAM Endothelial leucocyte adhesion molecule
ELAM-1 Endothelial leucocyte adhesion molecule-1
ELF Respiratory epithelium lung fluid
ELISA Enzyme-linked immunosorbent assay
EMS Eosinophilia-myalgia syndrome
ENS Enteric nervous system
EO Eosinophil
EOR Early onset reaction
EPA Eicosapentaenoic acid
EPO Eosinophil peroxidase
EpDIF Epithelial-derived inhibitory factor
EpDRF Epithelium-derived relaxant factor
EPO Epithelial peroxidase
EPX Eosinophil protein X
ER Endoplasmic reticulum
ESP Eosinophil stimulation promoter
ESR Erythrocyte sedimentation rate
ET Endothelin
ET-1 Endothelin-1
ETYA Eicosatetraynoic acid

FA Fatty acid
FAB Fast-electron bombardment
Fab Antigen binding fragment
factor B Serine protease in the C3 converting enzyme of the alternative pathway
factor D Serine protease which cleaves factor B
factor H Plasma protein which acts as a co-factor to factor I
factor I Hydrolyses C3 converting enzymes with the help of factor H
FBR Fluorescence photobleaching recovery
Fc Crystallizable fraction of immunoglobulin molecule
FcR Receptor for Fc region of antibody

FcₑRI High affinity receptor for IgE
FcₑRII Low affinity receptor for IgE
FCS Fetal calf (bovine) serum
FEV₁ Forced expiratory volume in 1 second
FGF Fibroblast growth factor
FID Flame ionization detector
FITC Fluorescein isothiocyanate
FKBP FK506-binding protein
FLAP 5-lipoxygenase-activating protein
FMLP *N*-Formyl-methionyl-leucyl-phenylalanine
FNLP Formyl-norleucyl-leucyl-phenylalanine
FSG Focal sequential glomerulosclerosis
5-FU 5-Fluorouracil

G6PD Glucose 6-phosphate dehydrogenase
GABA γ-Aminobutyric acid
GAG Glycosaminoglycan
GALT Gut-associated lymphoid tissue
GBM Glomerular basement membrane
GC Guanylate cyclase
GC-MS Gas chromatography mass spectroscopy
G-CSF Granulocyte colony-stimulating factor
GDP Guanosine 5'-diphosphate
GEC Glomerular epithelial cells
GF-1 Insulin-like growth factor
GFR Glomerular filtration rate
GH Growth hormone
GH-RF Growth hormone releasing factor
GI Gastrointestinal
GIP Granulocyte inhibitory protein
GMC Gastric mast cell
GM-CSF Granulocyte-macrophage colony-stimulating factor
GMP Guanosine monophosphate (guanosine 5'-phosphate)
GMP-140 Granule-associated membrane protein-140
GP Glycoprotein
GPIIb-IIIa Glycoprotein IIb-IIIa, a platelet membrane antigen
GRP Gastrin-related peptide
GSH Glutathione (reduced)
GSSG Glutathione (oxidized)
GTP Guanosine triphosphate
GTP-γ-S Guanarine 5'*O*-(3-thiotriphosphate)
GTPase Guanidine triphosphatase
GVHD Graft-versus-host-disease
GVHR Graft-versus-host-reaction

H₁ Histamine receptor type 1
H₂ Histamine receptor type 2
H₂O₂ Chemical symbol for hydrogen peroxide

H₃ Histamine receptor type 3
HA Histamine
Hag Haemagglutinin
Hag-1 Cleaved haemagglutinin subunit-1
Hag-2 Cleaved haemagglutinin subunit-2
H & E Haematoxylin and eosin
hIL Human interleukin
Hb Haemoglobin
HBBS Hank's balanced salt solution
HDC Histidine decarboxylase
HDL High-density lipoprotein
HEL Hen egg white lysozyme
HEPE Hydroxyeicosapentanoic acid
HEPES N-2-hydroxylethyl-piperazine-N'-2-ethane sulphonic acid
HES Hypereosinophilic syndrome
HETE 5, 8, 9, 11 and 15 Hydroxyeicosatetraenoic acid
HETrE Hydroxyeicosatrienoic acid
HEV High endothelial venule
HFN Human fibronectin
HGF Hepatocyte growth factor
HHT 12-hydroxy-5,8,10-heptadecatrienoic acid
HHTrE $12(S)$-Hydroxy-5,8,10-heptadecatrienoic acid
HIV Human immunodeficiency virus
HLA Human leucocyte antigen
HMG CoA Hydroxylmethylglutaryl co-enzyme A
HMW High molecular weight
HMT Histidine methyltransferase
HMVEC Human microvascular endothelial cells
HNC Human neutrophil collagenase (MMP-8)
HNE Human neutrophil elastase
HNG Human neutrophil gelatinase (MMP-9)
HODE Hydroxyoctadecanoic acid
HPETE Hydroperoxyeicosatetraenoic acid
HPETrE Hydroperoxytrienoic acid
HPODE Hydroperoxyoctadecanoic acid
HPLC High-performance liquid chromatography
HRA Histamine-releasing activity
HRAN Neutrophil-derived histamine-releasing activity
HRf Homologous-restriction factor
HRF Histamine-releasing factor
HRP Horseradish peroxidase
HSA Human serum albumin
HSP Heat-shock protein
HS-PG Heparan sulphate proteoglycan
HSV Herpes simplex virus
HSV-1 Herpes simplex virus 1
³HTdR Triitiated thymidine

5-HT 5-Hydroxytryptamine *also known as* Serotonin
HUVEC Human umbilical vein endothelial cell
[Hyp³]–BK Hydroxproline derivative of bradykinin
[Hyp⁴]–KD Hydroxproline derivative of kallidin

I_{sc} Short-circuit current
Ia Immune reaction-associated antigen
Ia+ Murine class II major histocompatibility complex antigen
IB₄ Anti-CD18 monoclonal antibody
IBD Inflammatory bowel disease
IBMX Isobutylmethylxanthine
IBS Inflammatory bowel syndrome
IC₅₀ Concentration producing 50% inhibition
ICAM Intercellular adhesion molecules
ICAM-1 Intercellular adhesion molecule-1
ICAM-2 Intercellular adhesion molecule-2
ICAM-3 Intercellular adhesion molecule-3
ICE IL-1β-converting enzyme
IDC Interdigitating cell
IDD Insulin-dependent (type 1) diabetes
IEL Intraepithelial leucocytes
IELym Intraepithelial lymphocytes
IFA Incomplete Freund's adjuvant
IFN Interferon
IFNα Interferon α
IFNβ Interferon β
IFNγ Interferon γ
Ig Immunoglobulin
IgA Immunoglobulin A
IgE Immunoglobulin E
IgG Immunoglobulin G
IgG1 Immunoglobulin G class 1
IgG₂ₐ Immunoglobulin G class 2a
IgM Immunoglobulin M
IGF-1 Insulin-like growth factor
IGSS Immuno-gold silver stain
IHC Immunohistochemistry
IHES Idiopathic hypereosinophilic syndrome
IκB NFκB inhibitor protein
IL Interleukin
IL-1 Interleukin-1
IL-1α Interleukin-1α
IL-1β Interleukin-1β
IL-1Ra Interleukin-1 receptor antagonist
IL-2 Interleukin-2
IL-2R Interleukin-2 receptor
IL-3R Interleukin-3R
IL-3 Interleukin-3
IL-4 Interleukin-4
IL-5 Interleukin-5

IL-5R Interleukin-5-receptor
IL-6 Interleukin-6
IL-8 Interleukin-8
ILR Interleukin receptor
IMMC Intestinal mucosal mast cell
INCAM Inducible cell adhesion molecule
INCAM110 Inducible cell adhesion molecule 110
i.p. Intraperitoneally
IP₃ Inositol triphosphate
IP₄ Inositol tetrakisphosphate
IPO Intestinal peroxidase
IpOCOCq Isopropylidene OCOCq
I/R Ischaemia-reperfusion
IRAP IL-1 receptor antagonist protein
IRF-1 Interferon regulatory factor 1
ISCOM Immune-stimulating complexes
ISGF3 Interferon-stimulated gene factor 3
ISGF3α subunit of ISGF3
ISGFγ γ subunit of ISGF3
IT Immunotherapy
ITP Idiopathic thrombocytopenic purpura
i.v. Intravenous

K Potassium
K_a Association constant
kb Kilobase
20KDHRF A homologous restriction factor; binds to C8
65KDHRF A homologous restriction factor, also known as C8 binding protein; interferes with cell membrane pore-formation by C5b C8 complex
K_d Equilibrium dissociation constant
kD Kilodalton
K_D Dissociation constant
KD Kallidin
Ki Antagonist binding affinity
Ki67 Nuclear membrane antigen
KLH Keyhole limpet haemocyanin
KOS KOS strain of herpes simplex virus

λ_max Wavelength of maximum absorbance
LAD Leucocyte adhesion deficiency
LAK Lymphocyte-activated killer (cell)
LAM Leucocyte adhesion molecule
LAM-1 Leucocyte adhesion molecule-1
LAR Late-phase asthmatic reaction
L-Arg L-Arginine
LBP LPS binding protein
LC Langerhans cell
LCF Lymphocyte chemoattractant factor
LCR Locus control region
LDH Lactate dehydrogenase
LDL Low-density lipoprotein

LDV Laser Doppler velocimetry
LECAM Lectin adhesion molecule
LECAM-1 Lectin adhesion molecule-1
LFA Leucocyte function-associated antigen
LFA-1 Leucocyte function-associated antigen-1; a member of the beta-2 integrin family of cell adhesion molecules
LG β-Lactoglobulin
LHRH Luteinizing hormone-releasing hormone
LI Labelling index
LIS Lateral intercellular spaces
LMP Low molecular mass polypeptide
LMW Low molecular weight
L-NOARG L-Nitroarginine
LP(a) Lipoprotein a
LPS Lipopolysaccharide
LT Leukotriene
LTA$_4$ Leukotriene A$_4$
LTB$_4$ Leukotriene B$_4$
LTC$_4$ Leukotriene C$_4$
LTD$_4$ Leukotriene D$_4$
LTE$_4$ Leukotriene E$_4$
L$_y$-1$^+$ (Cell line)
LXA$_4$ Lipoxin A$_4$
LXB$_4$ Lipoxin B$_4$
LXC$_4$ Lipoxin C$_4$
LXD$_4$ Lipoxin D$_4$
LXE$_4$ Lipoxin E$_4$

M3 Receptor Muscarinic receptor subtype 3
M-540 Merocyanine-540
α_2-M α_2-macroglobulin
mAb Monoclonal antibody
mAB IB4 Monoclonal antibody IB4
mAB PB1.3 Monoclonal antibody PB1.3
mAB R 3.1 Monoclonal antibody R 3.1
mAB R 3.3 Monoclonal antibody R 3.3
mAB 6.5 Monoclonal antibody 6.5
mAB 60.3 Monoclonal antibody 60.3
MAC Membrane attack molecule
Mac-1 Macrophage-1 antigen; a member of the beta-2 integrin family of cell adhesion molecules
MAF Macrophage-activating factor
MAO Monoamine oxidase
MAP Monophasic action potential
MBP Major basic protein
MBSA Methylated bovine serum albumin
MC Mesangial cells
M cell Microfold or membranous cell of Peyer's patch epithelium
MCP Membrane co-factor protein
M-CSF Monocyte colony-stimulating factor

MC$_T$ Tryptase-containing mast cell
MC$_{TC}$ Tryptase- and chymase-containing mast cell
MDA Malondialdehyde
MDGF Macrophage-derived growth factor
MDP Muramyl dipeptide
MEA Mast cell growth-enhancing activity
MEL Metabolic equivalent level
MEM Minimal essential medium
MG *Myasthenia gravis*
MHC Major histocompatibility complex
MI Myocardial ischaemia
MIF Migration inhibition factor
mIL Mouse interleukin
MI/R Myocardial ischaemia/reperfusion
MIRL Membrane inhibitor of reactive lysis
MLC Mixed lymphocyte culture
MLymR Mixed lymphocyte reaction
MLR Mixed leucocyte reaction
MMC Mucosal mast cell
MMCP Mouse mast cell protease
MMP Matrix metalloproteinase
MMP1 Matrix metalloproteinase 1
MNA 6-methoxy-2-napthylacetic acid
MNC Mononuclear cells
MO Macrophage (also abbreviated to Mac)
MPO Myeloperoxidase
MRI Magnetic resonance imaging
mRNA Messenger ribonucleic acid
MS Mass spectrometry
MSS Methylprednisolone sodium succinate
MT Malignant tumour
MW Molecular weight

Na Sodium
NA Noradrenaline *also known as* norepinephrine
NAAb Natural autoantibody
NAb Natural antibody
NADH Reduced nicotinamide adenine dinucleotide
NADP Nicotinamide adenine diphosphate
NADPH Reduced nicotinamide adenine dinucleotide phosphate
L-NAME L-Nitroarginine methyl ester
NANC Non-adrenergic, non-cholinergic
NAP Neutrophil-activating peptide
NAP-1 Neutrophil-activating peptide-1
NAP-2 Neutrophil-activating peptide-2
NC1 Non-collagen 1
N-CAM Neural cell adhesion molecule

NCEH Neutral cholesteryl ester hydrolase
NCF Neutrophil chemotactic factor
NDGA Nordihydroguaretic acid
Neca 5'-(N-ethyl carboxamido)-adenosine
NED Nedocromil sodium
NEP Neutral endopeptidase (EC 3.4.24.11)
NF-AT Nuclear factor of activated T lymphocytes
NF-κB Nuclear factor-κB
NGF Nerve growth factor
NGPS Normal guinea-pig serum
NIMA Non-inherited maternal antigens
Nk Neurokinin
NK Natural killer
Nk-1 Neurokinin receptor subtype
Nk-2 Neurokinin receptor subtype
Nk-3 Neurokinin receptor subtype
NkA Neurokinin A
NkB Neurokinin B
L-NMMA L-Nitromonomethyl arginine
NMR Nuclear magnetic resonance
NO Chemical symbol for nitric oxide
NPK Neuropeptide K
NPY Neuropeptide Y
NRS Normal rabbit serum
NSAID Non-steroidal anti-inflammatory drug
NSE Nerve-specific enolase
NT Neurotensin
N terminus Amino terminus of peptide

O$_2^-$ Oxygen free radical
OA Osteoarthritis
OAG Oleoyl acetyl glycerol
OD Optical density
ODC Ornithine decarboxylase
ODS Octadecylsilyl
·OH Chemical symbol for hydroxyl radical
OVA Ovalbumin
ox-LDL Oxidized low-density lipoprotein

P Probability
P Phosphate
P$_a$O$_2$ Arterial oxygen pressure
P$_i$ Inorganic phosphate
P150,95 A member of the beta-2-integrin family of cell adhesion molecules
PA Phosphatidic acid
pA$_2$ Negative logarithm of the antagonist dissociation constant
PADGEM Platelet-activation dependent granule external membrane
PAF Platelet-activating factor
PAGE Polyacrylamide gel electrophoresis

PAI Plasminogen activator inhibitor
PAM Pulmonary alveolar macrophages
PAS Periodic acid–Schiff reagent
PBA Polyclonal B cell activators
PBC Primary biliary cirrhosis
PBL Peripheral blood lymphocytes
PBMC Peripheral blood mononuclear cells
PBS Phosphate-buffered saline
PC Phosphatidylcholine
PCA Passive cutaneous anaphylaxis
PCNA Proliferating cell nuclear antigen
PCR Polymerase chain reaction
p.d. Potential difference
PDBu 4α-phorbol 12,13-dibutyrate
PDE Phosphodiesterase
PDGF Platelet-derived growth factor
PE Phosphatidylethanolamine
PECAM-1 Platelet endothelial cell adhesion molecule-1
PEG Polyethylene glycol
PET Positron emission tomography
PEt Phosphatidylethanol
PF$_4$ Platelet factor 4
PG Prostaglandin
PGA Polyglandular autoimmune syndrome
PGE$_2$ Prostaglandin E$_2$
PGF Prostaglandin F
PGI Prostacyclin
PGI$_2$ More standard abbreviation of above
PGD$_2$ Prostaglandin D$_2$
PGE$_1$ Prostaglandin E$_1$
PGF$_{2\alpha}$ Prostaglandin F$_{2\alpha}$
PGF$_2$ Prostaglandin F$_2$
PGG$_2$ Prostaglandin G$_2$
PGH Prostaglandin H
PGH$_2$ Prostaglandin H$_2$
PGI$_2$ Prostaglandin I$_2$
PGP Protein gene-related peptide
Ph^1 Philadelphia (chromosome)
PHA Phytohaemagglutinin
PHI Peptide histidine isoleucine
PHM Peptide histidine-methionine
PI Phosphatidylinositol
P$_i$ Inorganic phosphate
PIP Phosphatidylinositol monophosphate
PIP$_2$ Phosphatidylinositol biphosphate
PK Protein kinase
PKA Protein kinase A
PKC Protein kinase C
PL Phospholipase
PLA Phospholipase A
PLA$_2$ Phospholipase A$_2$
PLAP Putative phospholipase activity protein
PLC Phospholipase C
PLD Phospholipase D
PLP Proteolipid protein
PLT Primed lymphocyte typing

PMA Phorbol myristate acetate
PMC Peritoneal mast cell
PMD Piecemeal degranulation
PML Polymorphonuclear leucocyte
PMN Polymorphonuclear neutrophil
PMSF Phenylethylsulphonyl fluoride
PNU Protein nitrogen unit
p.o. *Per os* (by mouth)
PPD Purified protein derivative
PRA Percentage reactive activity
PRD Positive regulatory domain
PRD-II Positive regulatory domain II
PR3 Proteinase-3
proET-1 Proendothelin-1
PRP Platelet-rich plasma
PS Phosphatidylserine
PTA$_2$ Pinane thromboxane A$_2$
PTCA Percutaneous transluminal coronary angioplasty
PTCR Percutaneous transluminal coronary recanalization
Pte-H$_4$ Tetrahydropteridine
PtX Pertussis toxin
PUFA Polyunsaturated fatty acid
PUMP-1 Punctuated metalloproteinase
PWM Pokeweed mitogen
PYY Peptide YY

Qa Genetic locus encoding a non-classical class I MHC molecule
q.i.d. *Quater in die* (four times a day)
QRS Segment of electrocardiogram

·R Free radical
R15.7 Anti-CD18 monoclonal antibody
RA Rheumatoid arthritis
RANTES Regulated on activation, normal T expressed and secreted
RAST Radioallergosorbent test
RBC Red blood cell
RBF Renal blood flow
RBL Rat basophilic leukaemia
RE RE strain of herpes simplex virus type 1
REA Reactive arthritis
REM Relative electrophoretic mobility
RER Rough endoplasmic reticulum
RF Rheumatoid factor
RFL-6 Rat foetal lung-6
RFLP Restriction fragment length polymorphism
rh- Recombinant human (prefix usually refers to peptide)
RIA Radioimmunoassay
RMCP Rat mast cell protease
RMCPII Rat mast cell protease II
RNA Ribonucleic acid
RNase Ribonuclease
RNHCl *N*-Chloramine
RNL Regional lymph nodes

ROM Reactive oxygen metabolites
ROS Reactive oxygen species
R-PIA *R-N*G-(1-methyl-1-phenyltheyl)-adenosine
RPMI 1640 Roswell Park Memorial Institute 1640 medium
RS Reiter's syndrome
RSV Rous sarcoma virus
RTE Rabbit tubular epithelium
RTE-a-5 Rat tubular epithelium antigen a-5
RW Ragweed

S Svedberg (unit of sedimentation density)
SALT Skin associated lymphoid tissue
SAZ Sulphasalazine
SC Secretory component
SCF Stem cell factor
SCFA Short chain fatty acid
SCG Sodium cromoglycate
SCID Severe combined immunodeficiency syndrome
sCR$_1$ Soluble type-1 complement receptors
SCW Streptococcal cell wall
SD Standard deviation
SDS Sodium dodecyl sulphate
SDS–PAGE Sodium dodecyl sulphate–polyacrylamide gel electrophoresis
SEM Standard error of the mean
SGAW Specific airway conductance
SHR Spontaneously hypertensive rat
SIRS Soluble immune response suppressor
SK Streptokinase
Sl Murine Steel mutation
SLE Systemic lupus erythematosus
SLe^x Sialyl Lewis X antigen
SLO Streptolysin-O
SLPI Secretory leucocyte protease inhibitor
SM Sphingomyelin
SNAP *S*-Nitroso-*N*-acetylpenicillamine
SNP Sodium nitroprusside
SOD Superoxide dismutase
SOM Somatostatin
SOZ Serum-opsonized zymosan
SP Sulphapyridine
S Protein vitronectin
SR Systemic reaction
SRBC Sheep red blood cells
SRIF Somatotrophin release-inhibiting factor (somatostatin)
SRS Slow-reacting substance
SRS-A Slow-reacting substance of anaphylaxis
Sub P Substance P

t$_{1/2}$ Half-life
T84 Human intestinal epithelial cell line

TauNHCl Taurine monochloramine
TBM Tubular basement membrane
TCA Trichloroacetic acid
T cell Thymus-derived lymphocyte
TCP Toxin co-regulated pilus
TCR T cell receptor (α/β or γ/δ heterodimeric forms)
TDI Toluene diisocyanate
TDID$_{50}$ Tissue culture infectious dose – 50%
TEC Tubular epithelial cells
TF Tissue factor
Tg Thyroglobulin
TGF Transforming growth factor
TGFα Transforming growth factor α
TGFβ Transforming growth factor β
TGFβ_1 Transforming growth factor-β_1
T$_H$ T helper cells
T$_{HO}$ T Helper o
T$_{HP}$ T helper precursor
T$_H$0, T$_H$1, T$_H$2 Subsets of helper T cells
Thy 1+ Murine T cell antigen
t.i.d. *Ter in die* (three times a day)
TIL Tumour-infiltrating lymphocytes
TIMP Tissue inhibitors of metalloproteinase
TIMP-1 Tissue inhibitor of metalloproteinases 1

Tla Thymus leukaemia antigen
TLC Thin-layer chromatography
TLP Tumour-like proliferation
Tm T memory
TNF Tumour necrosis factor
TNF-α Tumour necrosis factor-α
tPA Tissue-type plasminogen activator
TPA 12-*o*-Tetradeconylphorbol-13-acetate
TPK Tyrosine protein kinases
TPP Transpulmonary pressure
Tris Tris(hydroxymethyl)amino-methane
TSH Thyroid-stimulating hormone
TTX Tetrodotoxin
TX Thromboxane
TXA$_2$ Thromboxane A$_2$
TXB$_2$ Thromboxane B$_2$
Tyk2 Tyrosine kinase

UC Ulcerative colitis
UDP Uridine diphosphate
UPA Urokinase-type plasminogen activator
UV Ultraviolet

VC Veiled cells
VCAM Vascular cell adhesion molecule

VCAM-1 Vascular cell adhesion molecule-1
VF Ventricular fibrillation
VIP Vasoactive intestinal peptide
VLA Very late antigen
VLA-3 Very late activation antigen-3
VLA-4 Very late activation antigen-4
VLA-5 Very late activation antigen-5
VLA-6 Very late activation antigen-6
VLDL Very low-density lipoprotein
V_{max} Maximal velocity
VP Vasopressin
VPB Ventricular premature beat
VT Ventricular tachycardia

W Murine dominant white spotting mutation
WBC White blood cell
WGA Wheat germ agglutinin

XO Xanthine oxidase

Y1/82A A monoclonal antibody detecting a cytoplasmic antigen in human macrophages

ZA Zonulae adherens
ZAS Zymosan-activated serum
ZO Zonulae occludentes

Key to Illustrations

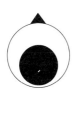 Helper
lymphocyte

 Suppressor
lymphocyte

 Killer
lymphocyte

 Plasma cell

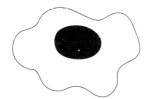 Bacterial or
Tumour cell

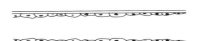 Blood vessel
lumen

 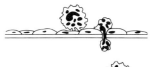 Eosinophil
passing through
vessel wall

 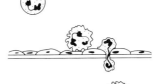 Neutrophil
passing through
vessel wall

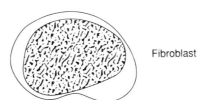 Fibroblast

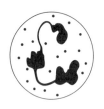

Resting
neutrophil

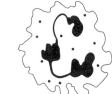

Activated
neutrophil

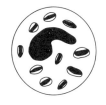

Resting
eosinophil

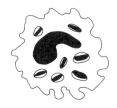

Activated
eosinophil

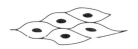

Smooth
muscle

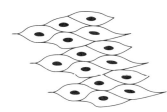

Smooth muscle
thickening

Smooth muscle
contraction

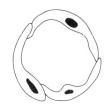

Normal blood
vessel

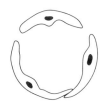

Endothelial cell
permeability

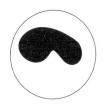

Resting
macrophage

Activated
macrophage

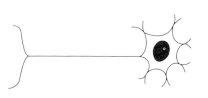

Nerve

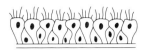 Intact epithelium

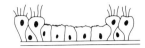 Damaged epithelium

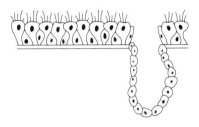 Intact epithelium with submucosal gland

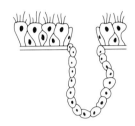 Normal submucosal gland

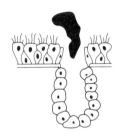 Hypersecreting submucosal gland

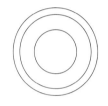 Normal airway

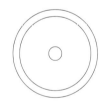 Oedema

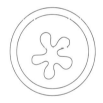 Bronchospasm

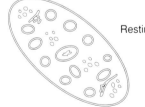 Resting platelet

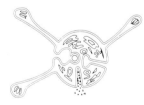 Activated platelet

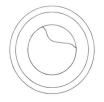 Airway hypersecreting mucus

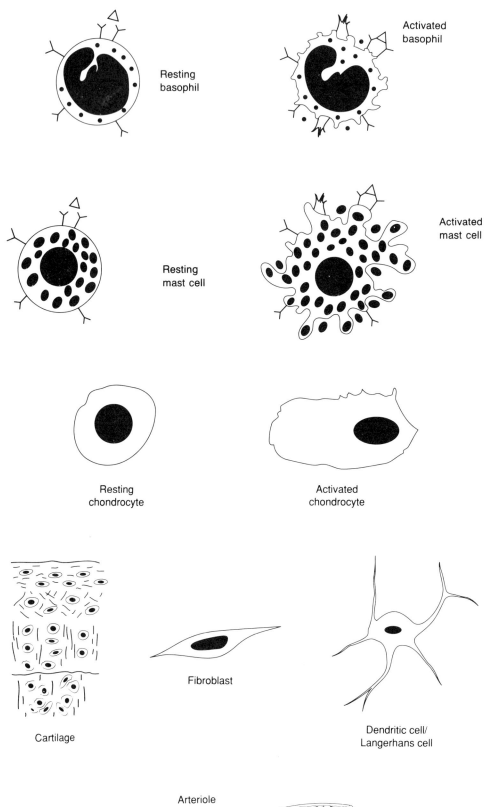

Resting
basophil

Activated
basophil

Resting
mast cell

Activated
mast cell

Resting
chondrocyte

Activated
chondrocyte

Cartilage

Fibroblast

Dendritic cell/
Langerhans cell

Arteriole

Venule

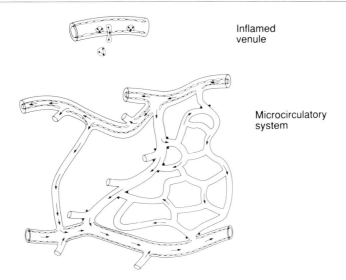

Inflamed
venule

Microcirculatory
system

Index